SAGINAW COMMUNITY HOSPITAL

Clinical Gerontological Nursing

A GUIDE TO ADVANCED PRACTICE

W. Carole Chenitz, R.N., Ed.D.
Formerly Associate Chief, Nursing Service for Research
Department of Veterans Affairs Medical Center
San Francisco, California

Joyce Takano Stone, R.N.C., M.S.
Clinical Nurse Specialist, Gerontology
Department of Veterans Affairs Medical Center
San Francisco, California

Sally A. Salisbury, R.N.C.S., M.S.
Program Coordinator
Geriatric Assessment Service, Institute on Aging
Mt. Zion Medical Center
San Francisco, California

1991
W.B. SAUNDERS COMPANY
Harcourt Brace Jovanovich, Inc.
Philadelphia   London   Toronto   Montreal   Sydney   Tokyo

W. B. SAUNDERS COMPANY
Harcourt Brace Jovanovich, Inc.

The Curtis Center
Independence Square West
Philadelphia, PA 19106

Library of Congress Cataloging-in-Publication Data

Chenitz, W. Carole

Clinical gerontological nursing: a guide to advanced practice /
authors, W. Carole Chenitz, Joyce Takano Stone, Sally A.
Salisbury.—1st ed.

p.   cm.

ISBN 0–7216–2299–2

1. Geriatric nursing.   I. Stone, Joyce Takano.
  II. Salisbury, Sally A.   III. Title.   [DNLM:
  1. Geriatric Nursing. WY 152 C518a]

RC954.C457 1991   610.73'65–dc20

DNLM/DLC   90–8556

Editor: Ilze Rader
Developmental Editor: Robin Richman
Designer: Joan Wendt
Production Manager: Ken Neimeister
Manuscript Editor: Karen Okie
Illustration Coordinator: Cecelia Kunkle
Indexer: Nancy Weaver
Cover Designer: Ellen Bodner

CLINICAL GERONTOLOGICAL NURSING: A GUIDE TO ADVANCED PRACTICE   ISBN 0–7216–2299–2

Printed in the United States of America.

Last digit is the print number: 9   8   7   6   5   4   3   2   1

This book is dedicated to our elderly patients, who have taught us about the aging process and life in old age and, most importantly, about life. As we complete this work, we are in the midst of an epidemic that is cutting short the lives of friends, colleagues, and members of our community. We dedicate this book to the memory of Kent Delventhal, R.N., and to all others who will never experience the joys and sorrows of old age.

CONTRIBUTORS

J. Elizabeth Bell, R.N.C., M.S., A.N.P.
Nurse Practitioner, Department of Veterans Affairs Medical Center; Auxiliary Faculty Member, College of Nursing, University of Utah, Salt Lake City, Utah
Physical Assessment: The Breast and the Pulmonary, Cardiovascular, Gastrointestinal, and Genitourinary Systems

Rebecca Lee Burrage, R.N.C., M.S., F.N.P.
Coordinator and Nurse Practitioner of Hospital-Based Home Care, Department of Veterans Affairs Medical Center; Auxiliary Faculty Member, College of Nursing, University of Utah, Salt Lake City, Utah
Physical Assessment: An Overview with Sections on the Skin, Eye, Ear, Nose, and Neck; Physical Assessment: Musculoskeletal and Nervous Systems

W. Carole Chenitz, R.N., Ed.D.
Associate Chief, Nursing Service for Research, Department of Veterans Affairs Medical Center; Assistant Clinical Professor, School of Nursing, University of California, San Francisco, San Francisco, California
An Overview of Gerontological Nursing; The Problem of Falls; Preventing Falls; Using Theory to Guide Nursing Interventions: A Case Study; Alcoholism in the Elderly

Juliet Corbin, R.N., D.N.Sc.
Research Associate, School of Nursing, University of California, San Francisco, San Francisco, California
Balancing Resources: Demand Against Supply

Linda Crossman, R.N., M.S.
Executive Director, Nursing Dynamics Corporation, San Anselmo; Clinical Associate in Nursing, Department of Mental Health, Community, and Administrative Nursing, School of Nursing, University of California, San Francisco, San Francisco, California
Nursing Dynamics: Community Care for the Elderly

Helen D. Davies, R.N.C.S., M.S.
Clinical Nurse Specialist, Psychiatry/Research, Geropsychiatry Rehabilitation Unit, Department of Veterans Affairs Medical Center, Palo Alto, and

v

Stanford University Alzheimer's Diagnostic and Resource Center, Stanford; Assistant Clinical Professor, School of Nursing, University of California, San Francisco, San Francisco, California
Dementia and Delirium

Anne J. Davis, R.N., Ph.D., F.A.A.N.
Professor, School of Nursing, University of California, San Francisco; Clinical Appointment, Nursing Service, University of California Hospitals, San Francisco, California
Ethical Issues in Gerontological Nursing

Lawrence Dixon, R.N.C., M.S., G.N.P.
Nurse Practitioner of Hospital-Based Home Care, Department of Veterans Affairs Medical Center; Auxiliary Faculty Member, College of Nursing, University of Utah, Salt Lake City, Utah
Physical Assessment: An Overview with Sections on the Skin, Eye, Ear, Nose, and Neck; Physical Assessment: The Breast and the Pulmonary, Cardiovascular, Gastrointestinal, and Genitourinary Systems

Lois K. Evans, R.N., D.N.Sc., F.A.A.N.
Geropsychiatric Nurse Consultant, The Hospital of the University of Pennsylvania; Associate Professor and Director, Geropsychiatric Nursing Section, School of Nursing, University of Pennsylvania, Philadelphia, Pennsylvania
Physical Restraint of the Elderly; The Sundown Syndrome: A Nursing Management Problem

Marilyn D. Fravel, R.N., N.H.A.
Executive Vice President, Easter Seal Society of Alameda County, Oakland, California
Program Planning and Development

Sato Hashizume, R.N.C., M.S., N.P.
Liaison Coordinator, Mt. Zion–University of California, San Francisco Home Care Program; Assistant Clinical Professor, School of Nursing, University of California, San Francisco; formerly Coordinator, University of California, San Francisco Home Care Program, San Francisco, California
A Nursing Model for Home Health Care

Judy R. Hensley, R.N.C.
Formerly Head Nurse, Medical-Oncology Unit, Department of Veterans Affairs Medical Center, San Francisco, California
A Protocol for the Management of Patients at High Risk for Pressure Sores

Theodore H. D. Jones, Ph.D.
Professor, Department of Chemistry, University of San Francisco, San Francisco, California
Parkinson's Disease

Jeanie S. Kayser-Jones, R.N., Ph.D., F.A.A.N.
Professor, Department of Physiological Nursing and Medical Anthropology Program, School of Nursing, University of California, San Francisco, San Francisco, California
Parkinson's Disease

Heather L. Kussman, R.N.C., M.P.A.
Instructor, Nursing Education, Department of Veterans Affairs Medical Center, San Francisco, California
Preventing Falls

Mary Lou Long, R.N.C., M.S.N.
Director of Senior Life, St. Luke's Regional Medical Center; Adjunct Faculty, Boise State University, Boise, Idaho
Managing Urinary Incontinence

Lois L. Miller, R.N., M.N.
Doctoral Student, School of Nursing, Oregon Health Sciences University; formerly Clinical Nurse Specialist, Gerontology, Department of Veterans Affairs Medical Center, Portland, Oregon
Models for Respite Care

Deborah Monicken, R.N., M.S.
Clinical Nurse Specialist, Rehabilitation, and Coordinator, Traumatic Brain Injury, Department of Veterans Affairs Medical Center; Adjunct Faculty, School of Nursing, University of Minnesota, Minneapolis, Minnesota
Immobility and Functional Mobility in the Elderly

Ginette A. Pepper, R.N., G.N.P., Ph.D.
Assistant Professor, School of Nursing, University of Colorado, Denver, Colorado
Monitoring the Effects of Anticholinergic Drugs

Linda R. Phillips, R.N., Ph.D., F.A.A.N.
Associate Professor and Associate Dean for Research, College of Nursing, University of Arizona, Tucson, Arizona
Social Support of the Older Client

Barbara L. Sater, R.N.C., M.S.N.
Clinical Nurse Specialist, Diabetes, Department of Veterans Affairs Medical Center, San Francisco, California
A Protocol for the Management of Patients at High Risk for Pressure Sores

Sally A. Salisbury, R.N.C.S., M.S.
Program Coordinator, Geriatric Assessment Service, Institute on Aging, Mt. Zion Medical Center; Assistant Clinical Professor, School of Nursing,

University of California, San Francisco, San Francisco, California
Cognitive Assessment of the Older Client; Preventing Excess Disability; Managing Behavioral Problems; Depression

Judith S. Schainen, R.N.C., Ph.D.

Clinical Nurse Specialist, Gerontology, Department of Veterans Affairs Medical Center; Clinical Faculty, School of Nursing, University of Washington, Seattle, Washington
Environments for Nursing Care of the Older Client

Doris Schwartz, R.N., M.A., F.A.A.N.

Senior Fellow, School of Nursing, University of Pennsylvania, Philadelphia, Pennsylvania
Physical Restraint of the Elderly

Yvonne A. Sehy, R.N.C., M.S., F.N.P./G.N.P.

Clinical Nurse Specialist, Medicine and Geriatrics, LDS Hospital; Auxiliary Clinical Instructor, College of Nursing, University of Utah, Salt Lake City, Utah
Physical Assessment: An Overview with Sections on the Skin, Eye, Ear, Nose, and Neck; Physical Assessment: The Breast and the Pulmonary, Cardiovascular, Gastrointestinal, and Genitourinary Systems; Functional Assessment

Neville E. Strumpf, R.N., Ph.D., F.A.A.N.

Associate Professor and Director, Gerontological Nurse Clinician Program, School of Nursing, University of Pennsylvania, Philadelphia, Pennsylvania
Physical Restraint of the Elderly

Joyce Takano Stone, R.N.C., M.S.

Clinical Nurse Specialist, Gerontology, Department of Veterans Affairs Medical Center; Assistant Clinical Professor, School of Nursing, University of California, San Francisco, San Francisco, California
An Overview of Gerontological Nursing; Managing Bowel Function; Pressure Sores; A Protocol for the Management of Patients at High Risk for Pressure Sores; The Problem of Falls; Preventing Falls; Preventing Physical Iatrogenic Problems; Managing Behavioral Problems

Marilyn P. Williams, R.N., M.S.

Assistant Clinical Professor, School of Nursing, University of California, San Francisco, School of Nursing, San Francisco, California
Functional Assessment

Jean F. Wyman, Ph.D., R.N.C., C.G.N.P.

Associate Professor and Director, Graduate Program in Gerontologic Nursing, School of Nursing, Virginia Commonwealth University, Richmond, Virginia
Incontinence and Related Problems

PREFACE

The purpose of this book is to assist gerontological nurses to fulfill their role in providing health care to older clients in all clinical settings. *Clinical Gerontological Nursing: A Guide to Advanced Practice* provides in-depth, research-based information and specific guidelines for nurses to effectively assess and manage the major clinical problems of older clients. It is designed for nurses specializing in the care of the aged: clinical specialists, students in graduate programs in gerontological nursing, nurse practitioners and nurse practitioner students, nurse educators, and gerontological nurses in all health care environments. It is also useful for nurses who work with the elderly in any setting.

This book is born of our experience as clinicians, researchers, and educators. The editors have combined their knowledge and experience to present a comprehensive text on the current state of practice. Contributors are nurses engaged in clinical practice, education, and research; they were invited to contribute to this book because of their expertise on a specific topic.

Several theoretical frameworks and practice models are presented in this book. This eclectic approach to theory both reflects the current clinical world and demonstrates the use of theory in practice. The reader does not have to embrace any specific theory or model in order to find this book useful. Throughout the text, research relevant to each topic is presented as it has been applied to practice. Research utilization is a theme that underlies *Clinical Gerontological Nursing*.

There are five major sections and 33 chapters in this book. It is designed to be used as a reference. The material is organized in a manner so that related chapters can be read together, or the reader may choose to read only selected chapters or to read each chapter in order. The extensive reference lists at the end of each chapter include the research base and encourage readers to further extend their knowledge on the subject.

In Unit I, the first chapter is devoted to tracing the historical perspective on care of the aged and the development of gerontological nursing. Chapter 2 focuses on ethics as it applies to care of the elderly.

Since accurate, thorough assessment is essential for appropriate care planning and intervention, the five chapters in Unit II are devoted to assessment. There are three chapters on physical assessment, a chapter on cognitive assessment, and a chapter on functional assessment. Each chapter contains pertinent questionnaires and interview guides useful in performing systematic assessments. These questionnaires are derived from gerontological research and are being used increasingly in clinical practice to provide a standard basis for assessment.

Unit III consists of 15 chapters concerned with nursing interventions for common clinical problems in the older client. This section includes chapters on subjects that are universal and prevalent and have great impact on the client's health and well-being, but that unfortunately are not often addressed in nursing textbooks. These subjects include incontinence, managing urinary incontinence and bowel function, immobility and functional mobility, pressure sores and a protocol for managing clients at high risk for pressure sores, falls and fall prevention, physical restraints in the elderly, and the sundown syndrome. These subjects are of great import to both the client and nurse and are presented in depth with a strong theoretical and research base. Each chapter focuses on approaches to intervention.

In Unit IV, the focus shifts to nursing care for selected health problems in the older adult. Most nurses practice in health care settings that are organized according to the traditional medical model. In these settings, the gerontological nurse assists clients and their families to manage and adapt to health problems. To be an effective member of the health care team, the nurse must have an understanding of current research in pathophysiology and treatment of health problems that are prevalent in an elderly population. The chapters in this section are organized to take into account encompassing knowledge of the health problem and the disease process, awareness of health care factors that impede diagnosis and treatment, and educational, supportive, and clinical nursing interventions across treatment settings. Clinical assessment questionnaires are included to facilitate accurate diagnoses. The health problems that comprise this section are depression, dementia and delirium, Parkinson's disease, and alcoholism. This section is not meant to be comprehensive and of necessity includes only selected health problems. Health problems chosen for inclusion in this section are those that are frequently underdiagnosed and not well understood. Each of these health problems causes functional disability that is primarily managed by the nurse.

In the last section, Unit V, our attention moves from the individual client and the family to examining the context of nursing care. Specifically, topics covered in this section include environments for nursing care, social support, balancing resources, a model for home health care, program planning and development, community care, and respite care. Each chapter presents related theory and research that have been applied to developing models for nursing practice. In this section, nurses illustrate their administrative and management functions to develop, implement, and direct programs for care. There is a growing demand for gerontological nurses to be sensitive to the changing needs of elders, their families, and the larger society and to develop cost-effective programs that meet these needs. This section provides the background and models to assist nurses to carry out this role.

Knowledge is the key to advancing and changing practice. Theory and research generate new knowledge that can then be applied to practice. The ultimate goal of all research, theory development, and knowledge in nursing is to improve care. Much has been done in the last two decades to improve nursing care of the aged. The authors hope that this text will serve to foster the ongoing development of gerontological nursing knowledge and improved health care for older adults.

W. CAROLE CHENITZ, R.N., Ed.D.
JOYCE TAKANO STONE, R.N.C., M.S.
SALLY A. SALISBURY, R.N.C.S., M.S.

ACKNOWLEDGMENTS

Many people are responsible for the existence of this book. We are grateful and take this opportunity to give special thanks:

To Ilze Rader, our editor at the W. B. Saunders Company, who saw the merit in the idea of an advanced clinical text and supported us with her ideas throughout the process of putting this book together.

To Nancy Strouse, R.N., M.N.Ed., Chief, Nursing Service, Department of Veterans Affairs Medical Center, San Francisco, who believes that nursing practice must be based on knowledge and who creates an administrative environment that fosters ideas and creativity within nursing service.

To our contributors, who enthusiastically gave of their time and knowledge on manuscripts that became the chapters in this book.

And thanks also to our reviewers: A. Gelene Adkins, B.S.N., M.S.N., Ph.D.; Virginia Brooke, R.N., Ph.D.; Margaret C. Brown, R.N.C., M.S.; Margaret Heitkemper, R.N., Ph.D.; Marilynn E. Koerber, B.S.N., M.P.H., Ph.D.; Janet K. Kuhn, B.S.N., M.S.N.; Claudia J. McCoy, R.N.C., M.S.N., C.D.E.; and Amie Modigh, R.N., M.S.N., G.N.P.-C.

CONTENTS

· · · · · · · · · · · · · U N I T II · · · · · · · · · · · ·

ASSESSMENT OF THE OLDER CLIENT

CHAPTER 5

Physical Assessment: Musculoskeletal and Nervous Systems .. 71

Rebecca Lee Burrage, R.N.C., M.S., F.N.P.

CHAPTER 6

Cognitive Assessment of the Older Client 91

Sally A. Salisbury, R.N.C.S., M.S.

· · · · · · · · · · · · · U N I T III · · · · · · · · · · · · ·

NURSING INTERVENTIONS FOR COMMON CLINICAL PROBLEMS IN THE OLDER CLIENT

CHAPTER 10

Managing Bowel Function 217

Joyce Takano Stone, R.N.C., M.S.

CHAPTER 11

Immobility and Functional Mobility in the Elderly 233

Deborah Monicken, R.N., M.S.

CHAPTER 12

Pressure Sores 247

Joyce Takano Stone, R.N.C., M.S.

CHAPTER 13

A Protocol for the Management of Patients at High Risk for Pressure Sores 267

Barbara L. Sater, R.N.C., M.S.N.
Judy R. Hensley, R.N.C.
Joyce Takano Stone, R.N.C., M.S.

CHAPTER 14

The Problem of Falls 291

Joyce Takano Stone, R.N.C., M.S.
W. Carole Chenitz, R.N., Ed.D.

CHAPTER 15

Preventing Falls 309

W. Carole Chenitz, R.N., Ed.D.
Heather L. Kussman, R.N.C., M.P.A.
Joyce Takano Stone, R.N.C., M.S.

CHAPTER 16

Physical Restraint of the Elderly 329

Neville E. Strumpf, R.N., Ph.D., F.A.A.N.
Lois K. Evans, R.N., D.N.Sc., F.A.A.N.
Doris Schwartz, R.N., M.A., F.A.A.N.

CHAPTER 17

The Sundown Syndrome: A Nursing Management Problem 345

Lois K. Evans, R.N., D.N.Sc., F.A.A.N.

CHAPTER 18

Preventing Physical Iatrogenic Problems 359

Joyce Takano Stone, R.N.C., M.S.

CHAPTER 21

Managing Behavioral Problems 403
Sally A. Salisbury, R.N.C.S., M.S.
Joyce Takano Stone, R.N.C., M.S.

CHAPTER 22

Using Theory to Guide Nursing Interventions: A Case Study 423
W. Carole Chenitz, R.N., Ed.D.

· · · · · · · · · · · · U N I T IV · · · · · · · · · · · ·

NURSING CARE FOR SELECTED HEALTH PROBLEMS IN THE OLDER ADULT

CHAPTER 25

Parkinson's Disease

Jeanie S. Kayser-Jones, R.N., Ph.D., F.A.A.N.
Theodore H.D. Jones, Ph.D.

CHAPTER 26

Alcoholism in the Elderly 507
W. Carole Chenitz, R.N., Ed.D.

··············· U N I T V ···············

THE CONTEXT OF NURSING CARE DELIVERY

CHAPTER 27

Environments for Nursing Care of the Older Client 523
Judith S. Schainen, R.N.C., Ph.D.

CHAPTER 28

Social Support of the Older Client
Linda R. Phillips, R.N., Ph.D., F.A.A.N.

CHAPTER 29

Balancing Resources: Demand Against Supply
Juliet Corbin, R.N., D.N.Sc.

CHAPTER 30

Home Health Care 557

Sato Hashizume, R.N.C., M.S., N.P.

CHAPTER 31

Program Planning and Development 577

Marilyn D. Fravel, R.N., N.H.A.

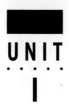

UNIT

I

GENERAL CONSIDERATIONS

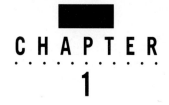

CHAPTER
1

An Overview of Gerontological Nursing

JOYCE TAKANO STONE, R.N.C., M.S.
W. CAROLE CHENITZ, R.N., Ed.D.

"When one has taken care of people and things and adapted to the disappointments and triumphs of life, a sense of order and meaning is attributed to one's life and one feels a sense of accomplishment and contribution to humankind."

Erik Erikson, 1963

Today, the first group of people to achieve advanced age in modern society is entering its ninth decade. The science of gerontology and the practice of gerontological nursing have undergone rapid development and growth as this cohort added another decade to the far limit of human life expectancy.

The role and practice of nurses in gerontological nursing have evolved as the population of elderly has grown and knowledge of their health care needs has emerged. The practice of nursing in this specialty, as in all nursing, is intrinsically linked with the needs of the consumers of care. Their health care needs and health problems become the concern of nurses. The identification and treatment of the health problems of older people have led to the development of gerontological nursing. Although gerontological nursing is relatively new, it is the fastest growing of all nursing specialties (ANA, 1981). Gerontological nursing does not exist as an entity by itself. It is part of the nursing profession, a part of the health care system, a part of the community, the society, and the world (Palmer, 1986). As such, the definition of nursing and gerontological nursing and the roles and functions of nursing specialists are influenced by multiple factors, including societal needs, conditions, and traditions.

In this chapter, we trace the development of gerontological nursing. Concepts of aging and the aged, the health care needs of the

3

aged, the system for health care, and philosophy of geriatric care are presented along with the development of this nursing specialty.

THE PAST

Social Thought on Aging

The history of mankind holds no precedent for the number of people that are defined as old today. In 1790 less than 2% of the population lived to age 65, whereas in 1985 11.5% were over 65 years old (US Bureau of the Census, 1986). The lifespan was shorter. In 1776 the average lifespan was one-third of what it is today (Fischer, 1978). Communicable diseases, infections, and epidemics were the major causes of mortality.

The demography of aging has changed, and along with it the social attitudes toward the elderly have also changed. In colonial America, elders were venerated. It was believed that to be an old person was a special sign from God of one's goodness; old age was a special gift from God. The old, during those times, were not only respected but also were exalted for their wisdom. During this time, behavioral norms and expectations of elders were clear. The old were to remain fully involved in all aspects of life, thereby giving youth the opportunity to benefit from their wisdom. Economics played a large part in the place of elders in society. Intergenerational relations were characterized by economic dependence of the young upon the old. In this agrarian society, land was the chief commodity. Elders held the land, and it wasn't until their death that their children achieved economic independence (de Beauvoir, 1972; Fischer, 1978).

Historically, for the old, though, age meant pain and infirmity. Yet, the aged were expected to behave in a serene and tranquil manner befitting one with wisdom and the grace of God. The pain of chronic ailments was suffered in isolation and loneliness. To be old and infirm was to be a subject of ridicule. The old attempted to preserve their appearance and place in society, and so they dealt with conditions such as gout, rheumatism, and arthritis in silence and with grace. It has been noted that every prominent American in early times left accounts of personal suffering and pain (Fischer, 1978).

Age veneration continued until after the American Revolution—the latter part of the eighteenth century. During this time, the population enjoyed new liberty and independence, and this spirit carried over to all social relations. A shift in the position and power of elders was seen, for example, as the first mandatory retirement laws were passed. Rest and disengagement became the tasks of old age (Fischer, 1978).

A strong youth bias developed in the years between 1790 and 1850, and the aged continued to lose power. By the mid-nineteenth century the aged were on the margins of society. By the end of the twentieth century, the marginal social status declined so that contempt for the old was the predominant social attitude. "Gerontophobia" is a term used to describe fear and contempt for the aged and aging. At the same time greater numbers of people were living into advanced age, and they often had no means of economic support (Achenbaum, 1978).

Old age was now defined as a social problem. In 1935, the Social Security Act was passed as a way to intervene on a national level to solve the economic problem (Achenbaum, 1978). During the remainder of the twentieth century, social views of the aged have grown ambivalent. On the one hand, there are positive images of certain old people in literature, politics, and social life. On the other hand, fear and loathing of aging and the aged continue (Covey, 1988). Rosow (1976) found that old people themselves hated to be old or considered aged. They would refuse to engage with other old people or accept themselves as aged. Throughout American history, there are several recurrent themes about the aged and aging that we can summarize and use to compare aging in the past with aging in modern American. These themes are: (1) the expectations of behaviors for elders in American society; (2) the changing roles of older people along with shifts in values, beliefs, economics, and power; and (3) power shifts among various segments of the population at different times in history. The focus is currently moving from youth to the aged. We are experiencing the "graying" of America, with older Americans becoming more politically aware and active.

Health Care of the Aged

For centuries, the aged were cared for by their families. However, as the population grew and people lived long, social thought and ideology changed, and formal institutions were established to care for the aged (Gold & Kaufman, 1970). The first of these institutions, the almshouse, was developed by churches to care for the indigent elderly without family. Later, in colonial America, county "poor farms," the first basic institution for housing the aged and infirm, served those without family. Geriatric care in times past can best be characterized as kind-hearted people giving shelter (Stone, 1969; Davis, 1983).

In the decades that followed, health care for the aged in this country was provided by families and family physicians. The development of hospitals meant there were new settings for medical care to be delivered. After the passage of the Social Security Act in 1935, the forerunners of modern nursing homes were formed. Typically, retired and widowed nurses converted their homes into boarding homes for the elderly needing assistance. City, county, and state hospitals were responsible for caring for the elderly who could neither remain at home nor live with family. During the 1940s, several states established minimal standards for nursing home care; licensing of these homes began. In 1965, Medicare was created and implemented. This federal act changed the health care system and created the mechanism for the development of the nursing home industry.

The Development of Gerontological Nursing

For the first half of the twentieth century, the goal of nursing care of the elderly was to keep the person clean, fed, and free of pain. During this time there was little interest in geriatric nursing. There were virtually no role models, and geriatric nursing as a specialty did not exist. However, there have always been nurses concerned specifically with the care of the aged. Highlights from this period illustrate concern among nurses for the sick aged population. In 1925, an editorial in the *American Journal of Nursing* suggested the formation of a specialty within nursing that focused on the care of the aged. It stated,

> Success in nursing the aged has, we believe, rarely been based on any finite body of knowledge of the subject. . . . The modern health movement is constantly increasing the span of life expectancy by its onslaught against preventable disease. . . . The nursing profession, therefore, must expect to care for larger and larger numbers of patients suffering from degenerative conditions. Is it perhaps time for nursing to consider another specialty? (AJN, 1925, p. 394)

In 1950, the first textbook on geriatric nursing was published. This book, *Geriatric Nursing*, written by Kathleen Newton and Helen Anderson, marked the unofficial beginning of geriatrics as a specialty within nursing. The first published research in geriatric nursing was done by Mack on "The Personal Adjustment of Chronically Ill Old People Under Home Care." This study was published in *Nursing Research* in 1952.

During the twenty-five years between 1950 and 1975 there were major changes in nursing and nursing education. A major goal of nursing during these years was to attain professional status. Nursing practice, previously based on tradition, intuition, and imitation, was now to be based on knowledge and theory derived from the basic and social sciences as they applied to nursing. Theory development and a body of knowledge unique to nursing would follow as the discipline moved along the course of professional development. The movement toward professional status sparked the identification and formation of specialty practice groups within the nursing discipline.

In 1962, 70 nurses met to form the first American Nurses' Association Conference Group on Geriatric Nursing. In 1966, the Division of Geriatric Nursing was created within the American Nurses' Association. By 1974, 26 state nursing associations reported conferences and special interest groups on geriatric nursing. This interest was fostered by the 1970 publication of the "Standards of Geriatric Nursing Practice" by the American Nurses' Association. These standards were based on the premise that "knowledge and theory when applied to practice should improve the care of the aged" (ANA, 1970, p. 4). Publication of these standards of practice marks the official recognition of geriatric nursing as a specialty within nursing.

The emergence of gerontological nursing as a specialty occurred during the time of prevalent negative societal attitudes toward aging and the aged. The new standards were an attempt to improve the quality of care given to the aged and to reestablish basic principles reflecting an attitude of acceptance of aging and the aged. This attitude would influence the behavior of nurses in practice. It was clearly stated in the original standards that the major issue distinguishing geriatric nursing was the effort by which its practitioners would seek to reverse negative cultural attitudes toward the aged. Therefore, the first standards related to the attitude of the nursing practitioner providing care to the aged client. Specifically, the nurse must

> . . . demonstrate understanding and appreciation of social and historic settings in which older people have developed and how these factors affect their behavior and values. This enables her to respect the older person as an individual (ANA, 1970, p. 4).

Nurses were urged to resolve their own conflicting attitudes toward aging, death, and dependency in order to care for the aged. Clearly, by these standards, nurses were to develop attitudes toward the aged that were different from those of the larger society. However, there were no clear prescriptions to help nurses change their attitude toward the aged or resolve their conflicting attitudes toward aging and death. The standards were ideals upon which quality care of the aged could be delivered.

Following the publication of the standards and the recognition of geriatric nursing, there was a period of growth and development of the specialty. In 1975, the *Journal of Gerontological Nursing* was published. In 1976, the Division of Geriatric Nursing was changed to the Division of Gerontological Nursing to reflect nursing's identification with health as a unifying concept and the emphasis of nursing on delivery of health care. The original standards were revised in 1973 and again in 1976 and renamed the "Standards for Gerontological Nursing Practice" (ANA, 1976). In 1980, the *American Journal of Nursing* began publication of *Geriatric Nursing*, the second journal devoted to nursing in this specialty.

During this period there was concern for the education of new gerontological nurses. In the late 1960s, there were few schools of nursing with curricula offering geriatric content. Gunter and Estes' book *Education for Gerontic Nursing* was published in 1979. The authors of this book identified competencies in geriatrics that could be expected of students at the baccalaureate level. It provided a basis for geriatric nursing to be included in the undergraduate nursing curriculum. By the mid 1970s, several basic textbooks appeared on the subject of care of the aged (Burnside, 1976). These highlights in the development of gerontological nursing are outlined in Table 1–1.

In spite of the growth and development of gerontological nursing and the fields of gerontology and geriatric medicine, negative attitudes toward the aged continued to be a problem plaguing nurses interested in this specialty. In 1976, Burnside wrote, . . . sometimes nurses view geriatric wards and units as the least desirable place to work. To be assigned to a geriatric unit is viewed as a punitive measure" (Burnside, 1976, p. 12). She recognized that ". . . all nurses are not prepared for this type of practice" (Burnside, 1976, p. 19) and pointed out that negative attitudes toward the aged were reflected on the nurses who chose to work with the aged. Burnside put forth the call for the acceptance of geriatric nursing within nursing. She wrote,

> . . . the negativistic attitude in the profession

Table 1–1. GERONTOLOGICAL NURSING HIGHLIGHTS: THE PAST

1904	First *American Journal of Nursing* article published on care of the aged
1925	*American Journal of Nursing* introduces idea of nurses forming a specialty in the care of the aged
1950	First textbook on geriatric nursing, written by K. Newton and H. Anderson
1950	Geriatrics emerges as a specialty within the nursing profession
1961–1962	American Nurses' Association recommends and forms a national geriatric nursing group
1966	American Nurses' Association creates the Division of Geriatric Nursing (emphasis on care of the aged ill)
1970	American Nurses' Association Standards of Geriatric Nursing Practice established
1973	Standards revised
1974	American Nurses' Association offers certification in gerontological nursing
1975	*Journal of Gerontological Nursing* first published
1976	American Nurses' Association changes name of division to Division of Gerontological Nursing Practice (emphasis on health)
1976	American Nurses' Association Standards for Gerontological Nursing Practice published
1979	The book *Education for Gerontic Nursing* written by L. Gunter and C. Estes
1980	*Geriatric Nursing* first published

is manifested in the subtle and not so subtle treatment of nurses who choose to work with the aged. For some time now, nurses who work in nursing homes, long term care facilities or geriatric units have stated they are tired of being treated as second class nurses (Burnside, 1976, p. 12).

THE PRESENT

Social Thought on Aging

The aging population continues to increase in number and proportion. This trend is expected to continue until the year 2010, when the "baby boom" generation reaches advanced age. Social changes have affected living patterns and care patterns in society. Since the women's movement of the 1960s, there has been an increase in the number of women working outside of the home. Generally, women enter motherhood today at a later age and have fewer children now than in previous generations. Divorce and the high cost of living have changed the "empty nest" of midlife to the "cluttered nest" as adult children and their children return to the parents' home. The middle generation has been termed the "sandwich generation," facing the needs of both their aged parents and their adult children. This has created new stress in midlife and intergenerational competition. Since women are no longer invariably providing family care, child and elder care is provided increasingly by social programs, services, and institutions (Aizenberg & Harris, 1982; Stone, Cafferta, & Sangl, 1987; Sussman, 1985; Treas, 1977).

During the past decade, gerontophobia as a social attitude has been fading; the natural limits of this movement may have been reached. Several powerful forces have brought this decline.

Political Power of the Aged. The increasing number of older Americans has created a growing political body. Today's elders are charting new territories and establishing new models for old age.

Advanced Knowledge of Aging. The study of the processes of aging reveals the complex, multifaceted nature of aging and the impact of psychosocial and biophysiologic factors on the way we age.

New Family Structures. Elders are now seen as part of an active, although different, family structure. The existence of the lineal family means that three or more generations, not necessarily living under the same roof, can provide aid and assistance to all family members.

Continuing Growth of the Aging Population. As the "graying" of America continues through the end of the baby boom generation, a major portion of society will continue to be affected by the "problems of aging."

Health Care of the Aged

The elderly are plagued by major illnesses more often chronic than acute in nature. Heart, cancer, and strokes take their toll, accounting for 80% of deaths in the over-65 age group (US Department of Health and Human

Services [USDHHS], 1987). Long-term care and rehabilitation are needed by those with hypertension, arthritis, diabetes, pulmonary diseases, or visual and hearing impairments. Other serious health problems include the dementing and disabling conditions, such as Alzheimer's disease. Also of concern are accidents and depression.

In 1956, the Commission on Chronic Illness defined chronic illness as follows:

> All impairments or deviations from normal which have one or more of the following characteristics: are permanent, leave residual disability, are caused by non-reversible pathological alteration, require special training of the patient for rehabilitation, may be expected to require a long period of supervision, observation, or care (Strauss, 1975, p. 1).

Chronic illness or long-term illness poses multiple problems, social and psychological as well as physical, for the older person who has one or more of these conditions. The person has to live with the illness; it will not disappear. The person is faced with trying to live as normal a life as possible; to manage the crises that occur; to handle the prescribed regimen; to control the symptoms; to tolerate disability, stigma, and social isolation; and to maintain adequate funds to support everyday living as well as necessary health care (Strauss, 1975).

The care of older persons with chronic or long-term illness presents problems beyond those of persons experiencing acute or short-term illnesses. The primary focus in long-term illness is not cure but rather prevention of complications, rehabilitation to the maximal level of function, and attainment of an optimal state of well-being.

The health care system is faced with increasing demands for services at a time of fiscal constraints. Health programs for the elderly have generally been expensive, poorly designed, and somewhat ineffective (Estes, 1988a; Mor & Spector, 1988).

The complexity and extended timespan of chronic illnesses involve many segments of the health care system. The movement in and out and throughout the segments of the health care system is not always a smooth flow for the older person. There is a great danger in a piecemeal approach to health care with its lack of continuity and coordination of care. Essential services may be nonexistent or overburdened with demands. Laura Reif (1975) identified the wide range of services and resources needed for the chronically ill and offered specific suggestions for planning policies and programs to meet their needs. These are illustrated in Table 1–2.

The Growth of Gerontological Nursing

The 1980s have been identified as the decade of decision in nursing (ANA, 1980). There are major changes occurring in the health field and in nursing, particularly in the area of the economics of health care. In terms of development, gerontological nursing has reached adolescence, that is, a period of change, turmoil, and fast growth as it moves with society and the health care system to meet the emerging needs and demands of the increasing number of older clients.

Currently, there are approximately 1.9 million registered nurses in the United States, of whom 78.7% are employed. Over two-thirds (68%) of employed nurses are practicing in hospitals, and the next largest group (7.7%) is practicing in nursing homes (ANA, 1987a). The elderly population has higher rates of hospitalization and longer average lengths of stay than younger population groups. In 1985, the elderly accounted for nearly one-third of all hospital discharges. The average length of stay for those over 65 years was 8.6 days, compared to 7 days for those between 45 and 65 years of age (USDHHS, 1986).

Approximately one-fourth of all older Americans will spend part of their lives in nursing homes. Nurse staffing in nursing homes is a problem for gerontological nursing. Most health care for the elderly takes place in the community, as shown by one study's results in which 75% of those over 65 had no days of hospitalization but only 10% to 20% had no health care visits (Koch & Havlik, 1987).

Table 1–2. SERVICES FOR PERSONS WITH CHRONIC ILLNESS

Counseling and Education
For sick person and associates on the medical/social/psychological aspects of chronic illness. Includes:
    Tailoring regimens to increase function
    Developing social skills to deal with visual disability, stigma, and social isolation
    Managing impact of illness on others
    Renegotiating responsibilities with family and employers
    Accounting for constraints of illness
    Managing the social, personal, and medical aspects of terminal illness
      legal counsel regarding manifestations

Revamping the Physical Environment
Designing/modifying living space, work areas, transportation to accommodate people with chronic illness

Funding/Money Management
Providing financial resources, budgeting for both direct and indirect costs of illness

Redesigning Social Arrangement
Providing the manpower to assist persons with chronic illness and their families. Includes:
    Task exchange networks
    Emergency back-up systems
    Social support arrangements

Supplying Technical Aid and Equipment
Providing new equipment and techniques to facilitate activities of daily living for those disabled by chronic illness

Medical Intervention
Medical and paramedical services. Includes:
    Dietary counseling
    Rehabilitation services
    Speech therapy

Daily Maintenance Services
Assistance with activities and tasks of daily living

Public Education and Informational Services
Education to increase sensitivity and understanding and decrease prejudice of those who encounter the chronically ill

Managerial Assistance
Broker to ensure access to necessary services. Includes:
    Obtaining information and services
    Assisting clients in decision making about services
    Coordinating services
    Ensuring quality care
    Facilitating feedback from consumers about services

(Data from Reif, L (1975). A policy perspective and its implications. *In* Strauss, AL: *Chronic Illness and the Quality of Life.* St. Louis, CV Mosby, 1975, 147–148.)

Nursing has struggled to make health a unifying concept for professional practice. In 1980, the American Nurses' Association's Social Policy Statement defined nursing practice as the diagnosis and treatment of human responses to health problems. Some of the human responses delineated form the core of gerontological nursing; for example, self-care limitations, impaired functioning, pain and discomfort, and strains related to life processes. According to the Social Policy Statement, the goal of nursing is to assist individuals, groups, and society to achieve wellness or an optimal state of well-being (ANA, 1980).

There has been a philosophical change in gerontological nursing from a disease-oriented approach to a health-oriented one (ANA, 1981). Emphasis is being placed on health promotion and self-care. Nursing, as a discipline, is concerned with the holistic nature of clients; that is, the interaction of health, clients, and environment for optimal health and wellness. Health is viewed as a dynamic process in which the potential of an individual is realized to the fullest extent possible (ANA, 1981).

Health or wellness is an optimal state of being. For nurses concerned with the care of elders, to achieve the goal of health and wellness requires that new definitions of health in advanced age be created. In recent times, models of coexistence of health with disability have been developed by nurses and are evidenced in the Model of Long-Term Care by the American Nurses' Association (ANA, 1982).

The ANA Nursing Model of Long-Term Care is proposed as appropriate for delivery of long-term care to older adults. The medical model, while appropriate for acute, short-term care, is inappropriate, as demonstrated by a comparison between the models on several salient points (see Table 1–3).

In 1987, the Standards for Gerontological Nursing Practice were revised again. The current Standards include process and outcome criteria for the evaluation of nursing practice, as well as sections delineating the roles of the gerontological nurse generalist and specialist (ANA, 1987b).

While nursing has identified with health and wellness, the relationship of nursing to the sick elderly is both a pragmatic and moral one. On a pragmatic level, the sick elderly require nursing care for survival. On a moral level, nursing, it has been said, ". . . is in some special sense responsible for being the conscience of the society on the particular issue of the care of the sick aged" (Yarling, 1977, p. 45). While nurses are responsible for the care of the sick aged, this responsibility did not come with authority nor was it accepted by the entire profession. Fateful circumstances, it has been said, rather than design, has given nurses de facto responsibility for the care of the sick aged in nursing homes, acute hospitals, psychiatric hospitals, and private residence (Yarling, 1977).

The ANA Social Policy Statement discussed specialization in nursing as a mark of advancement of the nursing profession. Gerontological nursing as a specialty has made considerable progress in the past decade. The negative image of gerontological nursing is changing. Certification by the American Nurses' Association has improved the image and status of gerontological nurses by recognizing this field as a specialty and by conferring a title to those who have demonstrated knowledge and expertise. Increasing numbers of nurses are being certified in gerontological nursing by the ANA (Fulmer, Ashley, & Reilly, 1986). As of January, 1988, 922 nurses were certified as gerontological nurse practitioners and 5,831 nurses were certified in gerontological nursing (Registered nurses, 1988). This places gerontological nursing third in the number of nurses holding certification, with 9,051 medical-sur-

Table 1–3. COMPARISONS BETWEEN THE MEDICAL MODEL AND THE NURSING MODEL

Factors	Medical Model of Care	Nursing Model of Care
Nursing and health needs	Secondary need	Major need
Medical needs	Major need	Secondary need
Setting for care delivery	Medical center/hospital	Any setting
Measurement of successful treatment	Number of diagnosed, appropriately treated, cured, or rehabilitated	Present level of physical, mental, social, and spiritual function compared to potential level of function
Treatment emphasis	Chief complaint: what's wrong; what's disabled; disability/illness orientation	Functional level: what's good; what's healthy; ability/health orientation
Focus of care	Individual organ, start with chief complaint	Holistic approach, total person, start where the person is
Duration of care	Episodic	Continuing
Role of the patient/client/family	Passivity, regressive-dependence	Active participation, progressive-independence

(Reprinted from American Nurses' Association: *A Challenge for Change: The Role of Gerontological Nursing.* Kansas City, Missouri, American Nurses' Association, 1982, p. 12.)

gical nurses and 10,225 psychiatric-mental health nurses holding certification.

While many nurses presently in gerontological nursing received their education through inservice education, continuing education, or on-the-job training, there has been an increase in the quantity and quality of these educational programs. The National League for Nursing, as the national accrediting body for schools of nursing, requires that gerontological nursing content be addressed in the curriculum (National League for Nursing, 1983). Educational programs in gerontological nursing have been and are still being established in graduate programs.

A recent survey of gerontological nurses in clinical settings identified a number of professional, clinical, and policy issues needing attention. Professional issues include continuing education and the ongoing development of gerontological nurses, developing and maintaining standards of nursing practice, and the educational preparation of gerontological nurses. Clinical issues of highest priority were confusional states, immobility, and sensory loss. Achieving an adequate number of gerontological nurses to meet the needs of the aged, financing health care for the aged, securing salaries and compensation of nurses, and enforcing standards of care through licensure and credentialing of agencies were considered the most important policy issues by the nurses (ANA, 1986). Highlights of current professional development in gerontological nursing are presented in Table 1–4.

THE FUTURE

Social Thought on Aging

John F. Kennedy once said, "It is not enough for a great nation to have added new years to life. Our objective must be to add new life to those years" (reprinted in Coni, 1977, p. 1).

It is anticipated that over 30 million people will be over 65 years of age by the year 2000. This number will continue to increase, eventually representing 15% to 18% of the total population by the year 2030 (US Bureau of the

Table 1–4. GERONTOLOGICAL NURSING HIGHLIGHTS: THE PRESENT

1980 American Nurses' Association: *Nursing: A Social Policy Statement*

1. Defines the nature and scope of nursing practice "Nursing is a self regulatory profession whose authority is based on a social contract between social and the profession" (ANA, 1980).

   "Nursing is the diagnosis and treatment of human responses to actual or potential health problems" (ANA, 1980).

2. Identifies specialization as a mark of advancement of the nursing profession; delineates criteria and roles and functions of specialist in nursing practice

1981 American Nurses' Association Division of Gerontological Nursing: *A Statement of the Scope of Gerontological Nursing Practice*

"Gerontological nursing practice focuses on assessing the health status of older adults, establishing a nursing diagnosis, planning and providing appropriate nursing and health care services, and evaluating the effectiveness of such care. Emphasis is placed on maximizing independence in the activities of daily living; promoting, maintaining, and restoring health; preventing and/or controlling disease; and maintaining life in dignity and comfort until death" (ANA, 1982).

1984 Division on Gerontological Nursing Practice becomes the Council on Gerontological Nursing.

Aim of the Council is to improve the quality of life and the quality of care for older persons in all settings (ANA, 1987b).

1986 American Nurses' Association publishes survey *Gerontological Nurses in Clinical Settings: Survey Analysis*

1987 American Nurses' Association: *Standards and Scope of Gerontological Nursing Practice*

1. "Standards call for quality care at a level beyond that required by minimal regulatory standards" (ANA, 1987b).

2. Standards may be used in quality assurance programs as a resource for assessment tools and plan for care, and peer review and evaluation of performance (ANA, 1987b).

3. Roles of the generalist and specialist in gerontological nursing practice are described (ANA, 1987b).

Census, 1986). Society is becoming age-irrelevant, that is, there are fewer clear-cut demarcations about age-specific behaviors and expectations. Older people go back to college, start new careers, and change life styles. They are challenging the old models of aging, creating new images of aging, and setting new possibilities for the final stage of life. The generation of old in the future will be better prepared for old age—better educated, financially more secure, and better prepared for leisure (Hagestad, 1987). The family will continue to be the main source of support for the elderly.

In the future, Fries and Crapo (1981) predict a "rectangularization" of the survival curve created by the continued decline in premature death and improved management of illness, allowing people to live well to the outer limit of the lifespan (Fries & Crapo, 1981). They envision that life will be physiologically, emotionally, and intellectually vigorous until shortly before its close. Others make more conservative predictions, stating that society will need to prepare for a number of ill, disabled, and frail elderly over the next four to five decades (Schneider & Brody, 1983; White et al., 1986). They also call for research on the many conditions that may decrease the length and quality of life (White et al., 1986).

There is a recognition in the health care system of the importance of long-term care (Estes, 1988b). If follows that we should see the achievement of equal status of long-term and acute care, with better financial support and professional talent invested in the long-term component of the health care system. We will continue to see a role for institutional care, but with an improved system (Gallagher, 1986; Mor & Spector, 1988). Creative, innovative programs will be designed to meet the changing health needs of society. Undoubtedly, there will be continued, if not accelerated, advancement in technology, resulting in new and improved methods of diagnosis and treatment of illnesses.

Health promotion, with its emphasis on the prevention of illness and disability, will continue to be the focus of our efforts. Health education will play an increasingly important role. Greater attention will be given to the quality of life.

Gerontological Nursing in the Future

Nurses need to be on the cutting edge of health care for the aged; nursing has been,

and is, an essential and critical component. Enthusiasm and excitement for geriatric care will continue among nurses. As scientific knowledge about aging advances, researchers in nursing will be contributors to the developing knowledge base. Gerontological nursing will need thinkers, planners, directors, and providers of care.

Gerontological nursing will reach full maturity in the very near future. Each generation of nurses has made numerous, valuable contributions to the development of this nursing specialty. In the years to come, gerontological nurses will continue to contribute to the overall advancement and improvement of care of the elderly. The improvement of practice and care is a collective endeavor.

Is our view of the future an optimistic and perhaps unlikely scenario? We think not. The energy that created and developed gerontological nursing as a legitimate specialty exists in today's generation of gerontological nurses. They will in turn pass it on to the next generation. We believe as Doris Schwartz, one of the pioneers of geriatric nursing, wrote in 1969, ". . . a predominant note that pervades this flood of writing for nurses is one of pervasive cheer. . .one reads the profession's endless enthusiasm, deep concern, and the will to improve" (Schwartz, 1969, pp. 90 to 91). It is this spirit that has created gerontological nursing. It is this spirit that will continue to advance and improve our practice.

References

Achenbaum, WA (1978): *Old Age in the New Land: The American Experience since 1790*. Baltimore, Johns Hopkins University Press.

Aizenberg, R, & Harris, RJ (1982): Family demographic changes: The middle generation squeeze. *Generations*, 7(2):5–7, 41.

American Nurses' Association (1970): *Standards of Geriatric Nursing Practice*. Kansas City, Missouri, American Nurses' Association.

American Nurses' Association (1976): *Standards of Gerontological Nursing Practice*. Kansas City, Missouri, American Nurses' Association.

American Nurses' Association (1980): *Nursing: A Social Policy Statement*. Kansas City, Missouri, American Nurses' Association.

American Nurses' Association (1981): *A Statement on the*

Scope of Gerontological Nursing Practice. Kansas City, Missouri, American Nurses' Association.

American Nurses' Association (1982): *A Challenge for Change: The Role of Gerontological Nursing.* Kansas City, Missouri, American Nurses' Association.

American Nurses' Association (1986): *Gerontological Nurses in Clinical Settings: Survey Analysis.* Kansas City, Missouri, American Nurses' Association.

American Nurses' Association (1987a): *Facts About Nursing 86—87.* Kansas City, Missouri, American Nurses' Association.

American Nurses' Association (1987b): *Standards and Scope of Gerontological Nursing Practice.* Kansas City, Missouri, American Nurses' Association.

Burnside, IM (1976): *Nursing and the Aged.* New York, McGraw Hill.

Coni, N, Davison, W, & Webster, S (1977): *Lecture Notes on Geriatrics.* Oxford, Blackwell.

Covey, HC (1988): Historical terminology used to represent older people. *Gerontologist,* 28:291–297.

Davis, BA (1983): The gerontological specialty. *J Gerontol Nurs,* 9:527–532.

de Beauvoir, S (1972): *The Coming of Age.* New York, GP Putnam's Sons.

Editorial (1925). *Am J Nurs,* 25:394.

Erikson, EH (1963): *Childhood and Society* (ed 2). New York, WW Norton.

Estes, CL (1988a): Cost containment and the elderly: Conflict or challenge? *J Am Geriatr Soc,* 36:68–72.

Estes, CL (1988b): Health care policy in the late 20th century. *Generations,* 12(3):44–47.

Fischer, DH (1978): *Growing Old in America.* New York, Oxford University Press.

Fries, JF, & Crapo, LM (1981): *Vitality and Aging.* San Francisco, WH Freeman and Company.

Fulmer, T, Ashley, J, & Reilly, C (1986): Geriatric nursing in acute settings. *In* Eisdorfer, C (ed): *Ann Rev Gerontol Geriat,* 6:27–80.

Gallagher, A (1986): A model for change in long term care. *J Gerontol Nurs,* 12(5):19–23.

Gold, JG, & Kaufman, SM (1970): Development of care of elderly: Tracing the history of institutional facilities. *Gerontologist,* 10:262–275.

Gunter, L, & Estes, C (1979): *Education for Gerontic Nursing.* New York, Springer.

Hagestad, GO (1987): Able elderly in the family context. *Gerontologist,* 27:417–422.

Koch, H, & Havlik, RJ (1987): Use of health care—ambulatory medical care. *In* U.S. Department of Health and Human Resources, Public Health Service, National Center for Health Statistics, *Health statistics on older persons. United States, 1986* (DHHS Publication No [PHS] 87-1409). Washington, DC, US Government Printing Office, 56–59.

Mack, MJ (1952): The personal adjustment of chronically ill and people under home care. *Nurs Res,* 1:9–30.

Mor, V, & Spector, W (1988): Achieving continuity of care. *Generations,* 12(3):47–52.

National League for Nursing (1983): *Criteria for the Evaluation of Baccalaureate and Higher Degree Programs in Nursing* (NLN Publication No. 15-1251,7). New York, National League for Nursing.

Newtown, K, & Anderson, HC (1950): *Geriatric Nursing.* St. Louis, CV Mosby.

Palmer, IS (1986): Nursing's heritage. *In* Werley, HH, Fitzpatrick, JJ, & Taunton, RL (eds): *Annual Review of Nursing Research,* 4:237–257. New York, Springer.

Registered nurses certified by ANA as of Jan. 1, 1988 (1988, September). *Am Nurs,* p 15.

Reif, L (1975): A policy perspective and its implication. *In* Strauss, AL (ed): *Chronic illness and the quality of life.* St. Louis, CV Mosby.

Rosow, IJ (1976): *Socialization to Old Age.* Berkeley, California, University of California Press.

Schneider, EL, & Brody, JA (1983): Aging, natural death, and the compression of mortality: Another view. *N Engl J Med,* 309:854–856.

Schwartz, D (1969): Aging and the field of nursing. *In* Riley, MW (ed): *Aging and Society,* vol. 2. New York, Russell Sage Foundation.

Stone, R, Caferata, GL, & Sange, J (1987): Caregivers of the frail elderly: A national profile. *Gerontologist,* 27:616–626.

Stone, V (1969): Nursing of older people. *In* Busse, EW & Pfeiffer, E (eds): *Behavior and Adaptation in Late Life.* Boston, Little, Brown, 313–321.

Strauss, AL (1975): *Chronic Illness and the Quality of Life.* St. Louis, CV Mosby.

Sussman, MB (1985): The family life of old people. *In* Binstock, RH, & Shanas, E (eds): *Handbook of Aging and the Social Sciences,* New York, Van Nostrand & Reinhold, 415–449.

Treas, J (1977): Family support systems for the aged: Some social and demographic considerations. *Gerontologist,* 17:486–491.

US Bureau of the Census (1986): *Statistical Abstract of the United States. 1987* (ed 107). Washington, DC, US Government Printing Office.

US Department of Health and Human Services, Public Health Service, National Center for Health Statistics (1987): *Health Statistics on Older Persons, United States. 1986* (DHHS Publication No. [PHS]. Washington, DC, US Government Printing Office, 1–79.

White, LR, Cartwright, WS, Cornoni-Huntley, J, & Brock, DB (1986): Geriatric epidemiology. *In* Eisdorfer, C (ed). *Ann Rev Gerontol Geriat,* 6:215–311. New York, Springer.

Yarling, R (1977): The sick aged, the nursing profession and the larger society. *J Gerontol Nurs,* 3:42–51.

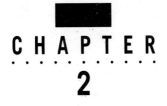

CHAPTER
2

Ethical Issues in Gerontological Nursing

ANNE J. DAVIS, R.N., Ph.D., F.A.A.N.

principles. The principle of respect for individuals says that we do not treat others merely as means but rather as ends in themselves. The principle of autonomy dictates that the individual has the right to make his or her own decisions. When we enter into specific situations of informed consent in the health care setting, these principles are brought to bear. We must take these ethical principles into the real and very complex world involving our interactions with patients and their families. Under informed consent, what does it mean to respect persons? Where, how, and to what extent does autonomy play its part?

INTRODUCTION

This chapter focuses on the problems of competency as it affects ethical and clinical issues with the elderly. Taking patients seriously and respecting their ethical positions, listening to patients and understanding that their values may differ from one's own, and acting on patients' decisions based on their values are important ethical issues in the clinical setting.

We put a great deal of stock in people making decisions about their lives and well-being in our society. Such a value has its philosophical grounding in at least two ethical

INFORMED CONSENT

Informed consent is an ethical and legal process that attempts to integrate delivery of health care with the principles of respect and autonomy. If a person is capable of consent, it is morally and legally impermissible to perform any procedure that involves touching or invading that person's body without specific written permission to do so. The person must not only give written consent without coercion, but must also understand what is being consented to. The first part of this requirement is fairly easy to satisfy with a signature on a consent form. It is the second aspect of this process that is difficult and gives rise to most ethical dilemmas in practice. This is really the heart of clinical ethics and law. The primary purpose of informed consent is the protection of individual autonomy.

The legal doctrine of informed consent is well grounded in the principle of autonomy. Justice Cardozo in Schloensdorff vs. Society of New York Hospital (1914) said: "Every human being of adult years and sound mind has a right to determine what shall be done with his own body; and a surgeon who performs an operation without his patient's consent commits an assault, for which he is liable in damages." In the 1960 case of Natanson vs. Kline, an even stronger view of autonomy is expressed: "Anglo-American law starts with the premise of thorough going self-determination. It follows that each man is considered to be master of his own body, and that he may, if he be of sound mind, expressly prohibit the performance of lifesaving surgery or other medical treatment."

An interesting aspect to these statements is the phase "of sound mind." Consent cannot be considered "informed" if the patient is not competent to make a decision. This means that this notion of competence is the foundation on which all other elements of consent rest. No matter how well we inform a person about proposed health care action, if he or she is not of sound mind the process of informed consent cannot proceed. And if someone is deemed to be incompetent, then a second-party consent must be obtained. This allows someone other than the patient to speak in the patient's best interest. This presumes yet another ethical principle—"do no harm" or nonmaleficence with its corollary of doing good or beneficence.

COMPETENCY

Competency is a complex notion that we need to understand if the patient is to be our primary ethical focus. Competency is a subject for the law as well as for ethics, but in the law a patient is judged incompetent in exceptional cases in order that a significant action may be

taken that opposes a person's expressed preference or when specific content would be required and is not forthcoming. But the ethical issue extends further and seeks to determine under what conditions a health care professional justifiably may deny a patient the opportunity to participate in all important decisions that affect treatment. A central and necessary starting point in examining competency is to ask: When is someone competent and when not?

One way to understand competency is to view it on a number of levels. We are all competent in some things and incompetent in others. For example, most of us are competent to manage our money but not to fix our cars. In general, most adults are deemed competent to make their own decisions. However, when these adults become patients they can be viewed as incompetent to make decisions about medical treatment. Such decisions as to the kind of treatment, if any, and the withholding and withdrawing of treatment become ethical dilemmas. These decisions can become even more crucial if the patient is elderly, because we tend to view older people as having less physical and mental ability. When elderly persons enter a hospital or other health care facility, they may be considered incompetent to sign a consent form even though they may understand the ramifications of procedures when explained in language at their level of comprehension. Sometimes, too, the level of competence varies over time; that is, a person may be competent to decide a matter today but not be able to decide in the future if the life situation changes.

Because competency is a multidimensional concept, varying from time to time and from situation to situation, Beauchamp and Childress (1983) have proposed the idea of intermittent or limited competency. This concept prevents a person being labeled either totally competent or totally incompetent, preserves a maximal amount of autonomy, and justifies declaring a person incompetent only in those areas in which competence is truly questionable. Therefore persons of limited intelligence could be considered competent to decide whether to consent to elective surgery because they could understand the risks and benefits, whereas they might not be competent to understand the details of financial arrangements made by their attorneys.

Declaring a person incompetent does not necessarily mean that this is so. Unless specific criteria are applied each time consent is required, an unfair evaluation of competency is likely to be made. Margot Fromer (1981), a nurse, gives an example of this. An attendant working in a large state mental hospital kicked a patient to such an extent that the patient died two days later of a ruptured liver. The attendant was indicted for first-degree murder but was not fired or even suspended from his job. The hospital administrator's rationale for permitting the attendant to continue his duties with patients was that he was sure that the attendant would be acquitted of murder charges. When someone mentioned that the event had been witnessed by many patients, the administrator replied that no one would take the word of a crazy person. With this response the administrator implied that because society had declared a person incompetent in one or more areas, he was automatically incompetent in other or all areas. Using the administrator's view of competency, these patients would not have been considered competent to sign a surgical consent form even though no criteria for competency in this area have been tested.

Like the mentally ill, the elderly are a vulnerable population. During a clinical ethics discussion focused on an elderly woman patient, the question arose whether to discontinue treatment. After much dialogue among the staff members, the question was asked whether the patient was physically and psychologically capable of making this decision. Some of the staff thought she was not capable because of her age. She was viewed as one in a category of patients, the elderly, and not as an individual person who happens to be elderly.

A leader in the Gray Panthers once said that in our society we tend to view old people as either senile or cute, and both of these descriptions have the possibility of reducing the older adult to a child in the eyes of others. And it goes almost without saying that old persons seen as children are not considered competent to make important decisions about their body, mind, life, and well-being in general. The elderly, especially those in institutions such as hospitals and nursing homes, can be viewed much as the mental hospital administrator viewed the patients in his institution.

Standards

When is someone competent and when not? In order to answer this question, we can attempt to apply standards. It is useful to divide these standards into three types. The first standard seeks to specify some minimal level of mental capacity that any patient must have in order to be judged capable of making or sharing in health care decisions. The notion of rationality is the most common term used in this connection. But the appeal to rationality is ambiguous. It receives its philosophical grounding in the familiar notion that persons are essentially rational agents and that it is this quality that confers on us the obligation to respect people's autonomy in a way that we are not obligated to respect that of other creatures. But in the health care context, where the emphasis is on a person's present and often changeable state rather than on underlying capacities, a patient's rationality is usually judged by whether sensible and realistic choices are being made. This practice increases the difficulty of determining what is required for a person to be considered minimally rational.

A second kind of standard for competency disavows the attempt to establish a minimal level of functioning for all persons. Instead it seeks to determine whether the person in his or her present state is expressing preferences that are continuous with those he or she has expressed in the past. If the patient is judged to be acting from a "true self," then on this standard the person is competent. The assumption is that the effects of disease and treatment often block the will of one's true self, perhaps only temporarily, thus justifying or even requiring someone else to make the patient's decisions. The living will, and the natural death act attempt to follow patients' own true desires at a time when they cannot express them. However, these mechanisms cover only life-and-death decisions and do not apply to the problematic cases where patients express a desire that is thought not to be their "real" one.

A third approach to competency is to consider an understanding of medical data a necessity and thereby to argue that paternalism is justified as a general policy on the grounds that most patients lack the expertise to make decisions about their health care.

Each of these approaches to defining competency poses substantial difficulties, and each sanctions a greater degree of paternalism on the part of the family or health professional than is considered acceptable outside the medical sphere. To require that a person choose rationally in order to be judged competent is to impose a heavier burden of proof for medical competence than that which we impose in other areas. Adults are not constrained from marrying unsuitable partners or wasting their money, however irrational these decisions may be. The health care professional who wishes to justify paternalistic behavior simply on the grounds that a patient's choice is irrational must present ethical reasons why rationality should be required in order for a *patient* to be entitled to act autonomously, whereas in nonmedical settings persons are not "protected from themselves" merely because their preferences are irrational.

There is, of course, the question of just what is a rational decision in a given situation. For example, the case study of a 92-year-old woman entering the hospital with an intestinal obstruction addresses this problem. The surgeon explained to her that she needed an operation and what this would entail, including putting her to sleep. He also explained that, given her age and general frailness, she might not make it through the surgery or might not recover fully. The woman asked to have time to think over her situation, and when she talked again with the surgeon she said that her decision was to forego the surgery. She wanted to be kept as comfortable as possible and allowed to die. The surgeon immediately asked the psychiatrist to come and evaluate the patient to determine whether she was competent to make a decision. Would the surgeon have asked the psychiatrist to evaluate the patient if she had said yes to the surgery? One might argue that agreeing to surgery could be considered an irrational decision under these circumstances. What this case study points out is how our own values come into play. When patients make decisions that go against the deeply held and sometimes unexamined values of health professionals, they may be viewed as incompetent or irrational.

Why must people be expected to display a higher level of competence in medical decisions? Many reasons have been advanced. However, many agree that physical limitation on expression is *not* a defensible ethical criterion for incompetency. Elderly patients often do not have the physical power to implement their wishes. The disabling effects of a patient's physical illness may make a person unable to implement decisions and less able to resist those of health care professionals.

Test for Competency

In the final analysis, the concept of competency is social, ethical, and legal, and not merely medical. In fact, there is nothing that is "merely" medical since that which is medical is always complex, never existing in a vacuum. Practitioners in the field of psychiatry have been grappling with this notion of competency for some time. In a 1977 issue of *The American Journal of Psychiatry*, Roth, Meisel, and Lidz say that several tests for competency have been proposed in the literature. Generally, they have identified four categories.

The first category is called "evidencing a choice." This test is set at a level low enough to grant maximal autonomy. Under this test the competent patient is one who evidences a preference for or against treatment. This test then focuses not on the quality of the patient's decision but on the presence or absence of a decision. This preference may be a yes, a no, or even the desire that the physician make the decision for the patient.

The second category is called "reasonable outcome of choice." This test of competency entails evaluating the patient's capacity to reach the reasonable, the right, or the responsible decision. The emphasis in this test is on outcome rather than on the mere fact that a decision has been reached. Patients are deemed incompetent if they fail to make decisions that a reasonable person in like circumstances would make. But, ultimately, because the test rests on the congruence of the patient's decision and that of a reasonable person or of the health care professional, it is biased in favor of decisions to accept treatment, even when such decisions are made by people who are incapable of weighing the risks and benefits of treatment. In other words, if patients do not decide the "wrong" way, the issue of competency probably will not arise. (Remember the example of the elderly woman who refused surgery.)

The third test, the ability of the patient to understand the risks, benefits, and alternatives to treatment, including no treatment, is probably the test most consistent with the law of informed consent. Decision-making need not be rational in either process or outcome. Unwise decisions are permitted. Nevertheless, at a minimum, patients must manifest sufficient ability to understand information about treatment, even if they weigh this information differently from health care professionals. What matters here is that the patient is able to comprehend the elements that are presumed by law to be part of treatment decision-making. Using this test, many questions arise: How sophisticated must understanding be in order that the patient be viewed as competent? There are considerable barriers, conscious and unconscious and intellectual and emotional, to understanding proposed treatment.

The fourth test is intended to measure actual understanding. Rather than focusing on competency as a requirement or an intervening variable in the decision-making process, the test of actual understanding reduces competency to an epiphenomenon of this process, that is, a secondary phenomenon accompanying another phenomenon and thought of as caused by it. The competent patient is, by definition, one who has provided a knowledgeable consent to treatment. Under this test the health care professional has an obligation to teach the patient and directly ascertain whether he or she has, in fact, understood. If not, according to this test, the patient may not have given informed consent. Depending on how sophisticated a level of understanding is required, this test delineates a potentially high level of competency, one that may be difficult to achieve.

Autonomy and Paternalism

Although an in-depth discussion of autonomy and paternalism is beyond the scope of this chapter, it must be mentioned. Miller (1981) proposes four senses of autonomy that are aligned with concepts outlined earlier. These four senses of autonomy are: Autonomy as free action, autonomy as authenticity, autonomy as effective deliberation, and autonomy as moral reflection. Miller's discussion points out that there is no single sense of autonomy. Whether to respect a refusal of treatment requires a determination of what sense of autonomy is satisfied by the patient's refusal. It also shows that there need not be a sharp conflict between patient autonomy and medical judgment. Sound decision-making need not run counter to patient autonomy; it can involve a judgment that the patient's refusal of treatment is not autonomous in the appropriate sense. Miller maintains that the conflict between the right of the patient to autonomy and the physician's medical judgment can be bridged if the concept of autonomy is given a more thorough analysis than it is usually accorded in discussions of the problem of refusal of lifesaving treatment. In some cases where medical judgment appears to override autonomy, the four different senses of autonomy have not been taken into account.

If a refusal of lifesaving treatment is not a free action, that is, is coerced or not intentional, then there can be no obligation to respect an autonomous refusal. It is important to note that if the action is not a free action then it makes no sense to assert or deny that the action was autonomous in any of the other senses. A coerced action can neither be one that was chosen in accord with the person's character and life plan, nor one that was chosen after effective deliberation, nor one that was chosen in accord with the person's considered moral standards. The point is the same if the action is not intentional. When a refusal of treatment is not autonomous in the sense of free action, the physician is obliged to see that the coercion is removed or that the person understands what he or she is doing. Is it possible that coercion cannot be removed or that the action cannot be made intentional? This could be the case with an incompetent patient who is not externally coerced but is subject to an internal compulsion, or one who lacked the capacity to understand the situation. The senile elderly woman who is suspicious of the physician and nurse who have done her no harm could be one example of this. For incompetent patients the question of honoring refusals of treatment does not arise; it is replaced by the issue of who should make decisions for these patients.

Decisions on Behalf of Incompetent Patients

An interesting and basic question arises as to who should determine patient competence. Obviously this is not merely a medical or nursing question, since it also deals with the position of an individual in a social system and that person's ability, according to that social position, to participate in decisions. In some situations, a person is so obviously incompetent that almost anyone can make that judgment. There are other times when such a decision is more problematic and complex, and a court may have to make the determination. Certainly, one reality we must take seriously is that the greater the potential impact of a competency decision on the patient and the more difficult the determination of competency, the greater the need for consultation and group decision.

Three common approaches have been developed to determine ethically how to treat incompetent patients, that is, how to make a decision on their behalf, whatever the source of incompetence (Jameton, 1984).

In the first approach—rational-person approach—one sets aside one's own and the patient's view, if any, and imagines what a rational or reasonable person would do in the patient's situation. The health professional's idea of what a rational person would do is limited; some of the difficult problems that patients encounter can be colored by our own personal experiences and notions of what constitues a rational decison. One may be able to set aside one's own view, but to say that a particular view is irrational or that another is more rational is not an objective position.

The second approach to making decisions on behalf of incompetent patients is called "substituted judgment." In this approach one puts aside one's own view and attempts to think of one's self in the place of this particular patient. The question here is: What would this particular person decide in this situation if he or she were competent and able to think about his or her state? The rational-person method works best for those who place respect for welfare over respect for choice in their respective positions. However, when there are few available facts about a patient's wishes (and this often is the case), then the substituted-judgment method tends to resemble the rational-person method.

The third approach in determining how to make a decision on behalf of incompetent patients is called the "durable statement of intent." This approach relies on the patient's last formally declared and written wishes on the issue. This method assumes that such a declared statement is available. It is a more formal version of substituted judgment, and it gives the health provider a strong basis on which to determine the patient's actual wishes. This approach has led to the development of the Living Will, fostered by a New York group, Society for the Right to Die, and others. An outgrowth of this approach is the Natural Death Act. In 1977, California became the first state to make such an act law; since then, many states have passed a natural death act. Both of these mechanisms exemplify efforts to encourage in citizens the foresight to determine their choices for care.

Living Wills are social contracts between the patient and health care professionals that indicate the patient's wishes regarding the end of his or her life. However, these wills do not always stand the rule of law. Sometimes, health professionals following the patient's wishes can be held legally liable and be sued by the patient's family. The Natural Death Act is a mechanism by which some states seek to legalize this social contract. In this case, patients make their wishes known; when health professionals follow the directives, they are protected by law. (States use these concepts in various ways. It is best to investigate what legal arrangements and language are valid in a given state.) Recently, many states have developed the Durable Power of Attorney process, allowing individuals to make decisions about the end of life. This is a simple document that does not require any legal advice or involvement.

Nurses will increasingly play an important role in educating the public in these matters. Usually the Living Will and the Natural Death Act are instituted once a person is diagnosed as having a terminal illness that will lead to death, regardless of treatment. The Durable Power of Attorney can be completed by any competent adult at any time. In order to educate the public, nurses need to be informed on these matters. While none of these documents is without problems, each can be helpful in respecting patients as people who have the right to make autonomous decisions.

Competency and the Older Patient

But what about those patients, especially older adults, who have not been a part of this recent open discussion of dying and death in our culture? It may be unlikely that they have dealt with the inevitability of their death and made their intent known in writing. In some instances, older persons have discussed with family members what their wishes are about the artificial prolonging of life.

Not all decisions that call into question the competency of people are life-and-death matters. In the film about nurses and ethics entitled "Code Gray," there is a poignant vignette that shows the following situation: An older woman in a nursing home wants to be allowed to walk in the halls by herself. The nurse tells the patient that if she does what she wants and walks alone she will fall and break a hip. Whereupon, the nurse restrains the patient by placing her in a chair and tying a sheet around her. The last camera shot is a close-up of this woman's face and her nonverbal communication speaks volumes . . . all negative. Ethically, this shows the dilemma between patient autonomy and the nurse's obligation to "do no harm." Clinically, one could argue that there are alternatives between walking alone with the risk of falling and being tied in a chair. The "real world" is complex and filled with problems such as staff shortages, complicating health workers' efforts to afford all patients autonomy. Sometimes it is easier for health professionals (not just nurses) to be callous rather than caring. The scene in the film raises the competency issue. It is easy to dismiss people and take them less seriously when we can define them as less than totally competent. And it is easy to define the elderly as less than competent.

How we perceive the other person, and especially the older other person, is important. Margaret Mead makes an interesting point in her autobiography, *Blackberry Winter* (1972). Margaret and her sisters and brothers were discussing their father, who was elderly at the time. One brother says that their father is getting senile because of certain behaviors he exhibits, but Margaret counters this statement by reminding them that father always engaged in that behavior. What this illustrates is that we have a tendency to see people within some social framework such as social status, gender, age, and so forth. When people are old we are more apt to view their behavior as senile or incompetent because of the social frame of age. The research study entitled *On Being Sane in Insane Places* (Rosenhan, 1973) supports this idea. In this study, people posing as patients called several psychiatric clinics and said that they were hearing voices. They then presented themselves to the clinics, where they were admitted. The professional staff saw these pseudo-patients as displaying ill behaviors or psychiatric symptoms. One nurse wrote in the nursing notes that the patient was engaged in compulsive writing while in reality the "patient," a researcher, was writing up field notes on the experience. It is interesting to read in this study that the "real" patients knew that these pseudo-patients were not really sick, but the staff was unable to recognize them. The social frame is a potent variable in coloring our vision of the other.

To return to the film "Code Gray" and the older woman tied in her chair, we must ask questions of how staff members view this patient and others like her. Is it because she is old that she is considered not competent to make a decision? Does it mean that because she is old she has fewer or different rights? How much risk and what kind should the staff permit? When we tie a patient in a chair to protect her, are we acting in her best interest? There are at least two sides to this patient's interests. To protect her from a potential fall is acting in her best interest, but to encourage her to be free to walk down the hall is also acting in her best interest. In reality, we probably also take into account our own best interest when we decide what we will do in these situations. If the patient is not accompanied down the hall and then falls, the nurse and possibly the institution may be in legal difficulties.

Some other problems arise with the older patient. These are not strictly ethical issues, but they play a part in the determination of competency. What occurs when the patient is blind or deaf or both? How do we as health professionals deal with informed consent in these cases? Do we equate these disabilities with incompetency? Because a person cannot see or hear do we say he or she cannot understand? In the informed consent literature there is evidence that some health professionals believe that most patients cannot understand the complex ideas necessary to give

consent. This is a statement being made about the typical adult patient, not necessarily about the elderly person. If this is the attitude of health professionals toward the general adult population, what is the attitude about the elderly adults' ability to understand and give informed consent? Is "understanding" the standard we must use?

A reverse side to this concern for elderly patients' decision-making rights is the problem of leaving the elderly alone with their rights. In the name of patient autonomy and the right to make a decision, we can in some ways abandon the patient. When we insist that a patient who cannot make a decision arrive at one anyway, we can be abandoning a patient psychologically or physically. The problem arises from the inability of someone, either family member or health professional, to see and understand the changes that have occurred in the older person. This then creates situations where older adults are assumed to be as they once were. It puts them into the position of making decisions about any number of matters that are beyond their ability to decide. One must be very careful with labeling a situation as "decisions beyond the ability" because such a label allows the one doing the labeling to act for the older person. It is certainly easier and less time-consuming to say that patients are not able to make decisions, but it also may be unethical. Conversely, *not* to make decisions for another person can also be unethical. This leads to the obvious. We have certain ethical and legal guidelines, and we have some ways of determining the competency of the individual, but each individual is just that . . . an individual. Few, if any, blanket rules can be applied without specific data about each case.

Along with the patient's rights and needs, the family has rights too. Perhaps a major one is the right to compassionate counseling and assistance during a time when the elderly person's best interest must be decided by the family because he or she is no longer able to make decisions. There has been a tendency in the recent past for health professionals to misjudge families who are dealing with their members who are elderly and incompetent, mentally retarded, or mentally ill. This misjudgment may have varying effects, but the outcome is usually the affixing of stigma. We tend to say in subtle and not so subtle ways to family members, "You are not good people and not good, loving relatives." Health professionals often say these things to family members but with little understanding of what the family members have been through in the past and are going through in the present.

SUMMARY

In summary, the following ethical issues have been raised and discussed. We have a legal and ethical tradition that allows competent adults to make reasoned decisions about their well-being, including the refusal of treatment. This tradition is grounded in the ethical principle of autonomy. The major question in clinical settings is when, if ever, is it ethically justifiable for paternalism to override patient autonomy.

The proposition that an incompetent patient should be afforded the same right of self-determination as the competent patient insofar as possible has been upheld by every court since the Quinlan case in New Jersey over ten years ago. Further, this proposition is upheld by the ethical principles of "do no harm" and "do good." Since by definition many incompetent patients are unable to exercise their own power of self-determination, this judgment must be made by someone else. Surrogates must make a good-faith effort to make the treatment decisions in the manner in which patients would have made them if they were competent. The decision-maker must focus on the patient's past expressed desires concerning treatment as the most critical factor in affording the newly incompetent patient the choices for his or her best interests. Obviously, in the absence of some prior expression by the patient, this judgment is subject to abuse.

In those cases in which it is not possible to accurately ascertain the patient's choice or preference, two avenues are open: either we adopt a rule that certain types of treatment can never be discontinued or we permit the discontinuance of all types of treatment under certain clearly specified conditions. The former alternative is too rigid and the other one must be carefully articulated to prevent potential abuses. The least restrictive alternative, one that says that we ought not use restrictive measures when something less restrictive can be found, is often a conflict between a patient's needs and rights. We might, for example, define a patient's need as maintaining health, and the patient may define his or her rights to include the freedom to walk alone down the hall of a nursing home. The questions for clinicians are: How do we meet both the needs and rights of the patient? And what do we do ethically if we cannot meet both when they are in total conflict?

In the discussion of competency, other questions arose. How is competency to be understood? How and by whom is it to be assessed reliably? Who is to decide for the individual who has been determined to be incompetent? According to what substantive standards or principles are decisions to be made? How are the burdens of caring for elderly incompetent individuals to be distributed fairly among families, social organizations, and various levels of government?

One basic guideline is to remember that competency is decision-relative and to be understood as decision-making capacity. Decision-making capacity encompasses three chief elements: (1) Communication and understanding, (2) a relatively stable set of values or a conception of the good, and (3) reasoning and deliberation. No single standard of competency is adequate for all decisions. The standard depends in large part on the risk and the complexity of the information involved.

Finally, two policy issues not discussed earlier will be simply mentioned here for further consideration. These policy issues are: (1) Whether increasing access to medical care for the nonelderly who currently lack it should take precedence over efforts to sustain current levels of Medicare coverage in the face of rising health care costs and a rapidly growing elderly population and (2) whether efforts should be made to achieve a reallocation of public resources for the elderly by shifting funds from medical care to long-term and supportive home care.

Nurses have a central role in all aspects of care for the elderly. Their understanding and input about the ethical issues involved in various issues of care are of vital importance. This chapter raises selected ethical questions so that nurses can better understand the issues and consider solutions to the ethical dilemmas confronting them and their elderly patients.

References

Beauchamp, TL, & Childress, JF (1983): *Principles of Biomedical Ethics* (ed 2). New York, Oxford University Press.

Code Gray (1983). Cambridge, MA, Fanlight Productions. Produced by Ben Actenberg and Joan Sawyer.

Davis, AJ, & Aroskar, MA (1983): *Ethical Dilemmas and Nursing Practice* (ed 2). Norwalk, CT, Appleton-Century-Crofts.

Fromer, MJ (1981): *Ethical Issues in Health Care.* St. Louis, CV Mosby.

Jameton, A (1984): *Nursing Practice: The Ethical Issues.* Englewood Cliffs, NJ, Prentice-Hall.

Mead, M (1972): *Blackberry Winter.* New York, Morrow.

Miller, BL (1981): Autonomy and refusing lifesaving treatment. *The Hastings Center Report,* 2:22–28.

Natanson vs. Kiline, 186 Kans. 393 (1960).

Natural Death Act (1976). California Health and Safety Code 7185–7195.

Rosenhan, DL (1973): On being sane in insane places. *Science,* 179(4070):250–258.

Roth, LH, Meisel, A, & Lidz, CV (1977): Test competency to consent for treatment. *Am J Psychiatr,* 134:279–284.

Schloensdorff vs. Society of New York Hospital, 211 NY 125 (1914).

Society for the Right to Die (1984): *Handbook of Living Will Laws.* 250 West 57th Street, New York, NY 10107.

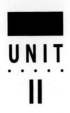

UNIT
II

ASSESSMENT OF THE OLDER CLIENT

CHAPTER
3

Physical Assessment: An Overview with Sections on the Skin, Eye, Ear, Nose, and Neck

REBECCA LEE BURRAGE, R.N.C., M.S., F.N.P.
LAWRENCE DIXON, R.N.C., M.S., G.N.P.
YVONNE A. SEHY, R.N.C., M.S., F.N.P./G.N.P.

INTRODUCTION

This chapter presents an overview of physical assessment of the elderly, with sections on assessment of the skin, eye, ear, nose, throat, and neck.

The basic techniques used in examining older adults are, for the most part, no different from those used in examining adults of any age. Therefore, only that which is unique to the assessment of the geriatric client is presented here. In addition, diseases and disorders commonly found in old age are presented under their respective system headings. The reader is referred to the geriatric medicine textbooks listed in the references for more comprehensive information on evaluation. General guidelines for client referral are offered because the referral process varies with each practice setting.

AN OVERVIEW OF THE PHYSICAL ASSESSMENT

General Considerations

Certain general considerations should be kept in mind while examining the geriatric client.

Beginning in the fourth decade, most body systems lose efficiency because of physiologic changes and disease. However, when a person is not stressed the changes due to normal aging usually are not significant enough to be clinically detected. Therefore, most symptoms cannot be attributed to age alone; the person's number of current diseases and medications is a better predictor of symptom prevalence than is age (Hale, Perkins, May, et al., 1986). The examiner should be hesitant to attribute signs and symptoms to aging, since to do so is to label as irreversible some deficit that might be amenable to treatment. There is evidence that the elderly themselves erroneously attribute symptoms to aging. Brody, Kleban, and Moles (1983) found that older people did not report half of their symptoms, in part because they attributed them to normal aging. A large number of elderly people attrib-

uted mild symptoms of long duration to normal aging, even when the symptoms had been labeled as disease by their physicians (Leventhal & Prohaska, 1986).

Older adults may not respond to diseases with the same signs and symptoms as younger persons. Instead, elderly persons with a variety of specific diseases may have nonspecific complaints such as falling, confusion, urinary incontinence, fatigue, weakness, or syncope. Alternatively, the elderly may not display signs and symptoms characteristic of certain diseases. For example, an older person with myocardial infarction, pneumonia, pulmonary embolism, perforated peptic ulcer, or acute cholecystitis may be pain-free (Caird, 1981). Older patients with pneumococcal bacteremia are more likely to be afebrile than are younger patients (Norman, Grahn, & Yoshikawa, 1985).

Because most elderly people have one or more chronic diseases, elderly clients frequently present with multiple complaints rather than one chief complaint. In studies of symptom prevalence, elderly subjects had an average of three to five symptoms (Brody, et al., 1983; Hale, et al., 1986). Consequently, the examiner should not necessarily try to find one diagnosis to explain all the symptoms, as is usually appropriate in younger clients. Symptoms may be due to a chronic disease, a synergistic effect of two or more chronic conditions, or an acute process superimposed on a chronic one. In addition, the symptoms of one disease may mask those of another. For example, elderly persons with worsening congestive heart failure may not experience dyspnea if their activity level is severely restricted by arthritis.

Medications are an important cause of symptoms in elderly persons. People 65 years of age and older account for only 11% of the population but take 25% of the prescription drugs and account for 50% of all adverse drug reactions (Brody, et al., 1983). Older adults also take large numbers of over-the-counter drugs. The health care provider should obtain a complete list of prescription and nonprescription medications when evaluating any client.

Since many chronic diseases are incurable or only partially remediable, it is extremely important to assess how a disease or disorder affects the client's ability to function. For example, the health care provider may benefit an arthritic client more by assessing how he or she gets up out of a chair than by counting the exact number of joints with deformity. In addition, non-life-threatening disorders such as urinary incontinence may have a devastating impact on the older person's ability to function.

Psychosocial factors may influence older people's health more than they do that of younger clients. For example, in evaluating weight loss, the examiner should consider social factors such as isolation, poor finances, and lack of transportation in addition to disease to explain undernutrition.

The prevalence of certain diseases and disorders varies with age. As a result, the examiner must often consider a different set of diseases in evaluating a similar symptom in clients of different ages. In addition, if it is known which diseases and disorders occur more frequently in old age, steps can be taken to prevent them, correct them, or at least mitigate their effects. For example, the examiner should routinely check for cerumen impaction, foot disorders, and visual and auditory impairment. These are frequently encountered disorders that can significantly affect function and are often correctable. Vaccines should be given for those diseases in which the benefits of reduced morbidity and mortality have been shown to outweigh the risks in taking the vaccine. Finally, the examiner should screen for those diseases with a higher incidence in elderly people, where early detection and treatment have been shown to have a significant impact on mortality. However, routine screening for rare diseases can be costly and entails risks without significant benefit. Early detection of diseases about which nothing can be done serves no useful purpose. Thus, routine ordering of a battery of tests, x-rays, and procedures in asymptomatic clients should not be done.

Height and Weight

A comparison of a client's height and weight with values from standardized tables indicates whether the person is above or below the weight level associated with the least mortality. Obesity or excess of fat, not weight alone, is most closely associated with a variety of health problems. Similarly, poor nutrition rather than low weight most likely accounts for the increased mortality associated with being underweight (Kent, 1982). Thus, weight is an easily measured but imperfect indication of degree of fatness and nutritional status. Weight is also a useful indicator of hydration status when compared with previous values and correlated with symptoms and physical findings.

Several studies have reported small but systematic errors in reported heights and weights (Palta, Prineas, Berman, et al., 1982). Although these errors were generally not large enough to be clinically significant, it is probably safer to measure height and weight rather than to rely on self-reported values.

The health implications of obesity were recently summarized at a national consensus conference (The National Institutes of Health [NIH], 1985). Not only is there a strong correlation between obesity and several risk factors for coronary artery disease (hypertension, hypercholesteremia, and diabetes), but recent evidence from the Framingham Study indicates that obesity may be an independent risk factor as well. In addition, excessive fatness is associated with colorectal and prostate cancer in men and with cancer of the gallbladder and biliary passages and certain reproductive cancers in women. While the prevalence of these forms of cancer is high, these studies did not include enough older subjects to conclusively determine the health effects of obesity in old age. At the very least, obesity can interfere with an older person's ability to function, especially if cardiac and pulmonary disease and osteoarthritis are present.

Determination of the health effects of obesity is also made difficult by the limitations of the standardized height/weight tables. The

Metropolitan Life Tables are the most widely used standard and have been criticized for not distinguishing between underweight and undernourished states (Kent, 1982), for not controlling for smoking and age, and for not including enough older subjects (NIH, 1985). Andres, Elahi, Tobin, Muller, and Brant (1985) reviewed the actuarial data used to determine the tables and concluded that they were probably too high for younger people and too low for older ones. They also questioned the applicability of the tables to so-called old-old clients. Therefore, definitive recommendations about obesity in the elderly await further studies.

Weight loss in the elderly can result from a variety of causes. These include social problems, such as isolation and lack of money or transportation, and psychological problems, such as depression. Medical conditions such as diabetes, tuberculosis, hyperthyroidism, cancer, and excessive diuretic therapy will also cause weight loss.

Vital Signs

Blood Pressure. Comparisons of indirect and direct intraarterial pressure readings reveal that the indirect method frequently, but not uniformly, overestimates diastolic blood pressure (DBP) in elderly people (Hla, Vokaty, & Feussner, 1985). Because the false elevation is in part due to severe sclerosis of large arteries, an attempt can be made to palpate a brachial or radial artery while occluding it manually or with a cuff. If the pulseless artery can be palpated, the blood pressure reading may be erroneous, and the client should be considered for intraarterial measurement (Messerli, Ventura, & Amodeo, 1985). Intraarterial measurement should also be considered in those patients with very high readings but with no end-organ damage. Another contributor to falsely elevated readings is exclusive use of a standard adult-size cuff (O'Callaghan, Fitzgerald, O'Malley, et al., 1983). When the large adult cuff was used appropriately, overestimation in older subjects was reduced (O'Callaghan, et al., 1983). Overestimation

may also occur if too few readings are taken because older adults exhibit a greater intraindividual variability in systolic blood pressure (SBP) than do younger people. For example, Gifford (1986) noted that up to 30% of cases of apparently isolated systolic hypertension (ISH) will disappear upon rechecking. Readings should be done on at least three different occasions before hypertension is diagnosed.

Initial readings should be taken in both arms, although in general there is no significant difference between right and left arm pressures in elderly people (Hashimoto, Hunt, & Hardy, 1984). Baseline readings should also be taken with the client lying, sitting, and standing. Robbins and Rubenstein (1984) reported that about 20% of people over 65 years of age have postural hypotension, defined as a drop in SBP of 20 to 30 mm Hg or more with a concomitant drop in DBP of at least 10 mm Hg for one to two minutes after standing. About half of this group is symptomatic. The incidence of orthostatic hypotension may increase up to 30% to 50% in people over 75 years of age and in ill elderly patients, and it may account for up to 20% of falls (Robbins & Rubenstein, 1984). Causes of postural hypotension include dehydration, anemia, autonomic dysfunction, and medications.

Blood pressure has also been found to drop postprandially in elderly subjects. This phenomenon was found in institutionalized elderly patients with and without a history of syncope (Lipsitz, Nyquist, Wei, et al., 1983), in hypertensive elderly people living at home, and even in some normotensive at-home older adults (Lipsitz & Fullerton, 1986). The examiner should be aware of this phenomenon in evaluating clients with a history of falls, dizziness, or syncope. Because of the frequency of both postural and postprandial hypotension and of falls in the elderly, the geriatric client should be counselled to get up slowly, especially in the morning and after meals.

Approximately 35% to 40% of people over 65 in the United States have SBP of 160 mm Hg or more and/or DBP at least 90 to 95 mm Hg; about two-thirds of these have ISH, defined as SBP of 160 mm Hg or more with a DBP less than 90 to 95 mm Hg (Chobanian,

1983). While ISH occurs in only 1% to 4% of people under 40 years of age, it occurs in 25% to 30% of those over 70, with the highest incidence in elderly women (Lichenstein, 1985). Both systolic and diastolic hypertension are significant risk factors for cardiovascular diseases in the older adult, including congestive heart failure, sudden death, myocardial infarction, and stroke (Chobanian, 1983).

The European Working Party on High Blood Pressure in the Elderly Trial found that treatment of diastolic hypertension was associated with a decrease in cardiovascular mortality, although total mortality was not significantly affected (Amery, et al., 1985). Although ISH is probably an even more important risk factor for cardiovascular disease in the elderly than is diastolic hypertension, the efficacy of treating it remains unproved. The Systolic Hypertension in the Elderly Program is currently under way to help determine this issue (Hulley, Feigal, Ireland, et al., 1986). Pending a definitive study, some experts recommend cautiously treating SBP greater than 180 mm Hg because substantial cardiovascular risk is associated with values in this range (Applegate, Dismuke, & Runyan, 1984; Chobanian, 1983; Rowe, 1983).

In evaluating elderly clients with elevated blood pressure readings, the health care provider should keep in mind that essential or primary hypertension usually begins before age 55 years, so emergence of diastolic hypertension at a more advanced age often has a secondary cause that needs to be determined (Gifford, 1986). A secondary cause, particularly renovascular disease, should also be suspected if the elevation is severe or refractory to medication (Chobanian, 1983).

Temperature. The elderly may have lower abnormal body temperatures and a greater variation in body temperature than do younger people. The diurnal variation in temperature, with higher readings obtained in the afternoon and lower ones at night, is not affected by age.

Although most elderly persons do respond to infections with fever, some, particularly the old-old, have minimal to no fever in response to at least some kinds of infections (Norman,

et al., 1985). When fever does occur in older people, it is more likely than in the young to be caused by serious diseases, in part because viral infections are less common and bacterial infections more common with advancing age (Keating, Klimek, Levine, et al., 1984). Fever of unknown origin can be a particular challenge for the examiner. In a survey of cases in the literature in which fever in elderly patients remained undiagnosed for at least a week, Esposito and Gleckman (1978) found the most common causes were infections such as abdominal abscesses, endocarditis, and tuberculosis; neoplasms such as lymphoma; and connective tissue diseases, particularly giant cell arteritis.

The incidence of hypothermia in older people is controversial. Although European studies have found up to 10% of elderly subjects with core temperatures at or below 35.5° C. (96° F.), one United States study of older adults supposedly at risk failed to discover a single case (Keilson, Lambert, Fabian, et al., 1985). When hypothermia does occur, causes include environmental exposure, metabolic causes such as hypothyroidism and hypoglycemia, drugs, and hypothalamic and central nervous system dysfunction (Reuler, 1978). Hypothermia may be missed if a rectal temperature is not checked or if a standard thermometer is not completely shaken down. If a client's temperature does not register on a standard thermometer, special low temperature thermometers are available.

Pulse. It is not clear whether resting heart rate changes with age. The heart rate response to exercise is blunted in the elderly, thereby reducing cardiovascular reserve (Kohn, 1977).

Respirations. Little data are available on the effects of age on respiratory rate (RR). Mc-Fadden, Price, Eastwood, and Briggs (1982) found that elderly institutionalized subjects without acute respiratory disease had an RR of 16 to 25 per minute, whereas elderly subjects with lower respiratory infections (LRI) consistently had an RR above that range. Because increased respirations were often present one to two days before the LRI was diagnosed, and because such increases did not occur with other types of infections, these investigators concluded that raised RR is a valuable physical sign that should not be ignored.

Laboratory Tests

In interpreting diagnostic laboratory tests, it is necessary to know how aging affects hematologic values. Blood urea nitrogen and creatinine increase with age due to the physiologic decline in plasma renal flow and glomerular filtration rate. Alkaline phosphatase also increases with age (Kelly, Munan, Petitclers, et al., 1979). In addition, fasting blood glucose increases by about 2 mg/dl/decade (Hale, Stewart, & Marks, 1983). Studies differ over whether calcium and phosphorus increase, decrease, or remain unchanged with age (Kelly, et al., 1979; Hale, et al., 1983; Caird, 1973). Although lower erythrocyte counts, hemoglobins, and hematocrits are frequently seen in old age, these changes reflect the presence of diseases rather than age-related physiologic decline. Most other values do not change with age (Hodkinson, 1981).

Elderly patients as a group also exhibit a wider range of variation of normal values than younger persons (Jernigan, Gudat, Blake, et al., 1980). Thus, a slightly abnormal value should not be taken as irrefutable evidence of disease. Likewise, because the blood work of some elderly patients does not change with certain diseases, a normal value does not necessarily rule out a disease.

Finally, any abnormal laboratory findings should be interpreted in light of the person's medications. Hale and associates (1983) found that older subjects taking medication had significantly different potassium, chloride, carbon dioxide, creatinine, and uric acid levels than subjects not taking drugs.

SKIN

Aging Changes

Dryness, wrinkling, laxity, uneven pigmentation, and a variety of proliferative lesions of the skin are due to normal aging, the genetic makeup of the individual, and environmental factors such as sun exposure. The dermoepidermal junction flattens with age, although the thickness of the epidermis and the stratum corneum remains unchanged. Dermal thickness declines by 20% in the elderly, and there is loss of subcutaneous fat. Age-related loss of normal elastic fibers may contribute to wrinkling. A reduced vascular bed results in reduced reflex vasodilation and vasoconstriction of dermal arterioles. A decrease in the number of active melanocytes makes skin more sensitive to sunlight. Eccrine and apocrine glands atrophy and decrease in function. Sebaceous glands do not appear to atrophy, although they too decrease significantly in function. Scalp hair generally becomes thinner and loses color, whereas facial hair increases in women. There is yellowing, thickening, and longitudinal ridging of nails (Gilchrest, 1984).

Common Disorders

An estimated 40% of Americans 65 to 74 years of age suffer from a skin disease that is severe enough for them to seek treatment. The most common skin disorders in the elderly are dermatitis, fungal infections, keratoses, and skin cancers (Johnson & Roberts, 1978). Table 3–1 presents common nonpathologic skin disorders, and Table 3–2 presents pathologic disorders.

Several types of dermatitis are frequently seen in the elderly. The most common type is caused by dry, xerotic skin. The incidence of seborrheic dermatitis steadily increases after the age of 50 years; it is recurrent and chronic and may occur with stressful events (Figure 3–1). It is well established that seborrheic dermatitis is much more severe and more difficult to treat in patients with Parkinson's disease than others. Its etiology is unknown (Orentreich & Orentreich, 1985). Dermatitis in the elderly may also be caused by hypoproteinemia, venous insufficiency, allergens or irritants, or underlying malignancy such as leukemia or lymphoma, or the dermatitis may be idiopathic (Waisman, 1979).

Table 3–1. NONPATHOLOGIC SKIN LESIONS FOUND IN THE ELDERLY

Lesion	Appearance
Xerosis (dry skin)	Dry, pruritic, scaly skin on the entire body, especially the lower legs
Solar elastosis (sun-damaged skin)	Leathery, lax, and wrinkled; facial areas of nodular thickening; periorbital cormedones; and small cysts
Senile (solar) lentigines	Hyperpigmented macular lesions resembling freckles on the dorsum of the hands and face, associated with fair complexion and sun exposure, "liver spots"
Acrochordon (skin tag)	Small (1 to 5 mm), soft, pedunculated papules of the eyelids, neck, trunk, axilla, and groin, with color and texture of normal skin
Actinic keratoses	Premalignant, slightly raised, scaly, pink, tan, red, or brown, irregular lesions on sun-exposed areas, especially in those with fair complexion; adherent scale, recurs when removed
Seborrheic keratoses	Raised, sharply circumscribed, wart-like and waxy growths with stuck-on appearance, tan, yellow, brown, or black color, often multiple, usually on the face, shoulders, trunk, and groin areas
Senile purpura	Irregular areas of ecchymosis after minimal trauma followed by hyperpigmentation on sun-exposed areas on backs of the hands and forearms
Senile angioma (cherry spot)	Bright or bluish red papules, 2 to 3 mm, usually found on the trunk
Telangiectasia	Dilation of capillaries or arterioles of the nose or face, often found as three or fewer characteristic spider angioma forms
Venous lakes	Small, flat, bluish blood vessels on backs of hands, ears, and lips; blanch with pressure
Lichenification	Well-circumscribed areas of cutaneous thickening and hardening, result of repeated rubbing or scratching

(Data from Gurevitch, 1983; Porth & Kapke, 1983; Tonnesen & Weston, 1982; and Sauer, 1985.)

Table 3–2. COMMON PATHOLOGIC SKIN LESIONS FOUND IN THE ELDERLY

Lesion	Appearance
Seborrheic dermatitis	Erythematous, scaling, yellow, greasy-appearing eruption of the scalp, face, upper chest, and groin
Contact dermatitis	Erythematous, scaling, fissuring, or vesicular eruption of skin directly exposed to an irritant or allergen; lesions form linear or sharp-bordered pattern limited to the site of contact
Psoriasis	Erythematous papules or plaques with thick silvery scales on the scalp, genitalia, umbilicus, elbows, knees; pitting, yellowing, and thickening of the nails may occur
Candidiasis	Macerated erythematous plaques with border satellite pustules and papules caused by *Candida albicans*; found in intertriginous areas
Dermatophytosis or tinea (ringworm)	Diffuse redness, scaliness, with center clear (ringing) and a raised, red scaly border; found anywhere on skin, hair, or nails
Herpes zoster (shingles)	Grouped, clear vesicles on an erythematous base with unilateral dermatonal distribution; may become pustular or hemorrhagic and then crust, resolving in about four weeks; hyperpigmentation or scarring may result
Bullous pemphigoid	Large tense bullae on erythematous or normal skin of the trunk and proximal extremities and occasionally the mouth; occasionally accompanied by pruritus
Basal cell carcinoma	Smooth, rounded papule or nodule with a rolled, pearly border, and telangiectasias; may have a central depression; usually on the face, but also on ear, upper chest, extensor surface on arms and hands
Squamous cell carcinoma	Erythematous, wart-like, scaly, indurated papule or nodule surrounded by a wide indurated border at sites of actinic keratoses on the hands, arms, ears, neck, and face or other scarred or ulcerated skin areas
Leukoplakia	White or gray keratotic dysplasia of the lips, buccal mucosa, tongue, or vagina; considered premalignant
Malignant melanoma	Irregular, thickened, or nodular lesion of varied colors of tan, brown, black, red, blue, gray, and white, often less than one cm in diameter; often developing from pigmented nevi, moles, or lentigo maligna

(Data from Gilchrest, 1984; Gurevitch, 1983; Sauer, 1985; and Tonnesen & Weston, 1982.)

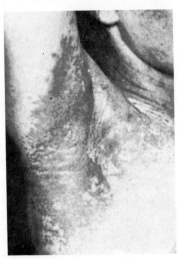

Figure 3–1. Seborrheic dermatitis. (From Domonkos, AO: Andrew's Diseases of the Skin, ed 7. Philadelphia, WB Saunders, 1982, p 220. Reprinted with permission.)

Dermatophytosis or tinea (ringworm infections) and candidiasis (monilial infections) are fungal infections. Candidiasis is the more common and occurs more frequently in females

and individuals who are obese or diabetic (Figure 3–2).

Actinic (solar) keratosis, also called senile keratosis, appears on sun-exposed areas such as the face, neck, forearms, and hands. The condition is seen in persons who work outdoors or who are actively involved in outdoor sports (Fitzpatrick, Polano, & Suurmond, 1983).

The incidence of skin cancers increases with age, especially between 50 and 80 years (Scotto & Fears, 1978). Approximately 80% of nonmelanoma skin cancers are basal cell carcinomas (Figure 3–3), and almost all the remainder are squamous cell carcinomas (Figure 3–4). Although the cure rate for nonmelanoma skin cancers is more than 95%, they account for more deaths each year in the United States than do melanomas (Scotto, Fears, & Fraumeni, 1981).

There are several other dermatologic conditions that are seen in older people. Drug eruptions are associated with multiple drug use. Systemic medications (such as penicillin, Keflin, and Dilantin) often cause generalized erythematous rashes, urticarial eruptions, and

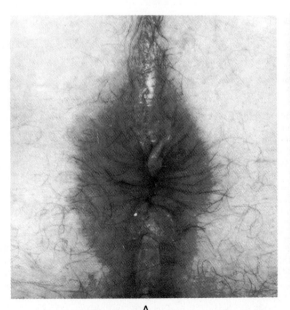

A

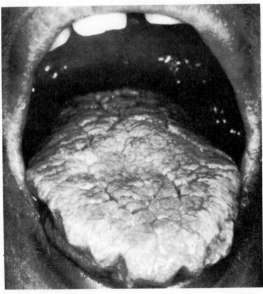

B

Figure 3–2. Candidiasis. *(A)* Perianal candidiasis, *(B)* oral candidiasis (thrush). (From Domonkos, AO: Andrew's Diseases of the Skin, ed 7. Philadelphia, WB Saunders, 1982, pp 366, 368. Reprinted with permission.)

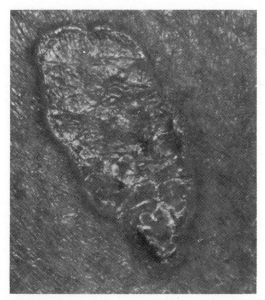

Figure 3–3. Basal cell carcinoma. (From Gilchrest, BA: Skin diseases in the elderly. *In* Calkins, E, Davis, PJ, and Ford, AB (eds). The Practice of Geriatrics. Philadelphia, WB Saunders, 1986, p 495. Reprinted with permission.)

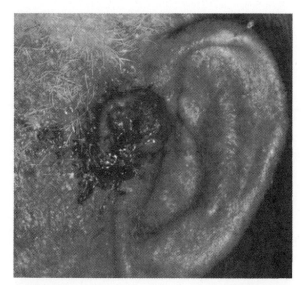

Figure 3–4. Squamous cell carcinoma. (From Gilchrest, BA: Skin diseases in the elderly. *In* Calkins, E, Davis, PJ, and Ford, AB (eds). The Practice of Geriatrics. Philadelphia, WB Saunders, 1986, p 496. Reprinted with permission.)

eczematous, vasculitic, and purpuric lesions. Individuals on thiazide diuretics or phenothiazine-type tranquilizers may experience a photosensitivity dermatitis (Anderson & Williams, 1983; Gilchrest, 1984).

Herpes zoster and bullous pemphigoid appear as blistering lesions. Herpes zoster or "shingles," caused by the reactivation of latent varicella virus, usually occurs in individuals older than 50 years of age (Figure 3–5). Bullous pemphigoid affects primarily those over 60 years of age and is probably an immune disorder. It is self-limiting but may last months to years and recur (Fitzpatrick, Polano, & Suurmond, 1983; Fitzpatrick & Haynes, 1983; Orentreich & Orentreich, 1985).

Leukoplakia, lichenification, and psoriasis

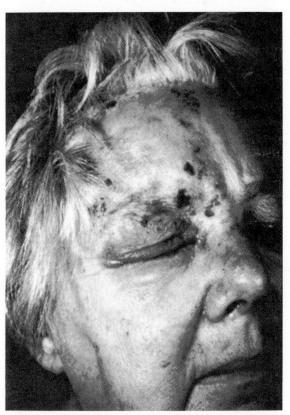

Figure 3–5. Herpes zoster. (From Sullivan, ND, and Basler, RSW: Geriatric dermatology. *In* O'Hara-Devereaux, M, Andrus, LH, and Scott, CD (eds). Eldercare: A Practical Guide to Clinical Geriatrics. New York, Grune & Stratton, 1981, p 283. Reprinted with permission.)

are other conditions seen in the elderly. Leukoplakia, a white patch or plaque in the mouth, is considered premalignant (Fitzpatrick, Polano, & Suurmond, 1983). Lichenification is caused by chronic irritation, such as scratching (Waisman, 1979). There is thickening of the skin with accentuated skin markings (Fitzpatrick, Polano, & Suurmond, 1983). Psoriasis has a strong genetic component and may have its onset in middle age or later. Approximately 8% to 10% of psoriasis may be associated with psoriatic joint disease (Tonnesen & Weston, 1982).

History

Although assessment of skin lesions is predominantly done by inspection, the history is often important in diagnosis and management. The history should include the onset and evolution of the skin condition, accompanying symptoms, past treatment, and past medical history. The medical history should include medications, allergies, family history of allergies, history of exposure to possible allergens, irritants and infectious diseases, and a selective review of systems.

Pruritus, pain, and paresthesia are the most common symptoms associated with skin lesions. However, symptoms of many acute and chronic diseases such as viral illnesses, arthritis, and diabetes may be the presenting complaints when associated lesions are found. For example, fever, malaise, and upper respiratory or gastrointestinal tract symptoms often accompany generalized macular and papular eruptions caused by viral illness (Lookingbill, 1985; Gilchrest, 1984).

Although many skin disorders cause pruritus, xerosis (dry skin) is the most common cause of generalized pruritus in the elderly. Systemic disease such as chronic renal failure, diabetes, hematologic malignancy, or hyperthyroidism may present as pruritus (Gilchrest, 1984). Pruritus vulva and pruritus ani have multiple etiologies, including atrophic and xerotic skin changes, poor hygiene, and use of enemas and cathartics (Waisman, 1979).

Almost any chemical coming into contact with the skin may cause dermatitis, no matter how long that product has been used. Soaps and topical medications are common offenders. The skin reaction may be allergic or irritant in nature and is usually pruritic. Contact dermatitis may begin insidiously, may generalize rapidly, and may resolve more slowly than in younger individuals (Orentreich & Orentreich, 1985).

The preherpetic neuralgia of herpes zoster may mimic angina, spinal cord compression, renal or biliary colic, or muscle strain. During the course of the disease, the reactivated virus causes neuritis, pain, and vesicle formation (Gilchrest, 1984). Severity and duration of postherpetic neuralgia increase with age, possibly affecting more than 50% of those infected (Gilchrest, 1984).

Habitual sun exposure is a major risk factor for both basal cell carcinoma and squamous cell carcinoma of the skin. Any skin lesions that are pigmented, vary in color, increase in size, or develop irregular borders, thickening, or nodularity should be evaluated for malignancy. Pigmented nevi (moles) and lentigo maligna, a solar lentigo that has enlarged and developed color variation, commonly develop into malignant melanomas. However, malignant melanoma may develop even on previously normal-appearing skin (Gurevitch, 1983; Fraser & McGuire, 1984; Orentreich & Orentreich, 1985). Metastatic tumors from other organ systems often develop as rapidly growing, inflamed, vascular nodules on the abdomen, chest, and scalp (Orentreich & Orentreich, 1985).

Examination

Several normal lesions of the aging skin do not necessarily indicate pathology but may require monitoring for prevention and treatment of pathological changes.

The morphology of the primary skin lesion is the most helpful diagnostic finding. Secondary lesions occur when the initial morphologic features have been altered, as by scratching, to cause excoriations and crusts. The arrangement or configuration and distribution on the body often indicate specific diagnoses. For example, herpes zoster classically erupts along the line of a dermatome in grouped lesions. The scalp is involved in both psoriasis and seborrheic dermatitis, but involvement of the extensor surfaces of the arms and legs is characteristic of psoriasis. Since some characteristics are shared by several skin disorders, it is the total constellation of findings that distinguishes each disorder (Lookingbill, 1985; Sauer, 1985).

Tests

Several examination techniques and diagnostic tests aid in diagnosis of skin lesions. Follicular plugging, fine telangiectasia, raised borders of basal cell carcinoma, and early color changes of lesions can be detected by a pocket magnifier (2 to 7X). Oblique lighting directed at skin lesions will reveal slight elevations or depressions. A microscope slide or clear plastic pressed over the skin lesion may reveal capillary dilatation and blanching of erythema or the unchanged color of purpura. Microscopic examination of scrapings treated with potassium hydroxide will differentiate fungal from other lesions. Material for culture may be obtained by scraping, aspiration, or biopsy of lesions.

Histologic examination by a pathologist on skin tissue obtained by biopsy is not necessary to diagnose the majority of skin disorders, but it is mandated to rule out malignancy and diagnose primary blistering disorders. For most skin lesions, a punch biopsy is adequate and convenient, although surgical excision and scissors biopsy may be necessary (Lookingbill, 1985).

EYE

Aging Changes

Mild loss of visual acuity occurs with age. Presbyopia, or the loss of the ability to focus on near objects, occurs around age 45 years. Presbyopia is caused by loss of elasticity in the lens, which then responds less readily to the action of the ciliary muscle. The ciliary muscle becomes less effective with age (Meltzer, 1983). Changes in the lens may cause opacities in the lens nucleus, the lens cortex, and the posterior subcapsule (Newell, 1986). Modifications in the endothelial layer of the cornea and the vitreous humor are minor causes of visual impairment (Corso, 1971). The light-sensing thresholds for both rods and cones are significantly affected, so adaptation from light to dark slows with aging. The loss of luteal pigment in the macular area occurs with age, causing a slight reduction in central acuity in the eighth and ninth decades (Keeney & Keeney, 1980). Color perception may be affected by yellowing of the lens and alterations in macular pigmentation (Rich, 1984).

Aging occurs in other structures as well, but with less functional significance. Tear production from the basic secretors is reduced with aging (Hawes & Ellis, 1963). Both excessive tearing and a dry eye are common in elderly persons. The vitreous body normally tends to shrink, become more liquid, contract onto itself, and detach from the retina. The eye recesses into the orbit as the fat cushion behind the eye atrophies. The skin of the eyelid becomes loose and the muscle tone decreases. Pupillary diameter decreases from the second to seventh decade, when it reaches its minimum size, and the iris becomes fibrotic (Keeney & Keeney, 1980).

Common Disorders

The incidence of potentially blinding diseases increases dramatically after the age of 65 (Rich, 1984). The Framingham Eye Study, in which 5262 people over 65 years of age were screened, demonstrated that the leading causes of blindness in elderly people are senile cataract (33.7%), senile macular degeneration (15.4%), diabetic retinopathy (3.0%), and glaucoma (2.9%) (Eifrig & Simons, 1983). In the same study, cataracts were found to have reduced visual acuity to 20/30 or less in 15% of people between ages 52 and 85 years. Senile macular degeneration is the result of degenerative changes in the posterior pole of the aging eye. These changes include permanent atrophic modifications in the retina and pigment epithelium due to loss of blood supply, primarily affecting the macular area. Although young people are more at risk for diabetic retinopathy than are aged individuals, 60% of all diabetics have retinopathy after 15 years of having diabetes (Nover, 1981). Acute angle-closure glaucoma is more common in the elderly person because as the lens thickens with age, it pushes the iris forward, blocking the flow of fluid. The incidence of chronic glaucoma also markedly increases with age (Graham, 1985).

History

Complaints related to visual acuity are helpful in determining the presence of disease. For example, a need for brighter-than-normal lighting may indicate corneal clouding, lens opacities, or macular degeneration. Vision may improve in dim light with cataracts because of pupil dilation. Individuals with cataracts complain of a gradual decrease in visual acuity without pain or inflammation of the eye. Other early symptoms of cataracts include double vision in one eye and the presence of colored halos around lights. Bright illumination and glare, as with night driving, cause constriction of the pupil and reduced visual acuity, especially with a posterior subcapsular cataract (Newell, 1986). Spots in the visual field may be present with cataracts, but unlike those resulting from vitreous floaters, the spots remain fixed instead of darting around (Newell, 1986).

Visual loss in chronic open-angle glaucoma is painless, so that early diagnosis by screening is crucial. The client with angle-closure glaucoma, which is less common, may experience blurred vision and colored halos associated with ocular pain in the early stages. Risk factors for glaucoma include a family history of glaucoma, history of eye trauma, or history of long-term treatment with systemic corticosteroids (Rodman, 1984).

The patient with reduced tear production may paradoxically present with a complaint of excessive tearing, which may occur as a reflex response to conjunctival and corneal irritation from dryness. Besides being uncomfortable, the dry eye is more susceptible to infection and corneal ulceration. Systemic illnesses associated with dry eye include Sjögren's syndrome and a neoplasm involving a lacrimal gland. Systemic medications that may produce dry eye include antihypertensives, antihistamines, anticholinergics, and sympatholytic agents (Ehrlich & Keates, 1978).

The history is also useful in determining the cause of excessive tearing. Drainage obstruction may be indicated by unilateral watering or severe and constant tearing. Local medications such as miotics or systemic medications such as 5-fluorouracil may occlude the puncta or canaliculi, causing obstruction of drainage. Increased tearing while eating may indicate seventh-nerve palsy. Other causes of excessive tearing include corneal or external eye disease and sinusitis or hay fever (Hawes & Ellis, 1983).

Examination

Lids and Adnexa. Malposition of the eyelids may cause discomfort or visual loss. Extremely flaccid upper eyelid skin folds sometimes cause obstruction of visual fields (Rich, 1984). Ectropion, or laxity of the lower eyelid with malposition, may lead to incomplete coverage of the globe, chronic irritation, and resultant complications. When relaxation of the lid causes the inner puncta to sag away from the globe, inadequate tear drainage occurs, with spilling of tears over the cheeks (epiphora) (Rich, 1984). Relaxation of the lids with obstruction of lacrimal passages may become more obvious when the patient leans forward about 20°, and may not be apparent in the supine or upright position. Such a maneuver may be useful in evaluating for the person who complains of tearing when reading (Hawes & Ellis, 1983).

Entropion, or inward turning of the eyelid margin onto the globe with resultant irritation of the eye by the lashes, is caused by either muscle atony or spasticity. The tendency toward entropion may be noted when the patient squeezes his eyelids tightly shut (Rich, 1984). Changes in the appearance of eyelids may also be caused by systemic disorders, such as proptosis in thyroid disease, or ptosis in nerve palsy or myasthenia gravis.

The eyelids should also be inspected for lesions, although it is often difficult to differentiate clinically between benign and malignant lesions. Basal cell epithelioma, the most common malignant lesion of the eyelids, is often seen in the elderly population and must be surgically removed. It may appear similar to many benign lesions, such as papillomas, keratocanthomas, and senile keratosis. Therefore, any pigmented lesion on the eyelid should be biopsied. Xanthelasma, a yellow, elevated lipid-infiltrated lesion most commonly occurring at the inner portion of the lids, is sometimes associated with an elevated blood lipid level.

Conjunctiva. Conjunctival tumors should be biopsied if they appear in a patient with a history of systemic malignancy or have recently changed in appearance. Common non-malignant growths in the elderly are pinguecula and pterygium. A pinguecula is a yellowish mass on the bulbar conjunctiva in the interpalpebral space, usually on the nasal side. A pterygium is a triangular fold of conjunctiva. It is only removed if it progresses onto the cornea and obstructs vision.

Visual Acuity. Adequate light should be provided when testing visual acuity. Dirty lenses and malaligned glasses affect visual acuity. For example, the line in bifocals may cause double vision if the glasses are malaligned. The test of distant vision is standardized at 20 feet. The test of near vision should be adapted to the patient's optimal reading distance, using conventional text to read rather than unrelated letters to identify. An individual with a visual acuity of 20/40 or less should be referred to an ophthalmologist to determine the cause (Wright & Henkind, 1983).

Tear Flow. The cornea is inspected for brightness, using oblique light. Spotty or diffused dullness suggests subnormal tear flow. Further examinations, such as the Schirmer test, identify impaired tear production through a standardized procedure in which filter paper is placed in the inferolateral lid border. Inadequate tear production is indicated by a strip that is wet to less than 10 mm in five minutes. The drainage system may be tested by placing a drop of fluorescein dye in the eye, which is cleared from the conjunctival cul-de-sac in five minutes in the normal eye.

Cornea. Arcus senilis, lipid deposits around the peripheral corneal stroma, which are very common in the elderly, is not normally associated with serum lipid abnormalities in this age group. Normally a bilateral and symmetrical condition, a less obvious arcus senilis may occur on the side of severely compromised carotid blood flow (Rich, 1984).

Anterior Chamber. The lens increases in thickness throughout life, resulting in progressive shallowing of the anterior chamber and the danger of acute closed-angle glaucoma. By directing the light of a flashlight from the temporal side, the depth of the chamber can be estimated. If the nasal aspects of the iris remain shadowed, there is probably dangerous shallowing, whereas if the entire iris plane is illuminated, depth is probably adequate (Keeney & Keeney, 1980).

Iris. The iris becomes less responsive to mydriatics with age (Keeney & Keeney, 1980). Miosis appears to be a normal variant, but it causes the ophthalmoscopic examination to be more difficult (Granacher, 1981).

Lens. The ophthalmoscopic examination of a person with cataracts may reveal a gross opacity that fills the pupillary aperture or an opacity with a red background (Newell, 1986), although only a slight loss of transparency on ophthalmoscopy may be present with early cataracts (Graham, 1985) (Figure 3–6). Dilation of the pupil is necessary to examine the lens well for evidence of the specific type of opacity (Newell, 1986). The clinician also looks for evidence of injury or inflammation. The general examination may reveal causes other than aging for the cataracts, such as diabetes mellitus, hypocalcemia, myotonic dystrophy, or toxins or drugs such as systemic corticosteroids (Newell, 1986).

Retina. The normal red light reflex is less

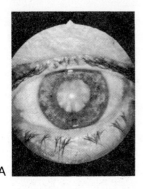

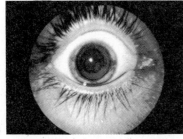

Figure 3–6. Cataracts. *(A)* Mature cataract, *(B)* cataract. (From Taisch, EA, Taisch, DA, and Metz, HS: Problems of the eyes. *In* O'Hara-Devereaux, M, Andrus, LH, and Scott, CD (eds). Eldercare: A Practical Guide to Clinical Geriatrics. New York, Grune & Stratton, 1981, p 268. Reprinted with permission.)

marked in the older person (Galloway, 1985). With the aging process, retinal arterioles normally show some sclerotic changes that would be considered pathologic in younger people. The vessels become straighter and more narrow (Galloway, 1985), and the visibility of the arteriolar wall light reflex increases (Rich, 1984) (Figure 3–7). Arterial venous (A/V) compression (the crossing of an artery over a vein, resulting in venous narrowing and constriction of the vein on either side of the crossing arteriole) is not an expected finding with age (Keeney & Keeney, 1980).

A thorough funduscopic examination by an ophthalmologist is essential if retinal detachment is suspected. Because treatment is often available to inhibit or improve diabetic retinopathy, the diabetic patient should have at least a yearly funduscopic examination (Nover, 1981) (Figure 3–8).

The optic disc is usually paler in the older person, which is not a sign of disease (Galloway, 1985). Pallor in the temporal area of the disc is a sign of glaucoma (Eifrig & Simons, 1983). The optic disc also appears paler following cataract surgery than prior to surgery.

Signs of glaucoma include an increase in ocular pressure, loss of visual field, and increased size of the physiologic cup compared to the optic disc. Screening for intraocular pressure is recommended for all patients over 40 years of age who have not had pressure readings done in the past two years (Rodman, 1984). Other clinicians recommend annual intraocular examinations (Wuest, Sayther, Carlson, et al., 1976) and regular examinations by an ophthalmologist for known glaucoma patients and for those with significant risk factors. Although the incidence of ocular hypertension (21 mm Hg and greater) does increase with aging (Eifrig & Simons, 1983), it is still recommended that this finding prompt a referral to an ophthalmologist (Wright & Henkind, 1983).

The ophthalmoscopic examination in early macular degeneration may reveal small, local-

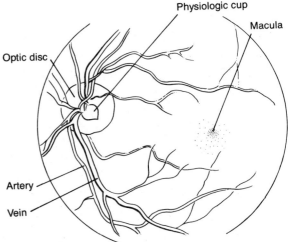

Figure 3–7. Normal ocular fundus. (From Swartz, M: Textbook of Physical Diagnosis: History and Examination. Philadelphia, WB Saunders, 1989, p 146. Reprinted with permission.)

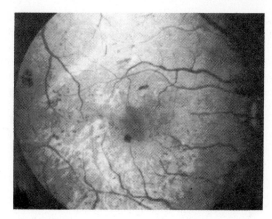

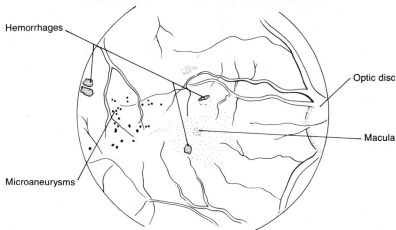

Figure 3–8. Ocular fundus in early diabetic retinopathy. (From Swartz, M: Textbook of Physical Diagnosis: History and Examination. Philadelphia, WB Saunders, 1989, p 153. Reprinted with permission.)

ized, and ill-defined yellow-white spots, known as colloid bodies or drusen, which may coalesce to forms areas of depigmentation (Graham, 1985). Dark pigmentary changes around the fovea centralis progress to clumping of the pigment and scarring (Meltzer, 1983). Usually only the macula is involved, causing a dense scotoma with normal peripheral vision in the worst cases.

EAR

Aging Changes

There are four types of presbycusis, or hearing loss due to age-related changes in the inner ear. They are sensory presbycusis (loss of hair cells in the cochlea), neural presbycusis (loss of neuronal cells of the spiral ganglion), strial presbycusis (atrophic changes in the cochlea), and cochlear conductive presbycusis (changes in the basilar membrane) (Mills, 1985).

Some disturbances of vestibular function, such as vestibular ataxia, may be related to the aging process (Mills, 1985). Vestibular lesions are common yet often go undetected without special testing (Bonikowski, 1983).

Common Disorders

Approximately one-third of people over 65 years of age have sufficient impairment to cause "unfavorable social consequences" (Mills, 1985). The older person may demonstrate conductive or sensorineural loss, or both. With conductive loss, there is a decrease in sensitivity to sound, particularly with low frequency tones, requiring increased volume. In sensorineural loss, the high frequencies are affected most. Perceived sound is distorted (Ruben & Kruger, 1983), especially with accelerated speech and the use of consonants such as s, z, t, f, and g, which have high frequency components to their sounds (Corso, 1971). Other common causes of hearing impairment in the elderly are cerumen impaction; exposure to the toxic effects of ototoxic drugs such as loop diuretics, aspirin, and aminoglycosides; cholesteatomas; and acoustic neuromas (Ruben & Kruger, 1983; Mader, 1984).

Twenty percent of the adult population complain of tinnitus, with the incidence increasing after 70 years of age. Although most of these elderly people also have a hearing loss, they report that the tinnitus is more disturbing.

History

Hearing Loss. Presbycusis usually presents with a negative history for previous ear disease or inner ear toxicity, although other auditory disorders may be superimposed upon presbycusis. The patient reports a gradual and progressive onset of bilateral deafness, with or without tinnitus, in the absence of other ear problems. The client may complain that everyone seems to mumble. Clients admit to having more difficulty hearing in crowds, large rooms, over the telephone, and in situations where background noise is present (Mader, 1984). In some cases, there is a reduced tolerance for loud sounds, including loud speech.

Often there is a marked difference between the measured hearing impairment and the resulting personal handicap (Riko & Alberti, 1984). Therefore, exploring the effect of the hearing loss on the person's life is necessary. Some studies argue against the consistent and predictably deleterious emotional effects of hearing loss (Thomas, et al., 1983). However, it is generally accepted that a moderate to severe degree of hearing loss (greater than 50

db) often results in both emotional and functional disturbances. This is caused by a breakdown in communication and resultant social isolation (Ruben & Kruger, 1983), particularly for those older individuals with serious physical handicaps (Jones, Victor, & Vetter, 1984). A number of questionnaires and scales are available to determine the attitudes, feelings, and abilities of people with hearing loss (Ruben & Kruger, 1983). Such tools are also useful in evaluating the effectiveness of an individual's progress in a rehabilitation program.

Tinnitus. Tinnitus is usually described as a rushing, buzzing, or ringing sound, although the type of sound does not help identify the etiology. Unilateral tinnitus may suggest an early developing acoustic neuroma (Mills, 1985). Sudden onset tinnitus, such as that due to a viral syndrome or noise exposure, is often accompanied by other symptoms such as hearing loss, pain, headache, ear fullness, vertigo, nasal congestion, otorrhea, or hyperacusis (Turner, 1982). Ototoxic drugs may also cause tinnitus, so a medical history is important. About 5% of people have objective tinnitus (evident to the examiner by auscultation) secondary to vascular disease (Turner, 1982). When a hearing loss is also present, a hearing aid may make the tinnitus less annoying.

Vertigo. Vertigo is a sense of spinning. True vertigo implies a disturbance in the vestibular system. An important consideration in older adults is the possibility that poorly fitting glasses or eye disease is providing adverse stimuli to the vestibular system (Senturia, Goldstein, & Hersperger, 1983). (Other causes of dizziness are discussed in Chapter 5.)

Otalgia. Complaints of pain in and around the ear are common in elderly people. Pain may be referred to the ear from almost any organ above the clavicle. A frequent cause of referred pain is temporomandibular joint dysfunction, which may be caused by poorly fitting or absent dentures.

Examination

Examination Techniques. When the patient complains of ear pain, almost all structures around the ear and above the clavicle should be carefully examined for possible sites of referred pain. For example, neck rotation may precipitate pain behind and below the ear via the cervical plexus secondary to cervical muscle spasm or arthritis. When pain is elicited by applying pressure over the temporomandibular joint as the patient opens and closes the jaw, arthritic changes in this joint may be the cause. Sometimes crepitus of this joint is associated with tinnitus. Infected teeth, usually the lower molars, may cause referred ear pain (Turner, 1982). Local pain or referred ear pain will be produced when the examiner taps gently along the axis of the affected teeth with a metal object such as the handle of an oral examining mirror or the end of a well-cleansed metal pen. The clinician should begin by tapping gently on healthy teeth so that the client can readily identify the difference when the diseased tooth is tapped.

Objective tinnitus is generally pulsatile in nature and vascular in origin (Turner, 1982). However, presence and amplitude of carotid bruits does not correlate well with the occurrence of tinnitus. In the person with tinnitus, inspection of the ear canal and surrounding area should include observation for a pulsatile mass.

In the person with hearing loss, the external auditory canals and tympanic membranes are inspected, using a pneumatic otoscope to delineate drum movement (Turner, 1982). The presence of infected fluid, impacted wax, foreign body, or disease of the middle or external ear may provide clues to the cause of pain, hearing loss, or tinnitus. Acute otitis media is an unusual finding in the elderly; chronic, painless middle ear infections are more common. Rare causes of ear pain include erosion from malignant disease, dural involvement by cholesteatoma, or expansion of an acoustic neuroma in the inner ear (Mills, 1985). Discharge produced by pathogens infecting the middle ear is usually mucopurulent and inoffensive in odor, whereas the discharge of otitis externa and cholesteatoma usually has an offensive odor. The presence of chronic discharge discolored by blood should suggest the possibility of a malignancy.

Tests

Of several tests that are available in screening for hearing impairment, the ticking watch and the whisper tests are not recommended. The sound of a ticking watch is probably too faint to be useful in quantitating a hearing loss; with the whisper test, whispers vary from examiner to examiner. Although bedside tuning fork tests are fairly nonspecific and insensitive, the Weber and Rinne tests can help determine whether the problem is equal bilaterally and whether it is most likely a conductive or sensorineural loss. It is recommended that two tuning forks, one of 256 cps and the other of 512 cps, be used for these tests (Carotenuto & Bullock, 1980).

The purpose of the Weber test is to determine lateralization of the hearing loss. The tuning fork is set into light vibration and placed on the middle of the patient's forehead. The patient is asked on which side the sound is heard better. The sound is not lateralized with normal hearing. In sensorineural deafness, the sound is heard better in the normal ear, and with conductive hearing loss, the sound is heard in the affected or deaf ear (Keith, 1984) (Figure 3–9).

The Rinne test differentiates between conductive and sensorineural deafness. The base of a vibrating fork is placed on the mastoid bone of the ear (bone conduction). When the sound is no longer heard, the fork is placed close to the external meatus (air conduction), and the patient is questioned as to ability to hear the sound. The location where the fork is heard longer determines the type of deficit. The normal response and that for sensorineural hearing loss (positive Rinne test) occurs when the patient first ceases to hear the sound on the mastoid and the vibrations at the meatus are still audible. A negative Rinne test indicates a conductive hearing loss. Bone conduction (mastoid bone) is heard louder than air conduction (ear canal) (Keith, 1984).

It is recommended that the elderly client with a hearing loss greater than 25 db who is also experiencing communication problems be referred to an audiologist. An otologist should be consulted if the history or examination

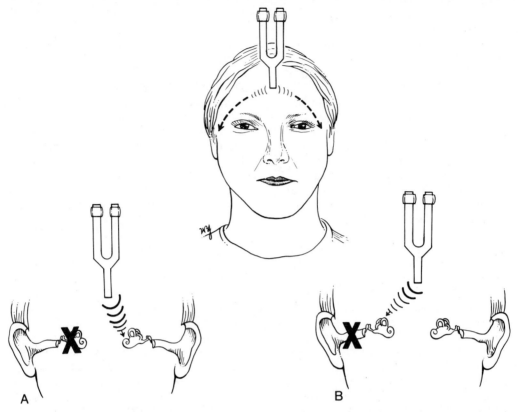

Figure 3–9. The Weber test. *(A)* Sensorineural deafness, *(B)* conductive hearing loss. (From Swartz, M: Textbook of Physical Diagnosis: History and Examination. Philadelphia, WB Saunders, 1989, p 176. Reprinted with permission.)

suggests a cause other than presbycusis for a hearing loss (Mader, 1984). Individuals with complaints and examination suggestive of vestibular disorders should be referred for an otoneurologic survey (Senturia, et al., 1983) (Figure 3–10).

NOSE

Aging Changes

Very limited information is available on the effects of aging on olfactory sense. Recent studies indicate a decreased sensitivity with age (Storandt, 1986).

Rhinologic disorders of older patients do not differ significantly from their presentation in younger patients. A common complaint in the older age group is dryness of the nasal vestibule (Price & Snider, 1983).

Epistaxis, or nosebleed, can be severe and difficult to treat in the elderly because bleeding occurs more commonly in the posterior portion of the nose. Causes of epistaxis include trauma, septal perforation, hypertension, blood dyscrasias, and tumors (Senturia, et al., 1983).

In atrophic rhinitis, nasal fossae are enlarged as a result of atrophic changes in the mucosa and underlying bone. The etiology of this progressive, chronic disease is unknown (Senturia, et al., 1983).

The acute loss of sense of smell may be due to acute coryza, whereas chronic loss is related to influenza-like viral infections, nasal polyps, crusty, or bloody. Whistling respirations may be due to abnormal blockage of the nose with drying and crusting (Prior, et al., 1981).

Examination

Examination is made for any deviation in the size, shape, or color of the nose and for flaring of the nares or discharge. Soft tissue of the nose is palpated for tenderness or masses. The patency of the nasal cavities is checked by asking the patient to close the mouth, close the nares with a finger, and breathe through the open nares. The olfactory nerve is tested by asking the patient to close the eyes and identify aromatic substances put to the nose. The nasal cavities are examined for polyps, swelling, exudate, and color of the mucosa. Tenderness over the maxillary and frontal sinuses is found in sinusitis (Malasonos, Barkauskas, Moss, et al., 1986).

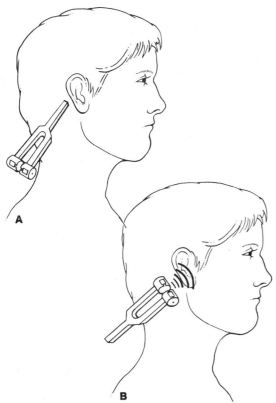

Figure 3–10. The Rinne test. (From Swartz, M: Textbook of Physical Diagnosis: History and Examination. Philadelphia, WB Saunders, 1989, p 175. Reprinted with permission.)

surgery, radiation, or high doses of drugs such as aspirin (Senturia, et al., 1983).

Perforations of the nasal septum result from trauma such as nasal fractures and picking of the nose. It is common to find nasal blockage, infection, bleeding, crusting, and drying with perforations (Senturia, et al., 1983).

History

A history is obtained about frequent colds, allergy, trauma, sense of smell, discharge, and obstruction (Prior, et al., 1981). Redness of the nasal mucosa indicates infection. Watery secretions may indicate an acute upper respiratory infection or an allergic rhinitis. Abnormal findings include secretions that are purulent,

NECK

Aging Changes

Kyphosis, an accentuation of the forward upper thoracic concave curve, is common in the elderly and may result in a forward curvature of the neck. The loss of muscle mass and subcutaneous tissues causes the neck to appear thin and wrinkled. In healthy elderly, range of motion remains unchanged. Although thyroid size does not change with age up to 90 years, nodular and impalpable glands are more frequently encountered. Likewise, thyroid hormone action is not affected by age (Hodkinson & Irvine, 1985).

Common Disorders

Illnesses that occur frequently in an elderly population and that present with signs and symptoms associated with the neck are cervical osteoarthritis, carotid arteritis, and thyroid disorders.

History

The symptoms of degenerative joint disease may be limited to mild headache or backache. More severe symptoms may be indicative of tumor or osteoarthritis with disc collapse (Pearson & Kotthoff, 1979). Patients with carotid arteritis may complain of pain in the side of the neck intensified by swallowing. Fever may or may not be present. Thyroid disorders in the elderly rarely present with the classic symptoms of the diseases in younger patients. Lethargy, slowed mentation, depression, and apathy are frequent complaints of patients with both hypo- and hyperthyroid conditions (Gregerman, 1985; Hodkinson & Irvine, 1985).

Examination

The examination of the neck of the elderly patient is the same as that for a younger patient. Common findings and their relevance to the common disorders of the elderly will be briefly described.

The neck is observed for asymmetry, swelling, and involuntary tension of the muscles. Active mobility is tested by asking the patient to perform the following movements: anteflexion, dorsiflexion, lateral right and left flexion, and rotation (Lodewick & Gunn, 1983). The cervical muscles and vertebrae are palpated and percussed, noting any tenderness. Passive range of motion is applied while palpating for crepitus. In cervical osteoarthritis, active and passive range of motion may be painless but may produce crepitus. When the patient's head is held in a position of neck extension, coughing may produce pain (DeGowin & DeGowin, 1987).

With the patient sitting at a 45° angle, the neck is observed for jugular venous distention. The carotid artery is palpated for thrills and ausculated for bruits. All lymph nodes are palpated. Patients who have had a long history of cigarette smoking often have shotty, palpable, submental and submandibular nodes. These are not clinically significant but must be distinguished from an acute lymphadenopathy.

In carotid arteritis the carotid artery may be tender, and digital compression of the artery may cause pain in the jaw, ear, and temple (DeGowin & DeGowin, 1987).

Hypothyroidism in the elderly is often insidious in onset, with or without a classic presentation. Certain manifestations of hypothyroidism may mimic other conditions commonly present in the elderly. Weight loss is more common than weight gain. A goiter or palpable thyroid gland is often absent. Pericardial and pleural effusion may be attributed to congestive heart failure. Synovial effusions may be attributed to osteoarthritis or rheumatoid arthritis, even though joint inflammation is absent. Hypothyroidism and hypertension often coexist. Treatment of hypothyroidism normalizes the blood pressure in about 40% to 50% of affected persons (Gilbert, 1981; Gregerman, 1985).

Blunted affect and slowed response to questioning may be found in elderly people with hyperthyroid disease. A mental status examination may differentiate the changes characteristic of hyperthyroidism from the true cognitive impairment of dementia. A normal sized or impalpable thyroid gland does not rule out hyperthyroidism, since about 10% to 20% of elderly with this condition do not have thyromegaly. When enlargement is present, it is nodular in almost three-fourths of the cases. Exophthalmus and proptosis are not often found in thyrotoxic elderly because Graves' disease is less common in this age group than in young adults (Gilbert, 1981; Gregerman, 1985). Although tachycardia is a classical finding in hyperthyroidism, about half of the elderly may have a normal pulse rate. Atrial fibrillation is the most common dysrhythmia and is seen in 20% to 40% of thyrotoxic elderly (Gilbert, 1981). Signs of heart failure are not uncommon, occurring in up to one-half of elderly hyperthyroid patients (Gregerman, 1985). Marked muscle wasting and weakness of the proximal muscles may be noted by observation and by testing the patient's ability to squat and return to standing and to lift the arms above the level of the shoulders with and without added small weights. Weight loss occurs in about half the cases and may exceed

20 pounds (Gilbert, 1981). Thyroid nodules that are new or growing, hard or fixed, solitary, or associated with hoarseness, bone pain, or cervical lymphadenopathy are suspicious for malignancy (Gilbert, 1981).

Tests

Cervical spine x-ray films are indicated in the presence of crepitus, particularly in women who are in the high risk group for osteoarthritic changes. Laboratory tests do not aid the diagnosis of carotid arteritis, but they are critical in the complete evaluation of thyroid function.

Diagnosis of hypothyroidism is confirmed by a low serum thyroxine (T_4) and an elevated thyroid-stimulating hormone (TSH) level. A T_4 level measured by radioimmunoassay that falls within the central 75% to 80% of the laboratory's reference interval does not warrant further testing in asymptomatic subjects. Serum triiodothyronine (T_3) concentration is less sensitive than T_4 in detecting hypothyroidism, since some hypothyroid patients may have decreased T_4 but normal T_3 concentrations. Measurement of T_4 level is significantly affected by coexisting illnesses such as cardiovascular, hepatic, and renal disease and concurrent drug therapy. Corticosteroids, estrogen and androgens, propranolol, L-dopa, propylthiouracil, and radiographic contrast media may alter T_4 and T_3 levels (Rock, 1985).

In hyperthyroidism, the serum T_3 is increased to a relatively greater extent than is the serum T_4. If the T_4 is elevated or there is clinical suspicion of hyperthyroidism, the T_3 should be measured by radioimmunoassay (T_3RIA) to confirm the diagnosis. Currently, most TSH assays are not sensitive enough to distinguish between low TSH levels of normal euthyroid individuals and those of hyperthyroid individuals whose TSH values are suppressed to below normal levels by the excess circulating T_4 and T_3 (Rock, 1985). Up to 30% of the elderly with hyperthyroidism have T_3 toxicosis in which T_3 is elevated while T_4 remains normal (Hodkinson & Irvine, 1985).

An ultrasound echogram will delineate whether the thyroid nodule is cystic or solid and whether the remainder of the thyroid is enlarged or nodular. Thyroid gland scanning with isotopes of iodide or pertechnetate will identify "hot nodules" associated with increased function and "cold nodules" associated with decreased function. Hot nodules are rarely malignant, whereas about 20% of cold nodules are malignant. Even "warm nodules," whose uptake is similar to the remainder of the gland, may be malignant. Definitive diagnosis depends upon biopsy for tissue identification (Gilbert, 1981).

SUMMARY

This chapter on physical assessment of the older client began with an overview of the assessment process. Particular attention has been paid to important points of clinical significance in the elderly client. Following this overview of the assessment process, sections that dealt with assessing the skin, eye, ear, nose, and neck were presented. In each section the changes that occur with age, the disorders commonly seen in the elderly, and pertinent areas related to history and examination were presented. If specific tests were available, they were included in the section.

References

Amery, A, Birkenhager, W, Brixko, P, et al. (1985): Mortality and morbidity results from the European Working Party on High Blood Pressure in the Elderly trial. *Lancet*, 1:1349–1354.

Anderson, F & Williams, B (1983): *Skin Disease. Practical Management of the Elderly* (ed 4). Oxford, Blackwell Scientific Publications, 285–292.

Andres, R, Elahi, D, Tobin, JD, et al. (1985): Impact of age on weight goals. *Ann Intern Med*, 103(Suppl):1030–1033.

Applegate, WB, Dismuke, SE, & Runyan, JW (1984): Treatment of hypertension in the elderly: A time for caution? *J Am Geriatr Soc*, 32:21–33.

Boniksowski, FP (1983): Differential diagnosis of dizziness in the elderly. *Geriatrics*, 38:89–104.

Brody, EM, Kleban, MH, & Moles, E (1983): What older people do about their day-to-day mental and physical health symptoms. *J Am Geriatr Soc*, 31:489–497.

Caird, FI (1973): Problems in interpretation of laboratory findings in the old. *Br Med J*, 4:348–350.

Caird, FI (1981): Physical examination of the elderly, problems and possibilities. *In* Reinders Folmer, ANJ & Schouten, J (eds): *Geriatrics for the Practitioner.* Amsterdam, Excerpta Medica, 3–7.

Callaghan, HG, Fitzgerald, DJ, & O'Malley, K, et al. (1983): Accuracy of indirect blood pressure measurement in the elderly. *Br Med J, 286:*1545–1546.

Carotenuto, R & Bullock, J (1980): *Physical Assessment of the Gerontologic Client.* Philadelphia, FA Davis.

Chobanian, AV (1983): Pathophysiologic considerations in the treatment of the elderly hypertensive patient. *Am J Cardiol, 59:*49D–53D.

Corso, JF (1971): Sensory processes and age effects in normal adults. *J Gerontol, 26:*90–105.

DeGowin, E & DeGowin, R (1987): *Bedside Diagnostic Examination* (ed 5). New York, Macmillan, 33.

Domonkos, AN, Arnold, HL & Odom, RB (1982): *Andrew's Diseases of the Skin* (ed 7). Philadelphia, WB Saunders.

Ehrlich, DR & Keates, RH (1978): What to do when the elderly patient complains of external eye problems. *Geriatrics, 33:*34–38, 43.

Eifrig, DE & Simons, KB (1983): An overview of common geriatric ophthalmologic disorders. *Geriatrics, 38:*55–77.

Esposito, AL & Gleckman, RA (1978): Fever of unknown origin in the elderly. *J Am Geriatr Soc, 26:*498–505.

Fitzpatrick, TB, Polano, MK, Suurmond, D (1983): *Color Atlas and Synopsis of Clinical Dermatology.* New York, McGraw-Hill.

Fitzpatrick, TB & Haynes, HA (1983): Alterations in the skin. *In* Petersdorf, RG, Adams, RD, Braunwald, E, et al. (eds): *Harrison's Principles of Internal Medicine* (ed 10). McGraw-Hill, New York, 249–265.

Fraser, MC & McGuire, DB (1984): Skin cancer's early warning system. *Am J Nurs, 84:*1232–1236.

Galloway, NR (1985): *Common Eye Diseases and Their Management.* Berlin, Springer-Verlag.

Gifford, RW (1986): Management of isolated systolic hypertension in the elderly. *J Amer Geriat Soc, 34:*106–111.

Gilbert, PD (1981): Thyroid function and disease. *In* Libow, LS & Sherman, FT (eds): *The Core of Geriatric Medicine.* St. Louis, CV Mosby, 246–279.

Gilchrest, BA (1984): *Skin and Aging Processes.* Boca Raton, Florida, CRC Press.

Gilchrest, BA (1986): Skin diseases in the elderly. *In* Calkins, E, Davis, D, & Ford, A, (eds): *The Practice of Geriatrics.* Philadelphia, WB Saunders, 495–496.

Graham, P (1985): The eye. *In* Pathy, MSJ (ed): *Principles and Practice of Geriatric Medicine.* London, John Wiley & Sons, 833–840.

Granacher, RP (1981): The neurologic examination in geriatric psychiatry. *Psychosomatics, 22*(6):486–499.

Gregerman, RI (1985): Thyroid diseases. *In* Andres, R, Bierman, EL, & Hazzard, WR (eds): *Principles of Geriatric Medicine.* New York, McGraw-Hill, 727–749.

Gurevitch, AW (1983): Dermatologic disorders. *In* Steinberg, FU (ed): *Care of the Geriatric Patient* (ed 6). St. Louis, CV Mosby, 199–215.

Hale, WE, Perkins, LL, May FE, et al. (1986): Symptom prevalence in the elderly: An evaluation of age, sex, disease, and medication use. *J Am Geriatr Soc, 34:*333–340.

Hale, WE, Stewart, RB & Marks, RG (1983): Haematological and biochemical laboratory values in an ambulatory elderly population: An analysis of the effects of age, sex, and drugs. *Age Ageing, 12:*275–284.

Hashimoto, F, Hunt, WC, & Hardy, L (1984): Differences between right and left arm blood pressures in the elderly. *West J Med, 141:*189–192.

Hawes, MJ & Ellis, PP (1983): Tearing in the geriatric patient: Causes and treatments. *Geriatrics, 38:*113–121.

Hla, KM, Vokaty, KA, & Feussner, JR (1985): Overestimation of diastolic blood pressure in the elderly. *J Am Geriatr Soc, 33:*659–663.

Hodkinson, HM (1981): Modern views about laboratory examination of the elderly. *In* Reinders Folmer, ANJ & Schouten, J (eds): *Geriatrics for the Practitioner.* Amsterdam, Excerpta Medica, 9–16.

Hodkinson, HM & Irvine, RE (1985): The endocrine system: Thyroid disease in the elderly. *In* Brocklehurst, JC (ed): *Textbook of Geriatric Medicine and Gerontology* (ed 3). New York, Churchill Livingstone, 686–714.

Hulley, SB, Feigal, D, Ireland, C, et al. (1986): Systolic hypertension in the elderly program (SHEP). The first three months. *J Am Geriatr Soc, 34:*101–105.

Jernigan, JA, Gudat, JC, Blake, JL, et al. (1980): Reference values for blood findings in relatively fit elderly persons. *J Am Geriatr Soc, 28:*308–314.

Johnson, MLT & Roberts, J (1978): Skin conditions and related need for medical care among persons 1–74 years. *Vital and Health Statistics,* Series 11, *212:*1–30.

Jones, DA, Victor, CR, & Vetter, NJ (1984): Hearing difficulty and its psychological implications for the elderly. *J Epidemiol Community Health, 38:*75–78.

Kasper, RL (1983): Eye problems of the aged. *In* Reichel, W (ed): *Clinical Aspects of Aging* (ed 2). Baltimore, Williams & Wilkins, 479–488.

Keating, HJ, Klimek, JJ, Levine, DS, et al. (1984): Effect of aging on the clinical significance of fever in ambulatory adult patients. *J Am Geriatr Soc, 32:*282–287.

Keeney, AH & Keeney, VT (1980): A guide to examining the aging eye. *Geriatrics, 35:*81–91.

Keilson, L, Lambert, D, Fabian, D, et al. (1985): Screening for hypothermia in the ambulatory elderly. The Maine experience. *JAMA, 254:*1781–1784.

Keith, RW (1984): The basic audiologic evaluation. *In* Northern, JL (ed): *Hearing Disorders.* Boston, Little, Brown & Co, 13–24.

Kelly, A, Munan, LM, Petitclers, C, et al. (1979): Patterns of change in selected serum chemical parameters of middle and later years. *J Gerontol, 34:*37–40.

Kent, S (1982): Body weight and life expectancy. *Geriatrics, 37:*149, 152, 154, 157.

Kohn, RR (1977): Heart and cardiovascular system. *In* Finch, CF & Hayflick, L (eds): *Handbook of the Biology of Aging.* New York, Van Nostrand Reinhold Company, 281–317.

Leventhal, EA & Prohaska, TR (1986): Age, symptom interpretation, and health behavior. *J Am Geriatr Soc, 34:*185–191.

Lichenstein, MJ (1985): Isolated systolic hypertension: How common? How risky? *South Med J, 78:*972–978.

Lipsitz, AS, Nyquist, RP, Wei, JY, et al. (1983): Postprandial reduction in blood pressure in the elderly. *N Engl J Med, 309:*81–83.

Lipsitz, LA & Fullerton, KJ (1986): Postprandial blood pressure reduction in healthy elderly. *J Am Geriatr Soc, 34*:267–270.

Lodewick, L & Gunn, ADG (1983): *The Physical Examination: An Atlas for General Practice.* Lancaster, England, MTP Press Limited.

Lookingbill, DP (1985): Principles of clinical diagnosis. *In* Moschella, SL & Hurley, HJ (eds): *Dermatology* (ed 2). Philadelphia, WB Saunders, 126–200.

McFadden, JP, Price, RC, Eastwood, HD, et al. (1982): Raised respiratory rate in elderly patients: A valuable physical sign. *Br Med J, 284*:626–627.

Mader, S (1984): Hearing impairment in elderly persons. *J Am Geriatr Soc, 32*:548–553.

Malasanos, L, Barkauskas, V, Moss, M, et al. (1986): *Health Assessment.* St. Louis, CV Mosby.

Meltzer, DW (1983): Ophthalmic aspects. *In* Steinberg, FU (ed): *Care of the Geriatric Patient* (ed 6). St. Louis, CV Mosby, 450–461.

Messerli, FH, Ventura, HO, & Amodeo, C (1985): Osler's maneuver and pseudohypertension. *N Engl J Med, 312*:1548–1551.

Mills, R (1985): The auditory system. *In* Pathy, MSJ (ed): *Principles and Practice of Geriatric Medicine.* London, John Wiley & Sons, 841–854.

National Institutes of Health (1985): Consensus Conference Statement: Health implications of obesity. *Ann Intern Med, 103*(Suppl.):1073–1077.

Newell, FW (1986): *Ophthalmology: Principles and Concepts* (ed 6). St. Louis, CV Mosby.

Norman, DC, Grahn, D, & Yoshikawa, TT (1985): Fever and aging. *J Am Geriatr Soc, 33*:859–863.

Nover, A (1981): *The Ocular Fundus* (ed 4). Philadelphia, Lea & Febiger.

O'Callaghan, WG, Fitzgerald, DJ, O'Malley, K, et al. (1983): Accuracy of indirect blood pressure measurement in the elderly. *Br Med J, 286*:1545–1546.

Orentreich, DS & Orentreich, N (1985): Alterations in the skin. *In* Andres, P, Bierman, EL, & Hazzard WR (eds): *Principles of Geriatric Medicine.* New York, McGraw-Hill, 354–371.

Palta, M, Prineas, RJ, Berman, R, et al. (1982): Comparison of self-reported and measured height and weight. *Am J Epidemiol, 115*:223–230.

Pearson, LJ & Kotthoff, EM (1979): *Geriatric Clinical Protocols.* Philadelphia, JB Lippincott.

Porth, C, & Kapke, K (1983): Aging and the skin. *Geriatric Nursing,* May/June, 158–162.

Price, LL & Snider, RM (1983): The geriatric patient: Ear, nose, and throat problems. *In* Reichel, W (ed): *Clinical Aspects of Aging* (ed 2). Baltimore, Williams & Wilkins, 489–497.

Prior, JA, Silberstein, JS, & Stang, JM (1981): *Physical Diagnosis,* (ed 6). St. Louis, CV Mosby.

Reuler, JB (1978): Hypothermia: Pathophysiology, clinical settings, and management. *Ann Intern Med, 89*:519–527.

Rich, LFF (1984): Ophthalmology. *In* Cassel, CK & Walsh, JR (eds): *Geriatric medicine: Volume 1.* New York, Springer-Verlag, 90–110.

Riko, K & Alberti, PW (1984): Rehabilitation of hearing impaired adults. *Otolaryngol Clin North Am, 17*:644–651.

Robbins, AS & Rubenstein, LZ (1984): Postural hypotension in the elderly. *J Am Geriatr Soc, 32*:769–774.

Rock, RC (1985): Interpreting thyroid tests in the elderly: Updated guidelines. *Geriatrics, 40*:61–68.

Rodman, WP: Glaucoma screening by the primary care physician (1984). *Postgrad Med, 76*:224, 227, 230.

Rowe, JW (1983): Systolic hypertension in the elderly (letter). *N Engl J Med, 309*:1246–1247.

Ruben, RJ & Kruger, B (1983): Hearing loss in the elderly. *In* Katzman, R & Terry, R (eds): *The Neurology of Aging.* Philadelphia, FA Davis, 123–147.

Sauer, GC (1985): *Geriatric Dermatology. Manual of Skin Diseases* (ed 5). Philadelphia, JB Lippincott, 343–352.

Scotto, J & Fears, TP (1978): Skin cancer epidemiology: Research needs. *Natl Cancer Inst Monographs, 50*:169–177.

Scotto, J, Fears, TP, & Fraumeni, JF, Jr (1981): Incidence of nonmelanoma skin cancer in the United States. DHHS Printing Office Publication No. NIH 82-2433.

Senturia, BH, Goldstein, R, & Hersperger, WS (1983): Otorhinolaryngologic aspects of geriatric care. *In* Steinberg, FU (ed): *Care of the Geriatric Patient* (ed 6). St. Louis, CV Mosby, 482–500.

Storandt, M (1986): Psychological aspects of aging. *In* Rossman, I (ed): *Clinical Geriatrics* (ed 3). Philadelphia, JB Lippincott, 606–617.

Sullivan, ND & Basler, RS (1981): Geriatric dermatology. *In* O'Hara-Devereaux, M, Andrus, LH, & Scott, CD (eds): *Eldercare.* New York, Grune & Stratton, 283.

Swartz, M (1989): *Textbook of Physical Diagnosis: History and Examination.* Philadelphia, WB Saunders, 98, 153, 146, 175, 176.

Taisch, EA, Taisch, DA, & Metz, HS (1981): Problems of the eyes. *In* O'Hara-Devereaux, M, Andrus, LH, & Scott, E (eds): *Eldercare.* New York, Grune & Stratton, 268.

Thomas, PD, Hunt, WC, Garry, PJ, et al. (1983): Hearing acuity in a healthy elderly population: Effects on emotional, cognitive, and social status. *J Gerontol 38*:321–325.

Tonnesen, MG & Weston, WL (1982): Aging of skin. *In* Schrier, RW (ed): *Clinical Internal Medicine in the Aged.* Philadelphia, WB Saunders, 296–304.

Turner, JS (1982): Treatment of hearing loss, ear pain, and tinnitus in older patients. *Geriatrics, 37*:107–118.

Waisman, M (1979): A clinical look at the aging skin. *Postgrad Med, 66*:87–97.

Wright, BE & Henkind, P (1983): Aging changes and the eye. *In* Katzman, R (ed): *The Neurology of Aging.* Philadelphia, FA Davis, 149–165.

Wuest, FC, Sayther, KD, Carson, CA, et al. (1976): The aging eye. *Minn Med, 59*(8):540–546.

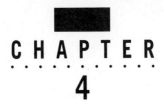

CHAPTER
4

Physical Assessment: The Breast and the Pulmonary, Cardiovascular, Gastrointestinal, and Genitourinary Systems

J. ELIZABETH BELL, R.N.C., M.S., A.N.P.
LAWRENCE DIXON, R.N.C., M.S., G.N.P.
YVONNE A. SEHY, R.N.C., M.S., F.N.P./G.N.P.

Introduction

The Breast

    Aging changes

    Common disorders

    History

    Examination

    Tests

Pulmonary System

    Aging changes

    Common disorders

    History

    Examination

    Tests and procedures

Cardiovascular System

    Aging changes

    Common disorders

    History

    Examination

    Tests

Gastrointestinal System

    Aging changes

    Common disorders

    History

    Examination

    Tests

Female Genitourinary System

    Aging changes

    Common disorders

    History

    Examination

    Tests

INTRODUCTION

This chapter focuses on the breast and the pulmonary, cardiovascular, gastrointestinal, and the genitourinary systems. It includes information on aging changes, common disorders, history, examination, and tests and procedures commonly used to clarify physical findings.

THE BREAST

Aging Changes

The replacement of fibrous tissue by fat, which occurs with aging, should enhance the identification of breast tumors by palpation. However, tumor palpation is difficult in large pendulous breasts and in patients receiving estrogen therapy when fibrous tissue may still be present (Moe, 1985). The elderly female generally has nipples that are less pigmented and smaller in size than those of younger women. The nipples may be retracted but should be easily retroverted with gentle pressure (Hafez, 1976).

Common Disorders

Breast cancer is the most common malignancy found in women and accounts for 2% of the deaths in those over 75 years. Nipple retraction and palpable masses are the most reliable indicators of cancer in this age group. Breast screening that includes breast self-ex-

amination, annual professional examination, and mammogram is the best diagnostic combination for women over 50 years. Early detection by this means has reduced mortality by one-third (Goodell, 1985). Furthermore, elderly women may have localized but advanced disease (Adami, Malker, Meirik, et al., 1985; Davis, Karrer, Moor, et al., 1985).

History

The patient should be questioned about the symptoms associated with breast cancer: pain, nipple discharges, the presence of a mass, and discoloration or abnormal shape of the breast. The examiner should also ask the patient about a family history of breast cancer or any other cancers, the use of estrogen or other drugs that affect the breast (digitalis, thyroid drugs, and antihypertensives), knowledge and practice of breast self-examination, and mammogram history. Commonly offered reasons for not practicing breast self-examination include lack of knowledge, ignorance of the importance of the procedure, fear, and anxiety (Keller, George, & Podell, 1980). The chapter authors found geriatric women willing to learn and practice breast self-examination. Indeed, Moe (1985) found that the geriatric female trained in breast self-examination practiced the procedure more than did the younger female.

Examination

The examiner should teach or review the technique of breast self-examination with those patients able to perform it. Breast self-examination detects 75% to 90% of breast masses (Baines, 1984). If the nipples are retracted they should be easily retroverted with gentle pressure. Any discharge should be considered abnormal, and a sample of the discharge should be placed on a slide for cytology screening. The breasts should be examined for superficial lesions and rashes. Women with large pendulous breasts may have fungal rashes on the underside of the breast and on the chest wall.

Tests

The elderly female is at risk for breast cancer. In this group the mammogram is very effective in screening for breast cancer because of the decreased density of breast tissue (Goodell, 1985; Moe, 1985). The importance of yearly mammography for women over 50 years cannot be stressed enough.

PULMONARY SYSTEM

Aging Changes

Several measurements of lung function change with age, due to normal aging, disease, and environmental factors. There is a 50% increase in residual volume (RV) between early adulthood and age 70 (King & Schwarz, 1982). Because a stiffer chest wall and other changes prevent an increase in total lung capacity, the increase in RV is accompanied by a corresponding decrease in vital capacity. Forced expiratory volume at 1 second decreases about 30 ml/year in males and 25 ml/year in females beginning in the third decade, with wide variation (Freeman, 1985). PO_2 decreases by about 4 mm Hg each decade, although PCO_2 is unchanged (King & Schwarz, 1982). Maximal oxygen uptake, an indication of aerobic exercise capacity, declines by a third between the ages of 20 and 60 years, although individuals vary greatly depending on past and present exercise training (Klocke, 1977).

Other aging changes include a less effective cough, impaired ciliary action, weaker respiratory muscles, and a blunted response to hypoxia and hypercapnia. These and other aging changes lessen elderly persons' exercise tolerance, predispose them to a variety of pulmonary diseases and disorders, and cause them to decompensate more easily when pulmonary disease is present.

Common Disorders

Pulmonary diseases seen frequently in older individuals include bronchogenic cancer, pneumonia, chronic obstructive pulmonary disease (COPD), pulmonary embolism, and tuberculosis. A brief discussion of the presenting symptoms of these diseases is included below.

History

The geriatric pulmonary history should address tobacco use, the usual questions about pulmonary symptoms asked of any adult, and the effect of chronic symptoms on function. Smoking remains a risk for coronary artery disease (CAD) and stroke in old age, and cessation of smoking decreases that risk. Excess risk of mortality from CAD declines within one to five years of tobacco avoidance (Jajich, Ostfeld, & Freeman, 1984), and cerebral blood flow significantly increases within one year of quitting smoking (Rogers, Meyer, Judd, et al., 1985). Elderly patients with chronic pulmonary disease should be asked about functional changes, such as the effect of dyspnea on activities of daily living. For example, how far can the client walk before becoming short of breath? Can he or she shop, prepare a meal, bathe, dress? Other areas to explore are whether the client's car bears handicapped license plates and whether the client knows the signs and symptoms of respiratory infection. The client should be able to use and clean a nebulizer, use oxygen safely, perform postural drainage, and read a thermometer.

The most common pulmonary symptoms in elderly people are dyspnea, cough, chest pain, and hemoptysis. A brief discussion of the implications of each follows.

Dyspnea. The decline in pulmonary function that occurs with aging usually is not severe enough to cause significant shortness of breath, so the examiner should not routinely attribute dyspnea to aging. In one study (Landahl, Steen, & Svanborg, 1980), 55% of elderly women and 77% of elderly men who complained of dyspnea had cardiac failure or pulmonary disease (mainly bronchitis, emphysema, or asthma). Other causes of dyspnea include chest wall dysfunction from neurologic or muscular diseases, metabolic acidosis, carbon monoxide poisoning, and anemia (Lillington, 1984).

Cough. If cough is present, the examiner should ascertain whether it is productive or nonproductive. A productive cough usually dominates the presentation of bronchitis, whereas dyspnea with or without cough is more common in emphysema. The amount and characteristics of any sputum should be determined to establish a baseline record. An increase in amount or change in color to yellow or green may indicate a bacterial infection.

Chest Pain. Chest pain is found in about 30% of elderly with pneumonia (Marrie, Haldane, Faulkner, et al., 1985) and in about 70% of older patients with severe pulmonary embolism (Wynne, 1979). It may also be caused by muscular strain from coughing. Chest pain is considered in more detail under the cardiovascular section.

Hemoptysis. If the client complains of coughing up blood, the examiner should try to determine by history and examination if the source is the nose, gastrointestinal tract, or the bronchial tree. In true hemoptysis, the mostly likely causes in people over 45 are bronchitis, bronchogenic cancer, tuberculosis, and pulmonary infarction (King & Schwarz, 1982).

Absence of Pulmonary Symptoms. The absence of pulmonary symptoms does not necessarily rule out pulmonary disease because pneumonia, pulmonary embolism, and tuberculosis may present in the elderly with few symptoms. One study found that older patients with pneumonia were less likely to complain of chills and myalgias than a younger group (Marrie, et al., 1985). Dyspnea may be present in only half of elderly patients with pneumonia (Freeman, 1985). Pneumonia may present itself by a nonspecific deterioration in health, slight cough, altered mental status, dehydration, and tachypnea. Similarly, the classic triad of pleuritic chest pain, sudden dyspnea, and hemoptysis is uncommon in the elderly patient with pulmonary embolism. Instead, the most common presentations are (1) acute onset of dyspnea with a normal chest x-ray, (2) cough or chest pain with infiltrate on chest x-ray, and (3) sudden development of acute cor pulmonale (Michael & Summer, 1985). Because of the frequency with which tuberculosis goes undetected, Nagami and Yoshikawa (1983) recommend that tuberculosis be considered in any elderly patient with vague pleuropulmonary symptoms or unexplained fever, loss of appetite, or weight loss.

Examination

Common normal findings in the elderly may be confused with signs of disease. A barrel chest, slight use of intercostal muscles, and slightly prolonged expirations may occur in normal elderly people and should not automatically be attributed to emphysema. Other sources of confusion are the scattered crackles in dependent lung segments of some elderly people; they may be mistaken for the rales of bronchitis or congestive heart failure. Physiologic crackles should decrease or disappear with coughing, which distinguishes them from those associated with pathology. Finally, a breathing pattern suggestive of Cheyne-Stokes respiration is sometimes seen in normal elderly people.

Physical Findings in Common Diseases. The physical examination of the elderly client with tuberculosis often reveals little, and diagnosis usually depends on the chest x-ray. The examination of an elderly client with a small or medium-sized pulmonary embolism may also reveal little, although a pleural friction rub, mild temperature elevation, and tachypnea and tachycardia may be found (King & Schwarz, 1982). In larger pulmonary emboli, there may be evidence of acute pulmonary hypertension, such as an accentuated pulmonic component of heart sound S2, a right ventricular heave, a right-sided S3 and S4, jugular venous distention, a hepatojugular reflex, and edema. The examiner should also look for signs of deep vein thrombosis in the lower extremities, such as unilateral calf enlargement of 1.5 cm or more, tenderness to palpation, erythema, and a positive Homan's sign. However, often the lower extremities may be normal or may merely show signs of chronic venous insufficiency (Michael & Summer, 1985). In one series, tachypnea was found in almost 90% of elderly patients with large pulmonary emboli, rales and an accentuated pulmonic component of S2 were found in 50%, tachycardia and fever in about 40%, and an S3 and S4 and phlebitis in about one-third (Wynne, 1979).

Authorities differ over the frequency of atypical presentations of pneumonia in the elderly. At least by anecdotal report, signs of consolidation may be absent, although they may become audible if the patient can be made to breathe deeply (Freeman, 1985). Fever and leukocytosis may also be absent. However, Marrie and associates (1985) found that rales, rhonchi, consolidation, and leukocytosis occurred at least as frequently in older people with pneumonia as in younger patients, and Fedullo and Swinburne (1985) reported no difference in body temperature when they compared younger and older patients with pneumonia.

In emphysema, particularly early in the disease, there may be few physical findings. In later stages the typical emphysemic patient is thin and anxious and uses pursed-lip breathing and accessory muscles. Breath sounds may be decreased and heart sounds faint if a barrel chest is present. Wheezing may be heard, especially if the client is asked to expire forcefully. The cardiac point of maximal impulse may be felt in the epigastric area, and lower than normal diaphragmatic levels may be percussed. The examination may be even less revealing in chronic bronchitis. Wheezes and rales may be heard, with either decreased or normal breath sounds. The examiner should look for cyanosis and evidence of right-sided heart failure.

The examination of the patient with COPD should include an assessment of exercise capacity and of ability to perform activities of daily living. The client should be asked to walk to the point of experiencing dyspnea, with vital signs and pulmonary assessment done before and after exercise to establish a baseline record. Observation during such activities as dressing, preparing a meal, and bathing may reveal whether a client could

benefit from using energy conservation techniques. If appropriate, the client should be observed using an inhaler.

Tests and Procedures

Most authorities do not recommend routine screening for pulmonary disease in asymptomatic clients. However, because of the atypical presentation of many diseases and the paucity and nonspecificity of physical findings, judicious use of diagnostic tests is mandatory in evaluating and managing many pulmonary complaints.

Pulmonary Function Tests (PFTs). PFTs are useful in confirming a diagnosis of obstructive or restrictive lung disease, in monitoring a client with an established diagnosis, and in evaluating therapy.

Tuberculin Skin Test. When tuberculosis is suspected, a purified protein derivative (PPD) should be placed intradermally, along with a test for anergy. A common delayed-hypersensitivity allergen such as mumps, *Candida*, *Trichophyton*, or streptokinase can be used for the latter. Greater than 5 to 10 mm of induration 48 to 96 hours after PPD injection indicates a positive result, depending upon geographic location and local standards. If the initial result is negative, the test should be repeated in a week to test for a boosted reaction, to avoid confusion later over whether a positive result is a new conversion or a booster effect. As many as 10% of clients with active tuberculosis may have negative tuberculin skin test results (Nagami & Yoshikawa, 1983).

Sputum. If the result of the tuberculin skin test is positive and tuberculosis is suspected from chest x-ray or symptoms, sputum for acid-fast bacilli should be obtained on three consecutive mornings. If tuberculosis is strongly suspected, even when the results of three tests are negative, as many as six to eight sputums should be obtained (Nagami & Yoshikawa, 1983). There is some controversy over whether sputum analysis is helpful in guiding treatment of pneumonias because of the high incidence of contaminants. Many authorities still recommend obtaining a sputum for

Gram's stain and culture. Marrie and co-workers (1985) found that sputum cultures had a better diagnostic yield than blood cultures, throat washings, or serologic studies, but the yield was still less than 40%.

Chest X-ray. A chest x-ray is helpful in diagnosing COPD, pneumonia, pulmonary embolism, tuberculosis, and bronchogenic cancer. The typical and atypical radiographic findings in elderly patients with these diseases are beyond the scope of this book but can be found in any of the geriatric medical textbooks listed in the references. The examiner should keep in mind that a negative chest x-ray does not rule out many pulmonary diseases. For example, only 40% of patients with moderate to severe emphysema in one series were diagnosed from an x-ray, and 10% of patients with pulmonary embolism have normal radiographic findings (King & Schwarz, 1982).

CARDIOVASCULAR SYSTEM

Aging Changes

Many structural and physiologic changes in the cardiovascular system commonly occur with aging. Amyloid deposition may lead to enlargement, with subsequent arrhythmias and congestive heart failure. Degenerative processes and sclerosis of the conduction system may lead to arrhythmias. However, there is no consistent change in cardiac mass with age. Body size and weight may correlate more strongly with cardiac mass than does advanced age (Hitzhusen & Alpert, 1984). There are also changes in specific structures of the heart; they are presented in Table 4–1.

Systole is prolonged, stroke volume decreases, and cardiac output decreases with subsequent decline of maximum coronary blood flow by 65% between the ages of 20 and 60 years (Eliopoulous, 1984). In addition, vasomotor tone decreases and vagal tone increases. The heart is more sensitive to carotid sinus stimulation, and baroreceptor sensitivity decreases. The maximal heart rate and maximal oxygen consumption during exercise decrease with age and parallel the decline in maximum

Table 4–1. STRUCTURAL CHANGES IN THE HEART WITH AGING

Structure	Change
Coronary arteries	Calcification of the media and elastic proliferation
Aorta and aortic branches	Dilation, elongation, becoming tortuous
Heart valves	Thickening and rigidity secondary to fibrosis and sclerosis
Sinoatrial node area	Fibroelastic thickening
Myocardium	Atrophy with loss of elasticity

(Data from Caird, Dall, & Williams, 1985; Hitzhusen & Alpert, 1984; Lindenfeld & Groves, 1982; Murphy & DeMots, 1984.)

work capacity (Lindenfeld & Groves, 1982). Physiologic changes at rest and with exercise are summarized in Table 4–2.

Atherosclerosis and arteriosclerosis occur in the arterial vascular bed with aging. Atherosclerosis, the accumulation of lipids and other products in the intima of arteries, increases with age. Its incidence correlates strongly with obesity, hypertension, hyperglycemia, and hyperlipidemia. Arteriosclerosis, the deposition of calcium in the medial layer of arteries, causes thickening and hardening of the arterial wall (Bierman, 1985).

Table 4–2. CARDIOVASCULAR PHYSIOLOGIC CHANGES WITH AGING

Resting
Heart rate—unchanged
Left ventricular stroke volume—decreased
Cardiac output—decreased
Left ventricular end-diastolic pressure—unchanged
Ejection time—increased
Systolic blood pressure—increased
Systemic vascular resistance—increased

Exercise
Maximal heart rate—decreased
Maximal oxygen consumption—decreased
AVO$_2$ difference—increased
Maximal cardiac output—decreased
Left ventricular end-diastolic pressure—increased
Systolic blood pressure—increased
Systemic vascular resistance—increased

(From Lindenfeld, J, and Groves, BM: Cardiovascular function and disease in the aged. In Schrier, RW (ed): *Clinical Internal Medicine in the Aged.* Philadelphia, WB Saunders, 1982, 87–123. Reprinted with permission.)

Electrocardiographic changes may include decreased voltage of all waves, slight prolongation of the P-R interval and left axis deviation due to cellular aging changes, fibrosis of the conduction system, and neurogenic effects (Mihalick & Fisch, 1974).

Common Disorders

Surveys by Kitchin, Lowther, and Milne (1973) and Kennedy, Andrews, and Caird (1977) have noted evidence of heart disease in 40% of 65 to 74 year olds and in 50% of those age 75 and over living at home. Ischemic heart disease, predominantly caused by atherosclerosis, is present in 20% of men and 12% of women over 65 years. Hypertensive heart disease is present in 8% to 13% of men and 12% to 16% of women over 65 years. Pulmonary heart disease and rheumatic heart disease have a much lower incidence.

Atrial and ventricular ectopic beats are more frequent in the elderly than in the young and may be due to cardiac disease, metabolic disorders, hypoxia, digoxin toxicity, tobacco use, or ingestion of caffeine or a heavy meal (Anderson & Williams, 1983). Frequently occurring abnormalities seen on electrocardiograms of the elderly include conduction disturbances such as first-degree atrioventricular (AV) block, fascicular and bundle branch block, atrial fibrillation, and premature systoles (Mihalick & Fisch, 1974).

Peripheral vascular disease, particularly occlusive vascular disease, aneurysm, and distal embolization, is caused predominantly by atherosclerosis and is probably accelerated by hyperlipidemia, cigarette smoking, and diabetes. Abdominal aortic aneurysms may be present in as many as 2% of the elderly. Only 5% of all aortic aneurysms extend above the renal arteries (Rubin & Goldstone, 1985). Elderly with venous thromboembolism and recurrent migratory superficial thrombophlebitis have an increased incidence of neoplasm (Finch, English, Dale, et al., 1985).

History

Since the elderly frequently have multiple system disorders, a detailed history of specific symptoms such as dyspnea and chest pain is necessary to identify the etiology. Dyspnea may indicate heart or pulmonary disease or may be caused by exertion in the deconditioned elderly in the absence of pathology. A history of associated symptoms and a physical examination that includes chest radiography, electrocardiogram, spirometric measurements, and selected laboratory tests may be necessary to diagnose the cause of dyspnea (Siefkin, 1985). Dyspnea may be the predominant presenting symptom of congestive heart failure and myocardial infarction. Paroxysmal nocturnal dyspnea and orthopnea remain classic findings in the elderly person with congestive failure, but they also may be seen in elderly with chronic obstructive pulmonary disease and restrictive pulmonary diseases (Siefkin, 1985). Dyspnea may also be associated with cardiac rhythm disturbances, angina, valvular disease, pericarditis or endocarditis, hypertension, and idiopathic hypertrophic subaortic stenosis. Lethargy, not dyspnea, may be the predominant presenting complaint in heart disease if musculoskeletal or neuromuscular disorders restrict activity (Anderson & Williams, 1983).

Chest pain usually accompanies myocardial ischemia and infarction in elderly individuals but was less frequently reported with increasing age in a group ages 65 to 100 with confirmed myocardial infarction (Bayer, Chadha, Farag, et al., 1986). Chest pain may also be caused by other cardiac diseases, such as mitral valve prolapse, pericarditis, dissecting aortic aneurysm, and idiopathic hypertrophic subaortic stenosis, and by pulmonary and gastrointestinal problems (Eliopoulous, 1984). Ischemic heart disease may present with dyspnea, fatigue, confusion, syncope, or stroke in the absence of chest pain (Bayer, et al., 1986). The Framingham Study found that 30% of recent myocardial infarctions in persons ages 30 to 92 were clinically unrecognized (Bayliss, 1985).

Valvular heart disease may present in the elderly as congestive failure, fatigue, syncope, dyspnea, palpitations, and anxiety (Cornell, 1985; Hunt, 1985). Persons with calcification of the mitral valve are usually asymptomatic but may develop mitral stenosis or regurgitation. In mitral stenosis and insufficiency, prognosis depends on the presence of congestive heart failure and atrial fibrillation (Gerstenblith, Weisfeldt, & Lakatta, 1985).

Ambulatory electrocardiogram recordings (Holter monitoring) of 1,238 inpatients ages 70 years and older revealed that chest pain, dizziness, and palpitations were common pre-Holter symptoms that occurred in only 13% of subjects during Holter monitoring. Syncope occurred during monitoring in only 1.6% of subjects. Chest pain that occurred during monitoring was usually not associated with arrhythmia; dizziness and palpitations were associated with arrhythmia 50% of the time, and almost 80% of patients reporting syncope had a recorded arrhythmia (Nelson, Ezri, & Denes, 1984).

Intermittent claudication or functional limb ischemia, predominantly of the lower extremities, is not uncommon in the elderly. Pain at rest is indicative of limb-threatening ischemia (Rubin & Goldstone, 1985). Lower extremity edema is often a sign of right-sided heart failure but may be related to chronic venous insufficiency, hypoproteinemia, liver disease, or sedentary lifestyle (Anderson & Williams, 1983).

Examination

Although their histories are often different, findings on examination of the cardiovascular system are very similar for the young and old. Only those physical findings specific to the elderly will be described.

The elderly often have kyphosis and an increased anterior-posterior diameter of the chest, which distorts the cardiac position (Figure 4–1). Palpitation and auscultation of the precordium may be possible only with the patient in the left lateral decubitus position or in the sitting position while leaning forward. A sustained left ventricular impulse is commonly indicative of left ventricular hypertrophy, although often it is a nonpathologic finding in the elderly. An audible fourth heart sound (S4) has no specific pathophysiologic

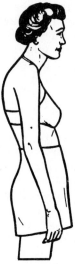

Figure 4–1. Kyphosis. (From Daniels, L, and Worthingham, C: Therapeutic Exercise for Body Alignment and Function. Philadelphia, WB Saunders, 1977, p 13. Reprinted with permission.)

importance in the elderly and probably reflects decreased compliance of the left ventricle contracting against increased peripheral resistance (Lindenfeld & Groves, 1982).

Arrhythmias may be detected on palpation and auscultation of the apical and peripheral pulses. The examiner may need to reevaluate the pulse more than once during the examination, since factors such as anxiety, position, and recent caffeine or tobacco use may be associated with cardiac arrhythmia. Normally, the pulse increases with a change in position from lying to sitting or from sitting to standing, but in the elderly this change is less noticeable (O'Brien, O'Hare, & Corrall, 1986). A pulse that remains constant or decreases with standing, especially if accompanied by hypotensive symptoms of lightheadedness or instability, may indicate baroreceptor insensitivity, autonomic dysfunction, cardiac pathology, or the effect of medications such as beta-adrenergic inhibitors (Halter, 1985).

Systolic ejection murmurs are found in 60% or more of the elderly (Hitzhusen & Alpert, 1984) and may be caused by aortic valve sclerosis, obstructive aortic stenosis, or mitral regurgitation. The murmur of aortic sclerosis is found at the apex or lower left sternal border and is a grade I to II flow murmur heard in mid-systole and does not radiate to the carotid arteries. In contrast, the pathologic murmur of aortic stenosis is a grade II to VI late systolic murmur heard loudest at the apex or the aortic area (right sternal border, second intercostal space) and commonly radiates to the carotid arteries. There may be a thrill over the aortic area and evidence of left ventricular hypertrophy. The murmur of mitral regurgitation is a systolic murmur of undiminished or increasing intensity heard best at the apex of the heart or along the sternal border; it may radiate to the left axilla. This murmur may be intensified with decreased cardiac output, in contrast to the systolic ejection murmurs, which are diminished with decreased cardiac output and intensified with increased cardiac output (Caird, 1976).

Peripheral arteries provide a wealth of information about the health of the heart and vascular system. The arterial pulse wave has a more rapid upstroke with a higher systolic peak in the elderly due to decreased elasticity of the large vessels. This may mask the slowly rising pulse of aortic stenosis or mimic the pulses of aortic insufficiency or idiopathic hypertrophic subaortic stenosis detected in the carotid arteries (Lindenfeld & Groves, 1982).

Arterial bruits are common signs of arteriosclerotic vascular disease, aneurysm, and vessel obstruction. Arterial bruits are commonly found at major arterial bifurcations and angulations such as those of the femoral arteries, the distal aorta below the renal arteries, and the carotid arteries at the common carotid bifurcation into the internal and external branches (Rubin & Goldstone, 1985). Asymptomatic carotid bruits are associated with increased incidence of cardiovascular morbidity and mortality, especially stroke, systolic hypertension, ischemic heart disease, and occlusive vascular disease of the lower extremities (Sutton, Dai, & Kuller, 1985). The abdominal aortic bruit of aortic aneurysm must be differentiated from a radiating systolic ejection flow murmur. Undue prominence of any of the peripheral arterial pulses may also indicate an aneurysm. Sudden onset of ischemic pain in

an extremity, accompanied by changes in temperature and sensation, may indicate thromboembolic occurrence often associated with a peripheral aneurysm.

Sclerotic peripheral arteries may be more easily palpable but are often associated with decreased blood flow to the extremities. Other signs of ischemia are loss of hair and the typically thin, shiny, atrophied skin of the distal leg and foot. Hypertrophic nails and skin ulceration at sites of frequent trauma are present in severe cases (Thiele & Strandness, 1985).

Findings of abnormal venous circulation are generally similar in the young and old. However, an elevation of left jugular venous pressure in the elderly that disappears on deep inspiration may be due to compression of the left innominate vein by the aortic arch. Acute onset or suddenly worsening peripheral edema may herald congestive heart failure. Chronic venous insufficiency is common in the elderly and is evidenced by distended tortuous veins, hair loss, hyperpigmentation, cool skin, and pretibial and pedal edema that worsens during the day and improves at night when the patient lies down to sleep (Eliopoulous, 1984). Stasis ulceration is rare with varicose veins but commonly occurs with chronic deep venous insufficiency (Spittell, 1983). Deep venous thrombosis and pulmonary embolism may occur without specific symptoms and physical signs, necessitating noninvasive tests such as Doppler studies and venography or pulmonary angiography to establish the diagnosis (Finch, English, Dale, et al., 1985).

Tests

Diagnostic tests of the cardiovascular system of the healthy elderly often demonstrate abnormal findings that are not associated with disease. These findings are summarized in Table 4–3.

Comparison of current and past chest x-ray films is helpful in detecting congestive heart failure, pulmonary edema, heart enlargement, enlarged pulmonary artery and aorta, tortuosity and elongation of the aorta, and calcific

Table 4–3. CARDIOVASCULAR TESTS OF
HEALTHY OLDER PERSONS

Electrocardiogram

Look for:

First-degree AV block
Isolated left axis deviation
Right bundle branch block
Nonspecific ST-T wave changes
Premature atrial beats
Atrial fibrillation
Premature ventricular contractions

Echocardiogram

Look for:

Increased aortic root diameter
Increased thickness of posterior left ventricular wall
Decrease in E-F slope of anterior mitral leaflet

Chest Roentgenogram

Look for:

Elongation of ascending part of aorta and tortuosity of
   descending part
Superior mediastinum (appears widened)
Calcification of aortic knob
Calcification of mitral annulus and aortic valve

(Data from Caird, Dall, & Williams, 1985; Hitzhusen &
Alpert, 1984; Lindenfeld & Groves, 1982; Murphy &
DeMots, 1984.)

changes in the vessels and heart valves. The
electrocardiogram allows identification of arrhythmias, conduction defects, evidence of
myocardial ischemia and infarct, ventricular
enlargement, voltage changes, ST-T wave
changes, axis deviation, metabolic disorders,
and the effect of medications. Holter monitoring is a 12- or 24-hour ambulatory electrocardiographic recording that identifies and quan-
tifies cardiac arrhythmias.

The exercise stress test is a standard screening tool for myocardial ischemia, in which the
electrocardiographic record is obtained during
graduations of aerobic exercise. The test is
60% to 90% sensitive and specific for ischemia
in young and middle-aged populations. Measurement of aerobic capacity and guidelines for
exercise prescription can be based on this test.
The exercise stress test is contraindicated for
elderly persons with symptoms of unstable
angina, second- or third-degree AV block,
congestive heart failure, acute cardiac and
noncardiac disease, aortic stenosis, and known
left main coronary artery disease. Modification
of the standard Bruce or Ellestad maximal
exercise protocols or use of the Naughton post-

myocardial infarction (MI) protocol may allow
elderly with decreased exercise capacity to
achieve near-maximal predicted heart rates
(Vasilomanolakis, 1985).

Enlargement of specific cardiac chambers,
increased thickness of the ventricular walls,
valvular dysfunction and disease, aortic root
diameter, pericardial effusion, and left ventricular function can be revealed by echocardiog-
raphy. Origin of heart sounds and identification of murmurs may be distinguished by
phonocardiography. A variety of devices using
ultrasound technology to detect and measure
blood flow and pressure enable noninvasive
diagnosis of peripheral vascular disease.

Arterial blood gases identify hypoxemia associated with cardiac or pulmonary disease.
Serial cardiac enzymes support diagnosis of
myocardial infarct.

GASTROINTESTINAL SYSTEM

Aging Changes

The aging gut may be characterized by decreased secretion, absorption, and motility.
The elderly are predisposed to xerostomia by
the reduction of saliva. Although gastrointestinal (GI) motility slows and abdominal muscles weaken with age, these changes alone
should not cause constipation. The liver decreases in size by 20% between the ages of 50
and 70 years; however, function is unaffected.
The elderly may have decreased gut absorption of iron, vitamin B_{12}, and folate, which
may cause anemia.

Common Disorders

The most common causes of severe abdominal pain in the elderly include gallbladder
disease (secondary to inflammation, obstruction, or cancer), small bowel obstruction, appendicitis, acute pancreatitis, mesenteric
thrombosis, infarction, or hemorrhage (Morgan, Thomas, & Schuster, 1981). The elderly
are at greater risk for gastric ulceration because
many of the medications routinely taken by

this group (nonsteroidal anti-inflammatory medications and steroids) are gastric irritants. Patients with gastric ulcers may present with severe acute abdominal pain or diffuse dull pain.

Diverticulitis is quite common in the elderly. In the early stages it may cause local irritation, slight fever, or change in bowel habits. In advanced states, patients with diverticulitis may present with an acute obstruction or bowel perforation and sepsis. The prevalence of colorectal cancer increases at 40 to 50 years of age, doubles every 10 years thereafter, and peaks at 75 to 80 years. The most common presentation of colorectal cancer is a change in bowel habits, pain, blood in the stool, and anemia (Chakravorty, 1983). Other causes of blood in the stool include hemorrhoids, fissures, and vascular ectasias. The latter are responsible for recurrent GI bleeding episodes in those over 60 years (Boley, Brandt, & Mitsudo, 1984).

Jaundice from either intrahepatic or extrahepatic obstruction may be related to carcinoma, cholelithiasis, drugs, alcohol, hepatitis, or cirrhosis (Smith, 1984). Gallbladder disease is common in the elderly. At autopsy, 30% of patients over 70 had gallstones and 5% had had a cholecystectomy (Berman & Kirsner, 1983).

History

Commonly encountered complaints related to the mouth are dryness of the mouth and difficulty chewing. The dryness may be further exaggerated by poor fluid intake or medication side effects from diuretics, antihypertensive medications, sedatives, and antidepressants. Difficulty chewing may be caused by factors from within or outside the mouth. Poorly fitting dentures are often the cause within the mouth. In one study (Hunt, Beck, Lemke, et al., 1985), 70% of those with dentures had not seen a dentist for five years and one-third of these patients reported painful, malfitting dentures. Arthritis of the temporomandibular joint may cause pain while chewing in the elderly (Bennett & Creamer, 1983).

Major esophageal symptoms involve problems with swallowing and pain. Difficulty swallowing liquids usually has a neurologic cause, whereas difficulty swallowing solids usually is caused by mechanical obstruction. Regurgitation without aspiration may be caused by hiatal hernia with the development of Schatzki's ring or esophageal diverticuli. Cricopharyngeal muscle failure may produce the sensation that food is stuck in the throat. Because this symptom also may be caused by hiatal hernia and esophageal diverticuli (Almay, 1985), endoscopic testing may be necessary to define the condition causing the symptom. Pain from esophageal spasm is difficult to differentiate from cardiac pain because both occur substernally, may be associated with eating, and may be relieved with nitroglycerin.

Bowel dysfunction is a common complaint of the elderly. Lack of adequate fiber and fluid in the diet and medication effect from diuretics, tranquilizers, and anticholinergics contribute to constipation (Bower & Patterson, 1985). Psychosocial stress and poor eating habits may add to the chance of ulceration. Atonic colon is often associated with chronic laxative abuse. Patients with fecal impaction may present with a history suggestive of overflow urinary incontinence. Diarrhea in the elderly may be present with fecal impaction, viral and bacterial diseases of the gut, or malabsorption syndromes. A thorough history of change in bowel habits, medications being taken (including over-the-counter preparations), and diet is most important in assessment of bowel dysfunction. The examiner should inquire about alcohol use, hepatitis, exposure to toxic chemicals, blood transfusions, and medications such as aspirin, acetaminophen, and methyldopa.

Examination

Mouth. Cheilosis at the angle of the lips may be observed in the edentulous person. The mouth may exhibit signs of the progressive oral dysfunction syndrome (increased plaque, poor oral hygiene, tooth loss, and poor nutrition) (Bennett & Creamer, 1983). The examiner should inspect the dentures for hygiene and damage after the client removes them. The gums and mucous membranes of the mouth should then be inspected for erosion, inflammation, and lesions. Sclerosis of the vessels to the tongue may cause a pale appearance. Leukoplakia, a white scaly patch, may be a cancer precursor. If the patient smokes or drinks, the area should be biopsied immediately. If the patient is not in this high risk group and an irritant causing the leukoplakia can be determined and removed, the patient may be observed and the area biopsied only if the leukoplakia recurs (Chakravorty, 1983). Any erythematous lesions seen on the tongue should be suspected as being cancerous unless they are observed bilaterally (Gordon & Jahnigan, 1983). The oral cavity should be palpated for masses that may not be visualized. The temporomandibular area should be palpated for tenderness and crepitation as the patient chews. Other aspects of the oral examination are covered in the neurologic assessment section of this text.

Abdomen. Inspection of the skin is important for lesions irritated by the rubbing of corsets or belts over the years. Fungal rashes may be observed in the skin folds of the obese elderly or in those who are incapacitated and unable to bathe.

Obstruction of the bowel may occur with diverticulitis, fecal impaction, mesenteric thrombosis, or cancer. Because bowel motility is decreased with age, listening for five minutes in each quadrant is required before determining the absence of bowel sounds (Burggraf & Donlon, 1985). Early in bowel obstruction, the pain may be well localized, and the bowel sounds proximal to the obstruction may appear hyperactive. As the obstruction persists, the abdomen becomes rigid and tympanic and the pain more diffuse as the peritoneum is affected. In this age group a palpable mass in the abdomen may be cancer or fecal impaction, and a thorough investigation is in order (Cope, 1972).

If abdominal pain is present the patient should point to the area with one finger because this gives more accurate information about the pain than does the history (Bailey, 1981). Adequate palpation may be difficult in the obese patient; this should be documented. Generally, though, the relaxed musculature of the abdomen in the elderly population enhances palpation (Burggraf & Donlon, 1985). Muscular pain and visceral pain are differentiated by palpating while the patient is supine and again while the patient tightens the abdominal muscles while doing a partial sit-up. If the pain is reproduced while the patient tightens the abdominal muscles and the examiner palpates lightly, a muscular reason exists for the pain. Conversely, if the pain is reproduced while the musculature is lax and during deep palpation, a visceral cause of pain is suspected. Generalized colon tenderness with splenic flexure tenderness may indicate functional bowel disease. Right lower quadrant pain may indicate appendicitis, and pain in the left lower quadrant is more common with diverticuli disease. Tenderness at the base of the xiphoid may reflect pathology of the stomach, hiatal hernia, or referred pain from the aorta. The aorta may be slightly tender to palpation and should measure less than 3 cm in diameter. Palpation of the size of the aorta is sufficient baseline screening for aneurysm in thin patients. Cardiac sounds may radiate into the abdomen and mimic a bruit. If a question exists about the findings, ultrasound and, if necessary, angiogram should be performed.

Rectum. This examination is important in any patient presenting with abdominal symptoms. The stool should be checked for occult blood. The examination is further described in the genitourinary sections of this chapter.

Tests

Screening for colorectal cancer is done by fecal occult blood testing, digital examination, and flexible sigmoidoscopy. In one study, up to 30% of patients had adenocarcinoma and 10% had other neoplasms when fecal occult blood testing was performed. The test had a 33% to 50% false negative result because polyps less than 2 cm in diameter may not produce enough blood to cause a reaction in the test. Also, colorectal cancers and polyps may bleed intermittently (Simon, 1985). Digital examination can detect 15% of colorectal cancers and should be done yearly (Swedberg, Driggers, & Deiss, 1986).

The American Cancer Society recommends testing of stools for occult blood every year and performance of sigmoidoscopy in asymptomatic individuals every three to five years after two consecutive annual examinations reveal negative results. A flexible sigmoidoscopic examination should be done because 50% to 60% of the tumors are above the 20 cm range of the rigidscope (Winawer, Miller, & Sherlock, 1984).

Recommendations for preparation for fecal occult stool testing vary. One study suggests avoidance of red meat, iron, nonsteroid antiinflammation medications, vitamin C, and high peroxidase foods for three days before and during the examination to avoid false positive results (Swedberg, Driggers, & Deiss, 1986). Another group recommends only the restriction of high dose vitamin C and red meat. If positive, the test may be repeated with the restrictive guidelines (Simon, 1985). Some patients may avoid the testing because of the restrictions unless they have been given an adequate rationale for the testing. Such a patient would be an arthritic person who requires daily nonsteroidal antiinflammatory medication for pain relief.

Because the elderly may present with atypical or minimal abdominal symptoms it may be more important to evaluate these patients more aggressively than younger patients with similar symptoms. The elderly patient may also require aggressive testing because symptoms for polyps, obstructive gastric bezoars (a mass of food or foreign materials), and cancer are similar, and many conditions may occur simultaneously. For example, it is not uncommon for an elderly patient with ulceration to have an underlying cancer.

Esophageal dysfunction is difficult to define with physical examination. If the history is positive, endoscopy or barium swallow is required. Because of the high incidence of gallbladder disease in the elderly the diagnosis must be pursued with ultrasound or oral cholecystogram or nuclear medicine scan if the patient is symptomatic. A patient whose fecal occult blood test is positive or one who has polyps on colorectal cancer screening should have a barium enema and colonoscopy. A history of liver or pancreatic dysfunction may be followed by ultrasound, nuclear scans, and evaluation of enzyme levels. The elderly may have decreased gut absorption of iron, B_{12}, and folate. A complete blood count with abnormal results should be followed by the appropriate iron studies and B_{12} and folate levels.

FEMALE GENITOURINARY SYSTEM

Aging Changes

Aging changes in the female genitourinary (GU) system are primarily the result of lack of estrogen and decreased muscle tone. Aging effects caused by estrogen deprivation include sparse pubic hair, decreased fat pad over the symphysis pubis, and friable mucosa with a pale appearance (Schiff & Wilson, 1978). Estrogen depletion also causes a decrease in the amount and an increase in the pH of Bartholin gland secretion, which provides a favorable environment for infection. Incontinence is more common in elderly females than in males. It should never be considered a normal aspect of aging. Stress incontinence is the most common form of incontinence in the female. Decreased muscle tone, cystocele, rectocele, uterine prolapse, and decreased bladder capacity contribute to this disorder.

Common Disorders

Women who are nulliparous, have taken estrogen not opposed by progesterone, or have experienced postmenopausal bleeding are at risk for endometrial cancer (Kase & Weingold, 1985). The prevalence of vulvar cancer peaks between the ages of 60 and 70 years (Kase & Weingold, 1983; Fuller, 1981). Uterine cancer has its peak incidence in women over 50 years. Incidence of ovarian cancer peaks in the 75 to 79 age group at a rate of 54 cases per 100,000 women. Most women are diagnosed with late stages of the disease (Yancik, Reis, & Yatos, 1986).

History

The patient should be questioned about loss of urine at rest or when straining, with coughing, or with exercise. If present, a careful history (including an incontinence record) and physical examination should be done to determine the etiology (Autry, Lauzon, & Holliday, 1984; Brink, Wells, & Diokno, 1983; Campbell, Reinkin, & McCosh, 1985). Frequency, urgency, and dysuria suggest infection, although estrogen deprivation may cause irritation of the urethra with secondary cystitis (Reid, 1985; Schiff & Wilson, 1978). Diabetes, congestive heart failure, and medications such as diuretics may contribute to incontinence. If symptoms recur after apparent problems are treated, or if the patient has symptoms of detrusor muscle instability, a urologic referral is needed. If cystocele or rectocele is present and stress incontinence is not reduced by Kegel exercises (isometric exercises of the pelvic muscles and urinary sphincter), then referral to a gynecologist is appropriate for evaluation (Pierson, 1984; Sier & Outslander, 1985).

Questions concerning the patient's reproductive years may suggest current problems. For example, the multiparous woman or one with a history of difficult labors is at greater risk for uterine prolapse. A thorough history of the menopausal years should include medications, treatment, and postmenopausal bleeding. The evaluation for postmenopausal bleeding includes ultrasound and dilation and curettage or endometrial sampling.

The patient should be asked if she ever had an abnormal Pap smear or was told that she had an abnormal pelvic examination. If the answer to either of these questions is affirmative, the patient should be asked if she received any treatment for the abnormality. Recommendations vary about the frequency of Pap tests. The American College of Obstetricians and Gynecologists recommends a yearly Pap and pelvic examination for all women. The American Cancer Society recommends yearly Pap tests from age 40 years to menopause. Annual Pap tests may be discontinued after two consecutive normal postmenopausal tests. The National Institutes of Health states that Pap tests can be discontinued at the age of 60 years after two consecutive negative tests (Bucher, 1983). However, none of these groups negates the need for an annual pelvic and rectal examination even when a Pap test is not needed.

Problems with sexuality can be elicited if the client is given permission to express her concerns. The clinician gives permission by asking questions about the presence of any problems with sexuality. The patient may need to be educated in the sex-related changes of the elderly male and female. The health care provider remains nonjudgmental and supportive (Davidson, 1985; Glover, 1978; Weg, 1985; Yeaworth & Friedman, 1975). Physical problems with intercourse may include dyspareunia and dryness secondary to estrogen depletion or positional problems secondary to other medical conditions such as hiatal hernia or arthritis. If the client has multiple partners she should be offered screening tests for venereal diseases.

Examination

Although the lithotomy position is preferable for examination, it may not be feasible for the client with orthopnea or arthritis. The client may be more comfortable with a pillow under her head and her legs supported by an assistant rather than in stirrups.

White lesions are most commonly leukoplakia but may be lichen sclerosis or malignancy. Biopsy of lesions is therefore indicated (Fuller, 1981; Kase & Weingold, 1983).

Muscle tone should be evaluated. Rectocele can be visualized by placing the spatula against the roof of the vagina and having the patient bear down. Conversely, by supporting the floor of the vagina with the spatula and having the patient bear down, a cystocele may be visualized. Uterine prolapse may also be visualized as the patient bears down. It was noted that 50% of patients with hysterectomy had vaginal vault prolapse (Glowacki, 1978).

Vaginal atrophy may limit the entry to one finger and necessitate a pediatric speculum. The geriatric cervix may exhibit retention cysts secondary to atrophy (Hafez, 1978). The geriatric vagina is most frequently atrophic, friable, and dry (Andrews, 1985). Any secretions should be prepared with saline and potassium hydroxide smears. The most common organisms found in the sexually active female are *Candida, Trichomonas,* and *Gardnerella* (Rice & Dale, 1984). With estrogen deprivation lactobacillus growth is inhibited, thereby causing an overgrowth of normal flora, including streptococcus, staphylococcus, diphtheroids, and coliforms (Schiff & Wilson, 1978). The presence of a foreign body (i.e., a pessary) may cause secondary infection.

On examination the postmenopausal uterus should be smaller than 3 × 2 inches, have a firm consistency, and remain freely movable and nontender to palpation. The ovary in the elderly female measures 1.5 × 0.75 × 0.5 cm and is therefore not palpable. Enlargement to the stage of palpation usually occurs in advanced disease (Carr & MacDonald, 1985). Any masses that are palpable should be noted for size, location, mobility, and tenderness, and the patient should be referred on for evaluation. It is unlikely that masses in the geriatric female are of the benign fibroid variety.

During rectal examination the posterior cervix is palpated. It should be freely movable, firm, and nontender. Any rectal masses should be described and the patient referred for further testing. Testing for colorectal cancer is identical for males and females.

Tests

Any abdominal or pelvic masses should be considered malignant until proved otherwise. Evaluation may require endometrial sampling, dilatation and curettage, endoscopy, and x-ray or ultrasound studies.

MALE GENITOURINARY SYSTEM

Aging Changes

Anatomic changes that make the elderly male prone to incontinence include a reduction by 500 to 950 ml in bladder capacity (Burggraf & Donlon, 1985), enlargement of the prostate, and an increase in bladder neck tone (Judson, Novotny, McAnich, et al., 1981). However, incontinence should never be considered a normal part of the aging process, and problems should be carefully evaluated.

Another common change with aging is a decrease in the size of the penis and testes due to sclerosis of the vessels (Harmon & Nanin, 1985). Sexual aging changes include an increased refractory time after orgasm (in which he is unresponsive to stimuli), decreased penile sensation and ejaculatory demand, decreased strength of pelvic striated muscles, and decreased force of ejaculation (Harmon & Nanin, 1985; Sieber, 1984). The patient or his partner may erroneously interpret these aging changes as impotence, thus causing performance anxiety.

Common Disorders

In the uncircumcised male, chronic balanitis may cause urethral stricture (Basso, 1978). Detrusor muscle instability may occur from a cerebrovascular event or medication (Eastwood & Smart, 1985). Benign prostatic hypertrophy (BPH) is common in men over 50 years. In the male, incontinence is usually due to infection or BPH. The mean age at diagnosis of prostate cancer is 73 years (Love, 1985). Prostate cancer is the third most lethal cancer in men. However, there is a 77% 5-year survival rate when the cancer is confined to the prostate (Chodak & Schoenberg, 1984). Rectal examination is the most efficient screening test for this cancer, and it is recommended annually for all men over 40 years (Citrin, 1983; Guinan, Bush, & Ray, et al., 1980).

History

The patient should be questioned about symptoms of BPH, such as a change in the urinary stream, difficulty starting the stream, dribbling, and the feeling that the bladder is not empty after voiding. He should be questioned for symptoms of infection such as frequency, urgency, and burning and for a history of nocturia, heart failure, kidney disease, diabetes, and use of medications such as diuretics and anticholinergics. If the examination is within normal limits, an incontinence record must be obtained.

If the client is not sexually active the nurse should determine if the cause is lack of sexual desire or physical dysfunction. The patient should be asked if he experiences physical desires and how he deals with them. He should be asked if he has morning erections and problems with erection, penetration, or ejaculation. If the patient has morning erections, the problem usually is not physical. If he has no morning erections, a physical cause such as diabetes, peripheral vascular disease, or medication effect should be considered. Regardless of the cause of sexual dysfunction, the patient and his partner should be offered referral for urologic or sexual counseling.

Examination

The patient may either stand or lie supine for the first part of the examination. For the rectal examination the patient may either stand or lean on the examination table or place himself in a side-lying position. The patient should stand for evaluation of a hernia. If this is impossible, the patient may lie supine and bear down. Any variation from the routine should be noted in the record.

If the patient is unable to retract the foreskin, his ability to perform proper hygiene is in question. A chairbound patient may develop swelling of the scrotum secondary to dependent edema. However, transillumination of the scrotum is required to differentiate hydrocele and hernia. Fungal rashes and se-

baceous cysts are not uncommon in this population.

The rectal examination attempts to detect rectal cancer, prostate cancer, prostatitis and prostate hypertrophy, and fecal impaction. The rectum is inspected for hemorrhoids, fissures, fistulas, lesions, and rashes. These abnormalities may produce a false positive fecal occult blood test. The absence of the bulbocavernous reflex (elevation of the penis in response to percussion of the dorsum of the penis) may indicate a neurologic cause of impotence (Rowe & Resnick, 1985). Stroking the anus with a cotton-tip swab should cause reflexive contraction of the rectal sphincter. The patient should then bear down so the muscle tone can be observed.

The normal prostate measures 3 to 4 cm in diameter and weighs 15 to 20 gm. Only 1.5 × 2 cm of the prostate can be palpated by rectal examination (Lapides, 1976). BPH should be considered if the consistency is normal and the median sulcus is not palpable. However, a patient with a normal examination but positive history deserves a urologic evaluation because a large area of the gland is not palpable and may be hypertrophied. A boggy prostate suggests congestion of the gland, and any tenderness suggests infection. If the examiner cannot palpate the gland thoroughly because of pain, the patient should be reexamined after treatment. Any firm mass should be considered a malignancy unless proved a cyst by biopsy (Chodak & Schoenberg, 1984) (Figure 4–2.)

Tests

Urinalysis is recommended by some authorities as part of the annual screening of elderly patients. In one study of elderly well adults, 44.4% had positive results and most were asymptomatic (Rubenstein, Josephson, Nichol-Seamon, et al., 1986). Basso (1978) recommends annual urinalysis, serum creatinine determination, and rectal examination. The results of these tests identify infection or renal damage in the asymptomatic patient.

Infection should be considered first in eval-

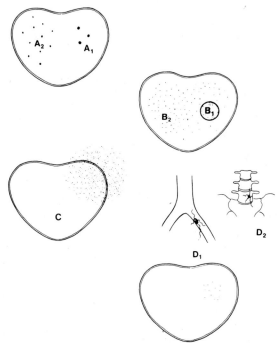

Figure 4–2. Stages of prostatic carcinoma. *Stage A.* Confined to the prostate, undetected clinically. *Stage B.* Confined to the prostate, clinically evident on rectal examination. *Stage C.* Extends to the prostatic capsule but has not metastasized. *Stage D.* Metastatic. (From Diokno, AC, and MacGregor, RJ: Prostate gland disease. *In* Calkins, E, Davis, PJ, and Ford, AB (eds). The Practice of Geriatrics. Philadelphia, WB Saunders, 1986, p 375. Reprinted with permission.)

uating incontinence. If present, it should be treated and then the incontinence reevaluated. The patient should keep an incontinence record. A post-voiding residual should be noted. The patient should be referred for urologic testing if there is a post-voiding residual of greater than 100 ml, unresolved hematuria, unresolved bacteriuria, or a question of detrusor instability (Sier & Outslander, 1985).

Several urologic tests are available to determine the presence of nocturnal erections. One easy and reliable test is the stamp test, in which a roll of 3 to 5 postage stamps are firmly wrapped around the base of the penis at night with the ends taped together. If the patient has an erection that is adequate to penetrate a vagina, the stamps will be broken at the per-foration; any other tear is considered to be due to movement (Sieber, 1984).

The patient who is sexually active and has multiple partners should be offered screening tests for sexually transmitted disease, including hepatitis B and the acquired immunodeficiency syndrome.

References

Adami, H-O, Malker, BM, Meirik, O, et al. (1985): Age as a prognostic factor in breast cancer. *Cancer, 56*:898–902.

Almay, TP (1985): Alteration in gastrointestinal function in old age. *In* Andres, R, Bierman, EL, & Hazzard, WR (eds): *Principles of Geriatric Medicine.* New York, McGraw-Hill, 297–310.

Anderson, F, & Williams, B (1983): *Heart Disease: Practical Management of the Elderly* (ed 4). Oxford, Blackwell Scientific Publications, 75–97.

Andrews, J (1985): Gynaecology of the elderly. *In* Pathy, MSJ (ed): *Principles and Practice of Geriatric Medicine.* London, John Wiley & Sons, 1107–1121.

Autry, D, Lauzon, F, & Holliday, P (1984): The voiding record: An aid in decreasing incontinence. *Geriatr Nurs, 5*:22–25.

Bailey, PA (1981): Clinical assessment of the elderly. *Top Clin Nurs, 3*:315–319.

Baines, C (1984): Breast self examination: The doctor's role. *Hosp Pract, 19*:120–127.

Basso, A (1978): The prostate in the elderly male. *In* Reichel, W (ed): *The Geriatric Patient.* New York, HP Publishing Company, 118–124.

Bayer, AJ, Chadha, JS, Farag, RR, et al. (1986): Changing presentation of myocardial infarction with increasing old age. *J Am Geriatr Soc, 34*:263–266.

Bayliss, RIS (1985): The silent coronary. *Br Med J, 290*:1093–1094.

Bennett, JS, & Creamer, HR (1983): Staging dental care for the oral health problems of elderly people. *J Oregon Dental Assoc 53*(1):21–24.

Berman, PM, & Kirsner, JB (1983): Gastrointestinal problems. *In* Steinberg, FU (ed): *Care of the Geriatric Patient* (ed 6). St. Louis, CV Mosby, 118–140.

Bierman, EL (1985): Aging and atherosclerosis. *In* Andres, R, Bierman, EL & Hazzard, WR (eds): *Principles of Geriatric Medicine.* New York, McGraw-Hill, 42–50.

Boley, SJ, Brandt, LJ, & Mitsudo, SM (1984): Vascular lesions of the colon. *Adv Intern Med, 29*:301–325.

Bower, FN, & Patterson, J (1986): A theory-based nursing assessment of the aged. *Top Clin Nurs, 8*:22–32.

Brink, C, Wellis, T, & Diokno, A (1983): A continence clinic for the aged. *J Gerontol Nurs, 9*:651–655.

Bucher, DA (1983): Cervical cancer. *In* Kahn, SB, Love, R, & Sherman, C et al. (eds): *Concepts in Cancer Medicine.* New York, Grune & Stratton, 463–472.

Burggraf, V, & Donlon, B (1985): Assessment of the elderly. *Am J Nurs, 9*:974–984.

Caird, FI (1976): Valvular heart disease. *In* Caird, FI, Dall, JLC, & Kennedy, RD (eds): *Cardiology in Old Age.* New York, Plenum Press, 231.

Caird, FI, Dall, JLC , & Williams, BO (1985): The cardiovascular system. *In* Brocklehurst, JC (ed): *Textbook of Geriatric Medicine and Gerontology* (ed 3). Edinburgh, Churchill-Livingstone, 230–267.

Campbell, AJ, Reinkin, J, & McCosh, L (1985): Incontinence in the elderly: Prevalence and prognosis. *Age Aging,* 14(2):65–70.

Carr, BR, & MacDonald, PC (1985): Menopause and beyond. *In* Andres, R, Bierman, EL, & Hazzard, WR (eds): *Principles of Geriatric Medicine.* New York, McGraw-Hill, 325–336.

Chakravorty, RC (1983): Colorectal cancer. *In* Kahn, SB, Love, R, & Sherman, C, et al. (eds): *Concepts in Cancer Medicine.* New York, Grune & Stratton, 437–461.

Chodak, GW, & Schoenberg, HW (1984): Early detection of prostate cancer by routine screening. *JAMA,* 252:3261–3264.

Citrin, DL (1983): Cancer of the prostate. *In* Kahn, SB, Love, R, Sherman, C, et al. (eds): *Concepts in Cancer Medicine.* New York, Grune & Stratton, 401–416.

Cope, Z (1972): *The Early Diagnosis of the Acute Abdomen* (ed 14). London, Oxford University Press.

Cornell, LV (1985): Mitral valve prolapse syndrome: Etiology and symptomatology. *Nurs Pract,* 10(4):25–29.

Daniels, L, & Worthingham, C (1977): *Therapeutic Exercise.* Philadelphia, WB Saunders, 13.

Davidson, JM (1985): Sexuality and aging. *In* Andres, R, Bierman, EL, & Hazzard, WR (eds): *Principles of Geriatric Medicine,* New York, McGraw-Hill, 337–353.

Davis, SJ, Karrer, FW, & Moor, BJ, et al. (1985): Characteristics of breast cancer in women over 80 years of age. *Am J Surg,* 150:655–658.

Eastwood, HD, & Smart, CJ (1985): Urinary incontinence in the disabled elderly. *Age Aging,* 14(2):235–239.

Eliopoulous, C (1984): *Health Assessment of the Older Adult.* Menlo Park, CA, Addison-Wesley, 53.

Fedullo, AJ, & Swinburne, AJ (1985): Relationship of patient age to clinical features and outcome for in-hospital treatment of pneumonia. *J Gerontol,* 40:29–33.

Finch, CA, English, E, Dale, D, et al. (1985): Hematological alterations with age. *In* Andres, R, Bierman, EL, & Hazzard, WR (eds): *Principles of Geriatric Medicine.* New York, McGraw-Hill, 372–386.

Freeman, E (1985): The respiratory system. *In* Brocklehurst, JC (ed): *Textbook of Geriatric Medicine and Gerontology* (ed 3). New York, Churchill Livingstone, 731–757.

Fuller, AF (1981): Role of the primary physician in the detection and treatment of gynecological cancer. *Prim Care,* 8(1):111–129.

Gerstenblith, G, Weisfeldt, ML, & Lakatta, EG (1985): Disorders of the heart. *In* Andres, R, Bierman, EL, & Hazzard, WR (eds): *Principles of Geriatric Medicine.* New York, McGraw-Hill, 515.

Glover, BH (1978): Sex counseling. *In* O'Hara-Devereaux, M, Andrus, LH, Scott, C, et al. (eds): *Eldercare: A Practical Guide to Clinical Geriatrics.* New York, Grune & Stratton, 125–133.

Glowacki, G (1978): Postmenopausal GYN problems. *In* Reichel, W (ed): *The Geriatric Patient.* New York, HP Publishing 102–108.

Goodell, BW (1985): Breast disease. *In* Andres, R, Bierman, EL, & Hazzard, WR, (eds): *Principles of Geriatric Medicine.* New York, McGraw-Hill, 636–646.

Gordon, SR, & Jahnigan, DW (1983): Oral assessment of the edentulous elderly patient. *J Am Geriatr Soc,* 31:797–801.

Guinan, P, Bush, I, & Ray, V, et al. (1980): The accuracy of the rectal examination in the diagnosis of prostate cancer. *JAMA,* 309:499–503.

Hafez, ES (1976): *Aging and Reproductive Physiology,* Vol II. Ann Arbor, Ann Arbor Science, 9–31.

Halter, JB (1985): Alterations of autonomic nervous system function. *In* Andres, R, Bierman, EL, & Hazzard, WR (eds): *Principles of Geriatric Medicine.* New York, McGraw-Hill, 218–230.

Harmon, SM, & Nanin, HR (1985): Alterations in reproductive and sexual function: Male. *In* Andres, R, Bierman, EL, & Hazzard, WR (eds): *Principles of Geriatric Medicine.* New York, McGraw-Hill, 337–353.

Hitzhusen, JC, & Alpert, JA (1984): The elderly heart: Special signs and symptoms to watch for. *Geriatrics,* 39:38–51.

Hunt, AH (1985): Mitral valve prolapse. Physical assessment, complications, and management. *Nurs Pract,* 10(4):15–21.

Hunt, RJ, Beck, JD, Lemke, JH, et al. (1985): Edentulism and oral health problems among elderly rural Iowans: The Iowa 65+ Rural Health Study. *Am J Public Health,* 85:1177–1181.

Jajich, CL, Ostfeld, AM, & Freeman, DH (1984): Smoking and coronary heart disease mortality in the elderly. *JAMA,* 252:2831–2834.

Judson, L, Novotny, T, McAnich, J, et al. (1981): Genitourinary system. *In* O'Hara-Devereaux, M, Andrus, LH, Scott, C, et al. (eds): *Eldercare: A Practical Guide to Clinical Geriatrics.* New York, Grune & Stratton 169–188.

Kase, N, & Weingold, A (1983): *Principles and Practices of Clinical Gynecology.* New York, John Wiley & Sons.

Keller, K, George, E, Podell, R (1980): Clinical breast examination and breast self examination: Experience in family practice. *J Fam Pract,* 11(6):887–893.

Kennedy, RD, Andrews, GR, & Caird, FI (1977): Ischemic heart diseases in the elderly. *Br Heart J,* 39:1121–1127.

King, TE, & Schwarz, MI (1982): Pulmonary function and disease in the elderly. *In* Schrier, RW (ed): *Clinical Internal Medicine in the Aged.* Philadelphia, WB Saunders, 124–128.

Kitchin, AH, Lowther, CP, & Milne, JS (1973): Prevalence of clinical and electrocardiographic evidence of ischemic heart disease in the older population. *Br Heart J,* 35:946–953.

Klocke, RA, (1977): Influence of aging on the lung. *In* Finch, CF, & Hayflick, L (eds): *Handbook of the Biology of Aging.* New York, Van Nostrand Reinhold, 432–444.

Landahl, S, Steen, B, & Svanborg, A (1980): Dyspnea in 70-year-old people. *Acta Med Scand,* 207:225–230.

Lapides, J (1976): *Fundamentals of Urology.* Philadelphia, WB Saunders.

Lillington, GA (1984): Dyspnea in the elderly: Old age or disease? *Geriatrics,* 39:47–52.

Lindenfeld, J, & Groves, BM (1982): Cardiovascular function and disease in the aged. *In* Schrier, RW (ed): *Clinical Internal Medicine in the Aged.* Philadelphia, WB Saunders, 67–123.

Love, RR (1985): The efficacy of screening for carcinoma of the prostate by digital examination. *Am J Prev Med,* 1:36–46.

Marrie, TJ, Haldane, EV, & Faulkner, RS, et al. (1985): Community-acquired pneumonia requiring hospitalization. Is it different in the elderly? *J Am Geriatr Soc,* 33:671–680.

Michael, JR, & Summer, WR (1985): Pulmonary vascular disease. *In* Andres, R, Bierman, EL, & Hazzard, WR (eds): *Principles of Geriatric Medicine.* New York, McGraw-Hill, 589–592.

Mihalick, MJ, & Fisch, C (1974): Electrocardiographic findings in the aged. *Am Heart J,* 87:117–128.

Moe, RE (1985): Breast diseases. *In* Andres, R, Bierman, EL, & Hazzard, WR (eds): *Principles of Geriatric Medicine.* New York, McGraw-Hill, 636–646.

Morgan, W, Thomas, C, & Schuster, M (1981): Gastrointestinal system. *In* O'Hara-Devereaux, M, Andrus, LH, Scott, C, et al. (eds): *Eldercare: A Practical Guide to Clinical Geriatrics.* New York, Grune & Stratton, 199–215.

Murphy, ES, & DeMots, H (1984): Cardiology. *In* Cassel, CK, & Walsh, JR (eds): *Geriatric Medicine.* New York, Springer-Verlag, 147–182.

Nagami, PH, & Yoshikawa, TT (1983): Tuberculosis in the geriatric patient. *J Am Geriatr Soc,* 31:356–363.

Nelson, RD, Ezri, MD, & Denes, P (1984): Arrhythmias and conduction disturbances in the elderly. *In* Messerli, F (ed): *Cardiovascular Disease in the Elderly.* Boston, Martinus Nijhoff, 83–107.

O'Brien, IAD, O'Hare, P, & Corrall, RJM (1986): Heart rate variability in healthy subjects: Effect of age and the derivation of normal ranges of autonomic function. *Br Heart J,* 55:346–354.

Pearson, RM (1983): Urology. *In* Steinberg, FU (ed): *Care of the Geriatric Patient.* St. Louis, CV Mosby, 360–372.

Pierson, C (1984): Assessment and quantification of urine loss in incontinent women. *Nurs Pract,* 9(12):18–27.

Reid, J (1985): Estrogen depletion urethritis. *Geriatr Nurs,* 6:42–43.

Rice, PA, & Dale, P (1984): Infections in the genitourinary tract in women: Selected aspects. *In* Stollerman, GH, Harrington, WJ, Lamont, JT, et al. (eds): *Advances in Internal Medicine,* Chicago, Year Book, 53–68.

Robbins, RE, & Lee, D (1985): Carcinoma of the breast in women 80 years of age and older: Still a lethal disease. *Am J Surg,* 149:606–609.

Rogers, RL, Meyer, JS, Judd, BW, et al. (1985): Abstention from cigarette smoking improves cerebral perfusion among elderly chronic smokers. *JAMA,* 253:2970–2974.

Rowe, JW, & Resnick, NM (1985): Disorders of the kidney and urinary tract. *In* Andres, R, Bierman, EL, & Hazzard, WR (eds): *Principles of Geriatric Medicine.* New York, McGraw-Hill, 614–628.

Rubenstein, L, Josephson, K, Nichol-Seamon, M, et al. (1986): Comprehensive health screening of elderly well adults: An analysis of a community program. *J Clin Gerontol,* 41(3):342–352.

Rubin, JR, & Goldstone, J (1985): Peripheral vascular disease: Treatment and referral of the elderly, Part 1. *Geriatrics,* 40(6):34–39.

Schiff, I, & Wilson, E (1978): Clinical aspects of aging of the female reproductive system. *In* Schneider, E (ed): *The Aging Reproductive System.* New York, Raven Press, 15–21.

Schrier, RW (1982): *Clinical Internal Medicine in the Aged.* Philadelphia, WB Saunders.

Sieber, SJ (1984): Impotence. *In* Stollerman, GH, Harrington, WJ, Lamont, JT, et al. (eds): *Advances in Internal Medicine,* Vol. 30. Chicago, Year Book, 359–375.

Siefkin, AD (1985): Dyspnea in the elderly: Cardiac or pulmonary? *Geriatrics,* 40(5):63–73.

Sier, H, & Outslander, J (1985): Urinary incontinence. *Geriatr Med Today,* 4:95–102.

Simon, JB (1985): Occult blood screening for colorectal carcinoma: A critical review. *Gastroenterology,* 88(3):820–837.

Smith, FW (1984): Gastroenterology. *In* Cassell, C, & Walsh, J (eds): *Geriatric Medicine.* New York, Springer-Verlag, 536–550.

Spittell, JA, Jr (1983): Diagnosis and management of leg ulcer. *Geriatrics,* 38(6):57.

Sutton, KC, Dai, WS, & Kuller, LH (1985): Asymptomatic carotid artery bruits in a population of elderly with isolated systolic hypertension. *Stroke,* 16(5):781–784.

Swedberg, J, Driggers, DA, & Deiss, F (1986): Screening for colorectal cancer. *Postgrad Med,* 79(3):67–74.

Thiele, BL, & Strandness, DE, Jr (1985): Disorders of the vascular system: Peripheral vascular disease. *In* Andres, R, Bierman, EL, & Hazzard, WR (eds): *Principles of Geriatric Medicine.* New York, McGraw-Hill.

Vasilomanolakis, EC (1985): Geriatric cardiology: When exercise stress testing is justified. *Geriatrics,* 40(12):47.

Weg, RW (1985): Sexuality in aging. *In* Pathy, MSJ (ed): *Principles and Practices of Geriatric Medicine.* London, John Wiley & Sons, 131–147.

Winawer, SJ, Miller, DG, & Sherlock, P (1984): Risk and screening for colorectal cancer. *In* Stollerman, GH, Harrington, WJ, Lamont, JT, et al. (eds): *Advances in Internal Medicine,* Vol. 30. Chicago, Year Book, 471–491.

Wynne, JW (1979): Pulmonary disease in the elderly. *In* Rossman, I (ed): *Clinical Geriatrics.* Philadelphia, JB Lippincott, 239–265.

Yancik, R, Reis, LG, & Yatos, JW (1986): Ovarian cancer in the elderly: An analysis of surveillance, epidemiology and end results. *Am J Obstet Gynecol,* 154:640–647.

Yeaworth, RC, & Friedman, JS (1975): Sexuality in later life. *Nurs Clin North Am,* 10:565–574.

CHAPTER
5

Physical Assessment: Musculoskeletal and Nervous Systems

REBECCA LEE BURRAGE, R.N.C., M.S., F.N.P.

INTRODUCTION

This chapter presents physical assessment of the musculoskeletal and nervous systems in the older client. The material for each system is organized to include changes related to aging, common disorders, history, physical examination, and diagnostic tests.

MUSCULOSKELETAL SYSTEM

Aging Changes

The loss of skeletal mass begins in the third and fourth decades of life and occurs at varying rates throughout the skeleton. Mandibular alveolar bone loss leads to loss of tooth support (Avioli, 1983). Shrinkage of the intervertebral discs and collapse of the osteoporotic vertebrae cause shortening of the spinal column, resulting in loss in height of up to 5 cm in females and 3 cm in males over age 50 years (Steinberg, 1983). Changes also occur in skeletal structure. Kyphosis of the thoracic spine leads to compensatory extension of the neck and forward displacement of the scapulae (Milne & Williamson, 1983). The normally lordotic curve of the lower back flattens. Both flexion and extension of the lower back are diminished. Varus deformities of the knees may result in a narrow-based, insecure gait. Changes in the placement of the femoral neck and shaft cause a valgus deformity of the hips.

Muscle strength decreases from 30% to 50% between ages 20 and 60 years as a result of advancing age, inactivity, and degenerative arthropathy (de Marchena & Brooke, 1983).

Common Disorders

Joint Disorders. Osteoarthritis, rheumatoid arthritis, gout, pseudogout, and septic arthritis are the most frequently occurring joint disorders in elderly people. Osteoarthritis, or degenerative joint disease, is characterized by deterioration of articular cartilage and formation of new bone at joint surfaces. It occurs in 83% to 87% of people between 55 and 64 years of age, although only 15% to 22% are symptomatic (Calkins & Challa, 1985). Predisposing factors include advanced age, trauma, mechanical stresses, and genetic predisposition (Hahn, 1983).

In rheumatoid arthritis, there is irreversible damage to the joint capsule and articular cartilage as a result of chronic inflammation of the synovial membrane. Most elderly people contract arthritis in their earlier years, but, occasionally, some elderly acquire acute arthritis, causing severe functional disability (Anderson & Williams, 1983; Gibson, 1985). New onset rheumatoid arthritis most frequently occurs among men between the ages of 60 and 69 and in women between 50 and 59 years (Calkins & Challa, 1985).

Gout results from the formation of microcrystals of monosodium urate in joints and surrounding tissues. The incidence of gout is highest in the fifth decade for males and the sixth decade for females. Pyrophosphate deposits (pseudogout), caused by crystals of calcium pyrophosphatedehydrate (CPPD) settling in the joints, occur more often in men and in older individuals.

Septic arthritis should be considered a potential diagnosis, especially in the case of a monoarthritis, when the etiology is unclear (Grahame, 1985). The infection of one joint occurs during the course of an infection affecting another area of the body (DeGowin & DeGowin, 1987). Septic arthritis occurs more frequently in patients with other types of arthritis or joint trauma (Hahn, 1983). It is more likely to occur in debilitated, immunosuppressed patients and in the presence of diseases such as diabetes mellitus, rheumatoid arthritis, and malignancy (Hammerman, 1986).

Neuromuscular Diseases. Polymyalgia rheumatica (PMR) is an inflammatory disorder of the muscles of unknown pathogenesis. It characteristically affects people over 55 years of age and occurs more often in women than in men. Another inflammatory disease of older people, temporal arteritis, is diagnosed by biopsy of the temporal artery, which reveals giant cell arteritis. Although the exact nature of the relationship between giant cell arteritis and PMR is unclear, 60% of patients with giant cell arteritis experience PMR either before or during the course of their disease (Healey, 1984).

Motor neuron disease (MND) is a broad term encompassing progressive muscular atrophy, progressive bulbar palsy, and amyotrophic lateral sclerosis. Although the disorders of progressive muscle weakness and wasting may begin at any age, presentation is more common in older age groups (Cheshire & Cumming, 1985). Other causes of muscle weakness in older adults include myasthenia gravis, cancer, drugs, and thyroid disorders.

Disorders of Bone. Osteopenia is a reduction in bone mass below that which is considered normal for the age, sex, and race of an individual (Avioli, 1983). Osteoporosis is a specific form of osteopenia in which bone mass is decreased and the smaller bone mass has normal calcification and chemical composition (Spenser, Sonntag, & Kramer, 1986). It occurs most frequently in postmenopausal women. An estimated 70% of women in the United States age 45 years and older who sustain fractures have osteoporosis (Avioli, 1983). Fractures of the femur, vertebral bodies, and distal radius and proximal humerus are particularly common in osteoporotic women (Lifschitz & Harmon, 1982).

Secondary osteoporosis may result from immobilization, Cushing's syndrome, hyperthyroidism, or diabetes mellitus, or from drugs such as corticosteroids, heparin, and aluminum-containing antacids taken in large amounts (Spenser, et al., 1986).

Osteomalacia indicates abnormal mineralization, with or without a change in bone mass. Although osteomalacia is unusual in the United States, it is seen among elderly individuals with vitamin D deficiency (Spenser, et al., 1986).

Other diseases that may be associated with skeletal demineralization in the elderly population include multiple myeloma, neoplastic bone disease, hyperparathyroidism, hyperthyroidism, excess vitamin D intake, and chronic alcoholism. Paget's disease occurs most often after age 40 and is characterized by excess bone resorption and deposition with subsequent sclerosis (Spenser, et al., 1986).

Commonly found disorders of the foot include heel pain (most commonly due to heel spurs), hallux valgus deformity (with bunions over the medial aspect of the first metatarsal head), metatarsalgia (resulting from atrophy of the plantar padding supporting the metatarsal head), and hyperkeratotic lesions such as corns, calluses, or ingrown toenails (Collett, Katzew, & Helfand, 1984).

History

Functional Information. Baseline information on mobility should include how much time is spent out of bed; how much time is spent standing, sitting, and walking; how far the client walks; and whether assistive devices are used. It is important to determine if falls occur and the circumstances surrounding them.

The clinician should determine what specific problems occur in each of the activities of daily living (ADL) and instrumental activities of daily living (IADL) and how much assistance is required for each activity (see Chapter 11).

Symptoms

Joint Complaints. In several studies, complaints of arthritis or other musculoskeletal problems ranked above distress from any other system (Calkins & Challa, 1985). Joint pain, stiffness, swelling, redness, heat, limited motion, and deformity are the symptoms most frequently associated with joint disease (Table 5–1). Gait or self-care limitations may be present. Table 5–2 provides a summary of the signs and symptoms of common arthritic conditions in the elderly. Table 5–3 outlines the typical presentation of gout and pseudogout. Septic arthritis is reviewed in Table 5–4.

Back Pain. Back pain is a common problem among elderly people. Frequent causes of spinal pain in the elderly person are osteoarthritis of the facets, disc degeneration, and soft tissue sprains. Back pain is usually intermittent; determining the specific underlying cause is difficult (Calkins, Papademetriore, & Challa, 1986; Judge, Zuidema, & Fitzgerald, 1982). Back pain from osteoarthritis is characterized as an ache that generally becomes more severe late in the day or after standing or sitting in one position for an hour or longer. Sudden onset of low back pain following a slight misstep off a curb may suggest a compression fracture. Malignancy or aneurysm causes a severe, deep, constant, boring back pain that is often more noticeable at night (Calkins, Papademetriore, & Challa, 1986; Judge, Zuidema, & Fitzgerald, 1982). Back pain in the presence of fever, weight loss, or anemia is suggestive of bone pathology of infective, metabolic, or neoplastic origin (Grahame, 1985).

Determination is made as to where the pain focuses and where it radiates (Calkins, Papademetriore, & Challa, 1986). Symptoms of pain radiating down the posterior or lateral leg, worsening with coughing or sneezing, are suggestive of radicular neurologic deficits. The patient with nerve compression may also complain of muscle weakness. A client with cauda equina syndrome, caused by massive compression on the cauda equina from a large midline disc herniation, tumor, or other mass, has symptoms of incontinence, difficulty in walking, or neurologic signs in both legs.

In the elderly person it is likely that the cause of back pain is a relatively serious disease, such as osteoporosis, osteomalacia, Paget's disease, infection of discs, vertebral osteomyelitis, myelomatosis, or cancer metastases (Gibson, 1985). Failure to improve within one month after onset of acute back pain is sugges-

Table 5–1. DEGENERATIVE JOINT DISEASE

History

Onset
Gradual

Pain, Stiffness
Brief morning stiffness, limbering with mild exercise, symptoms worsened with use, relieved with rest

Number of Joints
Few joints, sometimes polyarticular (mostly in hands)

Common Joints
Lower extremities predominate: hip, knee, first metatarsophalangeal joint (great toe)
Hands: distal interphalangeal (DIP); proximal interphalangeal (PIP); metacarpophalangeal (MCP) and wrist involvement uncommon
Cervical, thoracic, lumbar spine

Specific Complaints
Hands: difficulty with fine movements (e.g., sewing)
Elbows: restricted extension; pain; paresthesia or hand weakness (with osteophyte encroachment on ulnar nerve)
Knees: pain with stairs; "knee let me down" (loss of extension and stability of joints)
Hips: mobility problems (e.g., standing up, climbing); involvement usually unilateral; stiffness in groin (sometimes in buttocks); hip pain: often referred to knee; often severe at night
Cervical spine: pain radiating into back of head, shoulders, arms, enhanced by certain neck movements; if compression of nerve roots: parasthesias, sensory loss, weakness, atrophy of arms and hands
Lumbar spine: severe pain, worse on prolonged standing, relieved by reclining; if lumbar disc prolapse or osteophyte involvement of nerve root foramina: acute pain or paresthesia to buttock or leg, accentuated by cough or strain

Examination

General Features
Pain with pressure or movement; inflammatory signs rare (possible mild heat, erythema, effusion, soft tissue swelling); crepitus; deformity, subluxation, bony hypertrophy in advanced stages

Specific Features
Hands: tenderness; possible bone swelling: Heberden's node (distal interphalangeal [DIP] joints; asymptomatic or intermittent pain, erythema, edema, possible expansion to cyst with mucous material), Bouchard's node (proximal interphalangeal [PIP] joints; similar to Heberden's); thenar wasting (due to involvement of thumb carpometacarpal joint); adduction deformity causing rectangular appearance; subluxation DIP, PIP joints
Wrist, elbow, shoulders: little deformity
Knees: quadriceps wasting; possible synovial thickening and effusion; varus or valgus deformities (suspect pseudogout if acute changes superimposed on DJD)
Hips: painful restriction hip movement (first internal rotation, then loss of extension with flexion deformity); quadriceps wasting; leg shortening (exclude inflammatory disease, metastatic malignancy)
Feet/ankles: rare except first metatarsophalangeal joint, with hallux valgus deformity or following fracture
Spine: loss of normal lumbar curve; restricted spinal movements; tenderness (of neck with cervical spine; over sacroiliac joints, buttocks with lumbarsacral spine); signs of nerve root compression absent (e.g., muscle wasting, weakness, diminished tendon reflexes; sensory changes; negative straight leg raise test)

Laboratory Tests
Normal unless additional disease

X-Ray
Narrowing of joint spaces; sclerosis of subchondral bone; bony hypertrophy at joint margins; subchondral bone cysts; deformities

(Data from Calkins & Challa, 1985; Gibson, 1985; Grahame, 1985; Hahn, 1983, Stevens, 1980.)

Table 5–2. RHEUMATOID ARTHRITIS

History

Onset
Usually insidous: one-fourth with acute onset; often preceded by, or accompanied by, malaise, fever, anorexia, weight loss, depression, myalgia vasomotor instability

Course
Variable: may be chronic (benign or aggressive) or have spontaneous remissions (older people with insidious onset have milder course and disabilities)

Pain/Stiffness
Morning stiffness lasting ½ to 5–6 hours; painful, swollen, warm joints, minimal symptoms possible in long-standing disease

Systemic Symptoms
Often present (consider septic arthritis with fever, mental status changes, leukocytosis)

Number of Joints
Many

Joint Distribution
Usually symmetrical

Common Joints
Small joints commonly involved early, followed by larger ones, hands, wrist, elbow, shoulder (common in older people); metatarsophalangeal joints of feet, hip, knee, ankle, spine (cervical spine common in older people); cricoarytenoid, cricothyroid joints (with hoarseness); ossicles of middle ear (with deafness); temporomandibular joint

Common Complications in Older Persons
Cervical spine involvement with subluxation and compression; ankylosis of involved joints; popliteal extension of joint effusions (Baker's cyst); septic arthritis

Non-Rheumatologic Disorders Resembling Rheumatoid Arthritis (RA)
Hypo/hyperthyroidism, menopause, metastatic malignancy, Parkinson's disease

Examination

Common Features
Heat, synovial thickening, tenderness, tendon sheath effusions (synovitis less striking in older person)
Symmetrical, additive joint involvement common; all peripheral joints may be involved chronically
Subcutaneous nodules near elbows and around tendon sheaths (nodules less common in older person)
Flexion contractures and deformities

Hand Features
Proximal interphalangeal (PIP), metacarpophalangeal (MCP) joints and wrists initially
Swan neck deformity: distal interphalangeal (DIP) flexion contractures; PIP extension contractures
Boutonnière deformity: DIP extension contracture; PIP flexion contractures
Ulnar deviation at the MCP joints
Weak hand grip

Laboratory Findings
Erythrocyte sedimentation rate (ESR): often used index of activity (ESR may be more elevated in older person with RA but may rise without disease; 30 mm in 1 hour considered abnormal)
Rheumatoid factor assay: usually positive with RA (nonspecificity of positive test for RA increases with age)
Lupus erythematosus (LE) factor occasionally positive (occurs more frequently with older population)
Complete blood count: mild anemia common; leukocytosis with very active disease and in conjunction with corticosteroid therapy; thrombocytosis with active disease

X-Ray
X-rays of small bones may help identify early changes; typical deformities and erosive changes in chronic phrases

(Data from Calkins & Challa, 1985; Gibson, 1985; Hahn, 1983; Hammerman, 1986; Stevens, 1980; Zizic, 1980.)

Table 5–3. GOUT AND PYROPHOSPHATE ARTHROPATHY (PSEUDOGOUT)

History
Family history common with gout; trauma often precedes onset; sudden onset, severe pain and disability, subsiding symptoms over several days; symptom-free interval (few weeks–years) with gradually increased frequency of attacks

Joint Distribution
1 to 2 joints common (multiple joints often in pseudogout); common joints are foot instep, ankle, knee (most common site of pseudogout), elbow, wrist, great toe (most common site in *gout*)

Examination
Acute phase: fever (lower in pseudogout) and leukocytosis common; hot, swollen, erythematous joints; effusions; periarticular involvement common (erythematous streaks may extend to soft tissue and mimic cellulitis); mimics rheumatoid arthritis, degenerative joints disease, septic arthritis
Chronic phase: hot, swollen, multiple joints; deformities common; tophaceous deposits (tophi) in ears, elbows, tendons (with gout); crystal deposits in joints only (with pseudogout)

Laboratory Tests
Uric acid; greater than 8 mg/100 ml in males (7 mg/100 ml in females) with acute gout and 33% of people with pseudogout (older people may have incidental hyperuricemia due to oral diuretics)
Synovial fluid: diagnosis established by identification of crystals in synovial fluid or soft tissue deposits

X-Ray
Soft tissue swelling around joints; punched out lesions in surrounding bone

(Data from Hahn, 1983; Newcombe, 1980.)

tive of an underlying systemic disease (Deyo, 1987).

Soft Tissue Problems. Pain in and around the shoulder joint is a frequently encountered problem. Shoulder pain is caused either by a disorder intrinsic to the shoulder joint (fractures, bursitis, tendinitis, synovitis, arthritis) or referred from visceral organs (such as from myocardial ischemia, shoulder-hand syndrome, gallbladder disease, and diaphragmatic irritation). It also may be referred from adjacent musculoskeletal structures, such as the cervical spine (Sundstrom, 1983). The rotator cuff muscles are responsible for internal and external rotation, abduction of the shoulder, and depression of the head of the humerus. The most common cause of the non-traumatic shoulder pain is rotator cuff tendinitis (shoulder impingement syndrome, the painful arc syndrome). Minimal stress, such as lifting a small load, often results in a tendon tear in people over the age of 60 years. Clinical features include a subacute onset, often without a history of excessive shoulder use, night pain, and aching over the shoulder and midhumerus (White, 1989).

Some of the conditions causing painful elbow symptoms are the following: Synovitis (due to trauma or arthritis); epicondylitis, or "tennis elbow" (inflammation of tendons at the lateral epicondyle); and olecranon bursitis.

Common sites for bursitis are the olecranon, ischium, trochanter, patella, and achilles tendon (Hahn, 1983). A complaint of pain on sitting, with tenderness over the ischial tuberosity, may indicate ischial bursitis. There is often a history of trauma such as a fall on the buttocks. Paget's disease and bone tumors give similar presentations and may be ruled out with pelvic x-ray films (Hahn, 1983). It is also important to exclude inflammatory diseases, such as tuberculosis and rheumatoid arthritis (Calkins & Challa, 1985). Trochanteric bursitis produces lateral hip pain of an aching nature, aggravated by motions such as stair climbing and lying on the affected side. Rarely, there is a history of trauma (Hahn, 1983). It is

Table 5–4. SEPTIC ARTHRITIS

Symptoms
Usually painful, acute onset; often fever, chills

Joints/Distribution
Mono- or oligoarthritis more common than polyarthritis; common site: large joints, such as knee

Examination
Joints very tender, erythematous, hot, swollen; cellulitis common (may resemble gout, pseudogout, rheumatoid arthritis)
General examination may reveal source of infection (e.g., pneumonia, skin lesions, urinary or gastrointestinal tract infection)

Laboratory Tests
Synovial fluid often diagnostic (culture, leukocyte count, glucose); arthrocentesis should be done if septic arthritis suspected
Leukocytosis common

(Data from Hahn, 1983; Hammerman, 1986; Stevens, 1980.)

important to explore the possibility of intrinsic hip pain, such as osteoarthritis or fracture, or a coexisting spinal condition.

The client should be questioned regarding the presence of muscle cramping, pain, or weakness. Cramps frequently occur spontaneously in muscles after a sudden forceful contraction and in the lower extremities during sleep. Cramps take on pathologic significance in the presence of symptoms associated with neuromuscular disease, motor neuron disease, metabolic disturbance, and peripheral neuropathy (Shields, 1985). In polymyalgia rheumatica (PMR), there is a sudden onset of severe pain and stiffness in the neck, shoulders, hip girdles, upper arms, and thighs. Aching may last one month or more, and symptoms of fatigue, weight loss, and low grade fever may accompany the discomfort. Muscle wasting may be due to neuromuscular disorders associated with malignancy or drugs, most commonly steroids. Muscle weakness is seen in myasthenia gravis and hyperthyroidism (Cheshire & Cumming, 1985; Shields, 1985).

Examination

Functional Assessment. Assessment of range of motion provides information on the person's ability for self-care. Clark (1984) determined the critical range of motion required to perform activities of daily living. For example, the ability to feed oneself is dependent on wrist flexion of 45°, extension of 30°, and forearm pronation and supination of 45°.

The ability to perform activities of daily living is evaluated during the examination. Examples include observing clients as they undress and dress for the examination and allowing them to do the buttoning as a measurement of fine motor dexterity. A wide variety of standardized rating scales is available to aid in improving the client's functional status (Steinberg, 1983; Clark, 1984). The reader is referred to Chapter 7, Functional Assessment. The assessment tools are helpful not only in assessing current function, but also in measuring subsequent progress or decline.

Gait and Mobility. The gait of a normal elderly male is characterized by slight anteroflexion of the upper body. The arms and knees are slightly flexed, the arm swing is decreased, and the step shortened. Researchers are finding that some of the most sensitive indices to gait pathology, increasing the likelihood of problems such as falls, are velocity of gait and stride length (Imms & Edholm, 1981) (Figure 5–1).

The client's mobility and ability to transfer should be observed, when possible. Movement in bed and transfers in and out of bed, bathtub, chair, and from toilet or car require maneuvering skills that can easily be observed during the examination. The patient should be observed turning from side to side, standing from a sitting position, pivoting or turning, and sitting again. Standing balance is checked, including the ability to counter a gentle sternal push successfully. Endurance can be assessed by having the person ambulate for a defined distance. If stair safety is an issue, a brief trial on a nearby staircase may provide worthwhile information. When a wheelchair is used for locomotion, the person's ability to maneuver the wheelchair and manage functions such as locking the brakes are noted.

If the individual is unable to ambulate safely, the reasons for difficulty should be determined. Many elderly people have multiple disorders that result in a gait abnormality, as summarized in Table 5–5 (Nutt, 1984). The musculoskeletal examination includes a complete evaluation for evidence of joint involvement, adequacy of muscle strength, and specific gait disorder. For example, walking may be difficult with even minimal arthritic changes because of knee and hip flexion deformities causing compensatory changes in other joints to maintain the center of gravity. An adequate degree of foot dorsiflexion must be present in order to place the feet flat on the floor without flexing the knees and hips (Lorentz, 1985). The feet are checked for lesions or deformities that could interfere with gait and mobility.

Muscle Strength Assessment. A screening test for an older person includes evaluation of strength of shoulder elevators and abductors, elbow flexors and extensors, gross hand grasp,

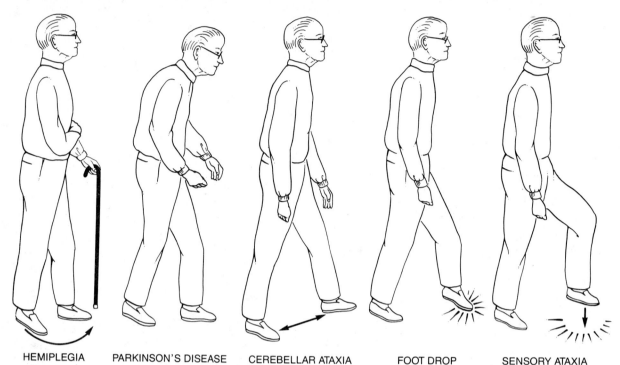

HEMIPLEGIA   PARKINSON'S DISEASE   CEREBELLAR ATAXIA   FOOT DROP   SENSORY ATAXIA

Figure 5–1. Common types of gaits. (From Swartz, M: Textbook of Physical Diagnosis: History and Examination. Philadelphia, WB Saunders, 1989, p 514. Reprinted with permission.)

thumb to index finger strength, hip and knee flexors and extensors, and ankle dorsiflexors (Clark, 1984). When muscles of the pelvic girdle are weak, resulting problems include exaggerated lumbar lordosis, waddling gait, and difficulty rising from chairs and managing stairs (Nutt, 1984).

Several factors influence the accuracy of the muscle strength assessment. If clients experience pain, they may give less than an optimal effort. Spasticity mimics greater than actual strength. Lack of cooperation or understanding of instructions often results in inaccurate findings (Clark, 1984).

The rating system shown in Table 5–6 provides a degree of objectivity for assessing muscle strength. The client is positioned to allow complete movement. Each muscle or group of muscles is assessed through a full range of motion as the examiner applies resistance against the client's movements. The grade of strength is a subjective measurement by the examiner.

Hand strength is fairly well maintained in spite of the thin, bony appearance of an older person's hands. Atrophy of the dorsal interosseus muscle, especially between the thumb and hand, leaves the marked guttering on the back of the hands (Locke & Galaburda, 1978). Loss of subcutaneous tissue in the hands is common with aging and may incorrectly be attributed to muscle wasting (Locke & Galaburda, 1978).

The thigh and calf muscles are other common sites of muscle wasting and loss of bulk, even in active people (Schaumberg, Spencer, & Ochoa, 1983). Fibrillation and fasciculation are not seen with normal aging changes; causes of muscle wasting other than aging should be sought. For instance, muscle wasting of the hands may be worsened by cervical spondylosis. Immobilized elderly individuals may develop muscle fibrosis, atrophy, and subsequent flexion of the legs as the muscles and tendons contract (Schaumberg, et al., 1983). Another condition, "senile muscle atro-

Table 5–5. CAUSES OF POSTURAL AND GAIT DISTURBANCES

| | | Sensory Abnormalities | |
Modality	*Lesion*	*Signs*	*Gait*
Proprioceptive	Peripheral nerves	Loss of position sensation, stocking glove sensory loss, decreased or absent DTRs,* positive Romberg sign	Ataxic
	Spinal posterior columns	Loss of position sensation Other signs of spinal cord dysfunction	Ataxic
Vestibular	Peripheral: labyrinth and vestibular nerve	Nystagmus, hearing deficits, past pointing	Weaving "drunken"
	Central: vestibular nuclei and pathways	Nystagmus, past pointing, cerebellar and other cranial nerve signs	Weaving or ataxic
Visual	Lens, vitreous, retina, extraocular muscles	Visual acuity, diplopia, or deficient downgaze	Tentative, uncertain

| | Motor Abnormalities | |
Lesion	*Signs*	*Gait*
Muscle	Proximal weakness, normal DTRs	Waddling
Distal motor nerve	Distal weakness, decreased DTRs	Slapping, foot drop, steppage
Proximal motor nerve or roots	Patchy weakness, proximal and distal	Waddling and/or slapping
Corticospinal tracts	Distal > proximal weakness, increased DTRs, increased tone, Babinski's sign	Circumduction, "spastic"

| | Central or Integrative Dysfunction | |
Lesion	*Signs*	*Gait*
Corticospinal tracts	Weakness, increased DTRs and tone	"Spastic," stifflegged, circumduction
Frontal lobes	Dementia, perseveration, hand and foot grasp reflexes	"Apractic"
Deep white and gray matter	Corticospinal tract signs, pseudobulbar palsy, history of "strokes"	Marche de petits pas
Basal ganglia	Tremor, rigidity, bradykinesia Choreic movements of face, trunk, limbs	Parkinsonian
Cerebellum	Limb dysmetria, intention tremor	Ataxic
Multiple central and peripheral sites	Absence of other significant central or peripheral disturbances to explain gait disorder	"Senile"

*DTRs—deep tendon reflexes
(From Nutt JG: Abnormalities of posture and movement. *In* Cassel, CK, & Walsh JR (eds): *Geriatric Medicine,* Vol. I. New York, Springer-Verlag, 1984, p. 51. Reprinted with permission.)

phy," is characterized by marked atrophy and fasciculation of the extremities (Schaumberg, et al., 1983).

Muscle tone is often difficult to assess in the elderly person. Joint disease may produce rigidity, which may appear secondary to a neuromuscular disease. Neurologic lesions in the muscle, in distal and proximal motor nerve roots, or in corticospinal roots result in weakness and alterations in muscle tone (Nutt, 1984). Proximal muscle is affected by primary muscle diseases, including dystrophy, myopathy, or myositis. *Gegenhalten* is fluctuating resistance of a muscle in response to passive range of motion. The patient is unable to cooperate and relax. Gegenhalten is seen in degenerative diseases such as Alzheimer's disease (Adams & Victor, 1989). It is different from the cogwheel rigidity associated with Parkinson's disease. With cogwheel rigidity, the examiner finds that when a hypertonic muscle is stretched (such as during dorsiflexion of the hand), there is a rhythmic ratchet-like resistance (Adams & Victor, 1989).

Joint Assessment. A limitation in passive range of motion may be caused by problems such as soft tissue contracture, osteophytes (bony outgrowths), or destruction of the joint. If passive range of motion is within normal limits, but active range is impaired, the prob-

Table 5–6. CRITERIA FOR RECORDING THE GRADES OF MUSCLE STRENGTH

Functional Level	Levett Scale	Grade	Percentage of Normal
No evidence of contractability	Zero (0)	0	0
Evidence of slight contractability	Trace (T)	1	10
Complete range of motion with gravity eliminated	Poor (P)	2	25
Complete range of motion with gravity	Fair (F)	3	50
Complete range of motion against gravity with some resistance	Good (G)	4	75
Complete range of motion against gravity with full resistance	Normal (N)	5	100

(Reproduced by permission from Malasanos, L, Barkauskas, V, Moss, M, et al.: Health Assessment (ed 3). St. Louis, 1986, The C. V. Mosby Co.)

lem may be muscle weakness or inflammation of the joint or periarticular structures (see Tables 5–1 to 5–4).

Figure 5–2 shows joint abnormalities of common arthritic conditions. The person with back pain due to the cauda equina syndrome has the following physical findings: loss of rectal sphincter tone, "saddle" anesthesia, and bilateral loss of leg strength or reflexes. Consultation should be made with a surgeon on an emergency basis for this disorder, and on a nonacute basis for other signs and symptoms of nerve impingement, such as caused by herniated disc, spondylolisthesis, or spinal stenosis. Muscle wasting or weakness, diminished knee or ankle reflexes, or sensory changes imply nerve root compression (Gibson, 1985).

Reflexes are sometimes reduced or difficult to elicit in the elderly person, even without the presence of a disease, sometimes making evaluation of nerve compression more confusing (see Neurologic Examination). The test for sciatic nerve root irritation, though not specifically for disc herniation, is the straight leg raise. The client lies in a supine position, and his straightened leg is lifted by the examiner. An abnormal finding is the presence of pain radiating down the posterior leg with thigh elevation of 60° or less (Deyo, 1987). The clinician should also examine for possible visceral or systemic sources of pain, such as breast or prostate cancer, which are common sources of spinal metastases, and for abdominal and femoral artery abnormalities, possible sites of aneurysm or dissection (Deyo, 1987).

Extraarticular Examination. Distinctive physical findings of common extraarticular conditions among elderly patients will be briefly discussed. Carpal tunnel syndrome is caused by compression of the median nerve in the carpal tunnel of the wrist. Pain and paresthesia usually occur in the thumb, forefinger, and middle finger but may sometimes radiate from the wrist to the elbow and shoulder. On examination there is decreased sensation in the thumb, forefinger, middle finger, and medial side of the ring finger. Atrophy of thumb abductors and the thenar eminence is present. When percussion over the carpal tunnel elicits pain or a tingling sensation from the wrist to the hand, it is a positive Tinel's sign. The Phalen's sign is positive when pain is experienced by the patient as he presses his flexed hands together (Hahn, 1983).

Examination of the patient with shoulder pain is facilitated by draping the patient so that both shoulders are exposed and easily compared. The shoulder is inspected for signs of swelling, redness, atrophy, and trauma. The shoulder is palpated systematically to identity the structures of the shoulder and sites of tenderness. The client is observed from behind while he takes his arms through complete active range of motion. Upward rotation of the scapula relative to the thorax should be smooth and coordinated from about 30° abduction to 180° abduction. Painful abduction, coarse shrugging of the shoulder, and tilting of the torso away from the affected shoulder occur with disorders such as rotator cuff tendinitis, glenohumeral arthritis, frozen shoulder, and acute calcific tendinitis. Rotator cuff tendinitis is suggested by a pain in the abduction arc between 40° and 120° in a patient with full range of motion. Pain usually occurs be-

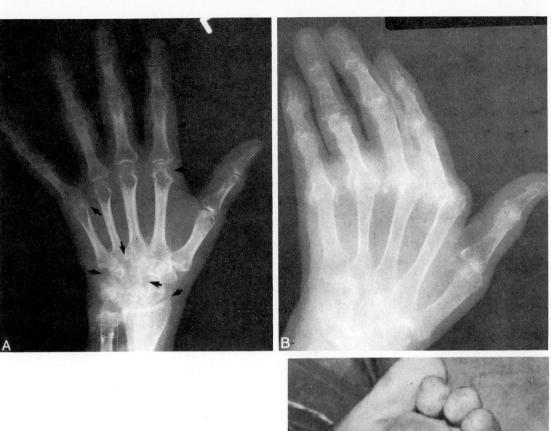

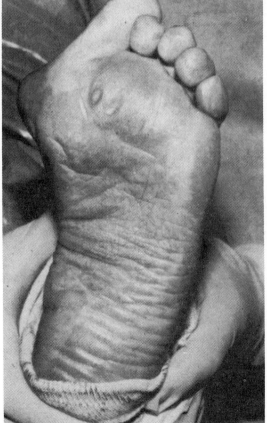

Figure 5–2. (A) Early and (B) late hand deformities in rheumatoid arthritis. (From Browner, AC: Arthritis in Black and White. Philadelphia, WB Saunders, 1988, pp 49, 447. Reprinted with permission.) (C) Rheumatoid foot. (From Gudas, CJ: Common foot problems in the elderly. *In* Calkins, E, Davis, PJ, and Ford, AB (eds). The Practice of Geriatrics. Philadelphia, WB Saunders, 1986, p 447. Reprinted with permission.)

tween 120° and 180° in patients with degenerative disease in the acromioclavicular joint. Active and passive range of motion are restricted in persons with a frozen shoulder (White, 1989).

Conditions producing painful elbow syndromes include arthritis and associated synovitis, epicondylitis, and olecranon bursitis. On examination of the elbow, epicondylitis, or "tennis elbow," demonstrates point tenderness near the lateral epicondyle, lack of inflammation, and pain elicited when the client extends the wrist against pressure. On physical examination of olecranon bursitis, there is a boggy swelling along the end of the ulna with mild inflammation (Hahn, 1983).

A significant finding in evaluation of hip pain is the presence of point tenderness along the greater trochanter, which is suggestive of trochanteric bursitis. In this condition pain is elicited by external rotation of the hip and abduction against resistance. There is no pain with internal rotation, flexion, and extension of the hips—a finding important in ruling out intrinsic hip disease (Hahn, 1983).

Tests

Specific tests for degenerative joint disease, rheumatoid arthritis, gout and pseudogout, and septic arthritis are listed in Tables 5–1 to 5–4. Radiography is indicated for back pain to detect compression fractures, malignancy, spondylolisthesis, or osteoporosis (Deyo, 1987). Computed tomography has replaced myelography in some centers in the evaluation of disc herniation that may require surgery. It is also useful in the diagnosis of spinal stenosis, osteomyelitis, paravertebral infections, and osteoporosis. Deyo (1987) recommends use of radionuclide bone scanning for patients whose clinical features suggest a high probability of cancer or infection, such as those who have either an abnormal x-ray or elevated erythrocyte sedimentation rate (ESR).

NERVOUS SYSTEM

Aging Changes

In the absence of disease most normal older adults demonstrate little change in the func-tion of information storage. They do experience a loss of speed in learning and processing new information and reaction to simple or complex stimuli (Katzman & Terry, 1983). Reaction time and time needed to perform certain activities increase with age. These changes may be due to delayed central processing time, changes in sensation or speed of execution, and decreased nerve velocity (Teravainen & Calne, 1983). The normal aging process does not result in disorientation, confusion, gross memory defects, paranoid ideation, hallucination, or depression (Jarvik & Neshkes, 1985).

There is a loss of sensory functions with aging. More than 80% of 80-year-olds have a major impairment in sensitivity to smell, probably because of degenerative processes in the olfactory epithelium and aging changes in the central neural pathways (Doty, Shaman, Applebaum, et al., 1984). After about age 60, taste sensitivity is diminished by changes such as loss in the number of taste buds, loss of elasticity in the mouth and lips, decreased saliva flow, and fissuring of the tongue (Corso, 1971). (Vision and hearing were discussed in Chapter 3.) It is generally believed that deep pain sensitivity decreases with age (Schaumberg, Spencer, & Ochoa, 1983).

Common Disorders

Approximately 75% of all cerebrovascular accidents occur in persons over age 65, at an annual incidence of 18 per 1000 individuals (Evans & Caird, 1982). Stroke is the second leading cause of death among persons over age 75 (Hardin, 1983).

Parkinson's disease is also more common with advanced age. The incidence is approximately 15 per 1000 at age 70, increasing to about 20 per 1000 persons at age 80 (Evans & Caird, 1982).

Studies indicate that the incidence of intracranial tumors peaks between ages 60 and 70. Researchers disagree whether the incidence of intracranial tumors decreases, increases, or stays the same after age 70 (Evans & Caird, 1982).

Infectious diseases of the central nervous system are associated with a high rate of morbidity and mortality in elderly people. For instance, pneumococcal meningitis has a mortality rate greater than 50% in this group. Herpes zoster occurs in 16.2% of patients over the age of 60, compared with an incidence of 5.4% in the average population (Roeltgen, 1983).

Diabetes mellitus, nutritional disorders of chronic illness, and alcoholism are the most frequent causes of neuropathy in the elderly. Trigeminal and post-herpetic neuralgia and facial nerve neuritis (Bell's palsy) are common causes of mononeuropathy (Hardin, 1983).

Delirium seems to occur more frequently in elderly people, possibly due to the high incidence of disease, medication use, and sensory deficits (Caird, 1982).

In a review of studies by Gurland and Cross (1982), dementia was found in 2% to 5% of the elderly population living in the community and in 30% to 50% of institutionalized elderly. The occurrence is higher in individuals over the age of 80 (20%) than in those between the ages 65 and 79 (less than 3%). Although most dementias are of the Alzheimer's or multi-infarct types, as many as 15% may be reversible. Reversible causes of dementia include metabolic encephalopathies (e.g., hyponatremia, hyperparathyroidism, hypoglycemia), endocrine disorders such as hypothyroidism, removable cerebral tumors such as meningioma, normal pressure hydrocephalus, deficiency disease (e.g., of B_{12} and folate), infections such as neurosyphilis, trauma, drugs, and depression.

Estimates of the incidence of depression in the elderly vary widely. Gurland and Cross (1982) report the occurrence of depression in 13% of community elderly. The rate of successful suicide in the elderly male is high, especially among those who are widowed, inactive, or depressed (Gurland & Cross, 1982).

History

The neurologic history of the elderly patient focuses on exploring presented symptoms and probing for information that relates to the common disorders of stroke, dementia, and depression and to the more uncommon disorders such as tumors and central nervous system infections. In a study of socially active well elderly, the most frequent neurologic symptoms were memory impairment, numbness and tingling of fingers and toes, headache, dizziness, light-headedness, and pain (Kokmen, Bossemeyer, Barney, et al., 1977). Alteration in acuity of the senses, weakness, and sleep disturbances are other frequently expressed concerns.

Memory Loss—Depression. The person initially presenting with dementia may describe vague symptoms such as irritability, nervousness, and anxiety, which do not fit into one of the major psychiatric syndromes. The multiple complaints may seem unrelated, and the client may have difficulty describing the problems. Information should be supplemented by another person to cover the following subjects: "general behavior, capacity for work, personality changes, language, mood, special preoccupations and concerns, delusional ideas, hallucinatory experiences, personal habits, and such faculties as memory and judgment" (Adams & Victor, 1989, p. 344).

Many older people with depression do not recognize it as such. Others do recognize the symptoms of depression but may fail to report the problem because of the stigma associated with mental illness. Symptoms of depression often occurring with old age include agitation, vague physical complaints, hypochondriasis, delusions of persecution and poverty, suicidal ideation, and confusion (Lehmann, 1982). Symptoms of depression may also include extreme difficulty falling asleep or early morning awakenings (Thompson, Moran, & Nies, 1983) and loss of appetite with accompanying weight loss.

Headache. Tension headaches are common in elderly persons and can frequently be linked to psychological factors, such as depression or anxiety, or to pathologic factors, such as osteoarthritis of the neck. The patient gives a history of mild to moderately severe pain with an aching, pressing, or squeezing quality. It is usually bilateral and diffuse, although it can be occipital, frontal, or bitemporal. It may also occur daily or several times a week and may be constant or recurring.

Cerebrovascular disease can cause intermittent severe headaches of a throbbing or steady nature. The patient with decreased cerebral blood flow secondary to carotid stenosis or vertebral-basilar stenosis develops headaches because of compensatory vasodilation. Headaches from vasodilation may also be caused by medications such as nitrates. Hypertension headaches may occur with a blood pressure above 180/110 mm Hg. Migraine headaches are rare in elderly persons, but cluster headaches may occur into the seventh decade. (The headache of temporal arteritis is discussed in the Musculoskeletal Assessment section.)

There are several other important common causes of headaches in elderly people. The headache symptoms of brain tumor are variable and usually do not fit any pattern, except that they usually worsen with time. They may be associated with nausea, vomiting, anorexia, confusion, and other neurologic symptoms. The patient with a subdural hematoma following a fall gives a history of unilateral severe headaches and neurologic symptoms such as changing levels of consciousness, slurred speech, or sensory or motor changes. Trigeminal neuralgia occurs in middle-aged or older patients and results in severe, lancinating pain on one side of the face, lasting from 30 seconds to 4 minutes (Rapoport, Sheftell, & Baskin, 1983). (Headaches due to temporomandibular joint (TMJ) syndrome are discussed in Chapter 3.)

Dizziness. A cerebellar or central nervous system etiology is suggested by such complaints as disequilibrium or unsteadiness and clumsiness. A history of a previous head injury, episodic vertigo, and cranial nerve symptoms may also implicate the nervous system. Some of the more common conditions causing dizziness in older people include the following: acoustic neuromas (and other neoplasms), vertebrobasilar insufficiency, cervical spine arthritis with cord compression, benign positional vertigo, vestibular neuronitis, toxin-induced labyrinthine disorders, acute bacterial meningitis and labyrinthitis, cholesteatoma, and Ménière's disease (Bonikowski, 1983).

Weakness. Weakness may result from diminished cardiovascular reserve, joint stiffness from arthritis, motor neuron disease, or primary muscle fiber disease. Patients may interpret as weakness disturbances of movement caused by impairment of the basal ganglia, forebrain, cerebellum, or suprasegmental motor neurons (Hardin, 1983). Neuropathy is also a common cause of perceived weakness of a body part.

Level of Awareness. Many elderly patients experience transient ischemic attacks or strokes associated with small vessel disease. These may go undiagnosed. Multiple thromboembolic infarcts that do not individually produce a clinical event may, in combination, cause significant cognitive impairment (Hachinski & Lasson, 1974). The clinician probes for any unreported fluctuations in alertness and periods of lethargy, somnolence, or confusion and disorientation, as well as amnestic episodes. Any difficulty in maintaining attention and concentration is also questioned.

Examination

Neurologic examination of the elderly may be complicated by the patient's inability to follow single or multiple step commands. The examiner may demonstrate the task performance or motor sequence being tested to assist patients in understanding what to do. Patients may be agitated, fearful, or uncooperative. If so, time spent reassuring them and gaining some measure of their confidence will facilitate subsequent aspects of the examination.

Cranial Nerves. A number of cranial nerve findings may be considered within normal range in the elderly population. Upward conjugate gaze and convergence may be limited in the normal aged client (Calne, 1983; Jenkyn, Reeves, Warren, et al., 1985). Other researchers have also reported impaired downward gaze. Impaired upward gaze with bilateral ptosis may be a sign of increased intracranial pressure (Caird, 1982) or myasthenia gravis, although onset of the latter is rare after age 70 (Adams & Victor, 1989). Normally smooth movements of the eye in following an object may become slow and irregular with age. This slowing of eye movements needs to be distinguished from nystagmus, a slow drift of the eye away from a position of fixation, corrected by quick jerky movements back. This may be indicative of brain tumors or midbrain lesions.

Sluggish pupillary constriction in response to light and of the convergency reflex is generally considered a normal finding with aging. The changes are probably due to a local ophthalmic abnormality rather than a cranial nerve defect (Carter, 1986). Miosis appears to be a normal variant (Granacher, 1981) and makes the ophthalmoscope examination more difficult.

The incidence of papilledema is a less common sign in the aged than in young people with hypertension and subdural hematoma (Caird, 1982) and is less commonly found in space-occupying lesions.

Granacher (1981) reports a decrease in gag reflex with aging. The gag response may be increased in individuals with multi-infarct dementia and bilateral cortical or subcortical disease, as a reflection of pseudobulbar palsy. This symptom is especially suggestive of disease if the patient also demonstrates dysphonia or dysphagia. Some clinicians have found there is no diminishment in the sensory function of the face or the corneal reflex (Caird, 1982). Others report that the corneal reflex should be present, but reaction time may slow (Calne, 1983).

The examiner asks the patient to smile, frown, and grimace, and observes for asymmetry. The patient is asked to squeeze the eyes shut and clench the jaws while the examiner palpates for muscle weakness and asymmetry in contractile strength.

The lower fibers of the facial nerve innervate the muscles of expression and the platysma muscle. Both muscles are weakened in facial paralysis due to an upper motor neuron or supranuclear lesion, such as stroke. It may be difficult in the edentulous patient to determine if drooping of the corner of the mouth during testing of the facial nerve is due to a mechanical or neurologic problem. The platysmas may be tested effectively, even without teeth, as a means of verifying the presence of an upper motor neuron lesion. The clinician observes for an asymmetric response as the patient draws down the angles of the mouth while tightening the neck muscles. In a supranuclear lesion, the voluntary movements of the facial muscles are affected more frequently than the emotional and associative movements, such as smiling, grimacing, or frowning. In addition, the lower facial muscles are usually more involved than those of the upper part of the face. In contrast, with a lower motor neuron lesion such as Bell's palsy, the voluntary, emotional, and associative facial movements are equally affected, as are the upper and lower facial movements (Bannister, 1985).

Sensory Position Sense. Vibration sensation in the feet and ankles diminishes in approximately one-half of elderly patients (Carter, 1986; Bender, 1974). Position sense abnormalities have been found in 15% to 30% of elderly patients (Carter, 1986; Wolfson & Katzman, 1983). Whether these changes in sensation, position sense, and vibration perception are normal or abnormal is unclear. It is important to rule out compression of the spinal cord secondary to arthritic changes, arteriosclerotic myelopathy, and metabolic problems such as diabetes with peripheral neuropathy (Bender, 1974; Sabin, 1982).

Position sense is tested by asking the patient to close the eyes and passively move one finger, then asking the patient to state whether the finger is flexed or extended. Also, the patient's lower extremities may be shielded from view, the great toe is dorsiflexed or plantar flexed and the patient is asked to tell whether the toe is pointing up or down. Vibratory sense is tested using a 128 cps tuning fork on the dorsal surfaces of the toes or feet. Tactile sense is tested by having the patient close the eyes while the examiner strokes the skin with gauze or paper; the patient then is asked to tell the area touched. It is important to include symmetrical body sections in performing this test.

Reflexes. Various studies have found an absent ankle jerk in from 27% to 40% of older people, with a larger percentage of areflexia as age increases. Care should be taken not to wrongly ascribe a peripheral neuropathy to the aging process when it is actually due to a pathologic condition such as diabetes, alcoholism, or malignancy. Impallomeni, Flynn, Kenny, and associates (1984) suggest that an absent reflex is often due to technique. The researchers were able to elicit the ankle jerk in 80% of subjects, possibly due to special efforts to reduce pain and anxiety. They recommend that the patient lie with the legs parallel as the examiner, using a percussion hammer, strikes his or her own fingers overlying the plantar surface of the patient's dorsiflexed foot. If the reflex if doubtful or absent, distractions such as having the patient clench the jaws may assist relaxation. It is vital that the reflex be tested as soon as the client is given the instruction to relax, because repeated attempts and impatient instructions to relax will probably be unsuccessful. Those with ankle areflexia may also lose knee and biceps responses. Superficial abdominal reflexes usually disappear with age (Wolfson & Katzman, 1983). The examiner may also experience difficulty in eliciting and interpreting the plantar response in the elderly person because of great toe deformities and hardening of the sole with decreased sensitivity (Carotenuto & Bullock, 1980).

Primitive frontal release reflexes are often present in cerebral injury or degenerative disease. Their significance in otherwise normal elderly individuals is unclear. The most commonly encountered of these reflexes in the elderly person are the snout (a pursing of the lips when the upper lip is gently tapped), the palmomental (a twitching of the chin when the thenar surface of the palm is scratched), and the corneomandibular (a lateral deviation of the mandible to the side opposite the side of the cornea stimulated by cotton wool). The presence of one or two of these reflexes is not an unusual finding in a normal elderly person. However, there is a possible correlation between the presence of all three reflexes and pathologic conditions (Isakov, Sazbon, Costeff, et al., 1984). The glabellar blink is most commonly associated with cortical or basal ganglia dysfunction (Granacher, 1981) and is elicited in the following manner: The examiner instructs the client to look at a point across

the room. The examiner then approaches the client from above the client's forehead and outside the field of vision. Using an index finger, the examiner rapidly taps the client's glabellar region (the smooth area on the frontal bone between the eyebrows) eight to ten times. Normally the lids blink several times in response to the taps and then remain open. A disinhibited, abnormal response is one in which reflex blinking continues throughout the tapping (Jenkyn, Reeves, Warren, et al., 1985).

Motor

Gait. The examination of the gait is discussed in this chapter, in the section on the musculoskeletal system.

Abnormal Movements. Fine fasciculation (small local contraction of muscles visible through the skin) in the calves, unless associated with weakness and atrophy, may be a normal finding in the elderly male (Granacher, 1981) but is rarely found in women (Caird, 1982). Cold exposure increases the occurrence of fasciculation. If fasciculations are numerous and there are signs of rapid muscle weakening, electromyographic studies should be obtained.

The tremor of Parkinson's disease and essential tremors (also known as idiopathic, senile, familial) are common forms in the elderly population. Characteristics of these tremors are summarized in Table 5–7.

Proprioception and Cerebellar Function. The tandem gait (walking heel to toe) remains

Table 5–7. COMMON TREMORS

Characteristics	Essential Tremor	Parkinsonian Tremor
Head involvement	Common	Rare
Voice involvement	Tremor	Microphonia
Hand involvement	Common	"Pillroll" movement
Foot involvement	Uncommon	Flexion/extension
Increased with	Voluntary action	Emotion; present at rest
Suppressed with	Alcohol	Voluntary action, sleep, conscious effort

(Data from Bannister, 1985; Gilmore, 1984.)

intact in normal elderly individuals (Potvin, Syndulko, Tourtellotte, et al., 1980). The ability to stand on one leg is frequently impaired, but there is speculation that this problem may be related to proprioceptive and sensory loss rather than to cerebellar dysfunction (Katzman & Terry, 1983). The finger-to-nose test is a test of the proprioceptive system. The examiner's finger is held about 18 inches away from the patient. The patient is instructed to repeatedly, and with increasing speed, alternate touching his nose and the examiner's finger, and then to repeat the process with his eyes closed. The test is generally accurate with elderly individuals if the client understands the instructions (Caird, 1982). Of 51 normal elderly people with no apparent proprioceptive loss who were given finger-to-nose test by Kokmen and associates (1977), 15% demonstrated an abnormal terminal tremor or hesitation. When one test of proprioception demonstrates an abnormality, other procedures may be done to verify the problem. The individual can be asked to run the heel of each foot down the shin of the opposite leg while lying down. It is also important to observe the client in action situations that require balance to complete the movement (Rijsdorp, 1981).

To test equilibratory coordination the patient is asked to stand with the feet close together. The examiner encircles the patient with the arms without touching. The patient is assured that the examiner will not let him or her fall. The patient is asked to close the eyes. The ataxia of the posterior column disease only appears or is worsened with the eyes closed. The direction of the fall gives an indication of the location of the cerebellar lesion (DeGowin & DeGowin, 1987).

Meningeal Irritation. Nuchal rigidity (stiff neck, tested by cervical flexing) is a test for meningeal irritation, which occurs with meningitis or subarachnoid hemorrhage. Although cervical spondylosis, a common disorder in the elderly, may make it harder to assess neck stiffness, there is still some forward flexibility at the atlanto-occipital joint with this orthopedic disorder. Therefore, if complete neck rigidity is found, meningeal irritation should be suspected (Carter, 1986). In another test for meningeal irritation, Brudzinski's sign, the patient is placed in a supine position and the examiner flexes the patient's head toward the sternum. With a positive sign, the patient resists the movement, usually complains of pain, and may flex the hips and knees. Kernig's sign for meningeal irritation does not involve neck mobility. To elicit Kernig's sign, the patient, supine with the leg flexed at the hip, is instructed to extend the lower part of that leg. A positive sign is the inability to extend the leg or the presence of resistance or pain with that movement (Malasanos, Barkauskas, Moss, et al., 1986).

Mental Status. The assessment of cognitive function and mental status is discussed in depth in Chapter 6. Given that many common disorders of the elderly are characterized by mental status changes, a mental status evaluation is a critical component of any neurologic examination. Cummings and Benson (1983) recommend incorporating a four-step examination that probes wide areas of mentation. These areas—awareness, language, learning, and visuospatial—were selected for their sensitivity and usefulness as screening tools. The patient is observed for any shifting of awareness, lethargy, or drowsiness. Attention can be quickly tested by asking the patient to count backwards from 20 or to name the months of the year backwards. Language is assessed by asking the patient to name common objects and write a sentence on command. Learning may be evaluated by simply asking for orientation to place, date, and time or by asking the patient to repeat three unrelated words immediately and then after a short diversion. Visuospatial skill is assessed by having the patient copy a three-dimensional design.

SUMMARY

This chapter and the previous ones described normal aging changes, common diseases and disorders, and frequently encountered findings in the examination and assessment of the older client. The physical assessment is a valuable tool for the gerontological nurse. Nurses can apply the data from the physical examination to improve their older clients' health and enable them to live as independently as possible.

References

Adams, RD, & Victor, M (1989): *Principles of Neurology* (ed 4). New York, McGraw-Hill, 53–75, 311–322, 449–456.

Anderson, F, & Williams, B (1983): *Practical Management of the Elderly* (ed 4). Oxford, Blackwell.

Avioli, LV (1983): Aging, bone & osteoporosis. *In* Steinberg, FU (ed): *Care of the Geriatric Patient* (ed 6). St. Louis, CV Mosby, 143–153.

Bannister, R (1985): *Brain's Clinical Neurology* (ed 6). London, Oxford University Press, 65–66.

Bender, MB (1974): The incidence and type of perceptual deficiencies in the aged. *In* Fields, WS (ed): *Neurological and Sensory Disorders in the Elderly*. New York, Stratton Intercontinental, 15–31.

Bonikowski, FP (1983): Differential diagnosis of dizziness in the elderly. *Geriatrics*, 38:89–104.

Brandt, KD, & Fife, RS (1986): Aging in relation to the pathogenesis of osteoarthritis. *Clin Rheum Dis*, 11:7–30.

Brower, AC (1988): *Arthritis in Black and White*. Philadelphia, WB Saunders, 49–50.

Caird, FI (1982): Examination of the nervous system. *In* Caird, FI (ed): *Neurological Disorders in the Elderly*. Bristol, Wright-PSG, 44–51.

Calkins, E, & Challa, HR (1985): Disorders of the joints and connective tissue. *In* Andres, R, Bierman, EL, & Hazzard, WR (eds): *Principles of Geriatric Medicine*. New York, McGraw-Hill, 813–844.

Calkins, E, Papademetriore, T, & Challa, H (1986): Musculoskeletal diseases in the elderly. *In* Calkins, E, Davis, PJ, & Ford, AB (eds): *The Practice of Geriatrics*. Philadelphia, WB Saunders, 368–430.

Calne, DB (1983): Normal aging of the nervous system. *In* Andres, R, Bierman, EL, & Hazzard, WR (eds): *Principles of Geriatric Medicine*. New York, McGraw-Hill, 231–235.

Carotenuto, R, & Bullock, J (1980): *Physical Assessment of the Gerontologic Client*. Philadelphia, FA Davis.

Carter, AB (1986): The neurologic aspects of aging. *In* Rossman, I (ed): *Clinical Geriatrics* (ed 3). Philadelphia, JB Lippincott, 326–351.

Cheshire, CM, & Cumming, WFK (1985): The musculoskeletal system: Skeletal muscle. *In* Brocklehurst, JC (ed): *Textbook of Geriatric Medicine and Gerontology* (ed 3). Edinburgh, Churchill Livingstone, 820–833.

Clark, GS (1984): Functional assessment in the elderly. *In* Williams, RF (ed): *Rehabilitation in the Aging*. New York, Raven Press, 111–124.

Collet, BS, Katzew, AB, & Helfand, AE (1984): Podiatry for the geriatric patient. *In* Eisdorfer, C (ed): *Annual Review of Gerontology and Geriatrics*, Vol 4. New York, Springer, 221–234.

Corso, JF (1971): Sensory processes and age effects in normal adults. *J Gerontol*, 26(1):90–105.

Cummings, JL, & Benson, DF (1983): *Dementia: A Clinical Approach*. Boston, Butterworth.

Davies, ADM (1985): The clinical psychology of the elderly. *In* Pathy, MSJ (ed): *Principles and Practice of Geriatric Medicine*. London, John Wiley & Sons, 603–625.

DeGowin, EL, & DeGowin, RL (1987): *Bedside Diagnostic Evaluation* (ed 5). New York, Macmillan.

DeMarchena, O, & Brooke, MH (1983): Muscle disease of the aged. *In* Steinberg, FU (ed): *Care of the Geriatric Patient* (ed 6). St. Louis, CV Mosby, 510–529.

Deyo, RA (1987): Reducing work absenteeism and diagnostic costs for backache. *In* Halder, NM (ed): *Clinical Concepts in Regional Musculoskeletal Illness*. Orlando, Grune & Stratton, 25–50.

Doty, R, Shaman, P, Applebaum, SL, et al. (1984): Smell identification ability: Changes with age. *Science*, 4680(226):1441–1444.

Evans, JG, & Caird, FI (1982): Epidemiology of neurological disorders in old age. *In* Caird, FI (ed): *Neurological Disorders in the Elderly*. Bristol, Wright-PSG, 1–15.

Gibson, T (1985): Disease of joints. *In* Pathy, MSJ (ed): *Principles and Practice of Geriatric Medicine*. London, John Wiley & Sons, 1059–1103.

Gilmore, R (1984): Movement disorders in the elderly. *Geriatrics*, 39(6):65–76.

Grahame, R (1985): The musculoskeletal system: Disease of the joints. *In* Brocklehurst, JC (ed): *Textbook of Geriatric Medicine and Gerontology* (ed 3). Edinburgh, Churchill Livingstone, 795–834.

Granacher, RP (1981): The neurologic examination in geriatric psychiatry. *Psychosomatics*, 22(6):486–499.

Geedas, C (1986): Common foot problems in the elderly. *In* Calkins, E, Davis, P, & Ford, A (eds): *The Practice of Geriatrics*. Philadelphia, WB Saunders, 447.

Gurland, BJ, & Cross, PS (1982): Epidemiology of psychopathology in old age. *Psychiatr Clin North Am*, 5(1):11–26.

Hachinski, VC, Lassen, NA, & Marshall, J (1974): Multi-infarct dementia: A cause of mental deterioration in the elderly. *Lancet*, 2:207–210, 1974.

Hahn, BH (1983): Arthritis, connective tissue disorders, and extra-articular rheumatism. *In* Steinberg, FU (ed): *Care of the Geriatric Patient* (ed 6). St. Louis, CV Mosby, 47–73.

Hammerman, D (1986): Rheumatic disorders. *In* Roseman, I (ed): *Clinical Geriatrics* (ed 3). Philadelphia, JB Lippincott, 513–521.

Hardin, WB (1983): Neurologic aspects. *In* Steinberg, FU (ed): *Care of the Geriatric Patient* (ed 6). St. Louis, CV Mosby, 462–481.

Healey, LA (1984): Rheumatology. *In* Cassel, CK, & Walsh JR (eds): *Geriatric Medicine: Vol 1*. Philadelphia, JB Lippincott, 288–298.

Imms, FJ, & Edholm, OG (1981): Studies of gait and mobility in the elderly. *Age Aging*, 10: 147–156.

Impallomeni, M, Flynn, MD, Kenny, RA, et al. (1984): The elderly and their ankle jerks. *Lancet*, 1(8378):670–672.

Isakov, E, Sazbon, L, Costeff, H, et al. (1984): The diagnostic value of three common primitive reflexes. *Eur Neurol*, 23:17–21.

Jarvik, LF, & Neshkes, RE (1985): Alterations in mental

functions with aging and disease. *In* Andres, R, Bierman, EL, & Hazzard, WR (eds): *Principles of Geriatric Medicine*. New York, McGraw-Hill, 237–247.

Jenkyn, LR, Reeves, AG, Warren, T, et al. (1985): Neurologic signs in senescence. *Arch Neurol, 42*:1154–1157.

Judge, RD, Zuidema, GD, & Fitzgerald, FT (1982): *Clinical Diagnosis* (ed 4). Boston, Little, Brown.

Jupiter, JB (1987): Approach to the patient with shoulder pain. *In* Goroll, AH, May, LA, & Mulley, AG (eds): *Primary Care Medicine*. Philadelphia, JB Lippincott.

Katzman, R, & Terry, R (1983): Normal aging of the nervous system. *In* Katzman, R (ed): *The Neurology of Aging*. Philadelphia, FA Davis, 15–50.

Kokmen, E, Bossemeyer, RW, Barney, J, et al. (1977): Neurological manifestations of aging. *J Gerontol, 32*(4):411–419.

Lehman, HE (1982): Affective disorders in the aged. *Psychiatr Clin North Am, 5*(1):27–44.

Lifschitz, ML, & Harmon, EE (1982): Musculoskeletal problems in the elderly. *In* Schrier, RW (ed): *Clinical Internal Medicine in the Aged*. Philadelphia, WB Saunders, 182–210.

Locke, S, & Galaburda, AM (1978): Neurological disorders of the elderly. *In* Reichel, W (ed): *Clinical Aspects of Aging*. Baltimore, Williams & Wilkins, 133–138.

Lorentz, EJ (1985): Rehabilitation in the elderly. *In* Andres, R, Bierman, EL & Hazzard, WR (eds): *Principles of Geriatric Medicine*. New York, McGraw-Hill, 930–950.

Malasanos, L, Barkauskas, V, Moss, M, et al. (1986): *Health Assessment* (ed 3). St. Louis, CV Mosby.

Milne, JS, & Williamson, JA (1983): A longitudinal study of kyphosis in older people. *Age Aging, 12*:225–233.

Newcombe, DS (1980): Gout and pseudogout. *In* Harvey, AM, Johns, RJ, McKusick, VA, et al. (eds): *The Principles and Practice of Medicine* (ed 20). New York, Appleton-Century-Crofts, 1153–1159.

Nutt, JG (1984): Abnormalities of posture and movement. *In* Cassell, CK, & Walsh, JR (eds): *Geriatric Medicine*, Vol. 1. New York, Springer-Verlag, 50–60.

Potvin, AR, Syndulko, K, Tourtellotte, WE, et al. (1980): Human neurologic function and the aging process. *J Am Geriatr Soc, 28*(1):1–9.

Rapoport, AM, Sheftell, FD, & Baskin, SM (1983): Geriatric headaches. *Geriatrics, 38*(5):81–87.

Rijsdorp, K (1981): Movement characteristics in the elderly. *In* Folmer, ANJ, & Schouten, J (eds): *Geriatrics for the Practitioner: Proceedings of a Seminar Held in Amsterdam*. Princeton, Excerpta Medica, 135–142.

Roeltgen, DP (1983): Infections and the nervous system in the elderly. *Geriatrics, 38*(2):105–116.

Sabin, TD (1982): Biologic aspects of falls and mobility limitations in the elderly. *J Am Geriatr Soc, 30*(1):51–58.

Schaumberg, HH, Spencer, PS, & Ochoa, J (1983): The aging human peripheral nervous system. *In* Katzman, R, & Terry, R (eds): *The Neurology of Aging*. Philadelphia, FA Davis, 111–122.

Shields, RW, Jr (1985): Disease of striated muscle. *In* Andres, R, Bierman, EL, & Hazzard, WR (eds): *Principles of Geriatric Medicine*. New York, McGraw-Hill, 857–861.

Spenser, H, Sonntag, SJ, & Kramer, L (1986): Disorders of the skeletal system. *In* Rossman, I (ed): *Clinical Geriatrics* (ed 3). Philadelphia, JB Lippincott, 523–537.

Steinberg, FU (1983): Rehabilitation medicine. *In* Steinberg, FU (ed): *Care of the Geriatric Patient* (ed 6). St. Louis, CV Mosby, 3–17, 530–550.

Stevens, MB (1980): The differential diagnosis of arthritis. *In* Harvey, AM, Johns, RJ, McKusick, VA, et al. (eds): *The Principles and Practice of Medicine* (ed 20). New York, Appleton-Century-Crofts, 1164–1180.

Sundstrom, WR (1983): Painful shoulders: Diagnosis and management. *Geriatrics, 38*(3):77–80, 85–86, 91, 96.

Swartz, M (1989): *Textbook of Physical Diagnosis*. Philadelphia, WB Saunders, 514.

Tervainen, H, & Calne, DB (1983): Motor system in normal aging and Parkinson's disease. *In* Katzman, R, & Terry R (eds): *The Neurology of Aging*. Philadelphia, FA Davis, 85–109.

Thompson, TL, Moran, MG, & Nies, AS (1983): Psychotropic drug use in the elderly. *N Engl J Med, 308*(3):134–138.

White, RH (1989): Diagnosis and management of shoulder pain. *In* Stultz, B, & Dere, W (eds): *Practical Care of the Ambulatory Patient*. Philadelphia, WB Saunders.

Wolfson, LI, & Katzman, R (1983): The neurologic consultation at age 80. *In* Katzman, R, & Terry, R (eds): *The Neurology of Aging*. Philadelphia, FA Davis, 221–244.

Wigley, FM, & Zieve, PD (1982): Rheumatoid arthritis. *In* Barker, LR, Burton, JR, & Zieve, PD (eds): *Principles of Ambulatory Medicine* (ed 2). Baltimore, Williams & Wilkins, 247–289.

Zizic, TM (1980): Rheumatoid arthritis. *In* Harvey, AM, Johns, RJ, McKusick, VA, et al. (eds): *The Principles and Practice of Medicine* (ed 2). New York, Appleton-Century-Crofts, 1135–1143.

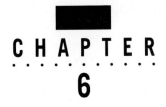

CHAPTER
6

Cognitive Assessment of the Older Client

SALLY A. SALISBURY, R.N.C.S., M.S.

PROLOGUE

A hospital room. Early morning.

    PSYCHIATRIST: How many children do you have?

    MOTHER: They're not children.

    PSYCHIATRIST: Who is President?

    MOTHER: Don't you know?

    PSYCHIATRIST: Where is your home?

    MOTHER: In the country behind a cluster of beautiful Australian pine trees. You're invited.

    PSYCHIATRIST: Who takes care of you?

    MOTHER: Who takes care of you?

Late afternoon of the same day.

    DAUGHTER: Mother, why did you fool that psychiatrist?

    MOTHER: What psychiatrist?

    DAUGHTER: The man who was in here after breakfast.

    MOTHER: Him? He didn't say so. Such a silly kid. Who sent him, anyway?

    DAUGHTER: I don't know. But, why didn't you cooperate?

    MOTHER: I wanted to have some fun with him. I confused him so. He couldn't figure it out.

    DAUGHTER: Oh, mother, you should see what he wrote down.

    MOTHER: Relax, dear. You're so much like your father. What could he write down? I gave him nothing.

INTRODUCTION

The following case was presented during a multidisciplinary treatment team conference on a geropsychiatric evaluation unit of an urban teaching hospital. The psychiatric resident, presenting the case of a 70-year-old patient admitted with diagnoses of depression and dementia, read the following excerpt from the neuropsychologist's evaluation:

> The patient is adequately oriented to place and time. Attention span is within normal limits. Visual perceptual ability on a matching model task is within normal limits. Immediate visual memory is defective and copying shows multiple errors. Recall of brief stories shows mild confabulation with normatively adequate information recall overall. Current background information on screening items is average but more complex testing shows retrograde amnesia with a temporal gradient. These findings are consistent with Korsakoff's syndrome. The patient's failure on visual memory items also is characteristic, as is the confabulatory reporting of recent history. The patient also exhibits lack of insight which leads to difficulty with reasoning and judgment. While the patient is not frankly demented by psychometric standards, the criteria for a diagnosis of Alcohol Amnestic Disorder are met.

Following this erudite summation, the patient's primary nurse interjected, "Yes, that's all very interesting, but can he zip up his fly?" Although flippant in tone, the question is clinically relevant. If cognitive assessment is to be meaningful for the practicing clinician, it must relate to clinical concerns of function and disability, disease process, and treatment response. The identification of a memory deficit in isolation has limited relevance for the practitioner.

This chapter defines cognitive assessment and links specific cognitive deficits to observed behavior. Factors that influence elderly patients' test performance will be discussed. Specific areas of mentation are defined, and formal test instruments, which have been selected for ease of administration and reliability and validity with elderly populations, are presented. Adjuncts to formal testing, assessment of

mental status, and neurologic and functional assessment also are addressed. The application of cognitive assessment skills allows the gerontological nurse to answer the question "Can he zip up his fly?" and effect a solution if one is required.

Cognitive Assessment: Definition and Purpose

Cognitive function refers to performance in intellectual tasks, such as thinking, remembering, perceiving, communicating, orienting, calculating, and problem-solving (Gurland & Cross, 1982). In its narrowest sense, cognitive assessment may be equated with cognitive testing. Cognitive tests are those that systematically measure an individual's ability to perform specific cerebral functions, performed sequentially or simultaneously by different areas of the brain, either consciously or unconsciously. The recent exponential growth of the fields of psychobiology (Restak, 1979) and neuropsychology (Reitan & Davison, 1974; Lezak, 1983) has greatly enhanced psychologists' ability to evaluate, through formal testing, the performance of specific cerebral functions and to identify areas of the brain that affect certain behaviors and perceptions. The tests used in this type of assessment are invaluable in the process of diagnosing specific deficits, in establishing normative values, and in measuring decline. Nurses in practice may consider all such testing within the realm of the neuropsychologist and fail to relate the results of formal neuropsychologic testing to patient behavior and possible interventions. The tendency of health care providers to intuit patient deficits and interventions results in an oversimplification of their observations, which is no more helpful than overspecification. Providers tend to describe patients as confused, disoriented, or combative. These terms have so many possible interpretations that they offer no guidelines to problem identification or solution.

In a broader sense, cognitive assessment involves evaluating how our cerebral functions enhance or limit our being in the world. We perceive, interpret our perceptions, relate them to our prior experiences, and store them in memory. As we are performing these functions we experience feelings, and we may or may not initiate motor responses. Subsequent stimuli may initiate the retrieval of previously stored information, or we may encode and store the new information separately. At some future time we might infer causality or similarity between new and previously stored information. These processes are dependent on our ability to attend to the world around us with selective attention and to perceive stimuli, verbal language, and sensory input in a way consistent with the perceptions of the majority of the other humans who make up our social field. (See Table 6–1 for a list of terms and definitions used in cognitive assessment.)

By way of example, consider a nursing home resident with Alzheimer's disease who formerly was a concert pianist. As he enters the day room, he is unable to focus his attention on the piano. An aide walks him to the piano, opens the keyboard, and seats him at the bench. The aide has focused the patient's attention on a selected stimulus. The act of sitting in a familiar position, in front of a familiar object, allows the patient's proprioceptor sense to enhance his retrieval of a long-term memory by forming an association. He plays part of a Chopin concerto with few errors. His auditory sense processes information and relates it to stored information, allowing him to recognize and correct his errors by executing fine motor movements. The encouragement and praise he receives from staff and residents in his audience help to sustain his attention and enhance his performance moti-

Table 6–1. DEFINITION OF TERMS

Term	Definition
Mood	A pervasive and sustained emotion that may markedly color a person's perception of the world. Examples of moods are depression, anxiety, elation.
Affect	A subjectively experienced feeling state or emotion that is expressed by observable behavior.
Speech	The use of language to express ideas and thoughts.
Thought content	The ideas, meaning, connection, and progression of a patient's mental process expressed by language.
Insight	The ability of a person to observe himself and his situation and to interpret this observation in a way that is consistent with the perceptions of others.
Judgment	As used in this chapter, the term refers to social judgment, that is, the ability to recognize social situations and the socially appropriate response in such situations, and to apply the correct response when faced with the real situation.
Memory	The intellectual function that registers stimuli, stores them as perceptions, and retrieves them at will.
Attention	The ability to focus in a sustained manner on one activity.
Concentration	The effortful, deliberate, and heightened state of attention in which irrelevant stimuli are deliberately excluded from conscious awareness.
Perception	The intellectual function that integrates sensory impressions into meaningful data and to memory. Perceptual functions include such activities as awareness, recognition, discrimination, patterning, and orientation.
Orientation	Awareness of where one is in relation to time, place, person, and situation.
Language	An expressive intellectual function through which information is communicated or acted upon.
Constructional praxis	The capacity to draw or construct two- or three-dimensional figures or shapes. This complex function depends on accurate visual perception, integration of perception into kinesthetic images, and translating the kinesthetic images into fine motor patterns that do the construction.

(Data from *Diagnostic and Statitical Manual of Mental Disorders*, DSM-III-R. Washington, DC, American Psychiatric Association, 1987, 391–405; Lezak, M: *Neuropsychological Assessment*. New York, Oxford University Press, 1983, 20, 25, 50–73; Strub, R, & Black, FW (eds): *The Mental Status Examination in Neurology*. Philadelphia, FA Davis, 1985, 100–101, 126.)

vation. This simple example illustrates how the cerebral process of attention, association, memory, and emotions interact with and respond to interpersonal and sensory stimuli to influence performance.

To be clinically relevant, cognitive assessment must include more than assessment of cognitive function. It must address function and mental status. Cognitive assessment includes perception, language, memory, construction, attention, concentration, orientation, and calculation. An evaluation of function determines a person's ability to perform necessary activities of daily living and instrumental activities of daily living, as well as ability to solve problems and to set and attain appropriate goals. Mental status evaluates a person's affect, mood, thinking, reasoning, judgment, and insight. Such an evaluation is within the purview of advanced clinical nursing practice and is essential for the provision of nursing care that is directed at correcting, compensating for, or preventing disability and enhancing health and well-being.

Assessment of cognition and mental status of the elderly must be done in the context of what is normal for the elderly in each of the aforementioned areas. In providing guidelines for the practitioner, instruments will be identified that have been age-adjusted for normal and have shown validity and reliability in clinical settings. Care has been taken to select instruments that can be administered in any setting and in a brief period of time. Methods that require elaborate instrumentation for their administration and scoring are omitted intentionally. The instruments presented in this chapter are those that the practicing nurse can use to identify deficits and measure small increments of change in a single patient or group of patients over time.

Factors Influencing Performance

When a patient has reached the point on the health-illness continuum where the nurse is doing a comprehensive assessment, some problem already exists. Cognition is seldom assessed unless abnormal results are expected.

Therefore, it is safe to assume that the patient being assessed may be fearful, disoriented, and unable or unwilling to cooperate. If the illness is a dementing type, the patient may be unaware of or deny any difficulties and may be brought in for treatment by family or community sources (Reifler, Cox, & Hanley, 1981). The assessment process is the beginning of the treatment process. Treatment can only produce positive outcome through the cooperative effort of patient and nurse. The primary goal of any treatment episode is to produce change in the desired direction.

The setting in which the assessment occurs is another critical variable that may affect patient performance. Ideally, elderly patients should be assessed in their home environment before admission to an inpatient setting to obtain an understanding of their overall baseline function (Lamont, Sampson, Mathias, et al., 1983).

Once in a health care institution, the elderly patient's functioning may be altered by interaction with the new environment. In long-term care settings, loss of personal control may decrease functional ability. In acute care settings, the stress of illness, unfamiliar surroundings, and immobility may produce functional loss. In one study, Roslaniec and Fitzpatrick (1979) found significant disorientation occurring after 4 inpatient days in a sample of 25 elderly patients. Research is needed to compare patients' performance on formal cognitive measures before, during, and after acute hospitalization.

The ability, perception, and objectivity of the person making the assessment, as well as the tools of measurement used, are other factors that influence performance. Rubenstein, Schairer, Wieland, and associates (1984) compared the scores on the Physical Self-Maintenance Scale, which hospitalized elderly persons gave themselves, with the scores on the same instrument that were given to the patients by their nurses and significant others. The patients rated themselves on self-report as functioning better than their significant others rated them. The nurses' scores fell between the high patient rating and the lower significant other rating. The inference is that systematic and objective ratings of ability and performance are needed to supplement the patient's and family's descriptions of function.

Characteristics of the patient as a person apart from the setting and the rater must be identified and considered to determine their possible influence on performance. Some of these are the presence and severity of active illness and the overall state of health, age, education, cultural and socioeconomic background, and motivation to interact with and influence the rater.

The administration of cognitive testing may be very threatening to a patient who is either denying the deficits or being made anxious by them. Raters should have an awareness of the mental status of the patient before beginning to test. It is important to time and frame the test appropriately. Learning to do this is part of the art of clinical practice and is difficult to elucidate, but the following suggestions may be useful. Some patients, such as those with good social skills and a sense of humor, do very well if the test is framed as a game or puzzle intended to help solve the riddle of why they are having difficulty with their memories. Anxious and fearful patients may need more focus on their successes, the tester again framing the test as a diagnostic tool that will give the treating personnel information to help ease the patient's difficulty. Such patients need time after the test to express their concerns. In telling patients how they did in testing, it is wise to follow an old axiom about telling the truth; that is, is it timely, is it kind, is it necessary? Other patients, particularly those who are depressed, will not respond because of inertia and a fear of being wrong. They generally improve their performance with coaxing and may respond well if their feelings are validated at the start by comments such as, "I know the last thing on earth you feel like doing right now is answer these nonsensical questions, but think of it as taking a pill, an unpleasant necessary part of your treatment here." Truly demented patients do not improve their performance with coaxing, and this distinction can be made by the time two items have been asked.

ASSESSMENT OF MENTAL STATUS

In psychiatry, the mental status examination is a basic assessment tool. In an assessment of cognitive function it is important that the practitioner, whatever the area of specialization, evaluate a person's present state of psychological functioning. Just as a physical examination follows a prescribed outline, mental status examinations review a patient's functioning in a systematic way. The nurse guides the interview, collecting information about the patient in the following areas: general appearance, emotional state, flow of speech and thought, content of thought, insight, and judgment (Adams, 1985).

Patients being interviewed for the purpose of mental status assessment will undoubtedly be anxious. In addition, elderly patients may be experiencing a sense of helplessness in a situation they have not actively sought. Patients may feel physically uncomfortable or may have perceptual or cognitive deficits that hinder their active participation in the interview process. The informal interview is the preferred way to elicit information. In an informal interview, the nurse questions the patient about specific areas while allowing the patient to guide the conversation and express concerns. It has the advantage of conveying to the patient that the interviewer is truly interested in the patient as a person and in learning the patient's perception of the problems. Gurland (1980) suggests setting mental health questions in the context of doing a thorough health and social problem interview to show concern for the patient and build confidence about the interviewer and the entire treatment team.

The Mental Status Examination

General appearance is the impression of overall physical health and a person's demonstrated ability to maintain grooming and hygiene and select appropriate clothing. A great deal can be learned about a patient's self-care ability by observation of the condition of the clothing, hair, nails, and other outward signs. Are there inappropriate aspects to the patient's attire, such as the wearing of several shirts or dresses? If so, a casual comment directed at the layered clothing may elicit a delusional statement, such as, "Yes, I wear layers to keep away the Beatles and dental decay." It may reveal that the patient is unaware of an idiosyncratic style of dressing. General appearance also addresses the patient's level of consciousness. Is the patient hypervigilant, startling at every unpredictable noise, or is the patient drowsy, stuporous, and seemingly unaware of the surroundings?

Emotional state is concerned with mood and affect. Mood is pervasive and lasting, not fleeting or transient, as is an emotional reaction. Well elderly, like all well people, will have a mood that is neither depressed nor overly cheerful. When asked how they feel, they will not complain of depression, agitation, or anxiety. While loneliness and isolation may be common in the elderly, the healthy person acknowledges their existence without dwelling on them. Well persons will describe an adaptation and a general satisfaction with daily life, a sense of peace with themselves. A prevailing mood that the patient describes as painful or troublesome, generally a depression, is termed "dysphoric."

"Affect" is the term used in psychiatry to describe the range of emotions that a person demonstrates in the interview. Affect is more transient than mood, and in the well person it fluctuates with both subject content and situation. In assessing affect, the examiner notes whether there is a range of expression and whether the feelings expressed are expected and related to the content and circumstance. Crying when describing the death of one's spouse and laughing at a joke in the same interview are indicators of an appropriate affect in both content and range.

Flow of speech and thought is the least precise area of the assessment. Conflicting definitions exist for the terms commonly used in this area, such as blocking, word salad, and circumstantiality. It is best to describe what patients say by using a few brief quotations from their speech. In general terms, the nurse can observe whether the speech is fluent or coherent. Do thoughts follow a logical progression or does the patient cling to one idea of thought and repeat it over and over (perseveration)? One patient, when asked why he had come to the hospital, succinctly replied that he had a coherence problem. In fact his self-assessment was most apt. Although verbally very fluent and cognitively intact, he was floridly psychotic.

The patient's thoughts are most easily explored in the context of an informal interview. A good place to begin is to ask about the events that led to the patient's being in a treatment situation. When the patient is reluctant to discuss major conflicts, the interviewer may begin by exploring more neutral topics, moving gradually toward more difficult conflict areas. This is an opportune time to gain a brief history, ascertain who is living in the patient's household, and learn what the patient's lifestyle is like. If the patient describes what sounds like an ideal active life, it is important to ask specifically when, for example, was the last visit to a friend, the last fishing trip, or the last visit from children.

While assessing a patient's thought content, one can examine problem-solving ability by asking situation questions. Examples of this are: What would you do if you woke up ill, home alone, in the middle of the night? What would you do in an airport in a strange city upon discovering that your money and airplane ticket were lost? These questions can be woven into conversation or framed as routine questions that one asks all new patients. The concept of futurity indicates a person's level of optimism and ability to set goals and think abstractly. This can be ascertained by asking, "What would you like to be doing a year from now?" People who are very depressed are often unwilling to think in terms of the future. People with cognitive impairment are often unable to do so.

Insight and judgment are critical areas that are easily assessed during a free-flowing conversation. Insight signifies that patients realize that they are ill (if they are), and that they understand the nature of their illness. It does not refer to the psychodynamics of the illness. Insight may be assessed by asking the following sorts of questions: Are you sick in any way?; What sort of illness do you have?; What do you think would be most helpful for your recovery?

Judgment is often best determined by history from informants, but it may be approximated by asking patients how they have handled their life and what recent decisions they made about their health care and living situation. Impaired insight and judgment may be found in patients with functional disorders or dementing illnesses, and the resultant behaviors may make patients seem more demented than they actually are.

For example, one patient was admitted to an acute-care psychiatric service after repeatedly attempting to leave his nursing home and assaulting the staff there. His most successful attempt at relocation had ended when the highway patrol picked him up traveling down the center of the interstate highway in his wheelchair. The patient had been diagnosed as having Alzheimer's disease and 6 months before had suffered a cerebrovascular accident, with right hemiparesis of upper and lower extremities. Shortly after admission he fell while getting out of bed and broke his right foot. Staff quickly became discouraged because he refused to help with rehabilitation activities. His moods fluctuated between tearful despondency and irritability. When tested, however, he scored 25 on the Folstein Mini Mental State Examination. (See Appendix 6–A.) When time was spent with him in informal conversation it became apparent that although he knew where he was and recalled recent and remote events well, he had absolutely no perception of himself as disabled. The man was enraged at his wife for not taking him home. He also could not understand why his wife, who was receiving radiation treatments for abdominal cancer, was unable to care for him, since in his perception he did not require care. He explained his wheelchair ride on the interstate as simply "going home" and could not understand why it had caused such a fuss. Rather than attempt to change these aberrant perceptions, the nurse focused on improving the patient's health status by using his intact cognition to bargain with him. The patient

was allowed to miss group therapy, which he abhorred, if he would practice self-care activities and ambulation during that time. Once the patient was ambulatory with a walker and was able to dress, groom, and feed himself, it was possible to place him in a more independent, albeit locked, setting rather than in a skilled nursing home. The irony was that the more physically rehabilitated the patient became, the more of an escapement risk he posed, since his insight and judgment remained severely impaired.

Selection of Instruments

Adept interviewing, to aid in making relevant clinical inferences from the information given, is part of the practitioner's art. Formal measurements are available to qualify, quantify, and compare emotional state and establish norms for the elderly. The Brief Psychiatric Rating Scale is an instrument that identifies psychiatric pathology. Overall and Beller (1984) have derived a factor structure for the Brief Psychiatric Rating Scale (BPRS) by analyzing intercorrelation among BPRS symptom ratings for patients in geropsychiatric populations and have found that they differed in important respects from factor structures most often reported from other populations. They included items from the Pfeiffer scale of social functioning for construct validation. In summary, they state that for a complete description of an individual geropsychiatric patient, it is necessary to characterize the presence and degree of the following major areas of psychopathology (the factor structure): cognitive dysfunction, depression, agitation, hostile suspiciousness, and psychotic distortion.

Depression can be assessed by the Zung Self-Rating Depression Scale, the Modified Beck Depression Inventory (Kane & Kane, 1981), and the Geriatric Depression Scale (Yesavage, Brink, Rose, et al., 1981). (See the chapter on depression, Chapter 23.) These instruments are self-report paper tools, and elderly patients may be unable to complete them. The Hamilton Rating Scale for depression uses an interview to determine the degree of depression present, but it is not intended as a screening tool. It has not been validated with use for elderly populations, and its usefulness is contingent on the skill of the interviewer (Hamilton, 1960; Hedlund & Vieweg, 1979).

For a more comprehensive description of available instruments and their appropriateness for specific situations the reader is referred to the following sources: *Assessing the Elderly: A Practical Guide to Measurement*, by Kane and Kane; *Assessment in Geriatric Psychopharmacology*, edited by Crook, Ferris, and Bartus; *Psychiatric Symptoms and Cognitive Loss in the Elderly*, edited by Raskin and Jarvik; and Chapter 23, Depression, in this book.

ASSESSING SPECIFIC COGNITIVE DOMAINS

Memory

Memory formation is dependent on the facilitation of synapses between the temporal lobe, the interpretive area of the brain, and the limbic system, which encodes information in terms of emotional feelings (Penfield & Jasper, 1954). Immediate memory is that which is first activated when a person recognizes and responds to a stimulus. The stored information is referred to as primary memory or immediate recall. This system has a very limited capacity. The normal for an adult is recall of nine forward digits. Immediate memory formation is partially dependent on rehearsal and is very distraction-labile. A person with a deficit in immediate memory may be able to remember only one of five digits forward. This person will not remember just taking medication or eating a meal. If asked to sit on a chair and wait for assistance with ambulation, the person may get up and fall in the time it takes a nurse to locate a wheelchair. Recent, or secondary, memory is not rehearsal-dependent. Information in recent memory is stored for a few minutes to a few hours. Tertiary, remote, or long-term memory formation requires the establishment of a relatively permanent neuronal change in the brain, which transfers information into a stable protein anagram. Patients may be unable to form immediate or recent memories but may recall material that was learned before the onset of their illness. An example is a patient with brain damage who enjoyed watching football. He still recognizes the plays as they are being made and is able to follow the action, although he does not recall which teams are playing or what the score is.

To understand a concept as complex as long-term memory, it is useful to think in terms of episodic and generic memory. Episodic memory is memory of a single event. Generic memories are formed from episodic memory, and each episodic memory is a potential generic memory, like "hot stoves burn" (Schonfield, 1980). Generic memories define concepts and relate to the environment. They are invaluable in assisting us to cope with our physical surroundings, make predictions, and plan appropriate responses. Episodic memory traces link to related generic memories and enable us to use the past to interpret the present. As traces are not used they become susceptible to disintegration. If the character and content of the new information change, appropriate changes can be made in the generic memory, even those that involve how we perceive ourselves.

The capacity and operations of memory have been demonstrated to change with aging. Total knowledge increases with age, and the old, in fact, retrieve information from a larger knowledge base than younger people (Fozard, 1980) and have been demonstrated to have a larger vocabulary than younger subjects (Bowles & Poon, 1985). However, older subjects process verbal information more slowly than younger subjects do (Wingfield, Poon, Lombardi, et al., 1985). Memory for language and the nuances of its use is that component of generic memory that is referred to as semantic memory. Spatial memory, that which acquires and retrieves information about actual physical environmental features, has been found to decline with age (Evans, Brennan, Skorpanich, et al., 1984).

Attention

The prefrontal area of the cerebral cortex enables an individual to maintain a focus of attention, concentrate on a sequence of memories or thoughts, and encode and classify incoming sensory information. Without the ability to maintain one's focus of attention, a person is distracted and loses the train of thought. Such a person may be able to do a one-step arithmetic problem but is unable to answer a serial question or a complex question. The prefrontal area and certain subcortical and right hemispheric areas enable us to maintain attention and perform executive functions of goal formulation, planning, and carrying out goal-directed plans and effective performance (Lezak, 1983). Patients with deficits in these areas may be incapable of volitional activity, even though they possess the cognitive and physical ability to act. Since the system of executive functions can break down at any one of the four components, it is important for the clinician to evaluate each component separately. Techniques will be included in the section on mental status testing and functional assessment.

Perception and Interpretation

All of the cognitive processes described thus far are dependent on accurate perception. Patients with posterior occipital lobe lesions have difficulty processing visual information. Patients with temporal lobe lesions may have impaired sound localization. Parietal lobe lesions may cause astereognosis, the inability to recognize objects through tactile stimulation; tactile localization may be affected.

Parietal lobe lesions or middle cerebral artery strokes may produce contralateral inattention, in which the patient does not attend to stimuli from the affected side, although he or she may be unaware of the deficit. The patient so affected may fail to dress or groom the affected side but is unaware that anything is amiss in this task performance. Lesions of the posterior temporal lobe and the angular gyrus and supramarginal gyrus, the general interpretive area, may cause patients to be unable to integrate sensory input from auditory, visual, or sensory receptive areas. Such a patient may hear, read, and retain sensation but may not recognize thoughts conveyed or the meaning of sensory stimuli (Boss, 1984).

A patient with bilateral temporal and frontal lobe involvement has a short attention span, is hyperreceptive to stimuli and easily distracted, and has a short-term and recent memory deficit and mixed aphasia. In addition, lacking interpretive and mitigating ability, behavior may be combative and impulsive. To attempt reasoning or problem-solving with this patient is nonproductive. Such a patient responds well to short sessions with input limited to concrete, discrete bits of information. The initial focus may be on limiting the assaultive behavior. Environmental manipulation that limits stimuli and firm limits repeated frequently, such as "It is *not* okay to hit people," are successful, particularly if a substitute for aggression is provided: "It *is* okay to hit the pillow." A system of negative or positive reinforcement is not effective, since the patient does not remember the causality. When asked if he had been assaultive on the previous day, such a patient replied, "If they say I hit someone, then I guess I did." After a month of repeated brief instructional sessions, this patient did learn to independently transfer his aggression to inanimate objects. Although he did not possess sufficient language or abstraction skills to communicate feelings spontaneously, he could give staff information about his emotional state if presented with a simple choice of questions: "Does the medicine make you feel the same or different, lively or peaceful, happy or sad, angry or friendly?"

Language

As used here, language refers to a system integrating sensory and motor cerebral centers, which enables people to communicate verbally and in writing. Approximately 90% of the population are right-handed and have a left hemisphere dominance for language.

Left-handed individuals generally have a mixed cerebral dominance pattern (Straub & Black, 1985). An evaluation of the language system involves spontaneous speech, comprehension, repetition, naming, and reading and writing (Strub & Black, 1985).

Spontaneous speech can be evaluated by asking uncomplicated open-ended questions, such as, "Tell me about why you are in the hospital," or "What do you do on an ordinary day?" The patient's ability to produce spontaneous speech should be evaluated, observing for mispronunciation and word-finding difficulty. Comprehension, a person's ability to demonstrate understanding of spoken language, is best tested by asking patients to demonstrate that they understand the examiner by a simple verbal or motor response. Asking questions that can be answered yes or no and having the patient point to common objects are ways to do this. If given more elaborate instructions, apraxia or memory deficits rather than lack of comprehension may cause the patient to fail.

Repetition is assessed by having the patient repeat a phrase or short list of words. Comprehension of writing can be assessed by asking the patient to read a short written command and do what it says. Writing is best tested by having the patient write to command and produce spontaneous written language. Table 6–2 summarizes some of the more common language disorders.

Selection and Use of Instruments

The Mental Status Questionnaire (MSQ) (Zarit, Miller, & Kahn, 1978) and the Short Portable Mental Status Questionnaire (SPMSQ) (Pfeiffer, 1975) are brief, easy-to-administer measures of memory and orientation. The SPMSQ also addresses attention and mental control by asking the patient to count backwards by threes from 20 to zero. (See Appendix 6–B.)

The SPMSQ consists of only ten questions. Ratings are made on the basis of errors: 0 to 2 means intact status, 3 to 4 means mild intellectual impairment, 5 to 7 means moderate impairment, and 8 to 10 means severe intellectual impairment. Because it requires no special training, is quickly administered and scored, and is well known, the SPMSQ is widely used. It does, however, have significant flaws. Nursing home residents or isolated elderly may experience each day as just like another and be unaware of day or date (Hays & Borger, 1985). This test was demonstrated to have good precision in differentiating functional psychiatric disorders from extremes of cognitive impairment in an inpatient psychiatric setting (Wolber, Romaniuk, Eastman, et al., 1984). However, it yielded a large number of false negatives when used with inpatients in psychiatric and neurologic departments (Dalton, Pederson, Bloom, et al., 1987; Nelson, Fogel, & Faust, 1986).

The Folstein Mini Mental State Examination (Appendix 6–A) is a more comprehensive instrument that measures orientation, recall, registration, attention, calculation, and language (Folstein, Folstein, & McHugh, 1975; Anthony, LeResche, Niaz, et al., 1982). It also tests praxis and copying of a graphic design. The advantages of this instrument are as follows: With a cooperative patient it can be administered in 10 minutes, with a demented patient it can be completed in 20 minutes. Its reliability has been established in samples of psychiatric and neurologic patients. Its scores correlate with age-adjusted scores on the WAIS. The Folstein Mini Mental State Examination was designed to be administered by health care personnel without special formal training in cognitive psychology. The disadvantage is that it does not address higher cognitive functions of judgment, problem-solving, abstract thought, or calculation. A score of 23 points or less out of a possible 30 in a person with more than 8 years of formal education is indicative of cognitive impairment.

The Cognitive Capacity Screening Examination (CCSE) (Jacobs, Bernard, Delgado, et al., 1977) contains 30 items and can be administered in 15 to 30 minutes by a health-care professional person without special training. Each item is scored one point, and a score of less than 20 is indicative of cognitive impair-

Table 6–2. LANGUAGE DISORDERS

Type of Aphasia	Manifestation	Affected Brain Area
Global	Spontaneous speech absent or limited to a few stereotyped words Comprehension reduced to patient's name or few words	Posterior and anterior cortical areas
Nonfluent aphasia	Telegraphic speech, conjunctions and pronouns not used Repetition and reading aloud impaired Naming may show paraphasias Auditory and reading comprehension intact Often have frustration agitation, depression	Anterior speech area Right-sided hemiplegia
Fluent aphasia	Severe disturbance in auditory comprehension Speech is well articulated but lacks meaningful content, is unrelated to questions, has paraphasias Patient seems unaware he does not make sense; reading and writing are impaired	Posterior language area
Conduction aphasia	Fluent, halting speech, word finding pauses, paraphasias Comprehension good, naming disturbed, reading unimpaired; writing shows errors in spelling, word choice, syntax	Supramarginal gyrus and arcuate fasciculus between anterior and posterior areas
Anomic aphasia	Word finding difficulty, inability to name objects on confrontation. Repetition good. May have alexia (inability to read) and/or agraphia (inability to write)	Can be caused by lesions in many parts of dominant hemisphere
Articulation disturbances (dysarthrias)	Buccofacial apraxia (inability to control muscles needed for speech) Dysfluency (stuttering or stammering)	Lesions between supramarginal gyrus and frontal lobe Etiology not known

(Adapted from Strub, R, & Black, FW (eds): *The Mental Status Examination in Neurology*. Philadelphia, FA Davis, 1985.)

ment. This test measures orientation, concentration, attention, mental control, language functions of repetition and concept formation, and short-term memory (Nelson, et al., 1986). It has an advantage in that it contains guidelines for further exploration if cognitive impairment is present. Many of the items are repetitious, however, and, like the Folstein test, its virtues are reliability and validity, not sensitivity, in that false negatives are frequent (Nelson, Fogel, & Faust, 1986).

The recently developed Neurobehavioral Cognitive Status Examination (NCSE) (Appendix 6–C) independently assesses multiple domains of cognitive function: level of consciousness, attention, concentration, constructions, memory, calculations, and reasoning. Lan-

guage is assessed in the areas of fluency, comprehension, repetition, and naming (Kiernan, Mueller, Langston, et al., 1987). The test has been validated and standardized on a geriatric population. Because it uses a screen and metric approach it can be completed by nonimpaired patients in 5 minutes and by most patients with impairments in 20 minutes. The two-page test booklet is accompanied by a training manual, and can be administered by professional health care providers after self-teaching. Although more difficult to use than other tests, the NCSE provides more patient information than the presence or absence of cognitive impairment (Kiernan, Mueller, Langston, et al., 1987). It has demonstrated more sensitivity than either the Folstein or the

CCSE (Schwamm, Van Dyke, Kiernan, et al., 1987). The NCSE can be obtained from the Department of Psychiatry, Veterans Administration Medical Center, San Francisco, California.

NEUROLOGIC ASSESSMENT

Physical assessment is not within the scope of this chapter, but the following neurologic tests, which are sensitive to cerebral damage, may be routinely included at the conclusion of the mental status examination. They are useful in separating psychotic functional states from pathophysiologic ones. The face-hand laterality test is performed by having patients close their eyes and touch their right and left cheek and back of right and left hand in a variety of ipsilateral and contralateral trials. Patients are asked where they feel the touch. No errors means that cerebral damage is unlikely (Sloane, 1980).

To test the integrative function of stereognosis, the ability to distinguish forms by touch, patients are asked to close their eyes and identify common objects placed in their hands, such as a pencil, coin, or keys. Astereognosis occurs in cortical disease and may be quite dramatic. One patient who chain-smoked cigarettes was unable to identify the cigarette in his hand with his eyes closed, yet superficially his functioning had appeared quite intact, and staff had felt that his fear of getting lost was a manifestation of his anxiety neurosis. He was subsequently diagnosed as having probable Alzheimer's disease.

Normal coordination includes the ability to arrest one motor impulse and substitute its opposite. Loss of this ability, called "diadochokinesia," is characteristic of cerebellar disease and may be tested by asking the patient to perform any type of rapid, alternating movements (DeGowin & DeGowin, 1969). The patient may be asked to raise his arms and rapidly rotate his wrists or to lay his hands on his lap and rapidly pronate and supinate his hands. It is possible to elicit cooperation from even demented patients with poor language comprehension for this test by simply having them imitate the examiner.

Mayer's reflex is absent in pyramidal tract disease. To elicit this reflex, the patient's supinated hand is laid lightly on the examiner's, with the patient's hand relaxed and the thumb abducted. The examiner grasps the patient's ring finger and with the other hand firmly and quickly flexes the patient's metacarpophalangeal joint. The normal response is adduction and apposition of the thumb.

ASSESSMENT OF FUNCTIONAL ABILITY

The mental status examination and cognitive testing give only a partial picture of the patient as a person who has a way of being in a world that may or may not be causing difficulty. To complete the picture, one needs to assess, not assume, actual functioning. An elderly female patient with Korsakoff's disease glibly described how she would call her daughter for help if she woke up ill in the middle of the night, when this question was asked on a mental status examination. When presented with a telephone task during a living skills evaluation, though, the patient was unable to dial the phone. The phone number she had given had belonged to the daughter at one time, but the daughter had moved out of state 6 years before. Disability does not refer to any anatomic defect but is only a descriptive means of inferring subnormal activity (Wolcott, 1981). Disability is not always measurable by objective methods but can be inferred from observing actual performance. Winograd (1984) found that patients in her study who did poorly on the SPMSQ were able to perform independent activities of daily living in a nursing home setting. This suggests that these activities involve areas of mental function—sequencing, sorting, and selection—that are not measured on the cognitive test. Kleban and associates (1976) demonstrated that among an institutionalized population, function, as defined by observed behaviors, declined at a slower rate than cognitive function measured by mental status questionnaire scores. In the community, successful performance in everyday life is more closely linked to the ability to perform complex social tasks, such as balancing a checkbook and paying attention to the news, than to the score on the more common mental status tests (Pfeiffer, 1975).

If a patient is in a protective total environment such as a hospital or long-term care institution, staff may assume disability and impose more assistance with self-care activities than is needed. On the other hand, health care providers may assume that the patient who lives alone must, by definition, be capable of independent function. Salisbury and Coleman (1987) found that systematized in-home assessment of community-dwelling patients evaluated at Alzheimer's centers revealed problems and risks that were not discernible from collateral information; from the psychiatric, neurologic, or physical examination; or from formal cognitive testing. If the patient lives at home, tightly scheduled outpatient visits may not afford the clinician the opportunity for observation. It is the responsibility of the clinician to construct situations for direct observation and to gather collateral information when needed. Is the patient able to independently make and keep an appointment? During the course of a routine physical examination one can observe the patient's ability to dress. Asking for a urine specimen and escorting the patient to the bathroom will reveal whether the patient can use the toilet. Does the patient remember to wash the hands and redress? Can the patient manipulate the faucet on an unfamiliar sink and find the way back to the examining room after using the bathroom without assistance? In inpatient settings one can devise many creative reasons for observing the patient showering and grooming. This initial assessment observation should not be relegated to nonprofessional staff unless the observers have been taught assessment criteria. When taken to the bathroom, does the patient recognize the purpose of the room? Can he initiate activities? Does the patient need encouragement or step-by-step instructions? Does the patient know what to do with a toothbrush placed in the hand?

When bathing does the patient ignore certain parts of the body? The same systematic observations can be applied to mealtime and, equally important, to unstructured time.

Accurate assessment of a patient's functional self-care abilities is needed to determine the existence of specific disabilities, set attainable rehabilitation goals, determine the level of nursing care that will meet these goals, and measure increments of change in a patient or groups of patients. Functional assessment is dealt with in detail in Chapter 7.

All of the material presented thus far has the clinician in the role of director of the assessment process. The clinician selects the line of inquiry and the approach to best obtain information. A refreshing and revealing change in routine is to allow patients to discuss areas in which they feel most comfortable, allowing them to tell about hobbies, show collections, or describe their most meaningful life event as they define it. In this way, the clinician has an opportunity to see patients at their best when they are relaxed and involved in communication about a topic that has relevance. Often, the affect range broadens, verbal production becomes more fluent, and thinking is more clear. If the patient is unable to narrate anything without structured elicitation, this too is revealing. More often, however, the clinician is rewarded with a glimpse of the patient at baseline functioning or a fleeting glimpse of a former baseline. It gives examiners an understanding of the complete person, one who is more than the sum of assessed deficits and abilities.

CLINICAL APPLICATION AND SUMMARY

Cognitive function in the elderly patient is not static. The process of cognitive assessment that has been described here is intended to be a framework within which the practicing nurse interacts with patients, using goal-directed, focused communication. The total assessment can be completed in increments. Certain areas should be repeated to measure the effects of treatment or the impact of illness. The main concept is that deliberative, systematic assessment is a prerequisite of professional nursing care.

If patients have a dementing illness with a recent memory deficit, they may not remember to take medication, or they may take it, forget that they have taken it, and repeat the dose. Simply writing the medication schedule on a card and putting the card in the patient's pocket will not be helpful. The same memory deficits that preclude patients from taking their pills will render them incapable of remembering to read their cue cards. Medication classes and individual patient teaching will not improve compliance with medications if memory loss is the problem. Suppose that while in the hospital, a patient demonstrates that he is capable of responding to environmental cues and learns to follow a ward routine. After meals he comes to the medication room without prompting. The inference can be made that this patient, who is medication-dependent, will be safely compliant in a residential care setting where medications are dispensed at mealtime. The patient can learn to associate meals with medications, provided that someone other than himself generates the cues, that is, meals. Nursing intervention for this patient should focus on arranging suitable placement and preparing the patient for placement, and not on providing medication instruction.

This intervention uses patients' known strengths to place them in the least restrictive setting in which they can maintain their state of health and perhaps avoid increased disability. In this way an accurate assessment forms the foundation for the practice of gerontological nursing.

References

Adams, S (1985): *Mental Status Examination, RN Skills Orientation to Inpatient Psychiatry.* Palo Alto, CA, Veterans Administration Medical Center.

Anthony, JC, LeResche, L, Niaz, U, et al. (1982): Limits of the mini mental state as a screening test for dementia and delirium among hospital patients. *Psycholog Med,* 12:397–408.

Boss, PS (1984): Acute mood and behavior disturbances of neurological origin: Acute confusional states. *J Neurosurg Nurs,* 14:61–68.

Bowles, NL, & Poon, LW (1985): Aging and retrieval of words in semantic memory. *J Gerontol,* 40:71–77.

Crook, T, Ferris, S, & Bartus, R (1983): *Assessment in Geriatric Psychopharmacology.* New Canaan, CT, Mark Powley Associates Inc.

Dalton, JE, Pederson, SL, Bloom, BE, et al. (1987): Diagnostic errors using the short portable mental status questionnaire with a mixed clinical population. *J Gerontol,* 42:512–514.

DeGowin, E, & DeGowin, R (1969): *Bedside Diagnostic Examination.* New York, Macmillan.

Evans, GW, Brennan, PL, Skorpanich, MA, et al. (1984): Cognitive mapping and elderly adults: Verbal and location memory for urban landmarks. *J Gerontol,* 39:452–457.

Folstein, M, Folstein, SE, & McHugh, P (1975): Mini mental state, a practical method for grading the cognitive state of patients for the clinician. *J Psychiatr Res,* 12:189–198.

Fozard, JL (1980): The time for remembering. *In* Poon, L (ed): *Aging in the 1980's.* Washington, DC, American Psychological Association.

Gurland, BJ (1980): The assessment of the mental health status of older adults. *In* Birren, JE, & Sloane, RB (eds): *Handbook of Mental Health and Aging.* Englewood Cliffs, NJ, Prentice-Hall.

Gurland, BJ (1987): The assessment of cognitive function in the elderly. *Clin Geriatr Med,* 3(1):53–63.

Gurland, BJ, & Cross, P (1982): The epidemiology of psychopathology in old age: Some clinical implications. *Psychiatr Clin North Am* 11–26.

Hamilton, M (1960): A rating scale for depression. *J Neurol Neurosurg Psychiatry,* 23:56–62.

Harbot, B & Libow, L (1980): The interrelationship of mental and physical status and its assessment in the older adult: Mind body interaction. *In* Birren, JE, & Sloane, RB (eds): *Handbook of Mental Health and Aging.* Englewood Cliffs, NJ, Prentice-Hall.

Hays, AM, & Borger, F (1985): A test in time. *Am J Nurs,* 85:1107–1111.

Hedlund, JL, & Vieweg, BW (1979): The Hamilton rating scale for depression: A comprehensive review. *J Operat Psychiatry,* 10:149–165.

Jacobs, JW, Bernard, MR, Delgado, A, et al. (1977): Screening for organic mental syndromes in the medically ill. *Ann Intern Med* 86:40–46.

Kahn, RL (1975): The mental health system and the future aged. *Gerontologist,* 15:24–31.

Kane, RA, & Kane, RL (1981): *Assessing the Elderly: A Practical Guide to Measurement.* Lexington, MA, Lexington Books.

Kiernan, R, Mueller, J, Langston, WJ, et al. (1987): The neurobehavioral mental status examination: A brief but differential cognitive assessment. *Ann Intern Med,* 197:481–485.

Kleban, MN, Lawton, MP, Brody, EM, et al. (1976): Behavioral observations of mentally impaired: Those who decline and those who do not. *J Gerontol,* 31:333–339.

Koshansky, GE (1979): Psychiatric rating scales for assessing psychopathology in the elderly: A critical review. *In* Raskin, A, & Jarvik, F (eds): *Psychiatric Symptoms and Cognitive Loss in the Elderly.* New York, Halstead.

Lamont, CT, Sampson, J, Mathias, R, et al. (1983): The outcome of hospitalization for acute illness in the elderly. *J Am Geriatr Soc*, 31:282–294.

Lezck, MD (1983): *Neuropsychological Assessment.* New York, Oxford University Press.

Nelson, A, Fogel, BS, & Faust, D (1986): Bedside cognitive screening instruments: A critical assessment. *J Nerv Ment Dis*, 174:73–83.

Overall, JE, & Beller, SA (1984): The brief psychiatric rating scale (BPRS) in geropsychiatric research: Factor structure on an inpatient unit. *J Gerontol*, 39:187–193.

Penfield, W, & Jasper, H (1954): *Epilepsy and the Functional Anatomy of the Human Brain.* Boston, Little, Brown.

Pfeiffer, E (1975): A short portable mental status questionnaire for the assessment of organic brain deficits in elderly patients. *J Am Geriatr Soc*, 23:433–441.

Reifler, BV, Cox, GB, & Hanley, RJ (1981): Problems of mentally ill elderly as perceived by patients, families and clinicians. *Gerontologist*, 21:165–170.

Reitan, RM, & Davison, LA (1974): *Clinical Neuropsychology: Current Status and Applications.* New York, Winston/Wiley.

Restak, RM (1979): *The Brain: The Last Frontier.* New York, Warner.

Roslaniec, A, & Fitzpatrick, J (1979): Changes in mental status in older adults with four days of hospitalization. *Res Nurs Health*, 12:177–187.

Rubenstein, LZ, Schairer, C, Wieland, GP, et al. (1984): Systematic biases in functional status assessment of elderly adults: Effects of different data sources. *J Gerontol*, 39:686–691.

Salisbury, S, & Coleman, J (1987): The value of in-home assessment of cognitively impaired elderly. Paper presented at the 40th Annual Scientific Meeting of the Gerontological Society of America, Washington, DC.

Schonfield, AED (1980): Learning, memory and aging. *In* Birren, JE, & Sloane, RB (eds): *Handbook of Mental Health and Aging.* Englewood Cliffs, NJ, Prentice-Hall.

Schwamm, LH, Van Dyke, C, Kiernan, RJ, et al. (1987): The neurobehavioral cognitive status examination: Comparison with the cognitive capacity screening examination and mini mental state examination in a neurological population. *Ann Intern Med*, 107:486–491.

Sloane, RB (1980): Organic brain syndrome. *In* Birren, JE, & Sloane, RB (eds): *Handbook of Mental Health and Aging.* Englewood Cliffs, NJ, Prentice-Hall.

Strub, R, & Black, PW (1985): *The Mental Status Examination in Neurology.* Philadelphia, FA Davis.

Wingfield, A, Poon, LW, Lombardi, L, et al. (1985): Speed of processing in normal aging: Effects of speech rate, linguistic structure and processing time. *J Gerontol*, 40:579–585.

Winograd, CH (1984): Mental status tests and the capacity for self-care. *J Am Geriatr Soc*, 32:49–55.

Wolber, G, Romaniuk, M, Eastman, E, et al. (1984): Validity of the short portable mental status questionnaire with elderly psychiatric patients. *J Consult Clin Psychol*, 52:712–713.

Wolcott, L (1981): Rehabilitation and the aged. *In* Keichel, W (ed): *Topics in Aging and Long-Term Care.* Baltimore, Williams & Wilkins.

Yesavage, J, Brink, TL, Rose, T, et al. (1983): Development and validation of a geriatric depression screening scale: A preliminary report. *J Psychiatr Res*, 17:37–49.

Zarit, SH, Miller, NE, & Kahn, RL (1978): Brain function, intellectual impairment and education in the aged. *J Am Geriatr Soc*, 26:58–64.

APPENDIX 6–A

Mini Mental State Examination

_____/30

correct

What is the year? _____ (1)

    season? _____ (1)

    month? _____ (1)

    date (#1)? _____ (1)

    day of the week? _____ (1)

    part of the day? _____

    time of day (+ 1 hour)? _____

What is the name of this place? _____ (1)

On what street is it? _____

What floor are we on? _____ (1)

How long have we been here? _____

What is the name of this city? _____ (1)

What is the name of this county? _____ (1)

What is the name of this state? _____ (1)

Please repeat the following three words. (SHIRT, BROWN, HONESTY)

I would like you to remember these three words.

What are they?   Immediate Recall _____ (111)

Repeat the three words until the patient learns all three.

What are they?   Number of trials _____

Spell the word "world" _____

Now spell the word "world" backwards _____ (11111)

Do you remember the three words I gave you a few minutes ago?

_____   _____   _____ (111)

What is this called?   (Pencil) _____ (1)

        (Watch) _____ (1)

Please repeat the following phrase.

I would like to go home ————————————————

No ifs, ands, or buts ————————————————(1)

Listen carefully, I want you to: (111)

(   ) Take the paper in your right hand

(   ) Fold it in half, and

(   ) Put it on the floor

Do what this says: "Close your eyes" (1)

Write a sentence. (1)

(If the patient cannot write a sentence spontaneously, dictate: "This is a very nice day.")

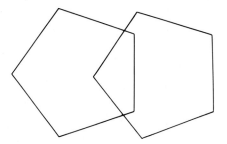

Copy a design: (1)

(From Folstein, M, Folstein, SG, & McHugh, P: Mini mental state, a practical method for grading the cognitive state of patients for the clinician. *J Psychiatr Res*, 1975, 12:189–198. Reprinted by permission.)

APPENDIX 6–B

Short Portable Mental Status Questionnaire (SPMSQ)

1. What is the date today? (month, day, year)
2. What day of the week is it?
3. What is the name of this place?
4. What is your telephone number?
4A. What is your street address? (Ask only if the patient does not have a telephone.)
5. How old are you?
6. When were your born?
7. Who is the President of the U.S. now?
8. Who was President just before him?
9. What was your mother's maiden name?
10. Subtract 3 from 20 and keep subtracting 3 from each new number, all the way down.

Instructions for Completion of the Short Portable Mental Status Questionnaire

Ask the subject questions 1 through 10 in this list and record all answers. All responses to be scored correct must be given by subject without reference to calendar, newspaper, birth certificate, or other aid to memory.

Question 1 is to be scored correct only when the exact month, exact date, and the exact year are given correctly.

Question 2 is self explanatory.

Question 3 should be scored correct if any correct description of the location is given. "My home," correct name of the town or city of residence, or the name of hospital or institution if the subject is institutionalized are all acceptable.

Question 4 should be scored correct when the telephone number can be verified or when the subject can repeat the same number at a different point in the conversation.

Question 5 is scored correct when stated age corresponds to date of birth.

Question 6 is to be scored correct only if the month, date, and year are all given.

Question 7 requires only the last name of the President.

Question 8 requires only the last name of the previous President.

Question 9 does not need to be verified. It is scored correct if a female first name plus a last name other than the subject's last name is given.

Question 10 requires that the entire series be performed correctly in order to be scored as correct. Any error in the series or unwillingness to attempt the series is scored as incorrect.

Scoring of the Short Portable Mental Status Questionnaire (SPMSQ)

For purposes of scoring, three educational levels have been established: (a) persons who have only a grade school education; (b) persons who have had any high school education or who have completed high school; (c) persons who have had any education beyond the high school level, including college, graduate school, or business school.

For white subjects with at least some high school education, but not more than high school education, the following criteria have been established:

0–2 Errors	Intact intellectual function
3–4 Errors	Mild intellectual impairment
5–7 Errors	Moderate intellectual impairment
8–10 Errors	Severe intellectual impairment

Allow one more error if subject has had only a grade school education.

Allow one less error if subject has had education beyond high school.

Allow one more error for black subjects using identical education criteria.

(From Pfeiffer E: A short portable mental status questionnaire for the assessment of organic brain deficit in the elderly patient. *J Am Geriatr Soc*, 23(10):433–441, 1975. Reprinted by permission.)

APPENDIX 6–C

The Neurobehavioral Cognitive Status Examination (NCSE)

NAME: _____   OCCUPATIONAL STATUS: _____

AGE AND DATE OF BIRTH: _____   DATE: _____

NATIVE LANGUAGE: _____   TIME: _____

HANDEDNESS (circle):   L   R   EXAMINER: _____

LEVEL OF EDUCATION: _____   EXAMINATION LOCATION: _____

Cognitive Status Profile*

	LOC	ORI	ATT	LANGUAGE			CONST	MEM	CALC	REASONING	
				COMP	REP	NAM				SIM	JUD
							--6--			--8--	--6--
†AVG. RANGE	-ALERT-	--12--	-(S)8-	-(S)6-	--(S)--	--(S)--	-(S)5-	--12--	-(S)4-	-(S)6-	(S)5-
					--12--	--8--					
		--10--	--6--	--5--	--11--	--7--	--4--	--10--	--3--	--5--	--4--
MILD	--IMP--	--8--	--4--	--4--	--9--	--5--	--3--	--8--	--2--	--4--	--3--
MODERATE		--6--	--2--	--3--	--7--	--3--	--2--	--6--	--1--	--3--	--2--
SEVERE		--4--	--0--	--2--	--5--	--2--	--0--	--4--	--0--	--2--	--1--
Write in lower scores											

ABBREVIATIONS:
ATT	– Attention	JUD	– Judgment	ORI	– Orientation
CALC	– Calculations	LOC	– Level of	REP	– Repetition
COMP	– Comprehension		Consciousness	S	– Screen
CONST	– Constructions	MEM	– Memory	SIM	– Similarities
IMP	– Impaired	NAM	Naming		

*The validity of this examination depends on administration in strict accordance with the NCSE Manual.

†For patients over age 65 the average range extends to the "mild impairment level" for Constructions, Memory, and Similarities.

Note: Not all brain lesions produce cognitive deficits that will be detected by the NCSE. Normal scores, therefore, cannot be taken as evidence that brain pathology does *not* exist. Similarly, scores falling in the mild, moderate, or severe range of impairment do not *necessarily* reflect brain dysfunction (see the section of the NCSE Manual entitled "Cautions in Interpretation").

(© Copyright 1983, 1988. The Northern California Neurobehavioral Group, Inc., P. O. Box 460, Fairfax, CA 94930. Reprinted by permission.)

THE NEUROBEHAVIORAL COGNITIVE STATUS EXAMINATION (NCSE)

Record patient's responses verbatim. _____

I. LEVEL OF CONSCIOUSNESS: Alert _____ Lethargic _____ Fluctuating _____
   Describe patient's condition: _____
   _____

II.   ORIENTATION (Score 2, 1, or 0.)

			Response	Score
A. Person	1.	Name (0 pts.)	_____	___
	2.	Age (2 pts.)	_____	___
B. Place	1.	Current location (2 pts.)	_____	___
	2.	City (2 pts.)	_____	___
C. Time	1.	Date: mo (1 pt.) ___ day (1 pt.) ___ yr. (2 pts.) ___		___
	2.	Day of week (1 pt.)	_____	___
	3.	Time of day within one hour (1 pt.)	_____	___

Total Score _____

III.   ATTENTION

A. Digit Repetition
   1. Screen: 8-3-5-2-9-1   Pass ___   Fail ___
   2. Metric: Graded digit repetition (Score 1 or 0; discontinue after 2 misses at one level.)

Score	Score	Score	Score
3-7-2 ___	5-1-4-9 ___	8-3-5-2-9 ___	2-8-5-1-6-4 ___
4-9-5 ___	9-2-7-4 ___	6-1-7-3-8 ___	9-1-7-5-8-2 ___

Total Score _____

B. Four Word Memory Task
   Give the four unrelated words from Section VI: robin, carrot, piano, green.
   (Alternate list: table, lion, orange, glove.) Have patient repeat the four words twice correctly (see Manual) and record the number of trials required to do this: _____.

IV. LANGUAGE
    A. Speech Sample
        1. Fishing Picture (Record patient's response verbatim.)

_____
_____
_____
_____

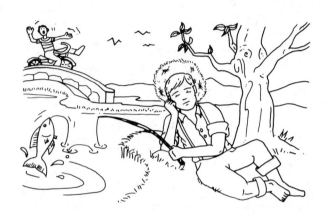

    B. Comprehension (Be sure to have at least 3 other objects in front of the patient for this test.) If a, b, and c are successfully completed, praxis for these tasks is assumed normal.
        1. Screen: 3-step command: "Turn over the paper, hand me the pen, and point to your nose."

                                            Pass _____   Fail _____

        2. Metric: (Score 1 or 0.) If incorrect, describe behavior.

	Response	Score
a. Pick up the pen.	_____	___
b. Point to the floor.	_____	___
c. Hand me the keys.	_____	___
d. Point to the pen and pick up the keys.	_____	___
e. Hand me the paper and point to the coin.	_____	___
f. Point to the keys, hand me the pen, and pick up the coin.	_____	___

                                                 Total Score _____

C. Repetition
   1. Screen: The beginning movement revealed the composer's intention

   Pass _____   Fail _____

   2. Metric: (Score 2 if first try correct; 1 if second try correct; 0 if incorrect.)

   Response   *Score*
      a. Out the window.   _____   ____

      b. He swam across the lake.   _____   ____

      c. The winding road led to the vil-   _____   ____
         lage.

      d. He left the latch open.   _____   ____

      e. The honeycomb drew a swarm of   _____   ____
         bees.

      f. No ifs, ands, or buts.   _____   ____

                                      Total Score _____

D. Naming
   1. Screen: a) Pen __   b) Cap or Top __   c) Clip __   d) Point, Tip or Nib __

   2. Metric: (Score 1 or 0.)   Pass _____   Fail __

	Response	*Score*			*Response*	*Score*
a. Shoe	_____	____	e. Horseshoe		_____	____
b. Bus	_____	____	f. Anchor		_____	____
c. Ladder	_____	____	g. Octopus		_____	____
d. Kite	_____	____	h. Xylophone		_____	____

                                      Total Score _____

a

b

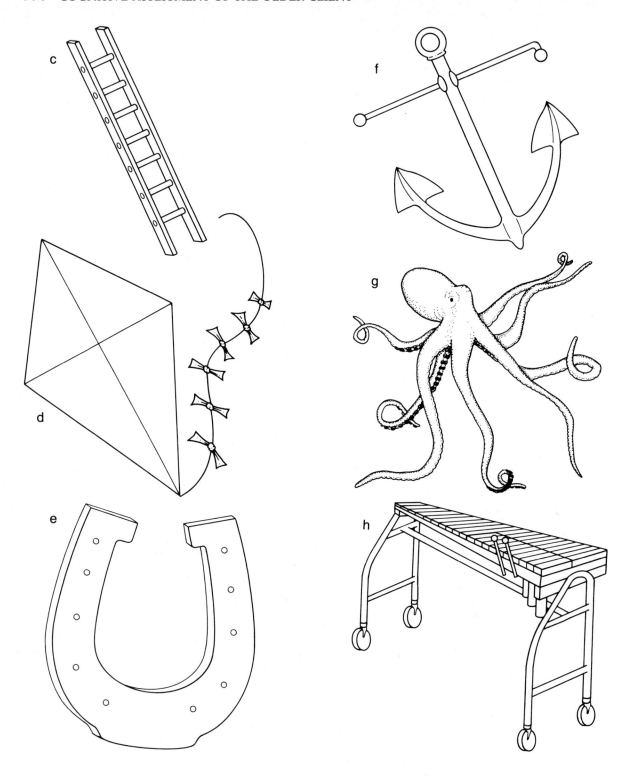

V. CONSTRUCTIONAL ABILITY

A. **Screen:** Visual Memory Task (Present stimulus sheet for 10 seconds, then have patient draw the two figures from memory. Must be perfect to pass. The examiner may wish to have patients who fail the screen copy the two figures.)

Pass _____   Fail _____

B. **Metric:** Design Constructions (Score 2 if correct in 0—30 seconds; 1 if correct in 31–60 seconds; 0 if correct in greater than 60 seconds or incorrect.)

Record incorrect attempts below   *Time*   *Score*

Place squares in front of patient as shown here:

1. Design 1:   ____   ____

2. Design 2:   ____   ____

3. Design 3:   ____   ____

Total Score _____

VI. MEMORY (Score 3 if recalled without prompting; 2 if recalled with category prompt; 1 if recognized from list; 0 if not recognized.) Check if correct.

Words	Check	Category Prompt	Check of Response	List (circle)	Score
Robin	_____	Bird	_____	Sparrow, robin, blue-jay	_____
Carrot	_____	Vegetable	_____	Carrot, potato, onion	_____
Piano	_____	Musical instrument	_____	Violin, guitar, piano	_____
Green	_____	Color	_____	Red, green, yellow	_____

Incorrect initial response: _____   Total Score _____

VII. CALCULATIONS
    A. Screen: 5 × 13   Response: _____   Time: _____ (Must be correct within 20 seconds.)

                                                   Pass _____   Fail _____

    B. Metric: (Score 1 point if correct within 20 seconds.) Problems may be repeated, but time runs continuously from first presentation.

	Response	*Time*	*Score*
1. How much is 5 + 3?	_____	____	____
2. How much is 15 + 7?	_____	____	____
3. How much is 39 ÷ 3?	_____	____	____
4. How much is 31 − 8?	_____	____	____
		Total Score	_____

VIII. REASONING
    A. Similarities Explain: "A hat and a coat are alike because they are both articles of clothing." If patients does not respond, encourage; if patient gives differences, score 0.)
        1. Screen: Painting-Music (Must be abstract—only "art," "artistic," or "forms of art" are acceptable.)

                                      Pass _____   Fail _____
        2. Metric: (Score 2 if abstract; 1 if imprecisely abstract or concrete; 0 if incorrect.) See manual for examples. Check if abstract.

	Check	*Abstract Concept*	*Other Responses*	*Score*
a. Rose-Tulip	_____	Flowers	_____	____
b. Bicycle-Train	_____	Transportation	_____	____
c. Watch-Ruler	_____	Measurement	_____	____
d. Corkscrew-Hammer	_____	Tools	_____	____
			Total Score	_____

    B. Judgment
        1. Screen: What would you do if you were stranded in the Denver Airport with only $1.00 in your pocket?

_____

_____

                                 Pass _____   Fail _____

        2. Metric: (Score 2 if correct; 1 if partially correct; 0 if incorrect.)
           a. What would you do if you woke up one minute before 8: a.m. and remembered an important appointment downtown at 8:00:

_____

_____

                                                   Score _____

b. What would do if you were walking beside a lake and you saw a two-year-old child playing alone at the end of a pier?

_____

_____

Score _____

c. What would you do if you came home and found that a broken pipe was flooding the kitchen?

_____

_____

Score _____

Total Score _____

IX. MEDICATIONS
List *all* current medications and dosages:
1. _____ 2. _____ 3. _____ 4. _____
5. _____ 6. _____ 7. _____ 8. _____

X. GENERAL COMMENTS
Note any known or observed motor, sensory, or perceptual deficits that may affect test performance (e.g., impaired visual or auditory acuity, tremor, apraxia, dysarthria):

_____

_____

_____

Note "process features" such as distractability, frustration, exhaustion, and nature of cooperation. The patient's impression of his or her performance should also be noted here.

_____

_____

_____

Space for Visual Memory Task

CHAPTER
7

Functional Assessment

YVONNE A. SEHY, R.N.C., M.S., F.N.P./G.N.P.
MARILYN P. WILLIAMS, R.N., M.S.

INTRODUCTION

Functional assessment is that part of a comprehensive health assessment that has as its focus those acts a person can and cannot do.

Generally, this is divided into two major categories: physical and social function.

Physical function includes the following domains: (1) general physical health or absence of illness; (2) activities of daily living (ADLs) or activities needed for self-care, such as bathing, dressing, or walking; and (3) instrumental activities of daily living (IADLs) or activities needed for independent living, such as cooking, shopping, and doing laundry. Social function includes social interactions and resources, subjective well-being and coping, and person-environment fit (Kane & Kane, 1981).

This chapter provides information on assessment of physical and social function, instruments to assess function in each of these categories, and instruments for multidimensional functional assessment.

REASONS FOR FUNCTIONAL ASSESSMENT

A review of the literature and clinical experience yields several reasons for incorporating systematic assessment of function into nursing practice.

First, assessment of functional status defines patient concerns. Illness for the majority of persons is characterized not by pathology or medical diagnosis but by the restriction of activity and/or presence of discomfort (White, Adjelkovic, Pearson, et al., 1967; White, Williams, & Greenberg, 1969). Illness, then, is defined by the patient as restricted activity and/or pain. The medical definition of illness, on the other hand, is viewed in terms of biological or psychological dysfunction. Thus the patient's definition of illness—patient-perceived morbidity—may or may not correlate with the medical definition of illness—clinical morbidity (Wilson-Barnett & Foraham, 1982). This can help to explain why the vast majority of elderly, despite multiple chronic conditions, continue to think of themselves as healthy—they can still do what they used to do.

Figure 7–1 illustrates the relationship between clinical morbidity and patient-perceived morbidity. First, although the goal in most traditional settings is to move patients from Group I to Group IV, often the goal, when working with the chronic problems of the elderly population, is to move patients from Group I to II; that is, persons still may have multiple health problems but regard themselves as healthy because they can still function as before.

Second, functional deficits may represent a manifestation of disease. Unlike ill younger persons, the older adult rarely presents with a single specific complaint that points to the system or organ in which disease occurs. Often, vague complaints, such as feeling weak or tired, lead to an impaired functional status and are the first indicators of a disease process, whether an acute illness or an exacerbation of a chronic disease (Besdine, 1982). Although the reasons for disease presenting first as loss of function in older patients are not well understood, it appears that disease causes a disruption in the homeostasis within the most vulnerable systems. Difficulties in ambulation,

cognition, nutrition, and continence, therefore, can signal disease in almost any system in the elderly (Besdine, 1983).

Third, assessment of functional status may support the decision to treat or not to treat. In the face of little or no functional limitation, treatment of laboratory abnormalities or abnormal test results may be withheld if the treatment carries with it substantial risk and greater discomfort (Besdine, 1983). Similarly, conservative treatment may be continued if it can be documented that the condition has not caused a decline in level of functioning.

Fourth, monitoring of functional status tracks changes in untreated conditions. If a decision has been made not to treat, as mentioned above, functional status must be monitored to determine changes that may indicate a need for reassessment. The patient with previously untreated mitral stenosis may become a candidate for surgery when fatigue or activity intolerance interferes with the level of functioning. Removal of cataracts may or may not be indicated, depending on how much the condition interferes with the person's normal functioning. The nurse using functional assessment to monitor change may advocate cataract removal based on different sets of data in the 80-year-old man who can no longer find his golf ball on the fairway and in the 75-year-old resident of a skilled nursing facility who can no longer find his room due to poor vision.

Fifth, describing remediable functional deficits assists in realistic goal-setting. Cure as a

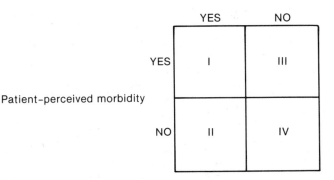

Figure 7–1. The relationship between clinical morbidity and patient-perceived morbidity. (From Wilson, BJ, & Foraham, M (1982): *Recovery From Illness.* New York, John Wiley & Sons.)

goal is often not appropriate when caring for the elderly person with chronic, irreversible conditions, and can lead to a sense of therapeutic impotence. An assessment of functional status can indicate strengths and define problem areas for further assessment. A return to or maintenance of functional status can then be reflected in the care plan, with appropriate interventions aimed at the source of the deficit. For example, the patient with a dementia who is hospitalized with a fractured hip after a fall may not be discharged ambulatory and cognitively intact. However, practical goals for discharge can be based on past abilities to perform ADLs. These goals would center around the maintenance of self-care activities prior to the fall. Not only will these goals be critical when planning discharge but also when giving daily nursing care. Knowledge of patients' functional ability prior to the acute illness will help the nurse determine what they can and should be doing for themselves and what are the appropriate discharge goals.

Sixth, focus on functional status decreases fragmentation within health care teams or in institutional settings by organizing the care plan according to functional status. Since the etiology of functional deficits in the elderly is frequently multifactorial, the expertise of a variety of disciplines is often required to plan and implement interventions aimed at the source of the deficits. It is not uncommon for a stroke victim to be seen by a physician, nurse, occupational therapist (OT), physical therapist (PT), speech therapist (ST), and social worker. Discipline-specific jargon not only hampers communication but interferes with coordination of care, leading to fragmented, discipline-specific goals. Degrees of independence in feeding, transfer, or ambulation are terms that are patient-oriented, measurable, and easily communicated within multidisciplinary settings.

Seventh, assessment of functional deficits assists in determining the need for services. Maddox (1981) emphasizes that services often do not have a beneficial effect for older adults. He cites the key issue as matching the care provided by the service to the specific impairment of the individual. This need for services is not determined by diagnosis alone but rather by specific functional deficits.

Equally important to defining the specific functional deficit is determining the etiological factor(s) of the defined deficits. For example, Mrs. Taylor is 85 years old, living alone, and losing weight because she is not eating. Depending on the etiology of the problem, Meals on Wheels may or may not be appropriate. If Mrs. Taylor is not eating because of difficulty in shopping or preparing food, then Meals on Wheels would be of value. If she is not eating because of anorexia, depression, or moderate dementia, Meals on Wheels will not be useful until these factors are addressed. First defining the functional deficit and then determining its etiology gives direction when attempting to locate appropriate community services.

Eighth, assessment of functional status assists in determining the need for placement. The decision to institutionalize an elderly person, particularly one who is cognitively impaired, is often made within the acute-care hospital at a time when family members are most vulnerable to the suggestions of health care professionals (Johnson & Grant, 1986). If discharge summaries are reflective of the information used to determine placement, it would appear that the decision to institutionalize is based on a list of diagnoses alone. Yet, many older people with long and impressive problem lists are still functioning independently within the community. Medical diagnosis alone is an inadequate indicator of the need for placement (Falcone, 1983). Rather, it is a deteriorating physical and formal support structure combined with the lack of available information that is most often associated with placement decisions.

To illustrate this point, one might attempt to determine the placement for 78-year-old Mr. Melton who was hospitalized 2 weeks ago and will be discharged with the following diagnoses: Left-sided cerebrovascular accident, arteriosclerotic heart disease, diabetes, degenerative joint disease. It will take only a short time before one realizes that major pieces of information regarding Mr. Melton's functional status and social support system are lacking.

Finally, assessment of deficits in function

can assist in ethical decision-making. As P. Jansen, a nursing colleague who works with elderly patients in a local acute-care hospital, so aptly said, "We must realize that when we see the patient on the floor, in the intensive care unit, or in the emergency room, we are seeing a snapshot of that person. What we need is the whole album." Knowing the person's capabilities regarding functional capacity and deficits prior to the illness provides valuable information regarding quality of life issues when making decisions regarding initiating or terminating treatment.

HOW TO CONDUCT A FUNCTIONAL ASSESSMENT

In almost any setting, the nurse is the health care professional who spends the most time with the elderly patient and is therefore in an ideal position to obtain data regarding functional ability.

Actual observation of the person performing the activity is obviously the most valid indicator of functional ability. The nurse in the skilled nursing facility or acute-care or home-care setting can obtain valuable information by simply taking time to watch a person eat, dress, ambulate, or bathe rather than intervening at the first sign of difficulty. Although appropriate for many ADLs, however, observation is most likely not the most efficient way to measure many IADLs. One must rely on report.

If relying on report to assess the person's ability to perform ADLs and IADLs, the nurse must assess the source as well as the reliability of the information. Information obtained from the patient (self-report) may be different from that obtained from a spouse, family member, or friend (proxy), and both may be different when compared to actual observation. Rubenstein and associates (1984) found in a small descriptive study of 24 patients that patients tended to overrate their functional abilities and family members tended to underrate the patient's functional abilities when compared to findings obtained from direct observation by a nurse.

Pinholt and associates (1987) found that although clinicians recognize severe functional impairments, sensitivity of clinical judgment was found to be poor in detecting moderate to mild functional impairments. In chart review studies, only about one-fourth of hospitalized patients with impaired cognitive function had documentation of the impairment (Cheah & Beard, 1980; McCartney & Palmatur, 1985). The ability to predict outcomes or to discriminate among different groups or domains based on scores derived from an assessment instrument may be the instrument's strongest evidence of validity (Kane & Kane, 1981).

The use of a formal tool to evaluate functional status allows the nurse to validate, monitor, and clearly communicate clinical impressions to other members of the health care team.

Functional Assessment Instruments

Instruments that measure function in the elderly have been developed in a variety of settings for a variety of purposes. Social gerontology is responsible for a wealth of research that has resulted in assessment tools. The rehabilitation and long-term care settings have been common sites of instrument development and testing. Since there is a need to more accurately assess the older individual in the clinical setting and the community, nurses and other health care providers are seeking and using functional assessment tools.

Choosing an Instrument

Instruments that assess function in the elderly should be chosen cautiously, based on the purpose of the measurement, the population being assessed, the role of the user, a knowledge of the instrument's content and value assumptions, and the history of the instrument's use (Applegate, 1987). Relevance of an assessment tool should be determined by the attributes of interest. Assessment tools have inherent assumptions or values that are either defined or implicit. For example, specific kinds of activities may be valued by the provider of long-term care services, but the activities available to an elderly individual in a nursing home setting may not meet that person's social needs or be valued by him. Therefore, a measure of participation in activities may be assessed as adequate for that individual as reported by the provider but assessed as quite inadequate by the resident's self-report.

Assessment instruments generally used in clinical settings may be classified as screening, assessment, or monitoring types. Screening for clinical purposes, or case finding, focuses on the likely population at risk and a threshold value such as eligibility for certain services. The specificity, or the extent to which individuals without a characteristic are accurately classified, is more important in screening than sensitivity, or the extent to which individuals who truly manifest a characteristic are accurately classified. This avoids falsely labeling elderly individuals who are not in need of interventions (Applegate, 1987). A screening tool should be brief, inexpensive, and appropriate for administration by nonprofessionals.

An assessment instrument used to diagnose or describe a condition should be capable of detecting increments of change in function. Assessment tools often require judgment of professionals or experts in specialized areas to determine criteria for appropriate measurement and to interpret data collected. Professionals may be required to perform actual data collection if significant judgment is required, although trained interviewers may collect data that are then interpreted or used as a resource by professionals (Kane & Kane, 1981).

Monitoring is rescreening or retesting of specific problem areas at specified intervals, especially following interventions. The frequency of monitoring is based on the expected frequency of change or on signs of actual change. For example, patients in a stroke rehabilitation setting may have ADLs assessed every 2 weeks to measure improvement related to the rehabilitation services.

Reliability and Validity. Issues of reliability and validity are of concern with all assessment instruments. Reliability is the degree to which results of repeated measures of an instrument are consistent or reproducible. Methods for testing reliability include internal consistency, test-retest reliability, and inter-rater reliability. Claims of reliability apply only if the instrument is used under similar conditions of setting, population, and procedure (Kane & Kane, 1981). Ware (1984) recommends instrument reliability scores of 0.90 or above for the purpose of making clinical decisions, although few assessment tools reviewed reported this high reliability. Self-administered questionnaires are more cost-effective than administered interviews, but they may be subject to low reliability levels due to misunderstanding of items, difficulty with accurate recall and reporting, physical frailty, or consensus reporting when others are helping fill out the form (Applegate, 1987).

Actual observation is not usually appropriate for abstract states such as depression, social supports, and shopping. It is most useful for areas of function than can be assessed in the clinical setting in a short time. Assessment instruments that rate abstract concepts such as depression and social support and instruments that require subjective, highly judgmental ratings are less likely to establish high inter-rater reliability (Applegate, 1987). Since the elderly commonly fluctuate in functional abilities within even short time frames, a change in a score due to a real change in status must be differentiated from low test/retest reliability. Also, lack of motivation or lack of the opportunity to perform an activity may be misinterpreted as lack of capacity.

Validity is the degree to which a measure reflects the attribute it is intended to assess. Types of validity are content, convergent, criterion, and predictive validity. Validity is difficult to establish with abstract concepts such as happiness and morale. Clinical judgment has been used to validate mental health measures, but it is not highly correlated with physical health or functional abilities (Kane & Kane, 1981).

The desire to give socially acceptable or personally advantageous responses is common with elderly respondents and is a threat to predictive validity of an instrument or assessment (Mangen, Peterson, & Sanders, 1982). The same threat occurs when elderly persons residing in institutions or otherwise dependent on the services of others feel inhibited in giving truthful responses because they are dependent on caregivers (Kane & Kane, 1981).

There is a need for assessment scores for the elderly that can be compared to allow evaluation of interventions, services, and programs. Multidimensional tools provide summary or composite scores that can meet this need. However, oversimplification in interpreting scores may occur if items or domains are not weighted by some determined value system (Kane & Kane, 1981). As multidimensional instruments are tested for use in clinical practice, modifications may result that promote shorter, less complicated assessments that are acceptable to the elderly and the providers of their care.

Criteria for Selection. The following criteria should be considered when choosing a functional assessment tool:

1. Comprehensiveness: The tool addresses all areas that may be relevant when seeking information to use when planning care to optimize functioning.

2. Acceptability: The most comprehensive tool may not be suitable for particular clinical settings because of length or time of administration. The Older American Resources and Services Center tool may include most information needed but is too lengthy for use in most clinical settings (Pfeiffer, Johnson, & Chiofolo, 1980).

3. Relevance: The data gathered must be useful to the clinical site. Acute-care and home-care sites may require information regarding ADLs as well as IADLs (Robinson & Gigg, 1983), whereas skilled nursing facilities may focus on ADLs alone (Katz, Ford, Moskowitz, et al., 1963; Linn & Linn, 1982; Mahoney & Barthel, 1965). Dichotomous ratings (independent versus dependent) may be appropriate for some sites. Most sites, however, may require more discrimination among levels of disability; often, even slight decrements in

functioning may be very significant in the frail elderly client. Some sites, however, particularly those where staff works with persons with dementia, may need further breakdown regarding assistance needed, that is, whether verbal cuing or actual physical assistance is necessary.

4. Longitudinal use: The key element in the use of any tool is that it tracks change over time. A functional assessment of a person in itself cannot give the critical information necessary to determine if a change has taken place. In long-term care, especially, recognition of a change in status may be more important than an actual observation at any one time (Kane & Kane, 1981).

5. Accessibility: The tool itself and the collected data must be readily accessible by other team members so that it can be used in planning, monitoring, or evaluating care. Information regarding functional status should become a regular part of all means of communication regarding the patient, using methods such as the Kardex, change of shift report, nurses' notes, multidisciplinary rounds, and case management records. Locating a consistent area within the permanent chart where this information is tracked is critical.

This chapter presents several functional assessment instruments. Selection was based on the needs of nurses specializing in care of the elderly in a variety of settings. Instruments were selected that were relatively brief, are of practical clinical interest, and have been tested in settings similar to ones in which nurse specialists and practitioners work. Physical, social, and multidimensional assessment tools are included. Assessment of mental function is presented in a separate chapter.

There are no specific recommendations for training to administer most of the functional assessment instruments included in this chapter. Some instruments indicate preferred characteristics of the test administrator, such as lay observer, interviewers familiar with medical terminology, or a staff member. A few instruments specify minimum criteria expected for training to ensure reliability and validity comparable to those established with previous use of the instrument.* Since potential administrators of assessment tools bring various strengths and weaknesses to the testing situation, supervised practice by experienced, competent administrators is recommended for all those doing assessments in order to strengthen reliability and validity of tests. It is hoped that by integrating use of assessment tools in practice, the body of appropriate measures for the elderly will grow and our nursing practice will be improved.

ASSESSMENT OF PHYSICAL FUNCTION

Measurement of physical health or physical functioning falls into three categories: general physical health or absence of illness, basic self-care activities or ADLs, and more complex activities associated with independent living or IADLs.

Instruments of General Physical Health

General physical health has been determined by utilizing medical diagnoses, physical measurements of health, evaluation of impairments, professional ratings of an individual's health, use of health services, and self-ratings of health. Although none of these methods gives a complete picture of an individual's health status, two instruments that measure physical health have been reported to be acceptable in reliability and validity.

The *Index of Illness* (Shanas, 1962) is a 5-minute, scored, self-report interview of elderly in which respondents report about illnesses experienced during the preceding 4-week period and current health problems from a body systems checklist. There is an open-ended assessment of past health problems and the

---

*OARS test training is available from staff of the Duke University Center for Study of Aging and Human Development, Durham, NC 27710. Functional Assessment Inventory training information is available from Dr. Eric Pfeiffer, University of Southern Florida, Division of Geriatric Psychiatry, 12901 North 30th Street, Tampa, FL 33612.

amount of restricted activity over the past 12 months. This index was reported as a reasonably adequate measure of general health in a national sample of noninstitutionalized elderly based on findings that "sicker" respondents had more complaints about health and were more likely recipients of public welfare money as a main source of income (Stahl, 1984). There is no report of reliability.

The *Older Americans Research and Service Center* (OARS) instrument developed at Duke University (1978) is a multidimensional tool with a section on physical health. (The OARS tool is presented in Appendix 7–A.) A global rating of physical health is obtained following descriptive anchors. It is the most widely used assessment tool that measures physical health for a community sample without physical examination and physiologic tests as part of the data base (Kane & Kane, 1981). The five OARS domains, including physical health, are administered in 1 hour. Test-retest and interrater reliability were reported as high. Consensual and criterion validity were based on professional judgments that correlated well with the instrument. The OARS also discriminates among elderly populations in the community, in outpatient clinics, and in institutional settings (Ernst & Ernst, 1984). The complete OARS tool appears in Appendix 7–A. Questions 37 to 55, 81, 82, and 96 pertain to physical health.

Instruments of Activities of Daily Living

Activities of daily living are those needed for self care—dressing, bathing, toileting, mobility, eating, and continence. Scores on ADL instruments are based on definitions of degree of independent function for each activity or the degree and type of assistance needed for the activity.

The *Katz Index of ADL* (Katz, Ford, Moskowitz, et al., 1963) is a Guttman scale allowing observation and rating of six ADL functions: bathing, dressing, toileting, transference, continence, and feeding. This index has also been adapted as a Likert-type scale to better define degree of dependence for each function measured. The index, which may be administered in about 5 minutes, was highly reproducible in elderly in home-care and sheltered-housing groups (Sherwood, Morris, Mor, et al., 1977). Evidence of concept validity is based on the scale's paralleling of human physical development. Overall ADL scores were correlated with range of motion and cognitive function (Katz, Downs, Cash, et al., 1970). The Katz Index is appropriate for patients in acute or long-term care or in community settings.

The *Barthel Index* (Mahoney & Barthel, 1965) includes 10 items: feeding, moving from a wheelchair to a bed and returning, performing personal toilet, getting on and off the toilet, bathing, walking on a level surface or propelling a wheelchair, ascending and descending stairs, dressing and undressing, maintaining continence of bowels, and controlling the bladder. Scoring takes account of the amount of assistance, if any, needed to perform an activity, and the measure is sensitive to change over time as the individual progresses or declines (Eustis & Patten, 1984). In rehabilitation settings, the Barthel Index correlates well with clinical judgment and is predictive of mortality (Wylie, 1967) and readiness for discharge to less restrictive settings (Granger & Greer, 1976). A Likert scale adaptation of the Barthel Index, called the Barthel Self-Care Rating Scale, includes more items and detailed descriptive anchor points for scoring. This scale appears to be internally consistent but has no test-retest reliabilities reported (Sherwood, Morris, Mor, et al., 1977). The Barthel Index and Self-Care Rating Scale are best suited to rehabilitation and long-term care settings where direct observation of performance can be made (Kane & Kane, 1981). Table 7–1 presents the Barthel self-care rating scale.

The *Kenny Self-Care Evaluation* (Schoening & Iversen, 1965) uses a Likert scale to rate performance in six categories of self-care: bed activities, transfers, locomotion, dressing, personal hygiene, and feeding. Trained observers rate the individual on 17 specific activities by the amount of assistance needed to perform the task. Iversen, Edwards, and Tjelta (1967) found high inter-rater reliabilities of scale ratings of 45 hospitalized rehabilitation patients. The scale is sensitive to changes in physical self-care status (Donaldson, Wagner, & Gresham, 1973).

The *OARS ADL section,* which includes bathing, dressing, toileting, transfers, continence, feeding, walking, and grooming, relies on self-report of the patient or a relative. A global score is obtained for both ADL and IADL function, which prohibits comparison to other ADL instrument scores. The OARS has been widely used in community-based gerontological research (Duke University, 1978). A shorter, 30-minute version of the OARS instrument, the Functional Assessment Inventory, distinguishes among elderly respondents in nursing homes, adult living facilities, adult day care centers, and senior centers (Pfeiffer, Johnson, & Chiofolo, 1980). The authors report reliability and validity similar to the OARS instrument if it is administered by trained interviewers. (See Appendix 7–A. Questions 63 to 70 pertain to ADLs.)

Instruments of Instrumental Activities of Daily Living

Instrumental activities of daily living, those needed to support independent living, generally include housekeeping, food preparation, use of the telephone, doing laundry, using public transportation, taking medicine, handling finances, shopping, mobility, and home maintenance. The same limitations of measuring physical functioning apply to IADLs as to ADLs.

Long-term care settings usually do not encourage IADL performance by the elderly. The choice of an IADL assessment tool should be based on expected performance in the least restrictive setting for the individual. Supportive organizations such as homemaker services or Meals on Wheels may allow an individual with other instrumental skills to live in the home.

The *Instrumental Activities of Daily Living Scale* developed at the Philadelphia Geriatric Center (Lawton & Brody, 1969) focuses on instrumental activities of the elderly necessary for successful community living. The Instrumental Activities of Daily Living Scale is presented in Table 7–2. The eight items on the scale, including food preparation, housekeeping, doing laundry, using a telephone, shopping,

Table 7–1. BARTHEL INDEX

Action	With Help	Independent
1. Feeding (if food needs to be cut up = help)	5	10
2. Moving from wheelchair to bed and return (includes sitting up in bed)	5–10	15
3. Personal toilet (wash face, comb hair, shave, clean teeth)	0	5
4. Getting on and off toilet (handling clothes, wipe, flush)	5	10
5. Bathing self	0	5
6. Walking on level surface (or if unable to walk, propel wheelchair)	0*	5*
7. Ascend and descend stairs	5	10
8. Dressing (includes tying shoes, fastening fasteners)	5	10
9. Controlling bowels	5	10
10. Controlling bladder	5	10

A patient scoring 100 BDI is continent, feeds himself, dresses himself, gets up out of bed and chairs, bathes himself, walks at least a block, and can ascend and descend stairs. This does not mean that he is able to live alone: he may not be able to cook, keep house, and meet the public, but he is able to get along without attendant care.

Definition and Discussion of Scoring

1. Feeding

10 = Independent. The patient can feed himself a meal from a tray or table when someone puts the food within his reach. He must put on an assistive device if this is needed, cut up the food, use salt and pepper, spread butter, etc. He must accomplish this in a reasonable time.

5 = Some help is necessary (with cutting up food, etc., as listed above).

2. Moving from wheelchair to bed and return

15 = Independent in all phases of this activity. Patient can safely approach the bed in his wheelchair, lock brakes, lift footrests, move safely from bed, lie down, come to a sitting position on the side of the bed, change the position of the wheelchair, if necessary, to transfer back into it safely and return to the wheelchair.

10 = Either some minimal help is needed in some step of this activity or the patient needs to be reminded or supervised for safety of one or more parts of this activity.

5 = Patient can come to a sitting position without the help of a second person but needs to be lifted out of bed, or if he transfers with a great deal of help.

3. Doing personal toilet

5 = Patient can wash hands and face, comb hair, clean teeth, and shave. He may use any kind of razor but he must put in blade or plug in razor without help as well as get it from the drawer or cabinet. Female patients must put on own makeup, if used, but need not braid or style hair.

4. Getting on and off toilet

10 = Patient is able to get on and off toilet, fasten and unfasten clothes, prevent soiling of clothes, and use toilet paper without help. He may use a wall bar or other stable object for support if needed. If it is necessary to use a bed pan instead of toilet, he must be able to place it on a chair, empty it, and clean it.

5 = Patient needs help because of imbalance or in handling clothes or in using toilet paper.

5. Bathing self

5 = Patient may use a bath tub, a shower, or take a complete sponge bath. He must be able to do all the steps involved in whichever method is employed without another person being present.

6. Walking on a level surface

15 = Patient can walk at least 50 yards without help or supervision. He may wear braces or prostheses and use crutches, canes, or a walkerette but not a rolling walker. He must be able to lock and unlock braces if used, assume the standing position and sit down, get the necessary mechanical aids into position for use, and dispose of them when he sits. (Putting on and taking off braces is scored under Dressing).

6a. Propelling a wheelchair

5 = If a patient cannot ambulate but can propel a wheelchair independently, he must be able to go around corners, turn around, maneuver the chair to a table, bed, toilet, etc. He must be able to push a chair at least 50 yards. Do not score this item if the patient gets a score for walking.

7. Ascending and descending stairs

10 = Patient is able to go up and down a flight of stairs safely without help or supervision. He may and should use handrails, canes, or crutches when needed. He must be able to carry canes or crutches as he ascends or descends stair.

5 = Patient needs help with or supervision of any one of the above items.

Table continued on following page

Table 7–1. BARTHEL INDEX *Continued*

Definition and Discussion of Scoring

8. Dressing and undressing

10 = Patient is able to put on and remove and fasten all clothing, and tie shoe laces (unless it is necessary to use adaptations for this). This activity includes putting on and removing and fastening corset or braces when these are prescribed. Such special clothing as suspenders, loafer shoes, dresses that open down the front may be used when necessary.

5 = Patient needs help in putting on and removing or fastening any clothing. He must do at least half the work himself. He must accomplish this in a reasonable time.

Women need not be scored on use of a brassiere or girdle unless these are prescribed garments.

9. Continence of bowels

10 = Patient is able to control his bowels and have no accidents. He can use a suppository or take an enema when necessary (as for spinal cord injury patients who have had bowel training).

5 = Patient needs help in using a suppository or taking an enema or has occasional accidents.

10. Controlling bladder

10 = Patient is able to control his bladder day and night. Spinal cord injury patients who wear an external device and leg bag must put them on independently, clean and empty bag, and stay dry day and night.

5 = Patient has occasional accidents or cannot wait for the bed pan or get to the toilet in time or needs help with an external device.

The total score is not as significant or meaningful as the breakdown into individual items, since these indicate where the deficiencies are.

Any applicant to a chronic hospital who scores 100 BDI should be evaluated carefully before admission to see whether such hospitalization is indicated. Discharged patients with 100 BDI should not require further physical therapy but may benefit from a home visit to see whether any environmental adjustments are indicated.

*Score only if unable to walk.

(From Mahoney, FI, & Barthel, DW (1965): Functional evaluation: The Barthel Index. *Maryland State Med J*, 14:62. Reprinted with permission.)

using transportation, taking medications, and handling finances, are based on an interview of an informant. A five- or six-item scale omitting food preparation, housekeeping, and sometimes doing laundry has been used for men to avoid sex bias. Lawton and Brody (1969) report reproducibility of 0.94 (Guttman scales) with a sample of 35 female applicants in a home for the elderly and 13 female family agency clients as well as high inter-rater reliability for 12 elderly rated individuals. Discriminant validity is supported by moderately high intercorrelations of the scale with four other measures of functioning in a sample of applicants to the Philadelphia Geriatric Center (Eustis & Patten, 1984).

The *Pilot Geriatric Arthritis Project Functional Status Measure* (PGAP) (Deniston & Jette, 1980) expands the repertoire of ADL and IADL items to include detailed activities in and out of the home. It includes ratings of the pain and difficulty involved in each activity. Although inter-rater reliability was high, the instrument scores did not correlate with professional ratings (Kane & Kane, 1981).

The *Performance Test of Activities of Daily Living* (PADL) requires the patient to actually perform selected and defined tasks that pertain to grooming and eating and a few instrumental activities of daily living necessary to sustain safe independent living (Kuriansky & Gurland, 1976).

The PADL takes about 20 minutes to administer by a paraprofessional using a portable prop kit. Scoring is done by determining proportion of tasks performed to the level of independence. Pilot study ratings by an interviewer and an observer produced an inter-rater reliability coefficient of 0.902. PADL results correlated more closely with informants' reports, psychiatric diagnosis, physical condition, and disposition than did self-reports of functional ability in a study of 100 hospitalized elderly psychiatric patients (Kuriansky & Gurland, 1976).

ASSESSMENT OF SOCIAL FUNCTION

Systematic assessment of social function provides an objective evaluation of an individ-

Table 7–2. INSTRUMENTAL ACTIVITIES OF DAILY LIVING SCALE

Action	Score
A. Ability to Use Telephone	
1. Operates telephone on own initiative—looks up and dials numbers, etc.	1
2. Dials a few well-known numbers	1
3. Answers telephone but does not dial	1
4. Does not use telephone at all	0
B. Shopping	
1. Takes care of all shopping needs independently	1
2. Shops independently for small purchases	0
3. Needs to be accompanied on any shopping trip	0
4. Completely unable to shop	0
C. Food Preparation	
1. Plans, prepares, and serves adequate meals independently	1
2. Prepares adequate meals if supplied with ingredients	0
3. Heats and serves prepared meals, or prepares meals but does not maintain adequate diet	0
4. Needs to have meals prepared and served	0
D. Housekeeping	
1. Maintains house alone or with occasional assistance (e.g., "heavy work-domestic help")	1
2. Performs light daily tasks such as dishwashing, bedmaking	1
3. Performs light daily tasks but cannot maintain acceptable level of cleanliness	1
4. Needs help with all home maintenance tasks	1
5. Does not participate in any housekeeping tasks	0
E. Laundry	
1. Does personal laundry completely	1
2. Launders small items—rinses socks, stockings, etc.	1
3. All laundry must be done by others	0
F. Mode of Transportation	
1. Travels independently on public transportation or drives own car	1
2. Arranges own travel via taxi, but does not otherwise use public transportation	1
3. Travels on public transportation when assisted or accompanied by another	1
4. Travel limited to taxi or automobile with assistance of another	0
5. Does not travel at all	0
G. Responsibility for Own Medications	
1. Is responsible for taking medication in correct dosages at correct times	1
2. Takes responsibility if medication is prepared in advance in separate dosages	0
3. Is not capable of dispensing own medication	0
H. Ability to Handle Finances	
1. Manages financial matters independently (budgets, write checks, pays rent, bills, goes to bank), collects and keeps track of income	1
2. Manages day-to-day purchases, but needs help with banking, major purchases, etc.	1
3. Incapable of handling money	0

(From Lawton, MP, & Brody, E (1969): Assessment of older people: Self-maintaining and instrumental activities of daily living. *Gerontologist*, 9:181. Reprinted with permission.)

ual's social functioning. Social functioning has been defined as the degree to which people function as members of the community (Donald, Ware, Brook, et al., 1978). Kane and Kane (1981) present three concepts of social functioning: social interactions and resources, subjective well-being and coping, and person-environment fit.

In general, there is no universal agreement on the components of models used to describe social functioning; therefore, measures for specific concepts differ. Norms are not available for many of the measures, and there are few longitudinal studies that correlate social scale scores to later outcomes (Kane & Kane, 1981). Cultural and socioeconomic background and the patient's environment define and limit social activities and relationships, making generalizability of social functioning scales questionable. The problems with reliability and validity of self-report instruments, common to other instruments, also plague social functioning assessment.

Instruments of Social Interactions and Resources

Measures of social interactions and resources include intergenerational support, professional ratings of social functioning, self-reported activity questionnaires, and diaries of daily activities.

Kerckhoff's Mutual Support Index (1965) includes six questions about help received or offered from children. Items are scored from 0 to 2, indicating the presence or absence of a need and whether it was met. A score for average geographic distance between respondent and child is combined with the supportiveness question scores to categorize the family as near or distant and as high or low mutual support. Reliability is questionable due to recall of data, but content validity has been reported (Mindel, 1982).

The *OARS Social Resources Scale* (Duke University, 1978) is the best known general social functioning measure for the elderly. This brief, scored, structured interview may be used for community-dwelling or institutionalized elderly to rate social resources, including family structure, patterns of friendship and visiting, availability of a confidant, and availability of a helper if needed. Appendix 7–A presents the section of the OARS on social resources. Questions 6 to 14, 73, 74, 87, and 88 pertain to social resources.

The *Bennett Social Isolation Scales* (Bennett, 1973a, b; Tec & Granick [Bennett], 1960) measure lifelong patterns of social isolation in the Adult Social Isolation Index; isolation prior to entering a congregate living facility in the Pre-entry Isolation Index; and recent isolation in the Past Month Isolation Index. The semistructured interview identifies the respondents' contacts with children, siblings, friends, rela-tives, spouse, parents, organizations, and the workplace. The scales have been used with groups of older persons from nursing homes, residential centers, geriatric wards of a state mental institution, and public housing apartment buildings, and community residents. Split-half reliability coefficients were 0.52 to 0.86 in various settings for the Adult Isolation Index and 0.10 to 0.62 for the Pre-entry Isolation Index (Nahemow & Bennett, 1967). The validity of the Adult Isolation Index is based on the assumption that the more categories of social contact the individual has, the less isolated he is (Kane & Kane, 1981).

The *Hebrew Rehabilitation Center for the Aged (HRCA) Reduced Activities Inventory* (Sherwood, Morris, Mor, et al., 1977) is a structured interview activity scale that measures interest and participation in eight activities in the institutional setting: reading, watching television, listening to the radio or music, engaging in hobbies, receiving and reading mail, writing letters, taking rides, and participating in informal group activities. Neither the method for combining values from the Likert-type scales to obtain a score nor reliability or validity was reported (Eustis & Patten, 1984).

Instruments of Subjective Well-Being and Coping

Although social well-being is difficult to define, Carp (1977) describes it as the inner aspect of coping, adaptation, or adjustment. Measures of social well-being have included subjective well-being, happiness, morale, life satisfaction, contentment, and personal adjustment. Subjective well-being is associated with positive mental health, so similar items may measure these two domains (Sauer & Warland, 1982).

Coping, or active problem-solving, has been measured with projective tests and responses to hypothetical situations, but a lack of longitudinal data and difficulty with interpretation make validity difficult to establish. The ability to cope depends on the environmental demands for coping, personality traits, and social-role modeling. Accurate prediction of the elderly person's ability to cope would enable more appropriate allocation of supportive resources (Kahana, Fairchild, & Kahana, 1982).

The *Philadelphia Geriatric Center Morale Scale* (Lawton, 1975), a 17-item scale interview or self-administered questionnaire, measures: agitation, attitude toward own aging, and lonely dissatisfaction. The initial version (Lawton, 1972) included five identified factors and had high reported test-retest reliability. Further revisions by Morris and Sherwood (1975) and Lawton (1975) resulted in the three-factor version. The instrument has reported predictive validity in that high morale correlated with such variables as physical health, participation in activities, satisfaction with social interaction, and mobility, but construct validity needs further testing. Coefficients of internal consistency, split-half reliability, and test-retest reliability were high for large samples of institutional, public housing, and community residents (Sauer & Warland, 1982).

The *Coping with Stress Sentence Completion Test* (Kahana & Kahana, 1978) was developed to assess the coping skills of an elderly person when presented with too few or too many environmental stimuli, conflict, restrictions in affective expression, and lack of continuity between current environment and past environment. The beginnings of 18 sentences are read to the respondent, who completes each statement, taking a total of 5 to 10 minutes for completion. Responses are then coded into one of five types of coping patterns. Reported inter-rater reliability is high, but validity is not reported (Kahana, Fairchild, & Kahana, 1982).

The *Geriatric Scale of Recent Life Events* (Kiyak, Liang, & Kahana, 1976) is a 55-item revision of the Holmes and Rahe Recent Life Events Schedule (Holmes & Rahe, 1967). Among the most stressful events for the elderly were, in descending order: death of a spouse, move to a home for the aged, going to jail, being victim of a crime, stopping driving, and friends and family turning away. Respondents indicate the degree of change required by a given event as well as whether the event has occurred in the previous 3 months. Administered in an interview format, the scale takes about 10 to 15 minutes to complete. This scale correlated with the Holmes and Rahe instrument, although its reliability and validity need further study, especially of construct validity (Kahana, Fairchild, & Kahana, 1982).

Instruments of Person-Environment Fit

Planning for long-term care requires an effort to predict or describe whether a particular care environment is compatible with an individual. The competencies as well as the expectations and preferences of an individual are important in selecting an appropriate environment (Kahana, 1974). Assessment of this area may also be appropriate in evaluating the current environment of community-dwelling elderly. A minimal level of safety, comfort, and courteous physical care is expected for an adequate environment, but subjective perceptions of the environment are probably more important in measuring well-being. Disclosure of negative comments about the environment requires protection of privacy and development of trust in the assessment situation.

The *Satisfaction With Nursing Home Scale* (McCaffree & Harkins, 1976) was developed to measure satisfaction with nursing home life. The 13-item structured interview schedule includes aspects of location, amenities, services, routines, and privileges that are rated as to personal importance and satisfaction to the respondent. Importance and satisfaction are each rated on a 3-point scale of 0 to 2, but only the satisfaction items are used for scoring because, in pilot testing, the single satisfaction scores were highly correlated with satisfaction scores weighted by the personal importance scores. Although there is no information about validity, test-retest reliability is reported high, with inter-rater reliability somewhat lower. The scale may be appropriate for an elderly population with a wide range of functional status and is recommended for further use in nursing homes (Eustis & Patten, 1984).

The *Sheltered Care Environment Scale* (Moos, Gauvain, Max, et al., 1979), part of the Multiphasic Environmental Assessment Procedure (Lemke & Moos, 1984), measures the social climate of a sheltered living facility. The scale taps contrasting staff and resident expectations and perceptions in seven areas: cohesion, conflict, independence, self-expectation, organization, resident influence, and physical comfort. The scale is a self-administered questionnaire with 63 yes-no items. The scale has reported acceptable internal consistency, and all scale items discriminated between skilled nursing facilities, retirement homes, and public housing units for the elderly, although there have been low response rates in settings with severely functionally impaired individuals (Eustis & Patten, 1984). Table 7–3 provides samples of items from this tool.

MULTIDIMENSIONAL ASSESSMENT INSTRUMENTS

Multidimensional measures provide information about functioning across a variety of domains to give a general idea of the overall status of the individual. These instruments are generally lengthy, requiring ½ to 1½ hours to complete and adequate staff training to administer and interpret, but they are considered valuable as initial screening tools that identify areas requiring in-depth assessment (Applegate, 1987).

A group of multidimensional instruments developed in the institutional setting relies on the judgment of caregivers to rate the functional status of patients. These include the Stockton Geriatric Rating Scale (Meer & Baker, 1966), the Parachek Geriatric Rating Scale (Parachek & Miller, 1974), and the Physical and Mental Impairment-of-Function Evaluation Scale (PAMIE) (Gurel, Linn, & Linn, 1972). Although these scales are much briefer and therefore more cost-effective than more extensive multidimensional tools, reliability is significantly weakened by their reliance on caregiver judgment. Although the Stockton Geriatric Rating Scale correlated highly with the OARS scale (Johnston & Stack, 1980), Kane and Kane (1981) recommend self-report and systematic observation over these scales to lessen reliability and validity problems.

The following multidimensional functional

Table 7–3. SHELTERED CARE ENVIRONMENT SCALE (SUBSCALE DESCRIPTIONS)

Relationship Dimensions

Cohesion	Measures how helpful and supportive staff members are toward residents and how involved and supportive residents are with each other.
Conflict	Measures the extent to which residents express anger and are critical of each other and of the facility. (Do residents ever start arguments?)

Personal Growth Dimensions

Independence	Assesses how self-sufficient residents are encouraged to be in their personal affairs and how much responsibility and self-direction they are encouraged to exercise. (Do residents set up their own activities?)
Self-exploration	Measures the extent to which the enviroment encourages residents to express and openly discuss their feelings and concerns. (Are personal problems openly talked about?)

System Maintenance and System Change Dimensions

Organization	Assesses how important order and organization are in the facility, the extent to which residents know what to expect in their day-to-day routine, and how explicit the rules and procedures are. (Are activities for residents carefully planned?)
Resident influence	Measures the extent to which the residents can influence and change the rules and policies of the facility and the extent to which the staff restricts the residents through regulations.
Physical comfort	Measures the extent to which comfort, privacy, pleasant decor, and sensory satisfaction are provided by the physical environment. (Can residents have privacy whenever they want?)

(From Moos RH, Gauvain, M, Max, SW, et al. (1979): Assessing the environments of sheltered care settings. *Gerontologist, 19:*77. Reprinted with permission.)

assessment instruments have had considerable testing with reported reliability and validity. But maintaining reliability and validity when using the instruments in a new setting requires adequate training of interviewers and optimizing of setting and respondent variables to allow accurate data collection.

The *Older Americans Resources and Services Group* (OARS) (Duke University, 1978) was developed for use in clinical research and program evaluation using a multidimensional functional assessment questionnaire (MFAQ), with 105 questions to be administered in about 1 hour. The OARS assesses function in five domains: social resources, economic resources, mental health, physical health, and activities of daily living. Judgment is then made to give an impairment score for each domain, which is then used to derive a cumulative impairment score. Reliability has ranged from low to high, depending on the domain tested, although there was good agreement among raters in assignment of comparative levels of functioning and close agreement on assignment of specific numerical rating (Fillenbaum, 1978). Consensual validity is claimed by the authors, and the OARS has demonstrated ability to discriminate among different populations. The OARS also includes a set of 24 types of services prescribed for respondents: basic maintenance services, supportive services, and remedial services. The services data have not been tested for reliability or validity but are reportedly well accepted by providers (Kane & Kane, 1981). A 30-minute version of the OARS, the *Functional Assessment Inventory* (Pfeiffer, Johnson, & Chiofolo, 1980), yields ratings on the same five domains with reported reliability and validity if administered by trained interviewers.

The *Comprehensive Assessment and Referral Evaluation* (CARE) (Gurland, Kuriansky, Sharpe, et al., 1978) was developed for clinical assessment of community-living elderly as well as institutionalized elderly to provide longitudinal and program-effectiveness data. It is a semistructured interview administered in an average of 90 minutes and is based on self-report, test items, observation, and global judgment. The tool integrates psychiatric, medical, and social items into the interview schedule to avoid stress and embarrassment caused by grouping of difficult or sensitive items. The interview has a standard format for branching to clarify certain items. Reported inter-rater reliability was highest on the psychiatric dimension and lowest on the medical-physical dimension in a 1974 version of the instrument. Interviewer and observer ratings were highly correlated in a cross-national study (Copeland, Kelleher, Kellett, et al., 1976). The authors claim face validity and validity of the instrument sources from which CARE items were derived (Kane & Kane, 1981).

The *Patient Appraisal and Care Evaluation* (PACE) (US Department of Health, Education and Welfare, 1978) was a joint project of Case Western Reserve University Medical School, Harvard University, Johns Hopkins University School of Hygiene and Public Health, and Syracuse University Research Corporation. A Patient Care Management version evolved, emphasizing quality of care assessment and client placement, although medical assessment is emphasized over psychosocial data. A patient care section identifies the need for a variety of services, including nursing, rehabilitation, education, and psychosocial interventions, and identifies those services already provided. Data for the PACE are derived from a variety of sources, including records, direct observations, and the identified respondent. There is no scoring method, since results are meant to be evaluated by a multidisciplinary provider team, with subsequent setting of treatment goals in conjunction with respondent and family. No overall reliability estimates are given, although a test of agreement on data collected from various sources by different investigators was reportedly high (Densen & Jones, 1976). The PACE variables—age, ADL status, number of medically defined conditions, and the presence of a diagnosis of cancer—correlated with survival rates to provide a crude test of predictive validity (Densen, 1976). Falcone (1979) developed a set of algorithms from an original version of the PACE to identify the need for services based on ratings on 22 assessment items. The algorithm correlated highly with recommendations from professionals and shows promise as a decision-making tool (Kane & Kane, 1981).

SUMMARY

Observational measures of physical functioning are best suited to clinical use with elderly individuals, whereas self-report measures such as the OARS ADL scale are more appropriate for large-scale population studies or as screening tools. Observation of performance of a function is always considered more accurate measurement than self-report or report offered by others. Kane and Kane (1981) emphasize that restricted environments with limited opportunity to perform will lead testers to overestimate disabilities, as will a person's failure to perform a function, for whatever reason, be considered a functional limitation.

Measures of social functioning are the least developed of the functional assessment measures. Important areas yet to be clarified are identifying clinically significant thresholds for interpreting social information, methods to accurately collect data on satisfaction with social environment, and longitudinal data describing social well-being over time (Kane & Kane, 1981).

Although multidimensional assessment instruments are more in demand in all geriatric settings, there are several concerns that need to be addressed when selecting one of these tools. The purpose of the assessment and the individuals and setting involved must be compatible with the multidimensional instrument. Selected dimensions of measurement taken from the multidimensional tools cannot be assumed to retain the same reliability and validity as reported in the original instrument. Since the quality of interviewing skills affects any instrument's reliability and validity, the longer multidimensional instruments, especially those that require judgment, require extensive interviewer training. If the instrument requires professional judgment to administer or interpret, assessment costs can be high (Kane & Kane, 1981). Summary rating

scores derived from the multidimensional instrument may allow evaluation or comparison of long-term care programs but may obscure meaningful interpretation for a specific individual. Testing and shortening of multidimensional assessment tools for use in the clinical setting may result in a more practical yet comprehensive assessment of the elderly (Applegate, 1987).

No single assessment instrument is ideal for every situation. The user is advised to select an instrument that has been used in a similar setting and has some indication of reliability and validity for measuring the attributes under evaluation. Applegate (1987) recommends pretesting instruments on a pilot group and performing inter-rater and test-retest reliability studies before using an assessment instrument. Emphasis on both theoretical concept development and psychometric testing of established assessment instruments is needed if measurements are to become more reliable and valid (Mangen, Peterson, & Sanders, 1982). Since each use of an assessment tool provides new information on its reliability and validity in similar or different settings with similar or different populations, clinical use will add to our knowledge of appropriate assessment tools for the elderly in various settings. Refinement and modification of assessment instruments for the elderly will result in more efficient and accurate measurement.

It seems that we have sufficient tools, but we lack efficient tools for the many demands for measurement in assessment of the elderly. Yet, assessment of functional abilities must become a required component of holistic health assessment if health care is to truly meet the needs of our elderly.

References

Applegate, W (1987): Use of assessment instruments in clinical settings. *J Am Geriatr Soc, 35:*45–50.

Bennett, R (1973a): Living conditions and everyday needs of the elderly with particular reference to social isolation. *Int J Aging Hum Dev, 4:*179–198.

Bennett, R (1973b): Social isolation and isolation-reducing programs. *Bull NY Acad Med, 49:*1143–1163.

Besdine, R (1982): The data base of geriatric medicine. *In*

Rowe, J, & Besdine, R (eds): *Health and Disease in Old Age*. Boston, Little, Brown, 1–14.

Besdine, R (1983): The educational utility of comprehensive functional assessment in the elderly. *J Am Geriatr Soc, 31*:651–656.

Carp, FM (1977): Morale: What questions are we asking of whom? In Nydegger, CSN (ed): *Measuring Morale: A Guide to Effective Assessment*. Washington, DC, Gerontological Society.

Cheah, KC, & Beard, OW (1980): Psychiatric findings in the population of a geriatric evaluation unit: Implications. *J Am Geriatr Soc, 28*:153–156.

Copeland, JRM, Kelleher, MJ, Kellett, JM, et al. (1976): A semi-structured clinical interview in the elderly: The geriatric mental state schedule: I. Development and reliability. *Psychol Med, 6*:439–449.

Deniston, OL, & Jette, A (1980): A functional status assessment instrument: Validation in an elderly population. *Health Serv Res, 15*:21–34.

Densen, PM (1976): *An Approach to the Assessment of Long-term Care: Final Report*. Boston, Harvard Center for Community Health and Medical Care.

Densen, PM, & Jones, EW (1976): The patient classification for long-term care developed by four research groups in the United States. *Med Care, 14*(Suppl):126–133.

Donald, CA, Ware, JE, Brook, RH, et al. (1978): *Conceptualization and Measurement of Health for Adults in the Health Insurance Study*, Vol. 4. Social Health (R-1978-4-HEW). Santa Monica, CA, Rand Corporation.

Donaldson, SW, Wagner, CC, & Gresham, GE (1973): A unified ADL evaluation form. *Arch Phys Med Rehabil, 54*:175–180.

Duke University Center for the Study of Aging and Human Development (1978): *Multidimensional Functional Assessment: The OARS Methodology*. Durham, NC, Duke University.

Ernst, M, & Ernst, NS (1984): Functional capacity. In Mangen, DJ, & Petersen, WA (eds): *Research Instruments in Social Gerontology*. Vol. 3. Minneapolis, University of Minnesota Press, 9–84.

Eustis, NN, & Patten, SK (1984): The effectiveness of long-term care. In Mangen, DJ, & Petersen, WA (eds): *Research Instruments in Social Gerontology*. Vol. 3. Minneapolis, University of Minnesota Press, 217–316.

Falcone, AR (1979): *Development of a Long-term Care Information System: Final Report*. Lansing, MI, Office of Services to the Aging.

Falcone, A (1983): Comprehensive functional assessment as an administrative tool. *J Am Geriatr Soc, 31*:642–650.

Fillenbaum, GG (1978): Validity and reliability of the multidimensional functional assessment questionnaire. *In Multidimensional Functional Assessment: The OARS Methodology*. Duke University Center for the Study of Aging and Human Development. Durham, NC, Duke University, 39–50.

Granger, CV, & Greer, DS (1976): Functional status measurement and medical rehabilitation outcomes. *Arch Phys Med Rehabil, 57*:103–109.

Gurel, L, Linn, MW, & Linn, BS (1972): Physical and mental impairment-of-function evaluation in the aged: The PAMIE scale. *J Gerontol, 27*:83–90.

Gurland, BJ, Kuriansky, J, Sharpe, L, et al. (1978): The comprehensive assessment and referral evaluation (CARE): Rationale, development and reliability. *Int J Aging Hum Dev, 8*:9–42.

Holmes, TH, & Rahe, RH (1967): The social readjustment rating scale. *J Psychosom Res, 11*:219–225.

Iversen, IA, Edwards, SN, & Tjelta, G (1967): *A Study of the Interrater Reliability of the Kenny Self-care Evaluation*. Mimeographed report. Minneapolis, American Rehabilitation Foundation.

Johnson, C, & Grant, S (1986): *The Nursing Home in American Society*. Baltimore, Johns Hopkins University Press.

Johnston, JC, & Stack, TF (1980, November): A comparison of the effectiveness of the OARS multi-dimensional assessment tool and the Stockton geriatric rating scale as a means of evaluating functional ability in the hospitalized elderly client. Paper presented at the meeting of the Gerontological Society of America, San Diego.

Kahana, E (1974): Matching environment to needs of the aged: A conceptual scheme. In Gubrium, JF (ed): *Late Life Communities and Environmental Policy*. Springfield, IL, Charles C Thomas.

Kahana, E, Fairchild, T, & Kahana, B (1982): Adaptation. In Mangen, DJ, & Petersen, WA (eds): *Research Instruments in Social Gerontology*. Vol. 1. Minneapolis, University of Minnesota Press, 145–193.

Kahana, E, & Kahana, B (1978): Strategies of coping in institutional environments. Summary Progress Report, NIH Grant Number MH 24959-02.

Kahana, E, & Kahana, B (1982): Coping with stress. In Mangen, DJ, & Petersen, WA (eds): *Research Instruments in Social Gerontology*. Vol. 1. Minneapolis, University of Minnesota Press, 161–162.

Kane, RA, & Kane, RL (1981): *Assessing the Elderly: A Practical Guide to Measurement*. Lexington, MA, Lexington Books, DC Heath.

Katz, S, Downs, TD, Cash, HR, et al. (1970): Progress in development of the index of ADL. *Gerontologist, 10*:20–30.

Katz, S, Ford, AB, Moskowitz, RW, et al. (1963): Studies of illness in the aged: The index of ADL, a standardized measure of biological and psychosocial function. *JAMA, 185*:914–919.

Kerckhoff, AC (1965): Nuclear and extended family relationships: A normative and behavioral analysis. In Shanas, E, & Streib, G (eds): *Social Structure and the Family: Generational Relations*. Englewood Cliffs, NJ, Prentice-Hall.

Kiyak, A, Liang, J, & Kahana, E (1976, August): *A Methodological Inquiry into the Schedule of Recent Life Events*. Paper presented to the American Psychological Association Meetings, Washington, DC.

Kuriansky, J, & Gurland, B (1976): Performance of activities of daily living. *Int J Aging Hum Dev, 7*:343–352.

Lawton, MP (1972): The dimension of morale. In Kent, D, Kastenbaum, R, & Sherwood, S (eds): *Research Planning and Action for the Elderly*. New York, Behavioral Publications, 144–165.

Lawton, MP (1975): The Philadelphia Geriatric Center morale scale. A revision. *J Gerontol, 30*:85–89.

Lawton, MP, & Brody, E (1969): Assessment of older

people: Self-maintaining and instrumental activities of daily living. *Gerontologist, 9:*179–186.

Lemke, S, & Moos, RH (1984): *Multiphasic Environmental Assessment Procedure (MEAP): Handbook for Users.* Palo Alto, CA, Social Ecology Laboratory and GRECC, Veterans Administration Hospital and Stanford University Medical Center.

Linn, M, & Linn, B (1982): The rapid disability rating scale—2. *J Am Geriatr Soc, 30:*378–382.

Maddox, G (1981): Measuring the well-being of older adults. *In* Somers, AR, & Fabian, DR (eds): *The Geriatric Imperative.* New York, Appleton-Century-Crofts, 117–136.

Mahoney, FI, & Barthel, DW (1965): Functional evaluation: The Barthel index. *Maryland State Med J, 14:*61–65.

Mangen, DJ, Peterson, AW, & Sanders, R (1982): Introduction. *In* Mangen, DJ, & Petersen, WA (eds): *Research Instruments in Social Gerontology,* Vol. 1. Minneapolis, University of Minnesota Press, 3–23.

McCaffree, KM, & Harkins, EB (1976): Final report for the evaluation of the outcomes of nursing home care. Seattle, Health Care Study Center, Battelle Human Affairs Research Centers.

McCartney, J, & Palmatur, L (1985): Assessment of cognitive deficit in geriatric patients: A study of physician behavior. *J Am Geriatr Soc, 33:*467–471.

Meer, B, & Baker, JA (1966): The Stockton geriatric rating scale. *J Gerontol, 21:*392–403.

Mindel, CH (1982): Kinship relations. *In* Mangen, DJ, & Petersen, WA (eds): *Research Instruments in Social Gerontology.* Vol. 2. Minneapolis, University of Minnesota Press, 187–229.

Moos, RH, Gauvain, M, Max, SW, et al. (1979): Assessing the environments of sheltered care settings. *Gerontologist, 19:*74–82.

Morris, SN, & Sherwood, S (1975): A retesting and modification of the Philadelphia Geriatric Center morale scale. *J Gerontol, 30:*77–84.

Nahemow, L, & Bennett, R (1967): *Attitude Change with Institutionalization of the Aged. Final Report.* New York, Biometrics Research, New York State Department of Mental Hygiene.

Parachek, JF, & Miller, ER (1974): Validation and standardization of a goal-oriented quick-screening geriatric scale. *J Am Geriatr Soc, 22:*278–283.

Pfeiffer, E, Johnson, TM, & Chiofolo, RC (1980, November): *Functional Assessment of Elderly Subjects in Four Service Settings.* Paper presented at the annual scientific meeting, Gerontological Society of America, San Diego.

Pinholt, EM, Kroenke, K, Hanley, JF, et al. (1987): Functional assessment of the elderly: A comparison of standard instruments with clinical judgment. *Arch Intern Med, 147:*484–488.

Robinson, B, & Gigg, L (1983, March): Functional dependency index. Paper presented at 29th Western Gerontological Society, Albuquerque, NM.

Rubenstein, L, Schairer, C, Wieland, G, et al. (1984): Systematic biases in functional status assessment of elderly adults: Effects of different data sources. *J Gerontol, 39:*686–691.

Sauer, WJ, & Warland, R (1982): Morale and life satisfaction. *In* Mangen, DJ, & Petersen, WA (eds): *Research Instruments in Social Gerontology.* Vol. 1. Minneapolis, University of Minnesota Press, 195–240.

Schoening, HA, & Iversen, IA (1965): *The Kenny Self-Care Evaluation.* Minneapolis, American Rehabilitation Foundation.

Shanas, E (1962): *The Health of Older People.* Cambridge, MA, Harvard University Press.

Sherwood, SJ, Morris, J, Mor, V, et al. (1977): *Compendium of Measures for Describing and Assessing Long-term Care Populations.* Boston, Hebrew Rehabilitation Center for the Aged.

Stahl, SM (1984): Health. *In* Mangen, DJ, & Petersen, WA (eds): *Research Instruments in Social Gerontology.* Vol. 3. Minneapolis, University of Minnesota Press, 85–116.

Tec, N, & Granick (Bennett), R (1960): Social isolation and difficulties in social interaction of residents of a home for the aged. *Social Problems, 7:*226–232.

US Department of Health, Education and Welfare (DHEW) (1978): *Working Document on Patient Care Management.* Washington, DC, US Government Printing Office.

Ware, JE (1984): Methodologic considerations in the selection of health status assessment procedures. *In* Wenger, NK, Mattson, ME, Furberg, CD, et al. (eds): *Assessment of Quality of Life in Clinical Trials of Cardiovascular Therapies.* New York, LeJacq Publishing, 87–111.

White, K, Adjelkovic, D, Pearson, R, et al. (1967): International comparisons of medical care. *N Engl J Med, 277:*516–522.

White, K, Williams, T, & Greenberg, B (1969): International comparisons of medical care. *N Engl J Med, 265:*885.

Wilson-Barnett, J, & Foraham, M (1982): *Recovery from Illness.* New York, John Wiley & Sons.

Wylie, CM (1967): Gauging the response of stroke patients to rehabilitation. *J Am Geriatr Soc, 15:*797–805.

APPENDIX 7–A

OARS Multidimensional Functional Assessment Questionnaire

Subject Number _____

Subject's Address _____
               Street & Number   *City*   *State*

Date of Interview _____

Time Interview Began _____

Interviewer's Name _____

Relationship of Informant to Subject _____

Place of Interview [SPECIFY HOME OR TYPE OF INSTITUTION.]

_____

Subject's Residence if Not the Place of Interview

[SPECIFY HOME OR TYPE OF INSTITUTION.]

PRELIMINARY QUESTIONNAIRE

[ASK QUESTIONS 1–10 AND RECORD ALL ANSWERS. (ASK QUESTION 4a. ONLY IF SUBJECT HAS NO TELEPHONE.) CHECK CORRECT (+) OR INCORRECT (−) FOR EACH AND RECORD TOTAL NUMBER OF ERRORS BASED ON TEN QUESTIONS.]

+	−

1. What is the date today? _____
                               Month   *Day*   *Year*

2. What day of the week is it? _____

3. What is the name of this place? _____

Older Americans Resources and Services Program of the Duke University Center for the Study of Aging and Human Development, Durham, North Carolina 27710. Eric Pfeiffer, M.D., Project Director. © April, 1975. Duke University Center for the Study of Aging and Human Development. All rights reserved. Reprinted with permission.

continued on next page

+	−

4. What is your telephone number? _____

    a. [ASK ONLY IF SUBJECT DOES NOT HAVE A PHONE.]
       What is your street address?

       _____

5. How old are you? _____

6. When were you born? _____
              Month   *Day*   *Year*

7. Who is the president of the U.S. now? _____

8. Who was the president just before him? _____

9. What was your mother's maiden name? _____

10. Subtract 3 from 20 and keep subtracting 3 from each new number you get, all the way down.

    _____

[CORRECT ANSWER IS: 17, 14, 11, 8, 5, 2.]

_____   Total number of errors.

---

1. Telephone number [IF SUBJECT IS RELIABLE TRANSFER FROM PRELIMINARY QUESTIONNAIRE; OTHERWISE, OBTAIN FROM INFORMANT OR LOOK ON TELEPHONE.] _____

2. Sex of Subject
    1   Male
    2   Female

3. Race of Subject
    1   White (Caucasian)
    2   Black (Negro)
    3   Oriental
    4   Spanish American (Spanish surname)
    5   American Indian
    6   Other
    —   Not answered

4. [GET FROM PRELIMINARY QUESTIONNAIRE IF SUBJECT IS RELIABLE; FROM INFORMANT IF NOT.]
    a. When were you born? _____
              Month   *Day*   *Year*

    b. How old are you? _____

5. How far did you go (have you gone) in school?
    1   0–4 years
    2   5–8 years
    3   High school incomplete
    4   High school completed
    5   Post high school, business or trade school
    6   1–3 years college
    7   4 years college completed
    8   Postgraduate college
    —   Not answered

SOCIAL RESOURCES

Now I'd like to ask you some questions about your family and friends.

6. Are you single, married, widowed, divorced, or separated?
    1   Single
    2   Married
    3   Widowed
    4   Divorced
    5   Separated
    —   Not answered

7. Who lives with you?
    [CHECK "YES" OR "NO" FOR EACH OF THE FOLLOWING.]

YES	NO	
		No one
		Husband or wife
		Children
		Grandchildren
		Parents
		Grandparents
		Brothers and sisters
		Other relatives [Does not include in-laws covered in the above categories.]

continued on next page

YES	NO
		Friends
		Non-related paid* helper [*Includes free room.]
		Others [SPECIFY.] _____

8. How many people do you know well enough to visit with in their homes?
   3   Five or more
   2   Three to four
   1   One to two
   0   None
   —   Not answered

9. About how many times did you talk to someone—friends, relatives, or others—on the telephone in the past week (either you called them or they called you)? [IF SUBJECT HAS NO PHONE, QUESTION STILL APPLIES.]
   3   Once a day or more
   2   2–6 times
   1   Once
   0   Not at all
   —   Not answered

10. How many times during the past week did you spend some time with someone who does not live with you, that is, you went to see them or they came to visit you, or you went out to do things together?
   3   Once a day or more
   2   2–6 times
   1   Once
   0   Not at all
   —   Not answered

11. Do you have someone you can trust and confide in?
   2   Yes
   0   No
   —   Not answered

12. Do you find yourself feeling lonely quite often, sometimes, or almost never?
   0   Quite often
   1   Sometimes
   2   Almost never
   —   Not answered

13. Do you see your relatives and friends as often as you want to or are you somewhat unhappy about how little you see them?
    1   As often as wants to
    2   Somewhat unhappy about how little
    —   Not answered

14. Is there someone who would give you any help at all if you were sick or disabled, for example your husband/wife, a member of your family, or a friend?
    1   Yes
    0   No one willing and able to help
    —   Not answered

    [IF "YES" ASK a. and b.]

    a. Is there someone who would take care of you as long as needed, or only for a short time, or someone who would help you now and then (for example, taking you to the doctor, or fixing lunch occasionally, etc.)?
       1   Someone who would take care of Subject indefinitely (as long as needed)
       2   Someone who would take care of Subject for a short time (a few weeks to six months)
       3   Someone who would help the Subject now and then (taking him to the doctor or fixing lunch, etc.)
       —   Not answered

    b. Who is this person?

    Name _____

    Relationship _____

ECONOMIC RESOURCES

Now I'd like to ask you some questions about your work situation.

15. Are you presently:
    [CHECK "YES" OR "NO" FOR EACH OF THE FOLLOWING.]

YES	NO	
		Employed full-time
		Employed part-time
		Retired
		Retired on disability

continued on next page

YES	NO	
		Not employed and seeking work
		Not employed and not seeking work
		Full-time student
		Part-time student

16. What kind of work have you done most of your life?

    [CIRCLE THE MOST APPROPRIATE.]

    1   Never employed
    2   Housewife
    3   Other [STATE THE SPECIFIC OCCUPATION IN DETAIL.] _____

    _____

    —   Not answered

17. Does your husband/wife work or did he/she ever work? [QUESTION APPLIES ONLY TO SPOUSE TO WHOM MARRIED THE LONGEST.]
    1   Yes
    2   No
    3   Never married
    –   Not answered

    [IF "YES" ASK a.]

    a. What kind of work did or does he/she do?
       [STATE THE SPECIFIC OCCUPATION IN DETAIL.] _____

    _____

    _____

18. Where does your income (money) come from (yours and your husband's/wife's)?

    [CHECK "YES" OR "NO" FOR EACH OF THE FOLLOWING AND IF "YES" ENTER THE AMOUNT AND CIRCLE "Weekly", "Monthly", OR "Yearly".]

YES	NO	IF YES HOW MUCH		
			Weekly Monthly Yearly	Earnings from employment (wages, salaries, or income from your business)

YES	NO	IF YES HOW MUCH		
			Weekly Monthly Yearly	Income from rental, interest from investments, etc. (Include trusts, annuities, & payments from insurance policies & savings.)
			Weekly Monthly Yearly	Social Security (Include Social Security disability payments but not SSI.)
			Weekly Monthly Yearly	V.A. benefits such as G.I. Bill, and disability payments
			Weekly Monthly Yearly	Disability payments not covered by Social Security, SSI, or VA. Both government & private, & including Workmen's Compensation
			Weekly Monthly Yearly	Unemployment compensation
			Weekly Monthly Yearly	Retirement pension from job
			Weekly Monthly Yearly	Alimony or child support
			Weekly Monthly Yearly	Scholarships, stipends (Include only the amount beyond tuition.)
			Weekly Monthly Yearly	Regular assistance from family members (including regular contributions from employed children)
			Weekly Monthly Yearly	SSI payments (yellow government check)
			Weekly Monthly Yearly	Regular financial aid from private organizations and churches

continued on next page

YES	NO	IF YES HOW MUCH		
			Weekly Monthly Yearly	Welfare payments or Aid for Dependent Children
			Weekly Monthly Yearly	Other

[IF COMPLETE INCOME AMOUNTS ARE OBTAINED IN QUESTION 18 SKIP TO QUESTION 19, BUT IF *ANY* AMOUNTS ARE MISSING ASK a.]

a. How much income do you (and your husband/wife) have a year?

[SHOW ANNUAL INCOME LADDER AND CIRCLE THE LETTER WHICH IDENTIFIES EITHER YEARLY OR MONTHLY INCOME CATEGORY.]

	YEARLY	MONTHLY
A.	0–$499	(0–$41)
B.	$500–$999	($42–$83)
C.	$1,000–$1,999	($84–$166)
D.	$2,000–$2,999	($167–$249)
E.	$3,000–$3,999	($250–$333)
F.	$4,000–$4,999	($334–$416)
G.	$5,000–$6,999	($417–$583)
H.	$7,000–$9,999	($584–$833)
I.	$10,000–$14,999	($834–$1249)
J.	$15,000–$19,999	($1250–$1666)
K.	$20,000–$29,999	($1667–$2499)
L.	$30,000–$39,999	($2500–$3333)
M.	$40,000 or more	($3334 or more)

19. How many people altogether live on this income (that is it provides at least half of their income)? _____

20. Do you own your own home?

    1   Yes

    0   No _____→ [IF "NO" ASK a. AND b. on next page.]

    —   Not answered
[IF "YES" ASK a. AND b below.]

    a. How much is it worth?
       1 Up to $10,000
       2 $10,000–$24,000
       3 $25,000–$50,000
       4 More than $50,000
       – Not answered

    b. Do you own it outright or are you still paying a mortgage?
       1 Own outright
       2 Still paying
       – Not answered

[IF 2 ASK (1).]

(1) How much is the monthly payment?
1   0–$59
2   $60–$99
3   $100–$149
4   $150–$199
5   $200–$249
6   $250–$349
7   $350 up
8   Not answered

a. Do you (and your husband/wife) pay the total rent for your house (apartment) or do you contribute to the cost, or does someone else own it or pay the rent?
1   Subject pays total rent
2   Subject contributes to the cost
3   Someone else owns it or pays the rent (Subject doesn't contribute)
—   Not answered

[IF 1 OR 2 ASK (1).]

(1) How much rent do you pay?
1   0–$59 per month
2   $60–$99 per month
3   $100–$149
4   $150–$199
5   $200–$249
6   $250–$349
7   $350 up
—   Not answered

b. Do you live in public housing or receive a rent subsidy?
1   No, neither
2   Yes, lives in public housing
3   Yes, receives a rent subsidy
—   Not answered

21. Are your assets and financial resources sufficient to meet emergencies?
1   Yes
0   No
—   Not answered

22. Are your expenses so heavy that you cannot meet the payments, or can you barely meet the payments, or are your payments no problem to you?
1   Subject cannot meet payments
2   Subject can barely meet payments
3   Payments are no problem
—   Not answered

23. Is your financial situation such that you feel you need financial assistance or help beyond what you are already getting?
1   Yes
0   No
—   Not answered

24. Do you pay for your own food or do you get any regular help at all with costs of food or meals?
1   Subject pays for food himself
2   Subject gets help
—   Not answered

continued on next page

[IF 2 ASK a.]

a. From where?
    [CHECK "YES" OR "NO" FOR EACH OF THE FOLLOWING.]

YES	NO	
		Family or friends
		Food stamps
		Prepared food (meals) from an agency or organization program [SPECIFY NUMBER OF MEALS PER WEEK.] _____

25. Do you feel that you need food stamps?
     1   Yes
     0   No
     —   Not answered

26. Are you covered by any kinds of health or medical insurance?
     1   Yes
     0   No
     —   Not answered

     [IF "YES" ASK a.]
     a.   What kind?

     [CHECK "YES" OR "NO" FOR EACH OF THE FOLLOWING.]

YES	NO	
		Medicaid
		Medicare Plan A only (hospitalization only)
		Medicare Plan A and B (hospitalization and doctor's bills)
		Other insurance: hospitalization only (Blue Cross or other)
		Other insurance: hospitalization and doctor's bills (Blue Cross and Blue Shield, major medical or other)

27. Please tell me how well you think you (and your family) are now doing financially as compared to other people your age—better, about the same, or worse?
[PROBE AS NECESSARY.]
    2   Better
    1   About the same
    0   Worse
    —   Not answered

28. How well does the amount of money you have take care of your needs—very well, fairly well, or poorly?
    2   Very well
    1   Fairly well
    0   Poorly
    —   Not answered

29. Do you usually have enough to buy those little "extras"; that is, those small luxuries?
    2   Yes
    0   No
    —   Not answered

30. Do you feel that you will have enough for your needs in the future?
    2   Yes
    0   No
    —   Not answered

MENTAL HEALTH

Next, I'd like to ask you some questions about how you feel about life.

31. How often would you say you worry about things—very often, fairly often, or hardly ever?
    0   Very often
    1   Fairly often
    2   Hardly ever
    —   Not answered

32. In general, do you find life exciting, pretty routine, or dull?
    2   Exciting
    1   Pretty routine
    0   Dull
    —   Not answered

33. Taking everything into consideration how would you describe your satisfaction with life in general at the present time—good, fair, or poor?
    2   Good
    1   Fair
    0   Poor
    —   Not answered

continued on next page

34. Please answer the following questions "YES" or "NO" as they apply to you now. There are no right or wrong answers, only what best applies to you. Occasionally a question may not seem to apply to you, but please answer either "Yes" or "No", whichever is more nearly correct for you.

    [CIRCLE "YES" OR "NO" FOR EACH.]

    (1) Do you wake up fresh and rested most mornings? .... yes NO

    (2) Is your daily life full of things that keep you interested? .... yes NO

    (3) Have you, at times, very much wanted to leave home? .... YES no

    (4) Does it seem that no one understands you? .... YES no

    (5) Have you had periods of days, weeks, or months when you couldn't take care of things because you couldn't "get going"? .... YES no

    (6) Is your sleep fitful and disturbed? .... YES no

    (7) Are you happy most of the time? .... yes NO

    (8) Are you being plotted against? .... YES no

    (9) Do you certainly feel useless at times? .... YES no

    (10) During the past few years, have you been well most of the time? .... yes NO

    (11) Do you feel weak all over much of the time? .... YES no

    (12) Are you troubled by headaches? .... YES no

    (13) Have you had difficulty in keeping your balance in walking? .... YES no

    (14) Are you troubled by your heart pounding and by a shortness of breath? ...... YES no

    (15) Even when you are with people, do you feel lonely much of the time? .... YES no

    Sum of Responses in Capital Letters _____

35. How would you rate your mental or emotional health at the present time—excellent, good, fair, or poor?
    3   Excellent
    2   Good
    1   Fair
    0   Poor
    —   Not answered

36. Is your mental or emotional health now better, about the same, or worse than it was five years ago?

    3   Better
    2   About the same
    0   Worse
    —   Not answered

PHYSICAL HEALTH

Let's talk about your health now.

37. About how many times have you seen a doctor during the past six months other than as an inpatient in a hospital?
    [EXCLUDE PSYCHIATRISTS.]

    _____ Times

38. During the past six months how many days were you so sick that you were unable to carry on your usual activities—such as going to work or working around the house?

    0   None
    1   A week or less
    2   More than a week but less than one month
    3   1–3 months
    4   4–6 months
    —   Not answered

39. How many days in the past six months were you in a hospital for physical health problems?
    _____ Days

40. How many days in the past six months were you in a nursing home or rehabilitation center for physical health problems?
    _____ Days

41. Do you feel that you need medical care or treatment beyond what you are receiving at this time?

    1   Yes
    0   No
    —   Not answered

42. I have a list of common medicines that people take. Would you please tell me if you've taken any of the following *in the past month.*

    [CHECK "YES" OR "NO" FOR EACH MEDICINE.]

continued on next page

YES	NO	
		Arthritis medication
		Prescription pain killer (other than above)
		High blood pressure medicine
		Pills to make you lose water or salt (water pills)
		Digitalis pills for the heart
		Nitroglycerin tablets for chest pain
		Blood thinner medicine (anticoagulants)
		Drugs to improve circulation
		Insulin injections for diabetes
		Pills for diabetes
		Prescription ulcer medicine
		Seizure medications (like Dilantin)
		Thyroid pills
		Cortisone pills or injections
		Antibiotics
		Tranquilizers or nerve medicine
		Prescription sleeping pills (once a week or more)
		Hormones, male or female (including birth control pills)

43. What other prescription drugs have you taken in the past month?

[RECORD THE "others". THEN ENTER THEM IN APPROPRIATE CATEGORIES ABOVE IF POSSIBLE.]
[SPECIFY.] _____

_____

_____

44. Do you have any of the following illnesses at the present time?
[CHECK "YES" OR "NO" FOR EACH OF THE FOLLOWING. IF "YES", ASK: "How much does it interfere with your activities, not at all, a little (some), or a great deal? AND CHECK THE APPROPRIATE BOX.]

[IF "YES", ASK:] How much does it interfere with your activities?

YES	NO	NOT AT ALL	A LITTLE	A GREAT DEAL	
					Arthritis or rheumatism
					Glaucoma
					Asthma
					Emphysema or chronic bronchitis
					Tuberculosis
					High blood pressure
					Heart trouble
					Circulation trouble in arms or legs
					Diabetes
					Ulcers (of the digestive system)
					Other stomach or intestinal disorders or gall bladder problems
					Liver disease
					Kidney disease
					Other urinary tract disorders (including prostate trouble)
					Cancer or leukemia
					Anemia
					Effects of stroke
					Parkinson's disease
					Epilepsy
					Cerebral Palsy

continued on next page

YES	NO	NOT AT ALL	A LITTLE	A GREAT DEAL	
					Multiple Sclerosis
					Muscular Dystrophy
					Effects of Polio
					Thyroid or other glandular disorders
					Skin disorders such as pressure sores, leg ulcers, or severe burns
					Speech impediment or impairment

45. Do you have any physical disabilities such as total or partial paralysis, missing or non-functional limbs, or broken bones?
    0   No
    1   Total paralysis
    2   Partial paralysis
    3   Missing or non-functional limbs
    4   Broken bones
    —   Not answered

46. How is your eyesight (with glasses or contacts), excellent, good, fair, poor, or are you totally blind?
    1   Excellent
    2   Good
    3   Fair
    4   Poor
    5   Totally blind
    —   Not answered

47. How is your hearing, excellent, good, fair, poor, or are you totally deaf?
    1   Excellent
    2   Good
    3   Fair
    4   Poor
    5   Totally deaf
    —   Not answered

48. Do you have any other physical problems or illnesses at the present time that seriously affect your health?
    1   Yes
    0   No
    —   Not answered

    [IF "YES" SPECIFY.] _____

    _____

SUPPORTIVE DEVICES AND PROSTHESES

49. Do you use any of the following aids all or most of the time?
     [CHECK "YES" OR "NO" FOR EACH AID.]

YES	NO	
		Cane (including tripod-tip cane)
		Walker
		Wheelchair
		Leg brace
		Back brace
		Artificial limb
		Hearing aid
		Colostomy equipment
		Catheter
		Kidney dialysis machine
		Other [SPECIFY.] _____

50. Do you need any aids (supportive or prosthetic devices) that you currently do not have?
     1   Yes
     0   No
     —   Not answered

[IF "YES", ASK a.]

   a. What aids do you need?   [SPECIFY.]

     _____

     _____

     _____

51. Do you have a problem with your health because of drinking or has your physician advised
     you to cut down on drinking?
     1   Yes
     0   No
     —   Not answered

continued on next page

52. Do you regularly participate in any vigorous sports activity such as hiking, jogging, tennis, biking, or swimming?
   - 1 Yes
   - 0 No
   - — Not answered

53. How would you rate your overall health at the present time—excellent, good, fair, or poor?
   - 3 Excellent
   - 2 Good
   - 1 Fair
   - 0 Poor
   - — Not answered

54. Is your health now better, about the same, or worse than it was five years ago?
   - 3 Better
   - 2 About the same
   - 0 Worse
   - — Not answered

55. How much do your health troubles stand in the way of your doing the things you want to do—not at all, a little (some), or a great deal?
   - 3 Not at all
   - 2 A little (some)
   - 0 A great deal
   - — Not answered

ACTIVITIES OF DAILY LIVING

Now I'd like to ask you about some of the activities of daily living, things that we all need to do as a part of our daily lives. I would like to know if you can do these activities without any help at all, or if you need some help to do them, or if you can't do them at all.

[BE SURE TO READ ALL ANSWER CHOICES IF APPLICABLE IN QUESTIONS 56. THROUGH 69. TO RESPONDENT.]

Instrumental ADL

56. Can you use the telephone. . .
   - 2 without help, including looking up numbers and dialing
   - 1 with some help (can answer phone or dial operator in an emergency, but need a special phone or help in getting the number or dialing),
   - 0 or are you completely unable to use the telephone?
   - — Not answered

57. Can you get to places out of walking distance. . .
    2   without help (can travel alone on buses, taxis, or drive your own car),
    1   with some help (need someone to help you or go with you when traveling)
    0   or are you unable to travel unless emergency arrangements are made for a specialized vehicle like an ambulance?
    — Not answered

58. Can you go shopping for groceries or clothes [ASSUMING SUBJECT HAS TRANSPORTA-TION]. . .
    2   without help (taking care of all shopping needs yourself, assuming you had transportation),
    1   with some help (need someone to go with you on all shopping trips),
    0   or are you completely unable to do any shopping?
    — Not answered

59. Can you prepare your own meals. . .
    2   without help (plan and cook full meals yourself),
    1   with some help (can prepare some things but unable to cook full meals yourself),
    0   or are you completely unable to prepare any meals?
    — Not answered

60. Can you do your housework. . .
    2   without help (can scrub floors, etc.),
    1   with some help (can do light housework but need help with heavy work),
    0   or are you completely unable to do any housework?
    — Not answered

61. Can you take your own medicine. . .
    2   without help (in the right doses at the right time),
    1   with some help (able to take medicine if someone prepares it for you and/or reminds you to take it),
    0   or are you completely unable to take your medicines?
    — Not answered

62. Can you handle your own money. . .
    2   without help (write checks, pay bills, etc.),
    1   with some help (manage day-to-day buying but need help with managing your checkbook and paying your bills),
    0   or are you completely unable to handle money?
    — Not answered

Physical ADL

63. Can you eat. . .
    2   without help (able to feed yourself completely),
    1   with some help (need help with cutting, etc.),
    0   or are you completely unable to feed yourself?
    — Not answered

continued on next page

64. Can you dress and undress yourself. . .
    2   without help (able to pick out clothes, dress and undress yourself),
    1   with some help,
    0   or are you completely unable to dress and undress yourself?
    —   Not answered

65. Can you take care of your own appearance, for example combing your hair and (for men) shaving. . .
    2   without help,
    1   with some help,
    0   or are you completely unable to maintain your appearance yourself?
    —   Not answered

66. Can you walk. . .
    2   without help (except from a cane),
    1   with some help from a person or with the use of a walker, or crutches, etc.,
    0   or are you completely unable to walk?
    —   Not answered

67. Can you get in and out of bed. . .
    2   without any help or aids,
    1   with some help (either from a person or with the aid of some device),
    0   or are you totally dependent on someone else to lift you?
    —   Not answered

68. Can you take a bath or shower. . .
    2   without help,
    1   with some help (need help getting in and out of the tub, or need special attachments on the tub),
    0   or are you completely unable to bathe yourself?
    —   Not answered

69. Do you ever have trouble getting to the bathroom on time?
    2   No
    0   Yes
    1   Have a catheter or colostomy
    —   Not answered

    [IF "YES" ASK a.]

    a.   How often do you wet or soil yourself (either day or night)?
         1   Once or twice a week
         0   Three times a week or more
         —   Not answered

70. Is there someone who helps you with such things as shopping, housework, bathing, dressing, and getting around?
    1   Yes
    0   No
    —   Not answered

[IF "YES" ASK a. AND b.]

a. Who is your major helper?

Name _____ Relationship _____
b. Who else helps you?

Name _____ Relationship _____

UTILIZATION OF SERVICES

71. Now I want to ask you some questions about the kinds of help you are or have been getting or the kinds of help that you feel you need. We want to know not only about the help you have been getting from agencies or organizations but also what help you have been getting from your family and friends.

TRANSPORTATION

(1) Who provides your transportation when you go shopping, visit friends, go to the doctor, etc.?

[CHECK "YES" OR "NO" FOR EACH.]

YES	NO	
		Yourself
		Your family or friends
		Use public transportation (bus, taxi, subway, etc.)
		Public agency [SPECIFY.] _____
		Other [SPECIFY.] _____

   a. On the average how many round trips do you make a week?
       0   None
       1   Less than one a week
       2   One to three a week
       3   4 or more
       —   Not answered

   b. Do you feel you need transportation more often than it is available to you now for appointments, visiting, social events, etc.?
       1   Yes
       0   No
       —   Not answered

continued on next page

SOCIAL/RECREATIONAL SERVICES

(2) In the past six months (since _____ [SPECIFY MONTH.]) have you participated in any planned and organized social or recreational programs or in any group
activities or classes such as arts and crafts classes? [EXCLUDE EMPLOYMENT-
RELATED CLASSES.]
   1   Yes
   0   No
   —   Not answered

[IF "NO" SKIP TO c.; IF "YES" ASK a., b., AND c.]

   a. About how many times a week did you participate in these activities?
       1   Once a week or less
       2   2–3 times a week
       3   4 times a week or more
       —   Not answered

   b. Do you still participate in such activities or groups?
       1   Yes
       0   No
       —   Not answered

   c. Do you feel you need to participate in any planned and organized social or
recreational programs or in any group activities or classes?
       1   Yes
       0   No
       —   Not answered

EMPLOYMENT SERVICES

(3) Has anyone helped you look for or find a job or counseled you in regard to getting
employment in the past six months (since _____ [MONTH])?
   1   Yes
   0   No
   —   Not answered

[IF "NO" SKIP TO b.; IF "YES" ASK a. AND b.]

   a. Who helped you?
       1   Family members or friends
       2   Someone from an agency
       3   Both
       —   Not answered

   b. Do you feel you need someone to help you find a job?
       1   Yes
       0   No
       —   Not answered

SHELTERED EMPLOYMENT

(4)   During the past six months have you worked in a place like a sheltered workshop which employs people with disabilities or special problems?
  1   Yes
  0   No
  —   Not answered

[IF "NO" SKIP TO b.; IF "YES" ASK a. AND b.]

  a.   Do you still work there?
    1   Yes
    0   No
    —   Not answered

  b.   Do you feel you need to work in a sheltered workshop?
    1   Yes
    0   No
    —   Not answered

EDUCATIONAL SERVICES, EMPLOYMENT RELATED

(5)   In the past six months have you had any occupational training or on the job training to further prepare you for a job or career?
  1   Yes
  0   No
  —   Not answered

[IF "NO" SKIP TO c.; IF "YES" ASK a., b., AND c.]

  a.   Was this full- or part-time training?
    1   Full-time
    2   Part-time
    —   Not answered

  b.   Are you still in classes or training?
    1   Yes
    0   No
    —   Not answered

  c.   Do you feel you need education or on the job training to prepare you for a job?
    1   Yes
    0   No
    —   Not answered

continued on next page

REMEDIAL TRAINING

(6) In the past six months have you had any remedial training or instruction in learning basic personal skills, for example, speech therapy, reality orientation, or training for the blind or physically or mentally handicapped?
[EXCLUDE PHYSICAL THERAPY.]
    1   Yes
    0   No
    —   Not answered

[IF "NO" SKIP TO c.; IF "YES" ASK a., b., AND c.]

    a. On the average about how many training sessions a week did you have over the past six months?
        1   Less than one a week
        2   One a week
        3   Two or more a week
        —   Not answered

    b. Are you currently receiving this type of training or instruction?
        1   Yes
        0   No
        —   Not answered

    c. Do you think you need remedial training or instruction in basic personal skills?
        1   Yes
        0   No
        —   Not answered

MENTAL HEALTH SERVICES

(7) Have you had any treatment or counseling for personal or family problems or for nervous or emotional problems in the past six months, that is, since _____ [SPECIFY MONTH.]?
    1   Yes
    0   No
    —   Not answered

[IF "NO" SKIP TO d.; IF "YES" ASK a., b., c., AND d.]

    a. Were you hospitalized for nervous or emotional problems at any time during this period? (Last six months)
        1   Yes
        0   No
        —   Not answered

b. During the past six months how many sessions have you had with a doctor, psychiatrist, or counselor for these problems (other than those when you were an inpatient in the hospital)?

    0   None, had treatment only as an inpatient
    1   Less than 4 sessions (only occasionally or for evaluation)
    2   4–12 sessions
    3   13 or more sessions
    —   Not answered

c. Are you still receiving this help?

    1   Yes
    0   No
    —   Not answered

d. Do you feel that you need treatment or counseling for personal or family problems or for nervous or emotional problems?

    1   Yes
    0   No
    —   Not answered

PSYCHOTROPIC DRUGS

(8) Have you taken any prescription medicine for your nerves in the past six months, like medicine to calm you down or to help depression?

    1   Yes
    0   No
    —   Not answered

[IF "NO" SKIP TO b.; IF "YES" ASK a. AND b.]

a. Are you still taking it?

    1   Yes
    0   No
    —   Not answered

b. Do you feel you need this kind of medicine?

    1   Yes
    0   No
    —   Not answered

PERSONAL CARE SERVICES

(9) In the past six months has someone helped you with your personal care, for example, helping you to bathe or dress, feeding you, or helping you with toilet care?

    1   Yes
    0   No
    —   Not answered

[IF "NO" SKIP TO d.; IF "YES" ASK a., b., c., AND d.]

continued on next page

a. Who helped you in this way?
    1   Unpaid family members or friends
    2   Someone hired to help you in this way or someone from an agency
    3   Both
    —   Not answered

b. On the average, how much time per day has this person helped you to bathe, dress, eat, go to the toilet, etc.?
    1   Less than ½ hour per day
    2   ½ to 1½ hours per day
    3   More than 1½ hours per day
    —   Not answered

c. Are you still being helped in this way?
    1   Yes
    0   No
    —   Not answered

d. Do you feel you need help with bathing, dressing, eating, or going to the toilet, etc.?
    1   Yes
    0   No
    —   Not answered

NURSING CARE

(10) During the past six months have you had any nursing care, in other words, did a nurse or someone else give you treatments or medications prescribed by a doctor? [EXCLUDE NURSING CARE WHILE IN THE HOSPITAL.]
    1   Yes
    0   No
    —   Not answered

[IF "NO" SKIP TO e.; IF "YES" ASK a., b., c., d., AND e.]

a. Who helped you in this way?
    1   Unpaid family members or friends
    2   Someone hired to help you in this way or someone from an agency
    3   Both
    —   Not answered

b. On the average, how many hours a day did you receive this help?
    0   Only occasionally, not every day
    1   Gave oral medicine only
    2   Less than ½ hour per day
    3   ½ to 1 hour per day
    4   More than 1 hour per day
    —   Not answered

c. For how long did you have this help within the past six months?
   1   Less than one month
   2   1–3 months
   3   More than 3 months
   —   Not answered

d. Are you still receiving nursing care?
   1   Yes
   0   No
   —   Not answered

e. Do you feel you need nursing care?
   1   Yes
   0   No
   —   Not answered

PHYSICAL THERAPY

(13) During the past six months have you received physical therapy?
   1   Yes
   0   No
   —   Not answered

   [IF "NO" SKIP TO d.; IF "YES" ASK a., b., c., AND d.]

a. Who gave you physical therapy or helped you with it?
   1   Unpaid family members or friends
   2   Someone hired to provide this or someone from an agency
   3   Both
   —   Not answered

b. On the average how many times a week did someone help you with your physical therapy activities?
   1   Less than once a week
   2   Once a week
   3   2 or more times a week
   —   Not answered

c. Are you still receiving physical therapy?
   1   Yes
   0   No
   —   Not answered

d. Do you think you need physical therapy?
   1   Yes
   0   No
   —   Not answered

continued on next page

CONTINUOUS SUPERVISION

(14) During the past six months was there any period when someone had to be with you all the time to look after you?

    1   Yes
    0   No
    —   Not answered

[IF "NO" SKIP TO c.; IF "YES" ASK a., b., AND c.]

  a. Who looked after you?

      1   Unpaid family members or friends
      2   Someone hired to look after you or someone from an agency
      3   Both
      —   Not answered

  b. Do you still have to have someone with you all the time to look after you?

      1   Yes
      0   No
      —   Not answered

  c. Do you feel you need to have someone with you all the time to look after you?

      1   Yes
      0   No
      —   Not answered

CHECKING SERVICES

(15) [IF SUBJECT HAS HAD CONTINUOUS SUPERVISION IN THE PAST SIX MONTHS, ASK ONLY c.]

[PERSONS WHO NEED CHECKING WHO ARE LIVING IN INSTITUTIONS OR WITH FAMILY MEMBERS MAY BE PRESUMED TO BE RECEIVING IT.]

During the past six months have you had someone regularly (at least five times a week) check on you by phone or in person to make sure you were all right?

    1   Yes
    0   No
    —   Not answered

[IF "NO" SKIP TO c.; IF "YES" ASK a., b., AND c.]

  a. Who checked on you?

      1   Unpaid family members or friends
      2   Someone from an agency, a volunteer, or someone hired to help you
      3   Both
      —   Not answered

b. Is someone still checking on you at least five times a week?
  1 Yes
  0 No
  — Not answered

c. Do you feel you need to have someone check on you regularly (at least five times a week) by phone or in person to make sure you are all right? [CIRCLE "NO", IF SUBJECT FELT HE NEEDED CONTINUOUS SUPERVISION, (14c.)].
  1 Yes
  0 No
  — Not answered

RELOCATION AND PLACEMENT SERVICES

(16) In the past six months have you had any help in finding a new place to live, or in making arrangements to move in?
[THIS INCLUDES PLACEMENT IN INSTITUTIONS.]
  1 Yes
  0 No
  — Not answered

[IF "NO" SKIP TO b.; IF "YES" ASK a. AND b.]

a. Who helped you with this?
  1 Unpaid family members or friends
  2 Other, such as someone from an agency
  3 Both
  — Not answered

b. Do you feel you need help in finding a (another) place to live?
  1 Yes
  0 No
  — Not answered

HOMEMAKER-HOUSEHOLD SERVICES

(17) During the past six months did someone have to help you regularly with routine household chores such as cleaning, washing clothes, etc.? That is, did your wife/ husband or someone else have to do them because you were unable to?
  1 Yes
  0 No
  — Not answered

[IF "NO" SKIP TO d.; IF "YES" ASK a., b., c., AND d.]

continued on next page

a. Who helped with household chores?
   1   Unpaid family members or friends
   2   Other, such as a paid helper or agency person
   3   Both
   0   Not answered

b. For about how many hours a week did you have to have help with household chores?
   1   Less than 4 hours a week
   2   4–8 hours a week (a half-day to a day)
   3   9 or more hours a week (more than one day a week)
   —   Not answered

c. Are you still getting this kind of help?
   1   Yes
   0   No
   —   Not answered

d. Do you feel you need help with routine housework?
   1   Yes
   0   No
   —   Not answered

MEAL PREPARATION

(18) During the past six months did someone regularly have to prepare meals for you? That is, did your wife/husband or someone else regularly cook because you were unable to, or did you have to go out for meals?
   1   Yes
   0   No
   —   Not answered

[IF "NO" SKIP TO c.; IF "YES" ASK a., b., AND c.]

a. Who prepared meals for you?
   1   Unpaid family members or friends
   2   Other, such as a paid helper or agency person
   3   Both
   —   Not answered

b. Is someone still having to prepare meals for you?
   1   Yes
   0   No
   —   Not answered

c. Do you feel that you need to have someone regularly prepare meals for you because you can't do it yourself?
1   Yes
0   No
—   Not answered

ADMINISTRATIVE, LEGAL, AND PROTECTIVE SERVICES

(19) During the past six months has anyone helped you with any legal matters or with managing your personal business affairs or handling your money, for example, paying your bills for you?
1   Yes
0   No
—   Not answered

[IF "NO" SKIP TO c.; IF "YES" ASK a., b., AND c.]

a. Who helped you?
1   Family members or friends
2   A lawyer, the Legal Aid Society, other agency personnel, or someone hired to help you?
3   Both
—   Not answered

b. Are you still getting help with legal matters or with managing your personal business affairs?
1   Yes
0   No
—   Not answered

c. Do you think you need help with these matters?
1   Yes
0   No
—   Not answered

SYSTEMATIC MULTIDIMENSIONAL EVALUATION

(20) In the past six months has anyone like a doctor or social worker thoroughly reviewed and evaluated your overall condition including your health, your mental health, and your social and financial situation?
1   Yes
0   No
—   Not answered

continued on next page

a. Do you think you need to have someone review and evaluate your overall condition in this way?
    1   Yes
    0   No
    —   Not answered

COORDINATION, INFORMATION AND REFERRAL SERVICES

(24) During the past six months did someone see to it that you got the kinds of help you needed? In other words, did someone give you information about the kind of help that is available or put you in touch with those who could help you?
    1   Yes
    0   No
    —   Not answered

    [IF "NO" SKIP TO c.; IF "YES" ASK a., b., AND c.]

a. Who was this person?
    1   A family member or a friend
    2   Someone from an agency
    3   Both
    —   Not answered

b. Is there still someone who sees to it that you get the kinds of help you need? In other words, is there someone who gives you information about the kind of help that is available or puts you in touch with those who can help you?
    1   Yes
    0   No
    —   Not answered

c. Do you feel you need to have someone organize or coordinate the kinds of help you need and make arrangements for you to get them?
    1   Yes
    0   No
    —   Not answered

---

72. QUESTION 71 WAS ASKED OF:
    1   Subject
    2   Informant
    3   Both

CONCLUDING STATEMENT TO THE SUBJECT

[MAKE A BRIEF CONCLUDING STATEMENT TO THE SUBJECT INDICATING THE CONCLUSION OF THE INTERVIEW AND EXPRESSING YOUR APPRECIATION FOR HIS COOPERATION.]

Questions to be Asked of an Informant Based on his Knowledge of the Subject

[IF THE SUBJECT IS UNRELIABLE THESE QUESTIONS *MUST* BE ASKED OF AN INFORMANT.]
[IF THE SUBJECT IS RELIABLE, THE QUESTIONS MUST BE ASKED IF AN INFORMANT IS AVAILABLE.]

SOCIAL RESOURCES

73. How well does _____ (Subject) get along with his/her family and friends—very well, fairly well, or poorly (has considerable trouble or conflict with them)?
    1 Very well
    2 Fairly well (has some conflict or trouble with them)
    3 Poorly (has considerable trouble or conflict with them)
    — Not answered

74. Is there someone who would help _____ (Subject) at all if he/she were sick or disabled, for example his/her husband or wife, a member of the family or a friend?
    1 Yes
    0 No
    — Not answered

    [IF "YES" ASK a. AND b.]

    a. [CIRCLE THE MOST APPROPRIATE.]
        Is there someone who would take care of him/her as long as needed, or only for a short time, or only someone who would help now and then (for example, taking him/her to the doctor, fixing lunch, etc.)?
        1 Someone who would take care of Subject indefinitely (as long as needed)
        2 Someone who would take care of Subject a short time (a few weeks to six months)
        3 Someone who would help him now and then (taking him to the doctor or fixing lunch, etc.)
        — Not answered

    b. Who is this person?

        Name _____

        Relationship _____

ECONOMIC RESOURCES

75. In your opinion are _____'s (Subject's) needs for the following basic necessities being well met, barely met, or are they not being met?

continued on next page

[CHECK THE APPROPRIATE BOX FOR EACH NEED.]

WELL MET	BARELY MET	NOT MET	
			Food
			Housing
			Clothing
			Medical care
			Small luxuries

MENTAL HEALTH

76. Does _____ (Subject) show good, common sense in making judgments and decisions?
    1   Yes
    0   No
    —   Not answered

77. Is _____ (Subject) able to handle (cope with) major problems which occur in his/her life?
    1   Yes
    0   No
    —   Not answered

78. Do you feel that _____ (Subject) finds life exciting and enjoyable?
    1   Yes
    0   No
    —   Not answered

79. How would you rate _____'s (Subject's) mental or emotional health or ability to think at the present time compared to the average person living independently—excellent, good, fair, or poor?
    3   Excellent
    2   Good
    1   Fair
    0   Poor
    —   Not answered

80. Is _____ (Subject's) mental or emotional health or ability to think—better, about the same, or worse than it was five years ago?
    3   Better
    2   About the same
    0   Worse
    —   Not answered

PHYSICAL HEALTH

81. How would you rate _____ (Subject's) health at the present time—excellent, good, fair, or poor?
    3   Excellent
    2   Good
    1   Fair
    0   Poor
    —   Not answered

82. How much do _____ (Subject's) health troubles stand in the way of his/her doing the things he/she wants to do—not at all, a little (some), or a great deal?
    3   Not at all
    2   A little (some)
    0   A great deal
    —   Not answered

[THE REMAINING QUESTIONS ARE TO BE ANSWERED BY THE INTERVIEWER IMMEDIATELY AFTER LEAVING THE INTERVIEW SITE.]

83. Length of interview _____
                        Minutes

84. Factual information obtained from:
    1   Subject
    2   Relative
    3   Other [SPECIFY.] _____
85. Factual questions (obtained from Subject and/or informant) are:
    1   Completely reliable
    2   Reliable on most items
    3   Reliable on only a few items
    4   Completely unreliable
86. Subjective questions (those in boxes, obtained from Subject only) are:
    1   Completely reliable
    2   Reliable on most items
    3   Reliable on only a few items
    4   Completely unreliable
    5   Not obtained

    [IF 5 ANSWER a.]

    a.   Why didn't the Subject answer the Subjective questions?
         [BE SPECIFIC.]

    _____

    _____

    _____

continued on next page

SOCIAL RESOURCES

87. Which of the following best describes the availability of help for the Subject if he(she) were sick or disabled?

[CIRCLE THE MOST APPROPRIATE.]

1   At least one person could and would take care of the Subject indefinitely (as long as needed).
2   At least one person could and would take care of the Subject for a short time (a few weeks to 6 months).
3   Help would only be available now and then for such things as taking him(her) to the doctor, fixing lunch, etc.
4   No help at all (except possible emergency help) would be available.

88. Which of the following best describes the Subject's social relationships?

[CIRCLE THE MOST APPROPRIATE.]

1   Very satisfactory, extensive
2   Fairly satisfactory, adequate
2   Unsatisfactory, of poor quality, few

ECONOMIC RESOURCES

89. In your opinion which of the following best describes the Subject's income?
1   Ample
2   Satisfactory
3   Somewhat inadequate
4   Totally inadequate
5   No income at all

90. In your opinion does the Subject have any financial reserves?
1   Yes, has reserves
0   No, has (little or) no reserves

91. In your opinion which of the following statements best describes the extent to which the Subject's needs are being met?
1   Food, housing, clothing, and medical needs are met; Subject can afford small luxuries.
2   Food, housing, clothing, and medical needs are met; Subject cannot afford small luxuries.
3   Either food, *or* housing, *or* clothing, *or* medical needs are unmet; Subject cannot afford small luxuries.
4   Two or more basic needs (housing, food, clothing, medical care) are unmet; Subject cannot afford small luxuries.

MENTAL HEALTH

92. Is it your impression that the Subject shows good, common sense in making judgments and decisions?
    - 1 Yes
    - 0 No
    - — Not answered

93. Is it your impression that the Subject is able to handle (cope with) major problems which occur in his/her life?
    - 1 Yes
    - 0 No
    - — Not answered

94. Is it your impression that the Subject finds life exciting and enjoyable?
    - 1 Yes
    - 0 No
    - — Not answered

95. During the interview did the Subject's behavior strike you as:

    [CHECK "YES" OR "NO" FOR EACH OF THE FOLLOWING.]

YES	NO	
		Mentally alert and stimulating
		Pleasant and cooperative
		Depressed and/or tearful
		Withdrawn or lethargic
		Fearful, anxious, or extremely tense
		Full of unrealistic physical complaints
		Suspicious (more than reasonable)
		Bizarre or inappropriate in thought or action
		Excessively talkative or overly jovial, or elated

continued on next page

PHYSICAL HEALTH

96. Is the Subject either extremely overweight, or malnourished and emaciated?
    - 0   No, neither
    - 1   Yes, extremely overweight
    - 2   Yes, malnourished or emaciated
    - —   Not answered

SOCIAL RESOURCES RATING SCALE

97. [RATE THE CURRENT SOCIAL RESOURCES OF THE PERSON BEING EVALUATED ALONG THE SIX-POINT SCALE PRESENTED BELOW. CIRCLE THE *ONE* NUMBER WHICH BEST DESCRIBES THE PERSON'S PRESENT CIRCUMSTANCES. SOCIAL RESOURCES QUESTIONS ARE NUMBERS 6–14, 73, 74, 87, AND 88.]

1. *Excellent Social Resources.*

   Social relationships are very satisfying and extensive; at least one person would take care of him(her) indefinitely.

2. *Good Social Resources.*

   Social relationships are fairly satisfying and adequate and at least one person would take care of him(her) indefinitely.
   OR
   Social relationships are very satisfying and extensive; and only short term help is available.

3. *Mildly Socially Impaired.*

   Social relationships are unsatisfactory, of poor quality, few; but at least one person would take care of him(her) indefinitely.
   OR
   Social relationships are fairly satisfactory, adequate; and only short term help is available.

4. *Moderately Socially Impaired.*

   Social relationships are unsatisfactory, of poor quality, few; and only short term care is available.
   OR
   Social relationships are at least adequate or satisfactory; but help would only be available now and then.

5. *Severely Socially Impaired.*

Social relationships are unsatisfactory, of poor quality, few; and help would only be available now and then.
OR
Social relationships are at least satisfactory or adequate; but help is not even available now and then.

6. *Totally Socially Impaired.*

Social relationships are unsatisfactory, of poor quality, few; and help is not even available now and then.

ECONOMIC RESOURCES RATING SCALE

98. [RATE THE CURRENT ECONOMIC RESOURCES OF THE PERSON BEING EVALUATED ALONG THE SIX-POINT SCALE PRESENTED BELOW. CIRCLE THE *ONE* NUMBER WHICH BEST DESCRIBES THE PERSON'S PRESENT CIRCUMSTANCES. ECONOMIC QUESTIONS ARE NUMBERS 15–30, 75, AND 89–91.]

1. *Economic Resources are Excellent.*

Income is ample; Subject has reserves.

2. *Economic Resources are Satisfactory.*

Income is ample; Subject has no reserves
OR
Income is adequate; Subject has reserves.

3. *Economic Resources are Mildly Impaired.*

Income is adequate; Subject has no reserves
OR
Income is somewhat inadequate; Subject has reserves.

4. *Economic Resources are Moderately Impaired.*

Income is somewhat inadequate; Subject has no reserves.

5. *Economic Resources are Severely Impaired.*

Income is totally inadequate; Subject may or may not have reserves.

continued on next page

6. *Economic Resources are Completely Impaired.*

Subject is destitute, completely without income or reserves.

[INCOME IS CONSIDERED TO BE ADEQUATE IF ALL THE SUBJECT'S NEEDS ARE BEING MET.]

MENTAL HEALTH RATING SCALE

99. [RATE THE CURRENT MENTAL FUNCTIONING OF THE PERSON BEING EVALUATED ALONG THE SIX-POINT SCALE PRESENTED BELOW. CIRCLE THE *ONE* NUMBER WHICH BEST DESCRIBES THE PERSON'S PRESENT FUNCTIONING. MENTAL HEALTH QUESTIONS ARE THE PRELIMINARY QUESTIONNAIRE, AND NUMBERS 31–36, 76–80, AND 92–95.]

1. *Outstanding Mental Health.*

Intellectually alert and clearly enjoying life. Manages routine and major problems in his life with ease and is free from any psychiatric symptoms.

2. *Good Mental Health.*

Handles both routine and major problems in his life satisfactorily and is intellectually intact and free of psychiatric symptoms.

3. *Mildly Mentally Impaired.*

Has mild psychiatric symptoms and/or mild intellectual impairment. Continues to handle routine, though not major, problems in his life satisfactorily.

4. *Moderately Mentally Impaired.*

Has definite psychiatric symptoms and/or moderate intellectual impairment. Able to make routine, common-sense decisions, but unable to handle major problems in his life.

5. *Severely Mentally Impaired.*

Has severe psychiatric symptoms and/or severe intellectual impairment, which interfere with routine judgments and decision making in every day life.

6. *Completely Mentally Impaired.*

Grossly psychotic or completely impaired intellectually. Requires either intermittent or constant supervision because of clearly abnormal or potentially harmful behavior.

PHYSICAL HEALTH RATING SCALE

100.   [RATE THE CURRENT PHYSICAL FUNCTIONING OF THE PERSON BEING EVALUATED ALONG THE SIX-POINT SCALE PRESENTED BELOW. CIRCLE THE *ONE* NUMBER WHICH BEST DESCRIBES THE PERSON'S PRESENT FUNCTIONING. PHYSICAL HEALTH QUESTIONS ARE NUMBERS 37–55, 81, 82, AND 96.]

1.   *In Excellent Physical Health.*

Engages in vigorous physical activity, either regularly or at least from time to time.

2.   *In Good Physical Health.*

No significant illnesses or disabilities. Only routine medical care such as annual check ups required.

3.   *Mildly Physically Impaired.*

Has only minor illnesses and/or disabilities which might benefit from medical treatment or corrective measures.

4.   *Moderately Physically Impaired.*

Has one or more diseases or disabilities which are either painful or which require substantial medical treatment.

5.   *Severely Physically Impaired.*

Has one or more illnesses or disabilities which are either severely painful or life threatening, or which require extensive medical treatment.

6.   *Totally Physically Impaired.*

Confined to bed and requiring full time medical assistance or nursing care to maintain vital bodily functions.

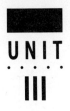

UNIT

III

NURSING INTERVENTIONS FOR COMMON CLINICAL PROBLEMS IN THE OLDER CLIENT

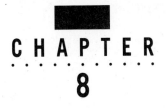

C H A P T E R
8

Incontinence and Related Problems

JEAN F. WYMAN, Ph.D., R.N.C., C.G.N.P.

INTRODUCTION

Incontinence, from either bladder or bowel, is a significant problem for many older adults.

Although urinary incontinence is more prevalent, fecal incontinence, which often occurs concomitantly with urinary incontinence, is more devastating to the individual and to caregivers. Both types of incontinence can seriously affect physical, psychological, and social well-being. Incontinence is associated with a decline in personal care, skin breakdown, urinary tract infection, and higher mortality rates, particularly among those institutionalized in long-term care settings (Donaldson & Jagger, 1983). Being incontinent can cause an individual to curtail daily activities and social contacts, thereby contributing to a loss of self-esteem, to social isolation, and to depression. The burden of caring for an older incontinent family member may result in institutionalization of the incontinent person. Nursing staff often report a "burnout syndrome" related to caring for incontinent patients (Ory, Wyman, & Yu, 1986). Costs associated with incontinence management are tremendous. Estimates for urinary incontinence management range from 2 billion dollars annually in nursing homes to 6 billion dollars in community settings (Hu, 1986). No estimates are available for fecal incontinence management.

Community-dwelling incontinent individuals are often reluctant to seek help, either because of extreme embarrassment or because they believe that it is a normal part of the aging process and nothing can be done to correct the problem. Even when directly questioned during health examinations, many older adults fail to report problems. Frequently when they do report problems, they do not receive the attention they deserve. In many instances, institutionalized incontinent patients also do not receive appropriate evaluation and treatment for their incontinence. Unfortunately, most nurses and physicians have had little preparation to help them evaluate and manage urinary and fecal incontinence. Many health care providers are unaware of recent advances in treatment methods. Although there is now sufficient literature on urinary incontinence in the elderly, there is a surprising lack of information on fecal incontinence even in geriatric care textbooks.

This chapter presents an overview of urinary and fecal incontinence and includes a description of the mechanism of continence, the pathophysiology associated with incontinence, and the diagnostic approach used in evaluation of incontinent patients. In addition, related problems such as urinary tract infection and constipation are also discussed.

URINARY INCONTINENCE

Prevalence

The International Continence Society has defined urinary incontinence as "involuntary urine loss which is a social or hygienic problem and is objectively demonstrable" (Bates, Bradley, Glen, et al., 1979). This definition is important because it points out that urinary incontinence is not a disease but a condition. It can range from the occasional loss of a few drops of urine to the loss of larger amounts of urine several times a day. Although frequently misperceived as an inevitable consequence of growing older, recent research has demonstrated that incontinence is not a normal part of the aging process.

The exact prevalence of urinary incontinence in older adults is unknown. Reported prevalence rates vary because of differences in survey methods and sampling techniques, study populations, definitions of incontinence, and data collection methods. Prevalence estimates range from 5% to 37% for community-dwelling elderly, 38% to 55% for individuals institutionalized in long-term care settings, and 19% for elderly admitted to acute-care hospitals (Mohide, 1986; Diokno, Brock, Brown, et al., 1986).

In general, prevalence research indicates that women are more likely to be affected than men. While there is a trend for increasing prevalence of incontinence with advancing age, the findings are inconsistent. Most studies support a relationship between incontinence and impaired cognitive and mobility function.

Mechanism of Continence

The lower urinary tract, consisting of the bladder and urethra, is considered one functional unit. Micturition has been divided into two distinct phases: a storage phase consisting of bladder filling and urine storage and an expulsion phase consisting of bladder emptying and urine evacuation. Normal function depends on several factors: (1) anatomic integrity of the lower urinary tract, (2) an intact neurologic system that provides voluntary coordinated control of micturition, (3) the pattern of urine production, and (4) the physical ability and psychological willingness to perform the tasks associated with toileting (Staskin, 1986).

The storage phase of micturition is dependent upon a stable detrusor muscle (the contractile portion of the bladder), which inhibits contractions as the bladder distends and accommodates increasing volumes of urine. In addition to a stable detrusor that does not contract involuntarily, the storage phase requires a competent "sphincter mechanism" of the urethra. This mechanism is considered physiologic and not anatomic in nature. Past terminology used to describe this mechanism—internal and external sphincters—is misleading. The sphincter mechanism consists of three parts: (1) an intrinsic urethral smooth muscle sphincter that extends from the bladder outlet through the pelvic floor, (2) a distal (external to the bladder neck) intrinsic urethral striated sphincter that surrounds the urethra and is separate from the pelvic floor, and (3) an extrinsic (external to the urethra) periurethral striated musculature located at the urogenital diaphragm (also known as the pelvic floor muscles) (Figure 8–1) (Gosling, 1979).

During bladder filling, the intraurethral pressure must exceed that of the bladder (intravesical pressure). The intrinsic urethral sphincter mechanism provides the necessary resistance that prevents urine from escaping. When high bladder pressures occur as a result of an increased intraabdominal pressure, such as with coughing or straining or because of an overdistended bladder, the resistance of the intrinsic urethral mechanism is strengthened by the pelvic floor musculature.

The emptying phase of micturition is dependent upon a voluntary detrusor contraction in coordination with active relaxation of the sphincter mechanism. During bladder emptying, the intravesical pressure must exceed the intraurethral pressure in order for voiding to result.

Micturition is coordinated through the central and autonomic nervous systems. Both the bladder and urethra are innervated by sympathetic and parasympathetic fibers. Parasympathetic stimulation can initiate bladder contraction and emptying. Stimulation of beta receptor sites in the body of the bladder and bladder outlet causes smooth muscle relaxation. Alpha-adrenergic receptor site stimulation causes contraction of the smooth muscle in the bladder neck, which in turn causes increased tone and resistance at the bladder

outlet. The pudendal nerve, part of the somatic nervous system, innervates the periurethral striated musculature or the extrinsic sphincter mechanism.

Micturition is primarily a spinal reflex activity that is mediated by the sacral micturition center (S2 to S4), which allows urine storage and emptying even when cortical micturition centers are not intact. Evidence for this is seen in infants who have not sufficiently developed neurologically and in spinal cord injury patients. As the bladder fills with urine, it stimulates stretch receptors in the bladder wall that send a signal to the sacral micturition center and brain via autonomic pathways. Centers in the brain can either facilitate or inhibit voiding. A pontine micturition center coordinates detrusor contraction with sphincter relaxation so they occur synchronously and voiding occurs. Centers in the basal ganglia and frontal lobes inhibit reflex detrusor contraction so that voiding can be delayed (Figure 8–2).

Continence is maintained as long as the intraurethral pressure is higher than the intravesical pressure. Under normal conditions, approximately 150 to 250 ml of urine can be stored before bladder pressure begins to increase and the first sensation of the urge to void is perceived. During this time, the sphincters increase their resistance, and central nervous system inhibition allows the bladder to continue to fill to a maximum capacity

Figure 8–1. Anatomy of the lower urinary tract. (Adapted from Gosling, 1979. From Wyman, J: Nursing assessment of the geriatric outpatient population. Nurs Clin North Am, 22:170, 1988. Reprinted with permission.)

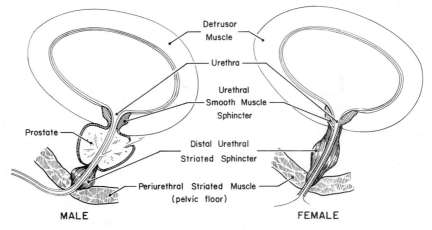

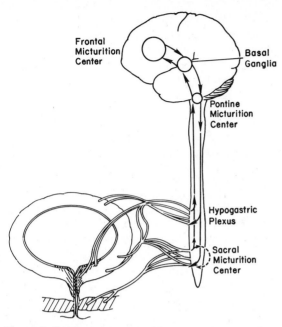

Figure 8–2. Neuroanatomy of lower urinary tract function. (From Wyman, J: Nursing assessment of the geriatric outpatient population. Nurs Clin North Am, 22:171, 1988. Reprinted with permission.)

of 350 to 550 ml. Voiding results when intravesical pressure exceeds intraurethral pressure. Central nervous system inhibition is released, which causes sphincter relaxation. Parasympathetic stimulation causes the bladder to contract and empty its contents.

Although age-related changes can alter bladder and urethral function, their impact on the maintenance of continence is unclear. While none of these changes alone causes incontinence, any can place a person at risk for its development. Changes that may occur include: decreased bladder capacity, making voiding more frequent; late onset of the desire to void, which makes it difficult to delay voiding; an increase in residual urine volume, which increases the risk of urinary tract infections; and an increased number of involuntary bladder contractions, which contributes to the symptoms of urgency, frequency, and incontinence. Decreased maximal urethral closing pressure may occur (Resnick & Yalla, 1985). Benign prostatic hypertrophy, a normal

change in older men, and atrophic vaginitis or urethritis resulting from the lack of estrogen in postmenopausal women are also associated with urinary incontinence. Other age-related changes that affect mobility, dexterity, and visual functions may make it more difficult to locate and reach a toilet and disrobe in time for voiding (Wells, 1980).

Pathophysiology of Urinary Incontinence

The pathophysiology of urinary incontinence involves dysfunctions occurring in either the filling and storage phase or the emptying phase of micturition (Figure 8–3). Failure to store urine may be caused by increased bladder contractility, also known as detrusor instability, or by decreased outlet resistance. Detrusor instability may result from damage to cortical and sacral micturition centers as a result of neurologic disease, such as cerebrovascular accident, Alzheimer's disease, or Parkinson's disease. It can also be caused by irritative symptoms associated with cystitis, bladder tumors, diverticuli, or stones. In early outlet obstruction, such as with benign prostatic hypertrophy in men, the bladder com-

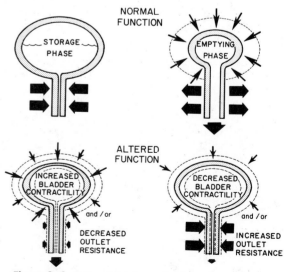

Figure 8–3. Pathophysiology of urinary incontinence.

pensates by increasing muscle mass and contractility. Decreased outlet resistance or sphincteric incompetence may result from pelvic muscle relaxation, which allows the proximal urethra and bladder neck to herniate through the urogenital diaphragm when abdominal pressure increases. This herniation can cause unequal abdominal pressure transmissions to the bladder and urethra, resulting in urine leakage during sudden increases of abdominal pressure such as with coughing, laughing, or physical exertion. In postmenopausal women, the decrease in estrogen that causes a thinning of urethral and vaginal tissues contributes to a decreased outlet resistance. Following prostatectomy surgery, men may have damage to their sphincter mechanism.

Failure to empty urine appropriately also can lead to incontinence. It can be caused by increased outlet resistance, which inhibits the passage of urine, or by decreased detrusor contractility. The most common cause of outlet obstruction that leads to overflow incontinence occurs with prostatic hypertrophy or urethral stricture in men. It is rare to find anatomic obstruction in women unless there is a large cystocele present. Increased outlet resistance can also result from spinal cord damage. Due to interruptions in nerve pathways that coordinate outlet opening with detrusor contraction, the outlet contracts rather than relaxes during bladder contractions, leading to outlet obstruction. Decreased detrusor contractility is associated with neuropathy resulting from diabetes mellitus and alcoholism and nerve damage to the bladder due to tumors or disc compression. In addition, myopathy related to chronic outlet obstruction can also cause the bladder not to empty normally.

Types and Causes of Urinary Incontinence

Urinary incontinence has been classified into two types: (1) acute or transient incontinence and (2) persistent or established incontinence. Acute or transient incontinence has a sudden onset, usually associated with an acute medi-

cal or surgical condition, and often resolves itself when the precipitating condition is resolved. Persistent or established incontinence may have a sudden onset with an acute condition or a gradual onset with no known precipitating cause, and it often increases in severity over time (Ouslander, 1981).

Acute Urinary Incontinence

The acute or reversible causes of urinary incontinence can be remembered by the mnemonic DRIP as coined by Kane, Ouslander, and Abrass (1984), with one addition by this author.

D = Delirium
R = Restricted mobility, retention (acute)
I = Infection, inflammation, impaction
P = Pharmaceuticals, polyuria, psychological

Delirium, an acute confusional state, interferes with the awareness of the need to void and the ability to get to a toilet in time. Restricted mobility, especially when urinary frequency and urgency are present, is a common cause of incontinence in the elderly. Acute urinary retention as a result of anticholinergic and narcotic medications that inhibit detrusor contraction can result in overflow incontinence. Any acute illness, including both systemic and symptomatic urinary tract infection, may precipitate incontinence. However, asymptomatic bacteriuria, which is common in older adults, usually does not cause incontinence. Fecal impaction, by obstructing the bladder outlet, causes urinary retention with overflow incontinence.

Many medications (Table 8–1), such as diuretics, sedatives/hypnotics (including alcohol), narcotics, antipsychotics, muscle relaxants, anticholinergics, alpha- and beta-adrenergic agonists or alpha antagonists, and calcium channel blockers can contribute to the development and exacerbation of incontinence. Endocrine or metabolic problems, such as hyperglycemia and hypercalcemia, which may produce polyuria, may occasionally cause incontinence. Psychological causes, such as depression, regression, anger, and hostility

Table 8–1. MEDICATIONS ASSOCIATED WITH URINARY INCONTINENCE

Drug Type	Effect on Function
Diuretics	Increase urinary volume and frequency
Sedatives/hypnotics, tranquilizers, narcotics	Decrease awareness of need to void
	Decrease conscious inhibition of voiding
	Decrease bladder contraction
	Decrease outlet resistance
Anticholinergics (psychotropics, antiparkinsonian, antispasmodics, antihistamines)	Decrease bladder contraction
	Increase outlet resistance
Alpha-adrenergic agonists	Increase outlet resistance
Beta-adrenergic agonists	Decrease bladder contraction
Alpha antagonists	Decrease outlet resistance
Calcium channel blockers	Decrease bladder contraction

toward caregivers, have also been linked to incontinence.

Persistent Urinary Incontinence

Several classification schemes have been devised to categorize the various types of established urinary incontinence. A useful method that is consistent with the nursing diagnoses approved through the North American Nursing Diagnosis Association (NANDA) is based on presenting symptoms: (1) stress incontinence, (2) urge incontinence, (3) overflow incontinence, and (4) functional incontinence (Table 8–2) (Ouslander & Uman, 1985). It is important to note that these types are not necessarily exclusive. Many older incontinent patients experience two of these types simultaneously. For example, stress and urge incontinence often occur together; this is referred to as mixed incontinence. Functional incontinence may also occur with the three other types of incontinence.

Stress incontinence is characterized by the loss of a small amount of urine usually occurring with sudden increases in intraabdominal pressure, such as with coughing, sneezing, laughing, lifting, or bending. The underlying etiology is sphincteric incompetence or the inability of the urethra to sustain adequate pressure under exertional conditions. With severe urethral sphincter damage, there may be a continuous loss of urine. Stress incontinence is more common in women, but it may also occur in men after prostatectomy surgery.

Urge incontinence is characterized by a strong urge to void occurring immediately prior to the loss of urine. Urine is usually lost in moderate to large amounts. Individuals relate that they cannot make it to the toilet before leakage occurs. Many of these patients also report micturition frequency and nocturia. The underlying etiology is an unstable bladder, also described as detrusor instability, uninhibited bladder, and hyperreflexic bladder. Urge incontinence is more common in men and older individuals.

Overflow incontinence is characterized by continuous dribbling of urine as a result of impaired bladder emptying due to bladder outlet obstruction or impaired detrusor contractility. In addition to constant urine leakage, these patients frequently void in small volumes and have a diminished urine stream and an impaired sensation of bladder fullness.

Functional incontinence is diagnosed when urine leakage occurs in spite of normal bladder and urethral function. It is associated with cognitive and physical impairments, psychological causes, and environmental factors that influence appropriate toileting. Functional incontinence can be caused by inaccessible toilets, unavailable caregivers to assist in toileting, depression, hostility, or impaired mental status.

Assessment of Urinary Incontinence

Urinary incontinence in the elderly results from multiple interacting causes, including physiologic, psychological, social, and environmental factors. Successful management of the problem is based on a thorough evaluation that characterizes the type of incontinence and, if possible, identifies the underlying etiology. Potentially reversible causes for the

Table 8–2. TYPES AND CAUSES OF PERSISTENT URINARY INCONTINENCE

Functional Type	Description	Associated Characteristics	Pathophysiology	Common Causes
Stress	Urine leakage associated with sudden increase in intraabdominal pressure (e.g., cough, sneeze, laugh, exercise) Urine loss, usually small to moderate amount	Occurs usually in daytime only; Infrequent nocturnal incontinence	Sphincter incompetence Urethral instability	Pelvic prolapse in women Sphincter weakness or damage, e.g., following prostatectomy surgery
Urge	Urine leakage preceded by strong desire to void; urine loss varies from moderate to large amount	Urinary frequency, nocturia, possible suprapubic discomfort	Detrusor overactivity (instability or hyperreflexia)	Central nervous system damage due to stroke, Alzheimer's disease, brain tumor, Parkinson's disease Interference with spinal inhibitory pathways due to spondylosis or metastasis; local bladder disorder such as bladder cancer, radiation effects, interstitial cystitis, or outlet obstruction
Overflow	Periodic or continuous dribbling of urine resulting from obstruction and/or overdistention of bladder	Hesitancy, straining to void, weak or interrupted urine stream; occurs day or night	Outlet obstruction or underactive detrusor	Obstruction: prostatic hypertrophy, bladder neck obstruction, urethral stricture Underactive detrusor: myogenic or neurogenic factors, e.g., herniated disc, or peripheral neuropathy from diabetes mellitus Anticholinergic/antispasmodic drugs
Functional	Urine leakage associated with inability or unwillingness to toilet appropriately because of cognitive or physical impairments, psychological factors, or environmental barriers	May be complicated by other medical problems, iatrogenic illness, adverse stimuli	Normal bladder and urethral function	Impaired mobility or cognitive status Inaccessible toilets Depression, anger, hostility, schizophrenia

(From Wyman, JF (1988): Nursing assessment of the geriatric outpatient population. Nurs Clin North Am, 22:169–187. Reprinted with permission.)

incontinence are ruled out. A comprehensive assessment consists of the following components: history and physical examination, a voiding diary or incontinence chart, laboratory and other tests, and, in selected instances, urodynamic evaluation. Key aspects of the evaluation of urinary incontinence are presented in Table 8–3.

Algorithm approaches useful in the diagnosis and management of urinary incontinence in the elderly have been developed (Hilton & Stanton, 1981; Ouslander, 1986).

Table 8–3. EVALUATION OF URINARY INCONTINENCE

History
Characteristics of the Incontinence
Onset, duration, frequency
Timing (diurnal or nocturnal, or both)
Amount and type of loss (spurt or stream, or both; continuous dribbling)
Precipitating circumstances (exertional, i.e., cough, sneeze, laugh, lifting, bending, exercise; position change; washing hands; stressful situations)
Associated symptoms (urgency; dribbling after urination; awareness of bladder fullness; inability to delay voiding; sensation of incomplete bladder emptying; obstructive symptoms, i.e., hesitancy, slow or interrupted stream, straining; UTI symptoms, i.e., dysuria, hematuria)
Use of pads (number of pads or clothing changes/ day)
Current and past management strategies (bladder training, pelvic floor exercises, drug therapy, surgery, preventive toileting, other)
Normal toileting patterns (diurnal, nocturnal)
Genitourinary History
Childhood enuresis
Females—Past childbirth (number, traumatic delivery)
Past surgery (pelvic or lower urinary tract)
Recurrent urinary tract infections
Bladder cancer
Renal disease
Neurologic History
Cerebrovascular accident
Parkinson's disease
Dementia
General Medical History
Acute illness
Diabetes mellitus
Cardiovascular disease (hypertension, congestive heart failure)
Bowel disorders (constipation, impaction, fecal incontinence)
Cancer
Psychological History
Depression
Mental illness
Medication Review
Including nonprescription medications
Functional Assessment
Mobility (use of assistive devices)
Dexterity

Patient's/Caregiver's Perceptions
Perception of cause and severity
Interference with daily activities
Motivation for continence
Expectations for cure
Environmental Characteristics
Accessible toilets
Distance to toilet
Need and use of toilet aids
Physical Examination
Neurologic Examination
Mental Status
Mood
Focal signs
Signs of Parkinson's disease
Gait, walking speed, and balance
Abdominal Examination
Distended bladder
Suprapubic discomfort
Masses
Genital Examination
Skin condition
Signs of infection
Bulbocavernous reflex
Females—Atrophic vaginitis, pelvic relaxation, or other abnormality
Rectal Examination
Sphincter tone
Fecal impaction
Masses
Males—prostatic enlargement
Other
Signs of congestive heart failure
Stress Test*
Voiding Record
Kept for 3–7 days
Laboratory and Other Tests
Post-void residual determination
Urine
Urinalysis (mid-stream, clean-catch specimen)
Urine culture and sensitivity (if indicated)
Blood test (glucose, urea nitrogen, creatinine)
Perineal pad test (outpatient populations)
Urodynamic Evaluation†
Uroflowmetry
Cystometry
Urethral pressure profilometry (females)
Cystourethroscopy

*Requires full bladder.
†In selected cases.

These are attempts to provide evaluation and treatment strategies without having to subject older patients to urodynamic evaluations. A potential problem in using algorithms is the number of patients with mixed urodynamic findings, which are important factors in the determination of appropriate treatment. Further clinical testing to document the validity of these algorithms needs to be conducted before there is widespread adoption of these approaches.

History

A detailed history should be obtained from the patient and caregiver to detail the nature and extent of the incontinence and identify influencing factors. Caution must be exercised in interpreting symptoms reported by older adults as being predictive of urethral or bladder dysfunction. Several studies have demonstrated through urodynamic testing that incontinence symptoms and actual lower urinary tract function do not necessarily correlate in elderly patients (Ouslander, 1986).

The history includes: an assessment of the incontinence; relevant genitourinary, neurologic, medical, and psychological data; medications; functional abilities; environmental characteristics; and attitudes of the patient and caregiver. The first part of the history focuses on identifying the type of incontinence—stress, urge, mixed, or overflow. Information regarding onset, duration, frequency, timing, and amount of urine loss with each incontinent episode and precipitating causes such as coughing, sneezing, lifting, bending, laughing, and washing hands is elicited. Associated symptoms, such as urgency, hesitancy, dysuria, hematuria, lack of sensation of a full bladder, dribbling after voiding, and straining to void, should be noted.

Normal toileting patterns should be determined. Although toileting patterns are variable among individuals, diurnal micturition frequency usually ranges from six to eight voidings per day, and nocturnal micturition frequency is usually not more than twice a night (Abrams, Feneley, & Torrens, 1983). It is also important to identify how long a patient can delay voiding once the first urge to void is perceived. This is critical in older adults with impaired mobility.

Information on the effectiveness of past and present management of the incontinence is important. This includes the use of pads or protective briefs and previous treatments, such as bladder training, drug therapy, or surgical intervention. Identification of past genitourinary surgery, such as repair of pelvic organ relaxation or prostatectomy, also is relevant.

A review of current and past medical problems along with medication use is helpful in determining their possible role in the development of incontinence. Both prescription and over-the-counter drugs should be assessed. Relevant problems to note are: bowel alterations, such as constipation, fecal impaction, or fecal incontinence; neurologic disorders, such as stroke, parkinsonism, and dementia; mobility problems, such as arthritis; metabolic disorders, such as diabetes mellitus and its control; genitourinary problems, such as childhood enuresis, frequency of past urinary tract infections, and bladder cancer; and cardiovascular disease, such as hypertension and congestive heart failure that require use of medications known to precipitate incontinence.

Functional assessment of dexterity and mobility is helpful, as is an evaluation of the environment—accessibility and distance to the bathroom, availability of caregivers, and need for and use of toileting aids. In addition, the patient's and caregiver's attitudes and psychological reaction toward the incontinence, how the incontinence interferes with daily activities, and expectations and motivation for cure are important considerations in determining the appropriate treatment approach.

Physical Examination

The physical examination includes abdominal, genital, rectal, and neurologic examinations, as well as a functional assessment. A mental status evaluation using a standardized 10-item test should be conducted to identify cognitive impairments that may be contributing to the incontinence. Observation of the patient's mood and motivation toward becoming continent is also important. Functional abilities in mobility and manual dexterity required in successful toileting should be assessed.

A brief medical examination should be performed to detect neurologic abnormalities, such as focal and parkinsonian signs and abnormal sensation, and physical findings indicative of congestive heart failure. An abdominal examination is completed to identify bladder distention, suprapubic discomfort or tenderness, and the presence of masses. The pelvic examination includes inspection of the genitalia, noting skin condition and signs of atrophic vaginitis, and palpation for pelvic organ relaxation—urethrocele, cystocele, urethrocystocele, enterocele, or rectocele. In the male, the genitalia should be inspected to note skin condition and any unusual swelling, lesions, nodules, or discharge. In both men and women, the bulbocavernous reflex should be tested to determine intact innervation. The reflex is present if there is an anal contraction in response to a cotton swab being lightly stroked against the glans of the penis in males or the skin near the clitoris in females. The rectal examination includes assessment of the sphincter tone and identification of possible obstructions, such as prostatic enlargement and fecal impaction.

A stress test in which the patient is observed for urine leakage during coughing is useful in diagnosing stress incontinence. This procedure should be performed on patients with a full bladder in both standing and supine positions.

Voiding Record

One of the most helpful assessment techniques is the voiding record (Figure 8–4). The voiding record (also known as a bladder chart or incontinence monitoring record) should be used for a 7-day period to obtain accurate data on the frequency and timing of voluntary micturitions and incontinent episodes. Several variations of a voiding record have been developed for use in institutions (Ouslander, Urman, & Uman, 1986; Autry, Lauzon, & Holliday, 1984) and in outpatient settings (Pierson, 1985; Wyman & Burgio, 1988; Wyman, 1988). Data obtained from the voiding record are helpful in characterizing the pattern and frequency of the incontinence, in determining the relationship between fluid intake and voiding patterns, and in establishing the appropriate management approach.

Laboratory and Other Tests

A clean-catch urine specimen to screen for infection should be collected. Ten or more white blood cells per high power field is suggestive of a urinary tract infection and warrants culture and sensitivity testing. Presence of red cells in the absence of pyuria or bacteriuria may indicate genitourinary pathology; this requires referral for further diagnostic evaluation. The urine pH level may help detect kidney disease and urinary calculus formation, both of which can be contributing factors in incontinence. Urine glucose and protein results may also reveal undetected diabetes and renal disease. Blood chemistry determination of glucose, urea nitrogen, and creatinine should be conducted to screen for uncontrolled diabetes and renal disease.

Documenting the postvoiding residual urine volume through a single sterile catheterization is valuable in ruling out overflow incontinence. Residual volumes of more than 100 ml may indicate significant obstruction or a hypotonic bladder.

Several techniques have been developed for objectively documenting the frequency of incontinent episodes or the severity of incontinence in terms of urine volume lost. These include electronic devices to record episodes of urine loss (Eadie, Glen, & Rowan, 1983) and a quantification test using a perineal pad technique. In general, pad tests involve the patient performing several activities while wearing a preweighed pad. Upon completion of the activities, the pad is reweighed to determine the amount of urine lost during the test. A weight gain of more than 2 gm is considered significant for the objective demonstration of incontinence. Both clinic and home tests have been developed (Sutherst, Brown, & Shawer, 1981; Pierson, 1985; Fantl, Harkins, Wyman, et al., 1987).

Urodynamic Evaluation

In selected patients, referral to a urologist or a urogynecologist for urodynamic evalua-

Time	Did you urinate in the toilet?	Did you have a leaking episode? L = large; S = small	Activity at time of leakage	Urge present	Amount/type fluid intake
12–1 AM					
1–2 AM					
2–3 AM					
3–4 AM					
4–5 AM					
5–6 AM					
6–7 AM					
7–8 AM					
8–9 AM					
9–10 AM					
10–11 AM					
11–12 N					
12–1 PM					
1–2 PM					
2–3 PM					
3–4 PM					
4–5 PM					
5–6 PM					
6–7 PM					
7–8 PM					
8–9 PM					
9–10 PM					
10–11 PM					
11–12 PM					

Figure 8–4. The voiding diary. (From Wyman, J: Nursing assessment of the geriatric outpatient population. Nurs Clin North Am, 22:182, 1988. Reprinted with permission.)

tion may be indicated after completion of the history, physical examination, and laboratory tests. Although urodynamic tests to evaluate urinary incontinence in the elderly have been questioned (Williams, 1983), most clinicians feel they are useful in specific situations (Castleden, Duffin, & Aswer, 1981; Resnick & Yalla, 1985; Diokno, 1986). Criteria for patient selection include: complex symptomatology, associated neurologic abnormalities, incomplete bladder emptying, previous incontinence surgery, behavioral or drug therapy failures with apparently simple or uncomplicated incontinence, and those scheduled for surgical correction of their incontinence (Diokno, 1986).

A basic urologic and urodynamic evaluation consists of uroflowmetry, cystometry, urethral pressure profilometry, and cystourethroscopy. Uroflowmetry is a simple, noninvasive test that is useful in the assessment of emptying phase dysfunctions. It is particularly helpful in the diagnosis of urethral obstruction in males. The test involves the patient voiding into a special toilet that is linked electronically to a strip chart recorder that measures the urine flow rate.

Cystometry is useful in the assessment of filling and storage dysfunctions. It provides information on bladder capacity, sensation of bladder filling, and the stability of the detrusor muscle during bladder filling and provocative maneuvers. Figure 8–5 illustrates a cystometric tracing of an uninhibited detrusor contraction.

Urethral pressure profilometry, used primarily in women, helps to determine the competence of the urethral sphincteric mechanism. The test is performed at rest and with coughing during withdrawal of a dual-tip catheter, which permits simultaneous measurement of intraurethral and intravesical pressure. This procedure provides information on the functional urethral length, the maximum urethral closure pressure, and the shape of the profile curve. When sphincteric incompetence is present, the urethral closing pressure becomes negative with coughing. Figure 8–6 illustrates three findings on the urethral dynamic profilometry. Cystourethroscopy allows direct visualization of the urethra and bladder. It is useful in determining the presence of abnormalities such as urethral stricture, tumors, fistulae, calculi, and diverticuli.

FECAL INCONTINENCE

Prevalence

Prevalence studies of fecal incontinence reveal that it occurs in 3% to 4% of the community-dwelling elderly (Thomas, Egan, Walgrove, et al., 1984; Campbell, Reinken, & McCosh, 1985) and in 10% of institutionalized older populations (Tobin & Brocklehurst, 1986). Fecal incontinence is usually associated with urinary incontinence (Gilleard, 1980). The prevalence of double incontinence (fecal and urinary incontinence) is estimated to be 10% to 13% in noninstitutionalized populations (Thomas, et al., 1984) and 20% in those elderly residing in institutions (Isaacs & Walkey, 1964). Fecal incontinence in older adults is often associated with cognitive impairments.

Mechanism of Continence

The maintenance of fecal continence involves the functioning of the internal and external sphincter and the puborectalis and levator ani muscles (Figure 8–7) in combination with nervous system control. Although the act of defecation is a reflex activity independent of the central nervous system, the desire to defecate and the ability to inhibit defecation are under central voluntary control through a center in the medulla.

The internal sphincter, composed of smooth muscle and regulated by the autonomic ner-

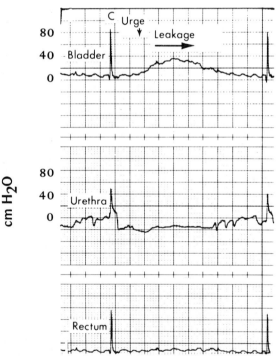

Figure 8–5. Cystometry tracing illustrating urge incontinence. An involuntary detrusor contraction occurred 10 seconds after a cough (C). There was a strong sensation of urge prior to the detrusor contraction, with evidence of urine leakage. (From Fantl, JA, Hurt, WG, and Dunn, LJ: Dysfunctional detrusor control. Am J Obstet Gynecol, 129:300, 1977. Used with permission.)

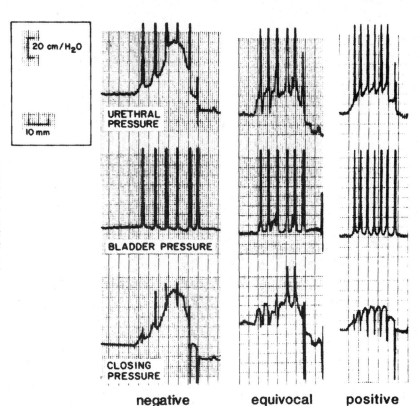

Figure 8–6. Dynamic urethral pressure profiles. These illustrate normal function (negative profile), equivocal function (equivocal profile), and abnormal function or sphincteric incompetence (positive profile). (From Fantl, JA, Hurt, WG, Bump, RC, et al: Urethral axis and sphincteric function. Am J Obstet Gynecol, *155*:555, 1986. Reprinted with permission.)

vous system, is under involuntary control. The external sphincter and the puborectalis and levator ani muscles are regulated by the somatic nervous system and thus are under voluntary control. The lumen of the anal canal in the normal resting state is occluded by the puborectalis muscle sling and by the resting tone of the internal and external sphincters.

The intake of food initiates the gastrocolic reflex and stimulates mass peristalsis in the small intestine and colon. Fecal contents progress toward the rectum, which becomes distended, leading to a transient relaxation of the internal sphincter and the feeling of an urge to defecate. This urge resolves as the rectum accommodates the increasing fecal mass. When the distention reaches 150 to 200 ml, the internal sphincter relaxes completely. Entry of fecal content into the anal canal causes reflex contraction of the external sphincter

with synchronous relaxation of the internal sphincter. If socially convenient, rectal contents are eliminated; if it is not convenient, the internal sphincter contracts again with inhibition of the desire to defecate (Smith, 1983). Voluntary inhibition of the defecation reflex returns stool to the sigmoid and descending colon.

Fecal continence is dependent upon four factors: (1) rectal sensation—the ability to perceive rectal distention, (2) ability to contract the external anal sphincter and puborectalis muscle, (3) motivation to make the appropriate response, and (4) ability of the rectum to serve as a reservoir for feces through adaptive compliance and accommodation (Wald, 1986). Alterations in cognitive function or the sphincter mechanism, or marked changes in fecal contents form the basis for the majority of cases of fecal incontinence.

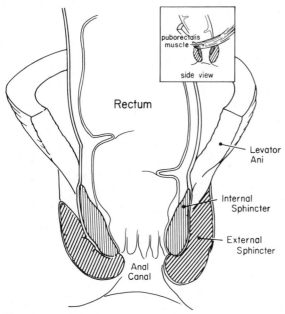

Figure 8–7. Structures involved in the maintenance of fecal continence.

Causes of Fecal Incontinence

Fecal incontinence is associated with four causes: (1) fecal impaction, (2) gastrointestinal disorders, (3) neurologic disorders, and (4) iatrogenic causes (Table 8–4) (Hamdy, 1984). The most common cause in the elderly is fecal stasis and impaction, which are often the result of chronic constipation. Contributing factors include immobility or lack of exercise, dietary causes associated with decreased intake of fibers and fluids, and painful anal conditions, such as hemorrhoids or fissures in which the patient postpones defecation to avoid pain. These patients usually present with continuous incontinence with loose stools. Although the majority of fecal impactions occur rectally and can be easily diagnosed by digital examination, this is not always the case. An x-ray film of the abdomen may reveal the presence of fecal impaction.

Gastrointestinal disorders that cause diarrhea can contribute to the development of incontinence, particularly in patients with reduced mobility or those with a loss of rectal sensation and feeling of the urge to defecate. Diarrhea can result from acute bowel infections, irritable bowel syndrome, and nonspecific inflammatory bowel conditions, such as diverticulitis, ulcerative colitis, or Crohn's disease. Tumors of the colon or rectum can also present as fecal incontinence. These usually occur with poor appetite, loss of weight, alternating bouts of diarrhea and constipation, and occult or frank blood in the stools.

Neurologic causes for fecal incontinence can be local or central in origin. Central causes are more common in the elderly and are related to the loss of inhibition of the defecation reflex, which occurs in patients with severe cognitive impairments. In these cases, there is once or twice daily passage of a formed stool into the bed or clothing usually following the intake of food when the gastrocolic reflex is stimulated. This type of incontinence can be more successfully managed than other types. Fecal incontinence can also occur in patients with inefficient local inhibitory reflexes, which make it difficult to constrict the sphincter adequately. Long-term laxative abuse, which can damage the colonic myenteric plexus, is a major contributory factor. Other factors are related to nerve damage associated with

Table 8–4. CAUSES OF FECAL INCONTINENCE

Fecal Impaction
Chronic constipation
    Decreased dietary fiber and fluids
    Decreased exercise
    Immobility
Gastrointestinal Disorders
Diarrhea
Diverticulitis
Infections
Ulcerative colitis
Crohn's disease
Proctitis
Rectal prolapse
Postoperative complications
Tumors of colon or rectum
Neurologic Disorders
Dementia
Autonomic neuropathy, e.g., diabetes mellitus
Inefficient local inhibitory reflexes
Spinal cord injury
Iatrogenic Causes
Chronic laxative or enema use
Drug-induced

stretching and compression of the nerves from prolonged straining at the stool, rectal prolapse, spinal cord injury, and pelvic floor descent (Smith, 1983). Diabetic neuropathy may also underlie fecal incontinence.

Iatrogenic causes for fecal incontinence are related to excessive use of enemas or drug use known to produce diarrhea or constipation (Table 8–5). Diarrhea-causing drugs include antibiotics, laxatives, and magnesium-containing antacids. Constipation-causing drugs include iron preparations, anticholinergics, narcotics, some diuretics, and aluminum-containing antacids.

Assessment of Fecal Incontinence

Assessment of the patient with fecal incontinence involves a careful history to identify possible contributing causes, a physical examination, a bowel record, and functional assessment. The prognosis for patients with double incontinence of long duration is worse than for patients with a recent onset of fecal incontinence associated with drug use or gas-

Table 8–5. MEDICATIONS ALTERING BOWEL FUNCTION

Drugs Inducing Diarrhea
Antibiotics
Magnesium-containing antacids
Stimulant laxatives, e.g., cascara, senna, bisacodyl
Lithium
Colchicine
Guanethidine
Drugs Inducing Constipation
Iron
Anticholinergics
   Antidepressants (tricyclics, monoamide oxidase
     inhibitors)
   Antiparkinsonian
   Antipsychotics, e.g., phenothiazines
   Antiarrhythmics
   Antispasmodics
   Antihistamines
Narcotics
Aluminum- and calcium-containing antacids
Muscle relaxants
Lomotil
Laxatives and cathartics (chronic use)
Diuretics
Sedatives

trointestinal symptoms such as diarrhea, abdominal colic, and tenesmus. Table 8–6 summarizes the key aspects in the evaluation of fecal incontinence.

History

The history includes a characterization of the incontinence, such as its onset, duration, frequency, timing, amount, and consistency, and associated symptoms, such as urgency, lack of warning, presence of blood, diarrhea, constipation, and straining to defecate. Normal bowel patterns and laxative use prior to the incontinence should be ascertained. An individual with chronic constipation who develops fecal incontinence is most likely to have an impaction, whereas a patient who has episodes of diarrhea alternating with constipation is likely to have either an underlying lesion of the lower gastrointestinal tract or a regimen of alternating laxatives and constipating agents. Fecal incontinence in patients with previously regular bowel movements could be related to a neoplastic lesion of the rectum or sigmoid colon, particularly if the feces contain a large amount of mucus. Relevant information should be collected on anorectal surgery or trauma, recent weight loss, diabetes, urinary incontinence, spinal surgery, immobility, dementia, neurologic disease, multiple childbirths, inflammatory bowel disease, and past pelvic radiation or trauma. A medication review should focus on identification of drugs known to induce constipation, such as anticholinergics, narcotics, iron, diuretics, and aluminum-containing antacids, and those known to induce diarrhea, such as cathartics, suppositories, enema preparations, and magnesium-containing antacids. A diet history with particular attention to adequacy of fiber and fluids, should be obtained as well as an activity history. Assessment of the environment for access to toileting facilities, availability of caregivers to assist in toileting, and difficulty with clothing fastenings should be conducted. Evaluation of the patient's motivation to be continent and the attitudes of the caregiver, if present, are also important con-

Table 8–6. EVALUATION OF FECAL INCONTINENCE

History	**Environmental Characteristics**
Characteristics of the Incontinence	Accessible bathrooms
Onset, duration, frequency	Use of bedside commode
Stool consistency (loose, formed, hard) and amount	Restrictive clothing
Timing (diurnal or nocturnal, or both; associated with meals)	Availability of caregivers
Associated symptoms (urgency, lack of warning, alternating bouts of diarrhea and constipation, straining to defecate, blood in stool)	**Physical Examination**
	Abdominal Examination
	Presence of masses
Normal bowel patterns (daily pattern, habits associated with defecation)	**Neurologic Examination**
	Mental status
Laxative (cathartics, suppositories) and enema use	Evidence of peripheral neuropathies
Relevant Medical History	**Rectal Examination**
Past surgery (anorectal, intestinal, laminectomy)	Condition of perineum (excoriation)
Past childbirths (number, traumatic delivery)	Anorectal conditions (fissures, hemorrhoids, prolapse, anal deformity)
Past pelvic trauma or radiation	Presence of anal gaping
Gastrointestinal disorders (bowel infection, irritable bowel syndrome, diverticulitis, ulcerative colitis, Crohn's disease, carcinoma, anorectal conditions)	External anal sphincter tone and voluntary contraction
	Fecal mass or impaction
	Prostatic enlargement
Neurologic disorders (dementia)	Bulbocavernous reflex
Metabolic disorders (diabetes mellitus)	Stool occult blood
Concomitant urinary incontinence	**Functional Assessment**
Medication Review	**Mobility Status**
(Include nonprescription drugs)	Ability to toilet self
Drugs inducing constipation	**Bowel Record**
Drugs inducing diarrhea	Keep 1 week
Diet History	**Laboratory and Other Tests***
Adequacy of fiber intake	Stool culture
Adequacy of fluid intake	Abdominal x-ray
Activity Patterns	Barium enema
Active versus inactive	Sigmoidoscopy
Patient's/Caregiver's Perceptions	
Perception of cause and severity	
Interference with daily activities	
Motivation for continence	
Burden on caregiver	

*If indicated.

siderations in determining the management approach.

Physical Examination

The physical examination includes abdominal palpation to determine presence of feces and a rectal examination to detect hemorrhoids or painful fissures, rectal prolapse, prostatic enlargement, fecal impaction or rectal mass, anal deformity or disease, and anal gaping. Anal gaping, or failure of the anal canal to contract after digital examination, indicates sphincter damage. In general, estimation of anal sphincter tone and strength on digital examination correlates poorly with objective tests (Wald, 1986). Any excoriation of the perineum should be noted.

Mental status testing should be conducted along with an exploration of the patient's awareness of the problem and motivation to become continent. In cases of severe dementia, the patient most likely has concomitant urinary incontinence and no awareness of either problem. A neurologic examination to screen for underlying contributory neuropathies and absent bulbocavernous reflex should also be completed. Mobility status and the ability to toilet oneself need to be determined.

Bowel Record

A bowel record (Figure 8–8) is useful in assessing the stool characteristics in relation-

DATE: _____

| TIME | BOWEL | | STOOL CONSISTENCY (Hard, Soft, Fluid) & Amount (Large, Small) | USE OF SUPPOSITORY (Number) or ENEMA | URINE | | FLUID INTAKE | FOOD INTAKE (Poor, Fair, Good) | PHYSICAL ACTIVITY (None, Poor, Fair, Good) |
	Incontinent	Normal			Incontinent	Normal			
12–1 AM									
1–2 AM									
2–3 AM									
3–4 AM									
4–5 AM									
5–6 AM								Breakfast	
6–7 AM									
7–8 AM									
8–9 AM									
9–10 AM									
10–11 AM									
11–12 AM								Lunch	
12–1 PM									
1–2 PM									
2–3 PM									
3–4 PM									
4–5 PM								Dinner	
5–6 PM									
6–7 PM									
7–8 PM									
8–9 PM									
9–10 PM									
10–11 PM									
11–12 PM									

Figure 8–8. Bowel record.

ship to variables known to influence bowel patterns. Data obtained from the bowel record are helpful in characterizing the pattern and frequency of the incontinence and the relationships among fluid and food intake, activity patterns, laxative use, and timing of bowel movements. This record will help determine the appropriate management approach.

Laboratory and Other Tests

Laboratory investigations may include tests for occult blood in the feces and a stool culture if the incontinence was of sudden onset, of short duration, and associated with diarrhea. Other tests might be indicated to rule out causes of contributory diarrhea or constipation. If indicated, patients may be referred for further medical evaluation, including radiographic studies of the abdomen and lower gastrointestinal tract and sigmoidoscopy.

URINARY TRACT INFECTION

Prevalence and Types

Older adults are at high risk for the development of urinary tract infections (UTIs). Prevalence estimates for bacteriuria range from 6% to 13% in community-dwelling elderly men and 7% to 33% in community-dwelling elderly women. Estimates in institutionalized elderly range from 17% to 26% in men to 23% to 27% in women. In hospitals, the incidence is approximately 33% for both men and women (Sourander & Kasanen, 1972; Akhtar, Andrews, Caird, et al., 1972; Brocklehurst, Dillane, Griffiths, et al., 1968). The incidence of UTI increases with advancing age and is associated with obstructive uropathy, high residual urine volumes, fecal and urinary incontinence, immobility, debilitating illnesses, diabetes mellitus, and institutionalization in either an acute-care hospital or nursing home. The risk of catheter-induced bacteriuria is especially high in the elderly.

Urinary tract infections include bacteriuria, cystitis, and pyelonephritis. Bacteriuria is the presence of 10^5 organisms per ml of urine or more. Cystitis is the presence of bacteriuria with lower urinary tract symptoms such as dysuria, urgency, and frequency. Pyelonephritis is bacteriuria with upper urinary tract symptoms, such as chills, fever, and flank pain.

Assessment of Urinary Tract Infections

The diagnosis of UTI in the elderly is complicated. Most older adults with UTIs are asymptomatic, particularly those with chronic bacteriuria. In addition, many elderly patients present with symptoms suggestive of infection, such as urgency and frequency, but they do not show laboratory evidence of UTI (Romano & Kaye, 1981). Other patients present atypically, perhaps with signs of confusion.

Assessment of UTI includes a history and laboratory tests. The history should focus on classic symptoms of infection, such as dysuria, urgency, frequency, incontinence, hematuria, pyuria, and suprapubic discomfort, as well as nonspecific symptoms, such as fever, vomiting, and mental changes.

Initial laboratory investigation includes a screening urinalysis using a clean-catch midstream urine specimen. If mobility or cognitive impairments prevent the collection of a midstream urine specimen, a catheterized specimen should be obtained. If 10 or more WBCs and/or positive nitrites are present, urine culture and sensitivity testing should be conducted. Positive diagnosis of UTI is made when there are at least 10^5 organisms per milliliter. Simple, economical dip-slide office culture kits are available that have good reliability for use in clinic and nursing home settings (Block, 1986). Men with documented UTIs should be referred for further urologic evaluation.

CONSTIPATION

Prevalence

Constipation is a common complaint of older adults. Although perceived to be an age-related problem, the frequency of bowel movements is not different in healthy old persons than in the young (Milne & Williamson, 1972). Transit time through the intestinal tract in mobile older people is similar to that in younger individuals (Brocklehurst, 1980). However, elderly persons are twice as likely to use laxatives than are younger people (Connell, Hilton, Irvin, et al., 1965). One explanation for this greater use of laxatives could be related to a latent constipation. According to Brocklehurst (1980), a more likely explanation is that many older adults were raised during the era of the medical notion of "autointoxication from the colon" in which daily bowel elimination was thought to be required for good health.

The definition of constipation is highly subjective. Constipation has been defined as insufficient frequency of defecation, deficient quantity of stool, or abnormally hard and dry stools (Benson, 1975). Determining insufficient frequency is difficult. A normal bowel pattern may range from three stools a day to a comfortable bowel movement once every 3 to 5 days.

Types and Causes of Constipation

Constipation may be classified into two types: spastic and atonic (Sklar, 1986). The spastic type is characterized by small hard stools and lower abdominal discomfort. Intermittent episodes of diarrhea are common. Rectal examination may reveal an empty ampulla. The underlying cause is excessive segmental contraction of the lower colon and an increase in sigmoid tone. This form of constipation is associated with fecal impaction.

The atonic type, the more common type, is characterized by soft, puttylike stool upon rectal examination. A dilated colon filled with feces is observed on abdominal x-ray film. This type of constipation is associated with a hypotonic colon. Laxative abuse is a common cause. Repeatedly ignoring the urge to defecate, which causes the rectum to accommodate, thus contributing to the loss of full rectal sensation, may also be a factor.

Several factors contribute to the development of constipation in the elderly. Decreased physical activity or immobility, inadequate intake of fluids and fiber, physical debility, and chronic use of laxatives and enemas are primary causes. Medications such as narcotics, anticholinergics, psychotropics, iron, and aluminum- or calcium-containing antacids may also cause constipation. Patients with painful rectal disorders such as anal fissures and hemorrhoids may postpone the urge to defecate, become constipated, and ultimately develop a fecal impaction. Gastrointestinal disorders such as diverticular disease, colorectal carcinoma, and colitis are causative factors. Metabolic disturbances, including diabetes mellitus, hypokalemia, hypercalcemia, and hypothyroidism, are other contributing factors. Psychological reactions, especially anxiety and depression, contribute to constipation. Neurologic disorders, including Parkinson's disease, autonomic neuropathy, and spinal cord abnormalities, are also associated with constipation.

Age-associated changes place an older person at risk for development of constipation. These include decreased intestinal motility, which causes a delayed transit time, and weakened abdominal muscles, which make it difficult to apply adequate pressure during defecation. In addition, diet alterations due to poor dentition, smell and taste changes, inadequate fluid intake related to decreased feeling of thirst, use of easy-to-prepare foods that are highly refined and low in fiber, and anorexia also contribute to the development of constipation. Psychological factors resulting from stress and depression accompanying the many personal losses an older person encounters may affect nutritional intake (Resnick, 1985).

Assessment of Constipation

Assessment of constipation involves a history, physical examination, and bowel record. The history should include the patient's definition of constipation along with a characterization of normal bowel function and associated symptoms, such as frequency of defecation, stool consistency and color, melena, difficulty in expelling feces, painful defecation, sensation of incomplete evacuation after a bowel movement, flatulence, and toileting habits related to defecation. Other symptoms that often accompany constipation should be noted: headache, foul breath, furred tongue, fatigability, irritability, and insomnia. The onset and duration of constipation should be determined. Strategies used by the patient to manage the constipation, including dietary changes and laxative and enema use, should be ascertained. Relevant information on past and present medical problems that could influence the development of constipation should be collected, such as anal fissures, hemorrhoids, ulcerative proctitis, diverticular disease, cancer, diabetes mellitus, and hypothyroidism. A review of medications focuses on drugs known to cause constipation. A careful diet history should be obtained and analyzed for adequacy of fiber and fluid intake and any recent changes in dietary patterns. Information on meal patterns and preferences should be obtained. Many older adults who live by themselves or have recently lost a spouse have difficulty eating alone. Activity patterns and recent changes should also be noted. The emotional state of the patient should be evaluated to determine if stress or depression may be a contributing factor.

The physical examination includes abdominal and rectal examinations. The abdominal examination notes increased or absent bowel sounds, abdominal distention or tenderness, and palpable masses. Absent or increased bowel sounds are associated with bowel obstruction. Tenderness may indicate diverticulosis. A palpated mass in the descending colon may be feces. The presence of an enlarged liver could be suggestive of a neoplastic process. A rectal examination is critical in the evaluation. The presence of anal fissures, hemorrhoids, and impaction should be noted, along with anal sphincter tone. A stool test for occult blood should be performed.

If simple causes for the constipation cannot be determined or if the clinical evidence such as recent onset of severe weight loss is suggestive of a pathologic process, the patient should be referred for further medical evaluation. This evaluation may incorporate additional tests, such as complete blood count and electrolyte determination, abdominal x-ray studies, barium enema, and proctoscopy or sigmoidoscopy examination.

SUMMARY

Incontinence is a common problem in gerontological nursing practice. Urinary incontinence is more prevalent in the elderly. When fecal incontinence does occur, it usually is associated with urinary incontinence. Both types of incontinence are amenable to management. The key to successful management lies in a thorough evaluation of the problem and identification of the underlying causes. Related problems that occur with incontinence are urinary tract infections and constipation. This chapter presented an overview of incontinence and related problems and described their assessment. Management will be presented in the following chapters.

References

Abrams, P, Feneley, R, & Torrens, M (1983): Patient assessment. *Urodynamics.* New York, Springer-Verlag, 6–27.

Akhtar, AJ, Andrews, GR, Caird, FI, et al. (1972): Urinary tract infection in the elderly: A population study. *Age Ageing,* 1:48–54.

Autry, P, Lauzon, F, & Holliday, PJ (1984): The voiding record: An aid to decrease incontinence. *Geriatr Nurs,* 5:22–25.

Bates, CP, Bradley, WE, Glen, ES, et al. (1979): The standardization of terminology of lower urinary tract function. *J Urol,* 121:551–554.

Benson, S (1975): Simple chronic constipation: Pathophysiology and management. *Postgrad Med,* 57(1):55–60.

Block, B (1986): Urinary tract infections. *Am Fam Physician,* 33:172–185.

Brocklehurst, JC (1980): Disorders of the lower bowel in old age. *Geriatrics,* 35(5):47–52.

Brocklehurst, JC, Dillane, JB, Griffiths, L, et al. (1968): The prevalence and symptomatology of urinary infection in an aged population. *Gerontol Clin,* 10:242–253.

Campbell, AJ, Reinken, J, & McCosh, L (1985): Incontinence in the elderly: Prevalence and prognosis. *Age Ageing,* 14:65–70.

Castleden, CM, Duffin, HM, & Aswer, MS (1981): Clinical and urodynamic studies in 100 elderly incontinent patients. *Br Med J, 282*:1103–1105.

Connell, AM, Hilton, C, Irvin, G, et al. (1965): Variations in bowel habit in 2 population samples. *Br Med J, 2*:1095–1099.

Diokno, AC (1986): Urinary incontinence in the elderly. *In* Calkins, E, Davis, PJ, & Ford, AB (eds): *The Practice of Geriatrics.* Philadelphia, WB Saunders, 358–369.

Diokno, AC, Brock, BM, Brown, MB, et al. (1986): Prevalence of urinary incontinence and other urological symptoms in the noninstitutionalized elderly. *J Urol, 136*:1022–1025.

Donaldson, LJ, & Jagger, C (1983): Survival and functional capacity: Three year followup of an elderly population in hospitals and home. *J Epidemiol Community Health, 37*:176–179.

Eadie, AS, Glen, ES, & Rowan, D (1983): The Urilos recording nappy system. *Br J Urol, 55*:301–303.

Fantl, JA, Harkins, SW, Wyman, JF, et al. (1987): Fluid quantitation test in women with urinary incontinence: A test-retest analysis. *Obstet Gynecol, 70*:739–743.

Fantl, JA, Hurt, WG, Bump, RC, et al. (1986): Urethral axis and sphincteric function. *Am J Obstet Gynecol, 155*:544–548.

Fantl, JA, Hurt, WG, & Dunn, LJ (1977): Dysfunctional detrusor control. *Am J Obstet Gynecol, 129*:299–303.

Gilleard, CJ (1980): Prevalence of incontinence in local authority homes for the elderly. *Health Bull, 38*:236–238.

Gosling, J (1979): The structure of the bladder and urethra in relation to function. *Urol Clin North Am, 6*:31–38.

Hamdy, RC (1984): Faecal incontinence. *In Geriatric Medicine: A Problem-Oriented Approach.* London, Bailliere Tindall, 150–165.

Hilton, P, & Stanton, SL (1981): Algorithmic method for assessing urinary incontinence in elderly women. *Br Med J, 282*:940–942.

Hu, T (1986): The economic impact of urinary incontinence. *Clin Geriatr Med, 2*:673–688.

Isaacs, B, & Walkey, FA (1964): A survey of incontinence in elderly hospital patients. *Gerontol Clin, 6*:367–376.

Kane, RL, Ouslander, JG, & Abrass, IB (1984): Incontinence. *In Essentials of Clinical Geriatrics.* New York, McGraw-Hill, 107–136.

Milne, JS, & Williamson, J (1972): Bowel habits in older people. *Gerontol Clin, 14*:56–60.

Mohide, EA (1986): The prevalence and scope of urinary incontinence. *Clin Geriatr Med, 2*:639–656.

Ory, M, Wyman, JF, & Yu, L (1986): Psychosocial factors in urinary incontinence. *Clin Geriatr Med, 2*:657–672.

Ouslander, JG (1981): Urinary incontinence in the elderly. *West J Med, 135*:482–491.

Ouslander, JG (1986): Diagnostic evaluation of geriatric urinary incontinence. *Clin Geriatr Med, 2*:715–730.

Ouslander, JG, & Uman, GC (1985): Urinary incontinence: Opportunities for research, education, and improvements in medical care in the nursing home setting. *In* Schneider, EL (ed): *The Teaching Nursing Home.* New York, Raven Press, 173–196.

Ouslander, JG, Urman, HN, & Uman, GC (1986): Development and testing of an incontinence monitoring record. *J Am Geriatr Soc, 34*:83–90.

Pierson, CA (1985): Pad testing, nursing interventions, and urine loss appliances. *In* Ostergard, DR (ed): *Gynecologic Urology and Urodynamics: Theory and Practice* (ed 2). Baltimore, Williams & Wilkins, 243–262.

Resnick, B (1985): Constipation: Common but preventable. *Geriatr Nurs, 6*:213–215.

Resnick, NM, & Yalla, SV (1985): Management of urinary incontinence in the elderly. *N Engl J Med, 313*:800–804.

Romano, JM, & Kaye, D (1981): UTI in the elderly: Common yet atypical. *Geriatrics, 36*:113–120.

Rosen, L, Khubchandani, IT, Sheets, JA, et al. (1986): Management of anal incontinence. *Am Fam Physician, 33*:129–137.

Sklar, M (1986): Gastrointestinal diseases. *In* Calkins, E, Davis, PJ, Ford, AB (eds): *The Practice of Geriatrics.* Philadelphia, WB Saunders, 555–575.

Smith, RG (1983): Fecal incontinence. *J Am Geriatr Soc, 31*:694–697.

Sourander, LB, & Kasanen, A (1972): A 5-year follow-up of bacteriuria in the aged. *Gerontol Clin, 14*:247–281.

Staskin, DT (1986): Age-related physiologic and pathologic changes affecting lower urinary tract function. *Clin Geriatr Med, 2*:701–710.

Sutherst, J, Brown, M, & Shawer, M (1981): Assessing the severity of urinary incontinence in women with perineal pads. *Lancet, 1*:1128–1129.

Thomas, TM, Egan, M, Walgrove, A, et al. (1984): The prevalence of faecal and double incontinence. *Comm Med, 6*:216–220.

Tobin, GW, & Brocklehurst, JC (1988): Faecal incontinence in residential homes for the elderly: Prevalence, aetiology and management. *Age Aging, 15*:41–46.

Wald, A (1986): Fecal incontinence: Effective nonsurgical treatments. *Postgrad Med, 80*(3):123–130.

Wells, T (1980): Promoting urine control in older adults: Scope of the problem. *Geriatr Nurs, 1*:236–240.

Williams, ME (1983): A critical evaluation of the assessment technology for urinary incontinence in older persons. *J Am Geriatr Soc, 31*:657–664.

Wyman, J (1988): Nursing assessment of the geriatric outpatient population. *Nurs Clin North Am, 22*:169–187.

Wyman, J, & Burgio, KL (1988): Advances in urinary incontinence management in the elderly. *Adv Clin Rehab, 2*:82–107.

CHAPTER
9

Managing Urinary Incontinence

MARY LOU LONG, R.N.C., M.S.N.

INTRODUCTION

Urinary incontinence is one of the most distressing health care problems facing the elderly. The physical and psychological effects of urinary incontinence contribute to feelings of hopelessness and low self-worth. They rob the elderly of their independence and dignity. Failure to properly diagnose and treat the problem leads to serious complications, including urinary tract infections, skin breakdowns, social isolation, and depression.

The economic burden is enormous when considering the resources required for direct care of the condition, plus the indirect costs of morbidity, disability, and mortality (Hu,

1986). The total economic impact is unclear due to the limited data on incontinence prevalence rates and relevant costs. Consequently, proper diagnosis and treatment have significant impact on elderly patients' health as well as on the health care system. This chapter identifies barriers to treatment and presents treatment options for specific types of urinary incontinence.

BARRIERS TO TREATMENT

Despite a growing body of knowledge about effective forms of treatment, urinary incontinence continues to be generally viewed by health professionals as an inevitable, untreatable result of aging. Barriers to treatment of urinary incontinence exist at all levels of the health care system: in the community, in hospitals, and in nursing homes. Three factors that contribute to the barriers in treatment of the incontinent person include the following (Long, 1985; Ouslander, Kane, Vollmer, et al., 1985):

1. Reluctance of both patients and caregivers to discuss the problem for fear of embarrassment and because of the misconception that it is an inevitable and untreatable condition.

2. Lack of knowledge on the part of health professionals about underlying causes, evaluation techniques, and treatment options.

3. Limited numbers of professionals and

203

financial resources available to treat patients, train other health care professionals, and carry out needed research on the condition.

TREATMENT OPTIONS

The overall goal of treatment of urinary incontinence is to restore continence or manage incontinence, thus keeping the patient dry and free of complications.

Selection of the most appropriate treatment for an elderly patient with urinary incontinence is dependent on a thorough evaluation of genitourinary, neurologic, psychological, and environmental factors. A thorough evaluation should result in a specific diagnosis for the type of incontinence and characteristics of the individual patient.

The treatment options discussed in this chapter are applicable for a specific type or types of incontinence. As illustrated in Table 9–1, more than one treatment option may be appropriate for any type of incontinence. The gerontological nurse's role as change agent, educator, and researcher plays a key part in combating the barriers to treatment. Nurses providing care to elderly persons in all settings must have knowledge and understanding of incontinence and its impact on the elderly patient in order to identify and implement appropriate treatment options. Nursing management consists of: (1) developing nursing standards, procedures, and patient teaching guides and (2) evaluating patient outcomes.

Drugs

Pharmacologic agents can be used to treat urge, stress, and overflow incontinence. The expected action(s) of drugs used to treat these types of incontinence are: strengthen bladder outlet, inhibit bladder contraction, and improve bladder emptying (Ouslander, et al., 1985). Drug therapy as an option must be based on a careful review of coexisting conditions in the elderly patient. Some drugs may elicit improvement of urinary incontinence but may cause cardiovascular, gastrointestinal, or

Table 9–1. TREATMENT OPTIONS FOR TYPES OF URINARY INCONTINENCE

Treatment Option	Type of Incontinence
Drugs	
Bladder relaxants	Urge
Alpha agonists	Stress
Estrogen	Stress
	Urge
Cholinergic agonists	Overflow
Alpha-adrenergic blockers	Overflow
Surgery	
Bladder neck suspension	Stress
Removal of obstruction or lesion	Overflow
Training Procedures	
Kegel exercises	Stress
Biofeedback	Stress
	Urge
Bladder and habit retraining	Urge
	Functional
Mechanical and Electrical Devices	
Artificial sphincters	Stress
Intravaginal electrical stimulation	Stress
	Urge
Anal electrical stimulation	Stress
	Urge
Catheters	
Intermittent and indwelling	Overflow
	Functional
External collection device	Functional
	Urge
Supportive Measures	
Environmental manipulation	Functional
Undergarments and pads	Functional
External collection devices	Functional

Data from Blaivas & Berger (1986); Burgio & Burgio (1986); Ouslander & Sier (1986); Schmidbauer, Chiang, & Raz (1986); Warren (1986).

respiratory complications. Table 9–2 summarizes the drugs commonly prescribed in treating urinary incontinence. Drug therapy is frequently used in combination with other treatment methods such as bladder retraining, biofeedback, and pelvic floor exercises. These treatment methods are discussed later in this chapter.

Bladder Relaxants. Detrusor instability and detrusor hyperreflexia (urge incontinence) have been reported to exist in 40% to 70% of incontinent elderly patients (Ouslander & Sier,

Table 9—2. DRUGS USED TO TREAT URINARY INCONTINENCE

Drugs	Dosages	Types of Incontinence	Potential Side Effects
Anticholinergic			
Propantheline	15–30 mg three times a day	Urge incontinence with uninhibited bladder contractions	Dry mouth Blurry vision
Imipramine	25–50 mg three times a day	Stress incontinence with uninhibited bladder contractions	Elevated intraocular pressure
Oxybutynin	25–50 mg three times a day	Stress incontinence with sphincter weakness	Constipation
Dicyclomine	10–20 mg three times a day	Stress incontinence with sphincter weakness	Postural hypotension, cardiac conduction disturbance (imipramine only)
Flavoxate	100 mg three to four times a day	Stress incontinence with sphincter weakness	Headache
Alpha-Adrenergic Agonists			
Pseudoephedrine	15–30 mg	Stress incontinence with sphincter weakness	Tachycardia
Phenylpropanolamine	50–75 mg twice a day		Elevation of blood pressure
Imipramine	25–50 mg three times a day		See Imipramine, above
Cholinergic Agonists			
Bethanechol	10–30 mg three to four times a day	Overflow incontinence with atonic bladder	Bradycardia, hypotension, bronchoconstriction, gastric acid secretion
Estrogens			
Oral	.625 mg per day	Stress incontinence/female	Endometrial cancer, elevated blood pressure, gallstones
Topical	.05–1 gm per application	Urge incontinence with atrophic vaginitis	

(From Ouslander, JG, & Sier, HC: Drug therapy for geriatric urinary incontinence. *Clin Geriatr. Med.*, 2:790, 1986.

1986; Resnick & Yalla, 1985; Williams & Pannill, 1982). Drug therapy for these conditions is aimed at reducing or blocking detrusor contractions.

Drugs with bladder relaxant properties, anticholinergic activity, or calcium channel blockade are frequently used to reduce detrusor contractions, thus improving the patient's condition (Ouslander & Sier, 1986; Williams & Pannill, 1982). Several drugs have bladder relaxant effect in addition to anticholinergic activity. The use of anticholinergic drugs to treat this type of incontinence has been frequently recommended; however, many side effects occur when they are taken by elderly patients. Such side effects include dry mouth, blurred vision, constipation, tachycardia, esophageal reflux, and mental status changes. Use of anticholinergic drugs in an elderly population should begin cautiously. (See Chapter 19 for a full discussion of anticholinergic drugs.)

Estrogen and Alpha-Adrenergic Agonists. Stress incontinence, characterized by sphincter weakness, is responsive to alpha-adrenergic agonists or estrogen. This pharmacologic intervention is directed toward increasing the resistance of the urethra by the use of the alpha agonists or the use of estrogen for women with atrophic vaginitis. Alpha-adrenergic agonists can be used alone as treatment for stress incontinence in both men and women (Diokno & Taub, 1975). Once again, because of side effects, alpha-adrenergic agonists must be used cautiously in elderly patients with cardiovascular disease, hypertension, or hypothyroidism.

Cholinergic Agonists. Treatment for overflow incontinence generally involves either surgery to remove the obstruction or intermittent or indwelling catheterization. In some situations, pharmacologic agents such as cholinergic agonists and alpha-adrenergic blockers are appropriate. Cholinergic agonists may be used on a short-term basis in patients with acute urinary retention or urinary retention secondary to tricyclic antidepressants (Ouslander & Sier, 1986). The action of cholinergic agonists is to increase the tonicity and contractibility of the bladder, thus increasing bladder emptying. Alpha-adrenergic blockers can be used to overcome outflow obstruction by decreasing the tone in the internal urethral sphincter (Shapiro, Mazouz, & Caine, 1981). The Ouslander and Sier (1986) review of drug studies does not show research findings supporting the use of these drugs as an effective long-term treatment for overflow incontinence.

Nursing Implications. Drug therapy is an effective treatment approach for urinary incontinence in the elderly and must not be overlooked as an option. Close monitoring of the responses to drugs is essential because of the elderly's sensitivity to drugs and potential problems related to multiple drug-taking (polypharmacy). As mentioned earlier, drugs are frequently used in combination with other therapies, such as bladder retraining, biofeedback, and pelvic floor exercises. The gerontological nurse has a major role in the implementation of combined therapies. The goal of combined therapies is to achieve optimal conditions to modify behaviors and strengthen weakened muscles contributing to incontinence. Guidelines for nursing management of the incontinent patient during drug therapy are presented in Table 9–3.

Surgery

Surgical intervention is an appropriate treatment for some patients with stress and urge incontinence, and it is essential for certain patients with overflow incontinence. Objectives of surgical interventions are to relieve obstruction, reposition the bladder neck and urethra, or correct other genitourinary pathology (Blaivas & Berger, 1986; Ouslander, et al.,

Table 9–3. GUIDELINES FOR NURSING MANAGEMENT OF INCONTINENT PATIENTS DURING DRUG THERAPY

Standard
Drug therapy for urinary incontinence.
Procedures/Interventions
Hospital and Nursing Homes
1. Clarify with patient and family the expected outcome of drug therapy.
2. Identify drugs the patient is currently taking that may pose high risk for interactions with the new drug(s).
3. Observe patients for both expected and unexpected effects, i.e., incontinence improved vs. urinary retention.
4. Maintain a bladder record to monitor change in incontinence patterns.
5. Monitor changes in blood pressure, mental status, and functional abilities.
6. Alert the physician to unexpected or potentially problematic outcomes that may be the result of, or affect, drug treatment.
Home Setting or Clinic
1. Clarify with patient and family the expected outcome of the drug therapy.
2. Provide a written list of possible adverse reactions or interactions that the patient should report to the physician.
3. Instruct patient on use of a bladder record to document any change in incontinence patterns.
4. Plan with the patient a time frame for followup.
Patient Teaching Guide
1. Expected outcome of drug therapy.
2. Specific instructions for drug administration, i.e., time, amount, and route.
3. Potential side effects or complications of drugs that the patient should report to the physician.
4. Potential interactions with other drugs or food.
Measurement Criteria for Evaluation
Patient will have:
1. Decreased or no incontinent episodes.
2. Complications or side effects of drugs less problematic than incontinence.

1985; Schmidbauer, Chiang, & Raz, 1986). Surgery should not be discounted as an option for the elderly simply on the basis of age. Improved anesthesia, better pre- and postoperative care, and improved operative techniques have made surgery a safer option for elderly patients.

Bladder Neck Suspension. The most common surgical intervention, bladder neck suspension, is appropriate for women with stress incontinence due to bladder neck incompetence. Fifty percent or more of elderly women have both bladder neck incompetence and urgency incontinence; thus, a combination of treatment options must be considered (Schmidbauer, et al., 1986).

Several types of surgical procedures may be performed, but the most frequently used are anterior colporrhaphy, retropubic transabdominal repair, and combined transvaginal and retropubic procedures.

Removal of an Obstruction or Lesion. Overflow incontinence caused by anatomic obstruction to urine flow requires surgery to relieve the obstruction. A urinary obstruction left untreated predisposes the patient to urinary tract infections that can lead to renal failure and death. The most common causes of obstruction, prostatism and urethral strictures, occur primarily in men. Surgical procedures most commonly done to relieve obstruction in men are transurethral prostatectomy or prostatotomy (Blaivas & Berger, 1986). If surgery is not feasible, intermittent or indwelling catheterization is the next treatment choice.

Surgical intervention is also indicated for incontinence that is the result of lower genitourinary tract pathology and that is causing irritation to the bladder or urethra. Such conditions include bladder tumors, bladder stones, and diverticuli of the bladder or urethra.

Nursing Implications. Elderly patients who require genitourinary surgery have similar risks for complications as younger persons. In most cases the surgery is elective rather than an emergency procedure; thus, there is ample time to do preoperative teaching and preparation for the expected outcomes. Guidelines for nursing management of the elderly patient undergoing genitourinary surgery are presented in Table 9–4.

Training Procedures

A wide variety of techniques called "training procedures," used alone or in combination with drugs or surgery, have been shown to be quite successful in managing urinary incontinence. The various training procedures include Kegel exercises, bladder retraining, habit

Table 9–4. GUIDELINES FOR NURSING MANAGEMENT OF PATIENTS HAVING GENITOURINARY SURGERY

Standard
Genitourinary surgery to relieve or improve urinary incontinence.

Procedures/Interventions
1. Prior to surgery, clarify with the patient/family expected outcomes of surgical intervention.
2. Monitor postoperative care, emphasizing adequate fluids and deep breathing.
3. Observe the patient for potential complications of genitourinary surgery, i.e., urinary tract infections postcatheterization, postoperative dehiscence, incisional hernia, hematuria, hematomas, and postoperative status changes.
4. Perform postoperative teaching appropriate for the type of surgery (verbally and written, including the family when appropriate).

Patient Teaching Guide
1. Clarify with patient and family the expected outcomes of surgery.
2. Orient to anesthesia and surgical procedure.
3. Explain postoperative pain and sensations.
4. Explain the general postoperative course including catheterization.
5. Provide discharge instructions, including physical limitations, signs of infection, or postoperative complications.
6. Discuss any limitations of sexual activity.

Outcome Criteria for Evaluation
Patient will have:
1. Decreased or no incontinent episodes.
2. Improved management of incontinence.

retraining, and biofeedback. These are useful treatments for stress, urge, and functional types of incontinence.

Kegel Exercises. Kegel exercises have been used for many years in the management of stress incontinence in females (Kegel, 1948). The goal of these exercises is to strengthen the pelvic, vaginal, iliococcygeus, and levator ani muscles. This form of treatment is most appropriate for postpartum or menopausal women. Most have experienced gross stretching of the pelvic floor muscles during childbirth. Weakened striated muscles can be retrained by use of Kegel exercises, but overstretched fascia requires surgical restoration.

Assessment and initial instruction are essential in successful treatment with this procedure. The muscles being strengthened are not visible, so a digital check or vaginal pressure gauge (periometer) reading should be used to assess strength of the muscles. If the pelvic floor muscle shows compression ability, pelvic exercises may be useful. Kegel instructions are presented in Table 9–5.

Kegel exercises can be used as treatment for elderly women if the patient has: (1) adequate cognitive function, (2) intact pelvic floor musculature, and (3) motivation to follow routine. Although these exercises are not a cure, they are useful adjuncts to therapies such as surgery, drugs, or electrical stimulation.

Biofeedback. Biofeedback has been used in the treatment of stress and urge incontinence in both men and women (Burns, Marecki, Dittmar, et al., 1985; Burton, 1984; Millard & Oldenburg, 1983; Taylor & Henderson, 1986). Biofeedback techniques can be used to: (1) measure the strength of muscles involved in voiding, (2) provide a "picture" of muscle activity, and (3) teach people how to strengthen appropriate muscles. Some women are able to effectively learn Kegel exercises from verbal or written instructions; however, many may have problems exercising properly and may be practicing these exercises without benefit. In this case, biofeedback devices can be used as an extension of the Kegel exercises by allowing for observation of exercise results.

In women, the biofeedback procedure involves placing a cone-shaped sensor device

Table 9–5. KEGEL EXERCISES

Find Your Pubococcygeus (PC) Muscle
1. Practice stopping your urine in midstream.
2. To feel the PC working, insert the periometer or your finger or a tampon partially into your vagina while it is contracting.
3. If your abdomen and buttocks move, you're using the wrong muscles.

Perform the Exercise
1. Contract your PC muscle and hold for 3 seconds, then release for 3 seconds. Repeat this routine nine more times (should take a minute).
2. Contract the PC muscle very quickly, then release. Try to do 100 of these (or any many as you can do) in 1 minute.

Time the Exercise
1. Perform the 2-minute routine three times a day.
2. Since no one will see you doing it, take advantage of free time to practice—waiting in lines, waiting at stop lights, during rest breaks at work, etc.

(Data from Burns, Marecki, Dittmar, et al., 1985; Kegel, 1948; and Taylor & Henderson, 1986)

(periometer) in the vagina. The patient is instructed to tighten the pelvic floor muscle around the sensor. Visual feedback on a monitor registers the strength of the contractions. This type of treatment requires specialized equipment and personnel and well motivated, cognitively intact patients. Biofeedback procedures have also been used for men with stress incontinence due to sphincter insufficiency after prostatic surgery (Burton, 1984).

Biofeedback procedures used in conjunction with other treatments require further study to confirm their efficacy in the treatment of urinary incontinence in the elderly patient.

Bladder and Habit Retraining. Bladder and habit retraining are behavioral interventions intended to combat incontinence by making alterations in the environment, such as establishing cues for voiding, scheduling voiding times, and altering toileting procedures. These nursing interventions are useful as a treatment option for urge and functional incontinence.

A variety of terms are used to describe retraining procedures (i.e., bladder training or retraining, habit training or retraining, bladder drill, or contingency management). Burgio and Burgio (1986) describe bladder retraining (also referred to as bladder training) as an intervention to restore a normal pattern of voiding and normal bladder function. This is accomplished by teaching the patient to empty the bladder at appropriate intervals so that the bladder does not reach the point where uninhibited bladder contractions occur.

Habit training or retraining (also referred to as bladder training, schedule toileting, bladder drill) is an intervention to diminish the number of incontinent episodes rather than to restore a completely normal pattern of voiding (Ouslander, et al., 1985). Continence resulting from habit retraining is attributed to the caregiver performing the procedure, rather than the patient relearning normal voiding patterns.

There are four nursing interventions that must be part of both types of retraining programs (Long, 1985):

1. Maintain the fluid intake.
2. Identify the most appropriate method of toileting.
3. Offer an appropriate toilet schedule.

4. Maintain an incontinence record.

All patients on retraining programs should attempt to drink 2000 to 3000 ml of fluid between 6:00 a.m. and 6:00 p.m. Some patients may have fluid restrictions (to 1500 ml) due to other medical conditions. Coffee, tea, and alcoholic beverages should be avoided at bedtime because of their diuretic effects. Allowing 2 hours between the last fluid intake and bedtime, controlling types of fluid intake, and having the patient void just prior to bedtime are methods intended to decrease the possibility of nocturia (Field, 1979).

The best method of toileting (i.e., in a urinal, bedpan, commode, or bathroom) should be selected based on each patient's functional capabilities, privacy, and comfort needs. Uncomfortable or unnatural methods of toileting can lead to deconditioned voiding reflexes, thus increasing detrusor instability.

A consistent, suitable toileting schedule is primary to the success of both bladder or habit retraining. Most retraining programs begin with a 2-hour toileting schedule. More frequent toileting causes chronic low-volume voiding, which reduces bladder capacity and increases detrusor tone and bladder wall thickness (William & Pannill, 1982). In a bladder retraining program, the 2-hour schedule is not fixed but rather is based on the actual time of the patient's last voiding (Long, 1985). The alternative method, habit training, uses a rigid regimen with a firm toileting schedule based on fixed times.

A crucial nursing intervention is accurate maintenance of a bladder retraining record. This record should be used to make observation about time intervals between voiding, amount of fluid intake, and episodes of incontinence. If drugs are also part of the treatment regimen, observations can be made about the drug effects on incontinence. Table 9–6 provides an example of a form to use as a bladder retraining record.

A criterion for a successful bladder retraining program is the patient's ability to maintain continence on a 3- to 4-hour voiding schedule and to regain normal function of the bladder. A successful habit retraining program results in the patient being toileted at scheduled in-

Table 9–6. BLADDER RETRAINING RECORD

Patient's Name:_____

Directions
Use the following abbreviations for recording:

I = Incontinent   V = Voiding
C = Continent   O = Did not Void

Date:

Time:	AM 1	2	3	4	5	6	7	8	9	10	11	PM 12
Intake												
Output												

tervals, thus maintaining continence. A trial program of 6 weeks should be allowed before determining success or failure of bladder retraining (Judson, Novotny, McAninch, et al., 1981).

Initially, both bladder and habit retraining programs are labor-intensive interventions. Staff must have a clear understanding of the plan of care and retraining technique. Bladder retraining is, in most cases, dependent on the patient having intact cognition or only slight mental impairment. Dependent physical function may not be a factor, depending on the caregiving situation. Habit retraining can be successful in patients with impaired mental status and physical function, since the emphasis is on the caregiver initiating the toileting procedure.

Nursing Implications. Management of urinary incontinence may be a difficult problem for the patient and caregivers. Successful training procedures have been reported in a variety of settings, such as in hospitals, nursing homes, and clinics (Brink, Wells, & Diokno, 1983; Long, 1985; Millard & Oldenburg, 1983; Overstall, Rounce, & Palmer, 1980). Common factors for success identified in these studies include:

1. A complete medical and nursing assessment to determine the appropriate type of treatment.

2. A plan of care incorporating the joint efforts of the health care team members (i.e., patient/family, physician, nurse, pharmacist, occupational therapist).

3. Willingness to employ key components of training options, including manipulation of the environment, use of knowledgeable caregivers, data collection, and communication of results to the team.

Guidelines for nursing management of bladder and habit training are presented in Table 9–7.

Mechanical and Electrical Devices

Several different approaches involving mechanical and electrical devices have been

Table 9–7. GUIDELINES FOR NURSING MANAGEMENT OF BLADDER AND HABIT TRAINING

Standard
Bladder and habit training to manage urinary incontinence.
Procedures/Interventions
1. Clarify with patient and family the plan and expected outcome. Allow 6 weeks for trial program.
2. Include in plan of care: prescribed fluid intake (2000–3000 ml/24 hours), method of toileting, toilet schedule, and maintenance of incontinence record.
3. Monitor incidence of incontinence and modify toilet schedule every 24 hours.
4. Provide positive feedback to patient, as appropriate.
5. Report results to health care team and modify plan of care accordingly, i.e., use of drugs, further diagnostics, discharge plans.
Patient Teaching Guide
1. Expected outcome of retraining.
2. Retraining plan, i.e., method of toileting, fluid intake, voiding schedule.
3. Type, amount, and time of fluid intake.
4. Explanation of any drugs used in combination with retraining program.
5. Discussion of any unusual pains or new problems that may arise during retraining, i.e., distended bladder, constipation, pain, and when to report.
Outcome Criteria for Evaluation
Patient will have:
1. Decreased or eliminated incontinence episodes.
2. Increased time between voiding to 4 hours.

tested over the last 20 years. The review of electrical stimulants and sphincter devices by Ouslander and associates (1985) outlines these treatment technologies. This category of treatment includes artificial sphincters, electrical stimulators, and external clamps for males and pessaries for females. External clamps and pessaries are used less frequently due to the availability of newer artificial sphincters. Mechanical and electrical devices are used to treat stress and urge incontinence.

Artificial Sphincters. Artificial sphincters are implanted devices primarily used to remedy weakness or total dysfunction of the bladder outlet and urethral sphincter mechanisms (stress incontinence). The entire device, used for males and females, is surgically implanted. The cuff is implanted around either the bladder neck or the bulbous urethra. The deflation bulb is placed within the labia or hemiscrotum, whereas the pressurized balloon is implanted into the perivesical space. The sphincter, designed to mimic the normal process of voiding, causes the urethra to close; this makes it possible for the bladder to store urine. To urinate, the patient opens the urethra by squeezing the device's pump, located in the scrotum or labium. After urination, the device automatically recloses the urethra. Most recent studies report a 50% to 90% success rate (Ouslander, et al., 1985). Potential complications are infection or malfunction of the device. This type of treatment requires elderly patients to be mentally and physically capable and motivated to manage the device or have a caregiver manipulate the device for them.

Electrical Stimulation. Three types of devices have been used: rectal, vaginal, and implantable stimulators. Electrical stimulation techniques work by either increasing the urethra resistance through stimulation of the pelvic floor musculature (as for stress incontinence) or by blocking uninhibited bladder contractions (as for urge incontinence).

Implantable devices have had limited success due to technical defects and movement of the electrodes. More successful outcomes have been seen with external techniques, which include anal plugs and pessary-like devices with electrodes. Recently developed electrical stimulators are inflated in the vagina to minimize electrode movement.

As in many of the other treatment options, patient selection is important to the success of the devices. Patients with stress incontinence must have intact pelvic floor musculature, and patients with unstable bladders must have an intact nervous reflex arc. This type of treatment is not appropriate for patients with disorders in which there is complete destruction of the peripheral nerves or lower spinal cord. As in the case with other electrical appliances, these devices cannot be used in patients who have pacemakers.

Nursing Implications. The gerontological nurse plays a key role in education and observation of the expected outcome. Guidelines for nursing management of mechanical and electrical devices can be found in Table 9–8.

Catheters

Catheterization is the most controversial and misused treatment for urinary incontinence. The three basic types of catheters—indwelling, intermittent, and external—offer a great convenience for hospital and nursing home staff. Catheters work effectively to keep the patient

Table 9–8. NURSING MANAGEMENT OF PATIENTS USING MECHANICAL AND ELECTRICAL DEVICES

Standard
Mechanical and electrical devices to manage urinary incontinence.
Procedures/Interventions
   1. Clarify with patient and family the expected outcomes and potential risks of procedure or prosthesis.
   2. Monitor signs of infection or malfunctioning device.
   3. Monitor postoperative voiding patterns.
Patient Teaching Guide
   1. General postoperative course.
   2. Understanding of how device functions.
   3. Management of sexual activity.
   4. Discharge instructions.
Outcome Criteria for Evaluation
Patient will have:
   1. Decreased or absent urinary incontinence.
   2. Improved management of incontinence.

and bed dry and, over the short term, are perceived by staff to save time. This time saving, however, is at the risk of costly and, for the frail elderly, life-threatening complications. The study of elderly nursing home patients by Ouslander and colleagues (1982) reported that 50% of the patients were identified as incontinent. Less than 5% of the elderly patients had a specific documented cause for their incontinence. Of the incontinent patients, 10% had external catheters and 28% had indwelling catheters.

Marron, Fillitt, Peskowitz, and associates (1983) studied the prevalence of bladder catheterization in a teaching nursing home. They reported a reduction in the number of patients catheterized, as compared to the number prior to the introduction of an education and research program in the nursing home environment.

Indwelling Catheters. Principal reasons for indwelling catheterization are (Kinney, Blount, & Dowell, 1980; Warren, 1986):

   1. Pre-/postoperative monitoring for surgeries requiring general anesthesia (short-term).
   2. Recovery from genitourinary surgery (short-term).
   3. Overflow incontinence due to obstruction (short- or long-term).
   4. Acute illness when input or output monitoring is crucial (short-term).
   5. Urine collection before leakage occurs in patients for whom all other forms of treatment have been unsuccessful (long-term).
   6. Urine collection before leakage occurs in patients requiring management of pressure sores (short- or long-term).

Catheterization is inappropriate when used without a complete medical and nursing assessment to diagnose the type of incontinence or when used as a convenience for staff.

If an indwelling catheter is the appropriate choice, consideration should be given regarding timespan. Soft latex catheters are comfortable for the short term, but may become encrusted after a few days. For long-term use, the silicone type is a better choice.

Complications associated with indwelling catheterization include urinary tract infections, renal and bladder stones, squamous cell carcinoma of the urethra, and, in males, epididymitis and penoscrotal complications. The more prevalent complication of indwelling catheterization is urinary tract infection. Measures taken to prevent or minimize infection include the following: avoid clamping the catheter, keep the collection bag below the level of bladder at all times, cleanse the perineal area daily, and empty the urine bag every 8 hours. Meatal care is frequently recommended; however, it has proved to influence the infection rate and may even contaminate the system. Unless the meatus is grossly dirty, washings should be avoided (Freed, 1982).

Intermittent Catheterization. If catheterization is the best treatment choice, the patient should first be assessed for benefits of intermittent over indwelling catheterization. Intermittent catheterization does not have as high a risk of infection as the indwelling method. The bladder has inherent antibacterial qualities that are effective if the bladder is usually empty and free of foreign bodies, such as an indwelling catheter.

Intermittent catheterization may be a short-term intervention for bladder retraining or a long-term treatment for bladder hypertonia. This procedure may be performed as either a sterile or a clean technique. If the patient is hospitalized and this treatment is considered, short-term sterile technique is suggested. Hospitalized patients have a greater chance of cross-contamination between patients. For long-term treatment with intermittent catheterization, a clean technique is recommended. There is no evidence that clean technique is harmful, and it encourages patient compliance because it is less complicated (Freed, 1982; Keegan & McNichols, 1982; Kinney, et al., 1980; Wahlquist, McGuire, Greene, et al., 1983).

Frequency of intermittent catheterization varies with fluid intake, voiding patterns, and the patient's or caregiver's daily schedule. Catheterization every 4, 6, or even 8 hours can be effective in maintaining an empty bladder and decreasing incontinence.

Elderly patients with poor vision, limited manual dexterity, impaired mental status, and physical limitations may not be able to catheterize themselves; however, spouses, family members, or friends can be taught the technique. The most important requirement is that the patient or caregiver have the interest and desire to learn.

External Catheters. External catheters or collection devices may be necessary when other techniques have been unsuccessful. Use of collection devices for women has not been widespread due to unsatisfactory design. The most common external device for men is a condom-type collector secured circumferentially proximal to the glans penis. The condom is attached to a tube that drains into a collection bag.

This type of device has no internal contact with the bladder; however, there are disadvantages to its use. Urine can collect in the condom where high concentrations of organisms are in contact with the urethra and skin of the penis. Complications such as skin irritation, maceration, and ulceration; urethral diverticulae and fistulae; and even gangrene of the penis are not uncommon (Golji, 1981; Hirsh, Fainstein, & Musher, 1979).

Safe use of external collection systems is dependent on careful application and maintenance of the condom and good skin care. Application procedures must avoid constriction of the glans penis. The collection system should be free of kinks to avoid backup of urine into the condom. The patient should be positioned to avoid twisting of the condom. Condom catheters should be removed at least daily, and for some patients twice daily, in order to wash and dry the underlying skin.

Nursing Implications. It is clearly documented that patients should not be catheterized for the convenience of the staff or if noninvasive treatments will control the incontinence. Once again, gerontological nurses play a key role in ongoing education of nursing staff as to appropriate reasons for catheters as treatment options and in the management of elderly patients with catheters. Table 9–9 presents nursing standards, procedures, teaching plans, and outcome criteria for nursing management of patients with catheters (Kinney, et al., 1980; Tortorello, Church, & Garis, 1984; Warren, 1986).

Table 9–9. GUIDELINES FOR NURSING MANAGEMENT OF PATIENTS WITH CATHETERS

Standard
Catheters (external, indwelling) to manage urinary incontinence.

Procedures/Interventions
1. Clarify with patient and family the purpose and outcome of catheterization.
2. Monitor signs and symptoms of infection or obstruction of catheter.
3. Modify clothing to accommodate catheter devices and allow for mobility, as appropriate.
4. Continue ongoing evaluation of catheterization as the safest and most appropriate option.

Patient Teaching Guide
1. Catheter care, i.e., cleaning, handwashing.
2. Proper application or placement.
3. Care of equipment, i.e., cleaning of tubing and bag.
4. Prescribed fluid intake 2000–3000 ml/24 hours.
5. Signs and symptoms of complications, i.e., infection, obstruction, catheter injury.

Outcome Criteria for Evaluation
Patient will have: Urinary incontinence managed without complications of infection or injury.

Supportive Measures

A variety of supportive measures can be used in conjunction with other treatment or as sole treatment for elderly patients when all other methods have failed. Supportive measures include environmental manipulation, and use of undergarments and pads.

Environmental Manipulation. A frequent cause of urinary incontinence is attributed to the elderly not being able to reach the toilet in time to avoid an accident (functional incontinence). Reasons for functional incontinence include musculoskeletal limitations, psychological problems, unfamiliar settings, lack of convenient toilet facilities, and iatrogenic factors (Williams & Pannill, 1982). Functional incontinence is frequently identified by thorough assessment of the following:

1. Patient's physical limitations (i.e., lack of dexterity, lack of flexibility, presence of restraints).
2. Environmental barriers to reaching the toilet (i.e., lack of handrails, distance from bathroom, toilet height).
3. Patient's mental limitations (i.e., depression, hostility, anger, dementia).
4. Iatrogenic factors (i.e., diuretics, sedatives, hypnotics, neuroleptics).
5. Dietary factors (i.e., fluid intake, caffeine, and diuretic-acting liquids).

Physical limitations can be overcome by using special clothing that make toileting easier for functionally dependent elderly people. Environmental barriers can be eliminated by establishing a setting with visual cues to the bathrooms, sufficient lighting, and specially designed height-adjustable toilet seats. Call systems in bathrooms are frequently not reachable by physically compromised elderly. Call lights can be made more accessible by simply using a dark-colored call cord so that it is visible against a light-colored wall and within reach.

Mental impairment due to depression, anger, and hostility can lead to incontinence as an attention-getting behavior. Recognition and treatment of underlying conditions are paramount in controlling this type of incontinence. Elderly persons with dementia respond to many environmental cues as well as to consistent, repetitive habit-retraining programs.

Iatrogenic factors must be considered causes for incontinence. Sedatives and hypnotics may dull the person's awareness of the need to void. Diuretics given at the wrong time can cause unnecessary incontinence during the night. In most cases, the degree to which the drug regimen is modified will likewise reduce incontinence.

As outlined in the bladder retraining program, decreased fluid may bring about chronic, low-volume voiding. Maintaining a 2000 to 3000 ml fluid intake in 24 hours and controlling the time and types of liquids given can eliminate incontinence for many elderly.

Undergarments and Pads. A variety of undergarments and pads are currently marketed. The products vary in price, comfort, style, reusable or disposable characteristics, and efficiency. Undergarments should be considered as aids to management of incontinence only until a specific diagnosis is determined or until all other treatments have been proved unsuccessful. Ideally, undergarments and pads are highly absorbent, nonallergenic, odor controlling, affordable, and easy to change by patients or caregivers. These products come in many forms, including disposable diaper-like briefs, reusable pants with disposable inserts, and mesh stretch briefs with inserts. Manufacturers of these products suggest that they bring considerable cost savings due to reduced laundry and labor needs (Ouslander, et al., 1985). These products offer comfort and convenience, thus decreasing the burden of caregivers when all other options have failed.

In addition to the undergarments, several products have been designed to protect bedding. Most are flat, disposable underpads with absorbent fillers and waterproof backing. These products are frequently used in institutional settings to protect beds and furniture. The absorbency characteristics of these products are very important. In the worst cases, they may keep the bed or chair dry but not absorb the wetness; thus, the urine is kept in contact with the skin.

Two self-help organizations, Help for Incontinent People (HIP) (P.O. Box 544, Union, SC 29739) and the Simon Foundation (P.O. Box 815, Wilmette, IL 60091), are valuable resources for the elderly and their caregivers. HIP publishes a *Resource Guide of Incontinence Aids and Services* (1985) and a quarterly newsletter, *The HIP Report*, which provides information about products, manufacturers, and other organizations and services available to people with incontinence. The Simon Foundation provides a variety of educational materials and a quarterly newsletter, *The Informer*.

Nursing Implications. It is the physician's responsibility to diagnose the type of incontinence, treat pathophysiologic conditions, and prescribe drug therapy. Effects of the medical diagnosis and prescribed treatment may have significant impact on the elderly person's management of daily living.

Nursing treatment regimens fall into two categories: those concerned with restoring continence and those that deal with managing the patient's daily living habits when incontinence is present (Specht, 1986). Supportive measures as treatment options for urinary incontinence relate to the latter, and they do not address the patient's recovery of continence.

Guidelines for nursing management of elderly patients with intractable urinary incontinence are presented in Table 9–10.

SUMMARY

Millions of elderly and their families are physically, mentally, socially, and financially affected by urinary incontinence. Barriers to treatment are of two types. First, patients and families may be too embarrassed to report problems, and second, health professionals have limited knowledge of assessment technique and treatment options. All may consider incontinence an inevitable effect of aging. Decisions about appropriate treatment options can only be made after a thorough assessment has been completed by the health care team, specifically by the physician and the nurse.

Once diagnosis and treatment decisions are made, the role of the nurse is to implement the treatment program and provide ongoing monitoring of the effects of treatment on incontinence and the elderly person's day-to-day living. While it is important that decisions to treat or not are not based on age alone, it

Table 9–10. GUIDELINES FOR NURSING MANAGEMENT OF PATIENTS WITH INTRACTABLE URINARY INCONTINENCE

Standard
Management of intractable urinary incontinence by use of undergarments, pads, and environmental manipulation.
Procedures/Interventions
1. Clarify with patient and family the purpose and expected outcome of treatment option.
2. Continue ongoing reevaluation of appropriateness of products being used.
3. Observe for skin breakdown or other injury from intervention.
Patient Teaching Guide
1. Instruct patient/family/caregivers on modifications of environment, i.e., use of handrails, proper lifting.
2. Instruct family/caregiver on cleaning or disposing of products.
3. Instruct family/caregivers about the variety of product options and when to purchase.
Outcome Criteria for Evaluation
Incontinence managed without skin breakdown, urinary tract infection, or other complications.

is important also to recognize when treatment may present more of a problem than the incontinence itself. Finding the delicate balance between effective and appropriate treatment options is a challenge faced by the entire health care team.

References

Blaivas, JG, & Berger, Y (1986): Surgical treatment for male geriatric incontinence. *Clin Geriatr Med*, 2:777–778.

Brink, C, Wells, T, & Diokno, A (1983): A continence clinic for the aged. *J Gerontol Nurs*, 9:652–655.

Burgio, KL, & Burgio, L (1986): Behavior therapies for urinary incontinence in the elderly. *Clin Geriatr Med*, 2:809–828.

Burns, PA, Marecki, MA, Dittmar, SS, et al. (1985): Kegel's exercises with biofeedback therapy for treatment of stress incontinence. *Nurs Pract*, 10(2):28, 33–35, 46.

Burton, JR (1984): Managing urinary incontinence: A common geriatric problem. *Geriatrics*, 39:46–62.

Diokno, AC, & Taub, M (1975): Ephedrine in treatment of urinary incontinence. *Urology*, 5:624–625.

Field, MA (1979): Urinary incontinence in the elderly: An overview. *J Gerontol Nurs*, 5:12–19.

Freed, SZ (1982): Urinary incontinence in the elderly. *Hosp Pract*, 17(3):81–94.

Golji, H (1981): Complications of external condom drainage. *Paraplegia*, 19:189–197.

Help for Incontinent People (HIP, Inc.), (Winter, 1985): Resource Guide of Continence Aids and Services (ed 2). HIP, Inc., Resource Guide, Union, SC.

Hirsch, DD, Fainstein, V, & Musher, DM (1979): Do condom catheter collecting systems cause urinary tract infections? *JAMA*, 242:340–341.

Hu, TW (1986): The economic impact of urinary incontinence. *Clin Geriatr Med*, 2:673–688.

Judson, L, Novotny, T, McAninch, J, et al. (1981): Genitourinary system. In O'Hara-Devereaux, M, Andrus, LH, & Scott, CD (eds): *Eldercare—A Practical Guide to Clinical Geriatrics*. New York, Grune & Stratton, 169–187.

Keegan, GT, & McNichols, DW (1982): The evaluation and treatment of urinary incontinence in the elderly. *Surg Clin North Am*, 62:261–274.

Kegel, AH (1948): Progressive resistance exercise in the functional restoration of the perineal muscles. *Am J Obstet Gynecol*, 56:238–248.

Kinney, AB, Blount, M, & Dowell M (1980): Urethral catheterization. *Geriatr Nurs*, 1:258–263.

Long, ML (1985): Incontinence: Defining the nursing role. *J Gerontol Nurs*, 11:30–41.

Marron, KR, Fillitt, H, Peskowitz, M, et al. (1983): The non-use of urethral catheterization in the management of urinary incontinence in the teaching nursing home. *J Am Geriatr Soc*, 31:278–281.

Millard, RJ, & Oldenburg, BF (1983): The symptomatic, urodynamic and psychodynamic results of bladder re-education programs. *J Urol*, 130:715–719.

Ouslander, JG, Hepps, K, & Raz, S (1986): Genitourinary dysfunction in a geriatric outpatient population. *J Am Geriatr Soc*, 34:507–514.

Ouslander, JG, & Kane, RL (1983): The costs of urinary incontinence in nursing homes. *Med Care*, 22:69–79.

Ouslander, JG, Kane, RL, & Abrass, IN (1982): Urinary incontinence in elderly nursing home patients. *JAMA*, 248:1194–1198.

Ouslander, JG, Kane RL, Vollmer S, et al. (1985): *Technologies for Managing Urinary Incontinence*. Library of Congress No. 85-600554. Washington, DC, US Government Printing Office.

Ouslander, JG, & Sier, HC (1986): Drug therapy for geriatric urinary incontinence. *Clin Geriatr Med*, 2:789–807.

Overstall, PW, Rounce, K, & Palmer, JH (1980): Experience with an incontinence clinic. *J Am Geriatr Soc*, 28:535–538.

Resnick, NM, & Yalla, SB (1985): Management of urinary incontinence in the elderly. *N Engl J Med*, 313:800–805.

Schmidbauer, CP, Chiang, H, & Raz, S (1986): Surgical treatment for female geriatric incontinence. *Clin Geriatr Med*, 2:759–776.

Shapiro, A, Mazouz, B, & Caine, M (1981): The alpha-adrenergic blocking effects of prazosin on the human prostate. *Urol Res*, 9:17–20.

Simon Foundation: *The Informer*. (Quarterly Newsletter) Wilmette, IL.

Specht, J (1986): Genitourinary problems. In Carnevali, DL, & Patrick, M (eds): *Nursing Management for the Elderly* (ed 2). Philadelphia, JB Lippincott, 447–466.

Taylor, K, & Henderson, J (1986): Effects of biofeedback and urinary stress incontinence in older women. *J Gerontol Nurs*, 12:25–30.

Tortorelli, BA, Church, J, & Garis, V (1984): Intermittent self-catheterization: A learning packet. *Rehab Nurs*, 9:31–32.

Wahlquist, GI, McGuire, E, Greene, W, et al. (1983): Intermittent catheterization and urinary tract infection. *Rehab Nurs*, 8:18–20.

Warren, JW (1986): Catheter and catheter use. *Clin Geriatr Med*, 2:857–871.

Williams, ME, & Pannill, FC (1982): Urinary incontinence in the elderly. *Ann Intern Med*, 97:895–907.

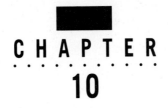

CHAPTER
10

Managing Bowel Function

JOYCE TAKANO STONE, R.N.C., M.S.

quency of their occurrence, the high degree of discomfort and distress they cause in the older person, their potential for complications, and the additional cost in time and material required for their treatment. Preventive measures and treatment modalities for constipation and fecal incontinence are discussed. In addition, information on equipment, pharmaceutical preparations, and supportive measures is included.

STEPS TO MAINTAIN NORMAL BOWEL FUNCTION

To maintain normal bowel function, prevent bowel dysfunction, and resolve a bowel problem, the basic elements of a bowel program must be considered: physical exercise, adequate fluids, high fiber foods in the diet, and prompt response to the urge to defecate or consistent toileting time (Cannon, 1981; Dudas, 1986; Okamoto, 1984; Stryker, 1977).

INTRODUCTION

The focus of this chapter is the maintenance of normal bowel function. Strategies for preventing bowel dysfunction and maintaining normal bowel function are presented. Two specific problems of bowel function, constipation and fecal incontinence, are of major concern in geriatric care because of the fre-

Physical Exercise

Exercise and activity are essential for normal bowel function. Even minimal activity, such as performing the activities of daily living or, in the case of the immobilized older person, having passive range of motion exercises performed, helps maintain the muscular system and physiologic bowel response. The ability to get to the toilet and to sit upright requires good muscle tone and strength (Cannon, 1981). Defecation requires good strength and tone of several muscle groups, primarily the abdominal, pelvic, and internal and external anal sphincter muscles (Cannon, 1981). The Valsalva maneuver, with inhalation followed by exhalation against a closed glottis and tightening of the abdominal muscles, starts the elimination process (Cannon, 1981).

Fluids and Food

Intake of sufficient amounts of fluid and a well balanced diet rich in high fiber foods is necessary to maintain a soft, formed stool. One and one-half to two liters of fluids a day are recommended for older persons (Dodge, Backman, & Silverman, 1988; Robinson, Lawler, Chenoweth, et al., 1986; Sklar, 1986; Smith, 1983; Winograd & Jarvik, 1986). Drinking warm fluids before a meal facilitates the gastrocolic and duodenocolic reflexes (Okamoto, 1984; Stryker, 1977).

The frequency and consistency of stool is determined by the foods consumed (Davies, Crowder, Reid, et al., 1986). The Western diet tends to be low in fiber, and the current average fiber intake of 11 gm daily is less than the optimal 20 to 30 gm, preferably in the form of cereal fiber (Burkitt, 1982; Eastwood, Fisher, Greenwood, et al., 1974; Pattee & West, 1988). Fiber binds water in the intestines, forms a gel, prevents the overabsorption of water from the large intestine, and ensures a bulky, soft stool (Burkitt & Meisner, 1979). The amount of fiber needed to keep the stool soft and prevent constipation varies considerably among individuals. Excessive fiber intake may lead to interference in the absorption of minerals and may also cause intestinal obstruction (Robinson, Lawler, Chenoweth, et al., 1986). Bowel dysfunction may result if there is inadequate fluid intake with increased fiber intake (Ellickson, 1988).

Foods with soluble fiber, such as cereals, are preferable to foods high in roughage, since soluble fiber has been found to be more effective in producing bulk (Borgman, 1981; Cannon, 1981). Foods high in dietary fiber include whole grain cereal and breads and, to a lesser degree, fresh fruit, green vegetables, and nuts (Burkitt & Meisner, 1979). The introduction of high fiber into the diet should be done slowly to prevent flatulence and abdominal cramping. Initially, whole grain bread and cereal, such as 1 teaspoon of flaked bran or one Wasa high fiber cracker, can be added to the diet. Cooked fruits and vegetables can be increased before progressing to raw fruits and vegetables (Robinson, Lawler, Chenoweth, et al., 1986; Williams, 1984; Winograd & Jarvik, 1986). Fruit juices, especially orange, lemon, and prune juice, can be included in the diet to keep the stool soft (Cannon, 1981; Stryker, 1977).

Bran has been promoted as an effective alternative or as a complement to laxatives in treating constipation. Several bowel program studies that included bran in the diet reported success in decreasing constipation and maintaining bowel function with its use (Battle & Hanna, 1980; Behm, 1985; Miller, 1985; Pattee & West, 1988; Resnick, 1985). However, caution is advised when using bran in constipated, bedfast patients because adding bulk to the distended colon may worsen the constipation (Rousseau, 1988a). The usefulness of bran has been limited by the difficulty in administering it in a palatable manner (Sandman, Adolfsson, Hallmans, et al., 1983). Suggestions to make bran more acceptable include adding it to meat loaf, apple sauce, juices, and other foods (Cannon, 1981; Miller, 1985).

Fluid and dietary adjustments may be the only changes the older person has to make to maintain good elimination. A nutritionist or dietitian may be consulted to evaluate the diet and provide suggestions for improvement. Acceptance of recommendations will be greater if the older person's food preferences, cultural beliefs, lifestyle, and economic resources are taken into consideration.

Toileting Time

Bowel evacuation occurs every day or every other day in most persons, and every 3 days in others. Timely response to the urge to defecate prevents problems of constipation. For those who are trying to regain continence, establishing a consistent routine or schedule for elimination is important. A specific time of day should be determined, based on the previous schedule or preferred time of the older person. To take advantage of the gastrocolic and duodenocolic reflexes, 30 to 40 minutes after a meal is often the best time for toileting (Cannon, 1981; Okamoto, 1984; Stryker, 1977).

Supportive Measures

Position. Proper positioning is important for defecation. The squatting position is the natural, optimal physiologic position for defecation, and toilets are designed to allow a position approximating squatting (Stryker, 1977). In the proper sitting position, the thoracoabdominal muscles can be used to help empty the rectum (Alterescu, 1986).

Equipment. For older patients, a toilet with a padded backrest and handrails at the side help with transfer, support, and comfort. An elevated toilet seat may make getting on and off the toilet easier. When the toilet seat is elevated, a footstool can be used to support the feet and raise the knees slightly higher than the hips, allowing for a natural squatting position (Cannon, 1981). A commode at the bedside is an alternative.

With illness and bedrest, the use of a bedpan may be necessary. The bedpan is uncomfortable at best, and its use should be temporary. If the patient is unable to use a bedpan, the sidelying position with the use of a kidney basin or incontinent pads is an alternative.

Disposable undergarments and pads are available to provide ease of care and to protect the patient from soiling clothes and bedding during the bowel training period. A fecal incontinence bag can be used to protect the skin when there is diarrhea or a frequent discharge of feces (Mowlam, North, & Myers, 1986).

Time and Privacy. Allowing enough time is essential so that the older person does not feel rushed or hurried. However, the amount of time the patient is left on the toilet, commode, or bedpan should not exceed 20 or 30 minutes (Stryker, 1977).

The provision of both visual and auditory privacy is important to help the patient relax and avoid embarrassment from the sounds and odors associated with defecation. If possible, the patient should be assisted to toilet in a bathroom and the door closed. If a bedside commode is used, it can be rolled into a bathroom or left at the bedside with the curtains pulled.

Patient and Family Education. Patients and their families often have misconceptions and incomplete knowledge about bowel function: what is a normal bowel pattern, what causes problems of elimination, and how should these problems be treated? Fecal incontinence tends to be under-reported and accepted as a way of life for elderly patients (Leigh & Turnberg, 1982; Smith, 1983). Unless a direct question is asked regarding incontinence, patients may not volunteer information that they have incontinence. For this reason, there is a need to include questions related to bowel function in the assessment of the older adult.

Confusion about the terminology used to describe bowel function is also common. For example, an older person may complain of diarrhea, meaning that he or she had one loose stool. The health care provider may use the term to mean frequent, loose, watery stools. To the elderly person, being constipated may mean fewer than the usual number of bowel movements per day or hard, dry stools or difficulty in having a bowel movement.

Self-prescribing of laxatives and self-imposed dietary restrictions are relatively common among the elderly. The consequences of inappropriate or prolonged laxative use and the undesirable addition or deletion of certain foods in the diet are important to stress in the patient education program. Factors affecting bowel function, such as activity and exercise, stress, muscle strength, diet, medications, and age-related changes, are discussed, with emphasis on their role in the prevention of elimination problems (Cannon, 1981). When a bowel problem is identified, information about the problem is provided, with specific instructions and explanations about its prevention and management. Patient and family education is essential to ensure the success of any treatment program.

CONSTIPATION

Constipation is a common complaint among the elderly. Several factors contribute to the high incidence of constipation: decreased physical activity; chronic illness; medications such as anticholinergics, narcotics, and antiparkinson drugs; poor nutrition with reduced intake of food and fiber; inadequate intake of fluids; and age-related changes in the gastrointestinal system (Rousseau, 1988a; Pattee & West, 1988). Other contributing factors are chronic laxative use (stemming from the misconception that at least one bowel movement a day is desirable) and a change in routine with missed meals, emotional stress, and episodes of acute illness (Pattee & West, 1988; Shane & McLane, 1988).

Treatment

A careful, comprehensive assessment of the patient is required to determine the underlying cause of constipation (see Chapter 8). Once the cause has been determined, appropriate treatment can be initiated. The goal of treatment is: (1) that the older person have a soft, formed stool within the range of three per day to one movement every 3 to 5 days (Benson, 1975) and (2) that complications such as abdominal distention, fecal impaction, idiopathic megacolon, and hemorrhoids are prevented (Brocklehurst, 1985).

Lubricants or stool softeners may be indicated if the stools are hard. If these are unsuccessful, osmotic agents such as lactulose or nonirritant enemas and suppositories can be administered (Rousseau, 1988a). Table 10–1 lists the steps in the treatment of constipation. Tables 10–2 and 10–3 list the types of laxatives,

Table 10–1. TREATMENT OF CONSTIPATION

1. Establish basic health maintenance measures.
   Establish a routine time for toileting
     Gastrocolic reflex after meals
     Prompt response to defecation urge
   Fiber in diet
   Minimum daily intake of 1500–2000 ml of fluids
   Daily physical exercise
2. Use pharmaceutical preparations on a temporary basis
   Mildest oral preparation at the lowest effective dose
     Oral lubricants/stool softeners
     Bulk forming agents
     Saline laxatives
     Stimulant laxatives
3. Administer suppositories and enemas if above measures not successful

(Data from Benson, 1975; Klein, 1982; Rousseau, 1988a.)

suppositories, and enemas available and their actions, preparations, dosages, and side effects. Documentation should include the number and times of bowel movements, the amount and consistency of stools, and administration of medications.

To prevent future occurrences of constipation, the patient's lifestyle, beliefs about bowel function, medication use, and dietary habits should be reviewed (Rousseau, 1988a). Recurrence of constipation may be prevented by instituting an individualized bowel program, including patient education on normal bowel function, prompt response to the urge to defecate, dietary measures to increase bulk and fiber in the diet, adequate intake of fluids, planned physical activity, and proper use of laxatives.

FECAL INCONTINENCE

Fecal incontinence is a distressing problem for the older person and for care providers. The older person who is incontinent suffers indignity, rejection, shame, and embarrassment, as well as discomfort from soiling and pain from skin irritation. The incontinent person at home often experiences an alteration in lifestyle with restriction of social activities. In addition, the increased burden for caregivers, especially if it causes interpersonal difficulties

Table 10–2. LAXATIVES

Type	Action	Preparation	Dose	Precautions/Side Effects
Bulk forming agents	Absorb water to form gelatin-like mass in the intestine, which distends the colon. Distention serves as a stimulus for intestinal activity. Laxative effect usually occurs within 12–24 hours; full effect may take 2–3 days.	Dietary bran Psyllium Methylcellulose	3–4 tablespoons/day 2.5–3.0 gm/day 4–6 gm/day	Flatulence and bloating may be experienced in first few days of treatment. Can harden stools and may lead to intestinal obstruction. Administered 1–3 times daily. Should be mixed with 240 ml of fluid, followed by an additional 240 ml.
Irritant or stimulant laxatives	Inhibit water and electrolyte absorption by altering intestinal mucosal permeability. Some stimulate peristalsis.			May produce abdominal discomfort, nausea, mild cramps. Adequate fluid intake should be ensured. Excessive purgation may result in dehydration and electrolyte disturbances. Chronic use may lead to laxative dependence and loss of normal bowel function. After years of abuse, cathartic colon with atony and dilation of the colon may result.
1. Anthraquinone laxatives	Mild laxative; 6–8 hours required for absorption and excretion. Act on colon to stimulate peristalsis.	Cascara segrada aromatic fluid extract Cascara tablet Senna	2–6 ml/day 0.3–1 gm 0.5–2 gm	Discoloration of urine (pink to red or brown to black) may occur.
2. Dehydrocholic acid	Mild laxative.	Dehydrocholic acid	250–300 mg, tid	
3. Diphenylmethane laxatives	Powerful stimulant of large bowel.	Bisacodyl (Dulcolax)	5–15 mg, hs	To prevent gastric irritation, the enteric-coated tablets should be taken whole, not crushed or chewed, or should not be taken within 1 hour of taking antacids or milk

Table continued on following page

Table 10–2. LAXATIVES *Continued*

Type	Action	Preparation	Dose	Precautions/Side Effects
	Acts directly or reflexly; increases activity of small intestine.	Phenolphthalein	30–270 mg	Discoloration of urine (pink to red) may occur. Allergy is manifested by dermal reaction, e.g., itching, fixed skin eruptions. Evacuation occurs in 6–8 hours. A single dose may produce laxation for several days.
4. Castor oil	Strong purgative. Extent of gastrointestinal absorption is unknown.	Castor oil	15 ml	Use should be reserved for total colonic evacuation. Emulsion preparation should be shaken before administering. Mix with 120–240 ml of fluid. Loose bowel movements occur within 2–3 hours.
Stool softeners	Lowers surface tension, permits water and lipids to penetrate fecal material. Softens stool to make passage easier. Laxative action is thought to result from stimulation of electrolyte and water secretion in the colon.	Docusate calcium Docusate potassium Docusate sodium	Range 15–360 mg, hs	Dosage varies widely. Doses should only be large enough to produce softening of the stools. May enhance absorption of co-administered drugs. Action enhanced if used with mineral oil. Combination should be used only for severe cases; should not be used for prolonged periods. Ensure adequate fluid intake.
Saline laxative	Exact mechanism not clear. Current thought, although unproved, is that nonabsorbable salts hold water in the small intestine in amounts to maintain isotonic concentration. The increased volume of intestinal contents indirectly stimulates stretch receptors and increases peristalsis.	Magnesium citrate	11–25 gm	Produces a semifluid or watery stool in 3–6 hours; may cause electrolyte imbalance. Minimum effective dose of magnesium preparations is 80 mEq of magnesium. Hypermagnesmia may occur in persons with decreased renal function.
		Magnesium hydroxide	30–60 ml 2.4–4.8 gm	
		Magnesium sulfate	10–30 gm	Dissolve in at least 240 ml of water.

Table 10–2. LAXATIVES *Continued*

Type	Action	Preparation	Dose	Precautions/Side Effects
		Sodium phosphate Dibasic Monobasic	3.42–7.5 gm 9.1–20.2 gm	Given as a single dose; dilute 30 ml of solution with 120 ml of water.
Lubricant	Retards absorption of water in intestines. Lubricates fecal matter and intestinal mucosa. Minimizes discomfort or effort to defecate.	Mineral oil	15 ml	Risk of aspiration in debilitated patients, especially those with impaired gag reflex. Chronic usage may cause malabsorption of fat soluble vitamins. Avoid routine, regular use. Precaution: Docusates may enhance mineral oil absorption.
Hyperosmotic	Draws water from tissues into feces by exerting a hygroscopic and/or local irritating action.	Sorbitol	25 gm daily	High oral doses are required for laxative action.
	Breakdown of synthetic sugar in colon. Produces lactic and pyruvic acids, which stimulate colonic secretions and motility. Osmotic effect of organic acid metabolites results in increased water content and softening of stool.	Lactulose	10–20 gm (15–30 ml) daily	Sweet taste of lactulose solution can be made more palatable by diluting with water or fruit juice. Frequent problem with abdominal discomfort, gaseous distention, belching, and flatulence during first few days of treatment. Diarrhea indicates a need for dose reduction. Effects of treatment occurs 24–48 hours after administration of drug. Serum electrolytes should be checked if the older person is on drug for more than 6 months. Laxatives should not be given with lactulose.

(Data from Cannon, 1981; Friesen, 1983; Gorbien, 1988; McEvoy, 1987; Peto & Skelton, 1983; Rousseau, 1988a; Stryker, 1977; Thompson, 1980.)

Table 10–3. SUPPOSITORIES AND ENEMAS

Type	Action	Preparation	Dose	Precautions/Side Effects
Irritant or stimulant	Strong stimulant that acts on mucous membrane to stimulate reflexes resulting in peristalsis.	Bisacodyl Fleet enema	10 mg/suppository 30 ml solution Bisacodyl 0.33 mg/ml	Proper administration is important. The suppository should be inserted beyond the internal and external sphincters and placed sideways against the colon wall. Contact with the colon wall is critical. Usually allow 15–20 minutes for results; may take up to 2 hours.
Lubricant	Lubricates fecal matter and intestinal mucosa.	Mineral oil	60–150 ml/enema	Pruritus ani may result from leaking oil.
Saline	Produces evacuation within 2–5 minutes.	Sodium phosphate Dibasic Monobasic Fleet enema	6.84–7.46 gm 18.24–20.16 gm 45 ml solution Dibasic 900 mg/5 ml Monobasic 2.4 gm/5 ml	Given as a single dose.
Hyperosmotic	Reflexly stimulates emptying of rectum.	Sorbitol 25–30% solution	120 ml/enema	Administer only at infrequent intervals in single doses.
		Glycerin	2–3 gm suppository 5–15 ml/enema	Evacuation occurs in 15–30 minutes. Adverse effects are rare. Glycerin may cause rectal discomfort, irritation, cramping pain.

(Data from Cannon, 1981; Friesen, 1983; McEvoy, 1987; Peto & Skelton, 1983; Rousseau, 1988a; Stryker, 1977; Thompson, 1980)

with family members, may lead to nursing home placement (Noekler, 1987; Smith, 1983). The costs to hospitals, nursing homes, and other health care centers are high in terms of expenses for supplies, laundry, and nursing time. Fecal incontinence can, for the most part, be prevented. If it occurs, it can be alleviated or controlled (Kane, Ouslander, & Abrass, 1984; Irvine, 1986; Tobin & Brocklehurst, 1986).

Treatment

As common and familiar as the fecal incontinence problem is, ignorance, negative attitude, confusion, and treatment inconsistencies are seen in the clinical setting (Davis, Nagelhout, Hoban, et al., 1986; Edgington, Shepherd, & Bainton, 1983; Moore, 1984). Nurses have a primary responsibility for management of fecal incontinence. In addition to possessing knowledge and technical skills required in the care of the incontinent patient, the nurse provides support, reassurance, and patient/family education so that continence is resumed and maintained whenever possible. Advanced clinicians are often called upon as consultants to assist in the management of the problem.

The success of a treatment program for the elderly person with incontinence depends on a thorough assessment and evaluation to determine the cause of incontinence, beliefs in the value of treatment, and the determination, effort, commitment, and patience of the incontinent person and the care providers (Alterescu, 1986; Tobin & Brocklehurst, 1986). Treatment of fecal incontinence begins with a careful assessment of the condition. This assessment includes a comprehensive history, physical examination, bowel record, functional assessment, and laboratory or diagnostic procedures (see Chapter 8). The capabilities of the patient and the caregivers are assessed. Once the cause of fecal incontinence has been determined and the contributing factors have been identified, a management plan can be developed and implemented.

The goal of the treatment program is to assist the older person to achieve fecal continence. If this is not possible, the goal is to manage the problem so that the patient will have predictable, planned elimination. The likelihood of success for any treatment program is increased when the patient and care providers understand and participate in the overall program of care from planning through implementation and evaluation. The goal is clearly stated and the objectives are outlined. The personal needs, lifestyle, finances, resources, and environment of the patient are taken into consideration (Bergstrom, 1968). The bowel program is a planned approach and must be consistent and practical if bowel regulation is to be achieved.

Careful documentation in the patient's chart or bowel record is essential. Key information to be kept for a bowel program includes medications, equipment, and techniques used; results; consistency, amount, and time of stools; and incontinent episodes. Evaluation is based on the results, and changes in the plan are made accordingly. A plan should be tried for a week before changes are made (Bergstrom, 1968). Any problems that arise, such as diarrhea or constipation, should be addressed immediately.

Types

Fecal incontinence is caused by a gastrointestinal disease, fecal impaction with overflow,

neurogenic disorders, or environmental and iatrogenic factors (Brocklehurst, 1985; Winograd & Jarvik, 1986). This section will describe the treatment modalities for each type of incontinence. A summary of treatment modalities can be found in Table 10–4.

Gastrointestinal Disorders. A change in normal bowel function resulting in diarrhea, constipation, or fecal incontinence may be the presenting sign of a number of conditions, including carcinoma of the colon or rectum, diverticulitis, or bowel infections (Dodge, Backman, & Silverman, 1988; Smith, 1983; Tobin & Brocklehurst, 1986). The underlying disease needs to be diagnosed and appropriate treatment initiated. For example, surgery is currently the preferred treatment for carcinoma of the colon and rectum. Diverticular diseases are treated with a high-fiber diet and bulk-forming agents (Borgman, 1981; Smith, 1983; Williams, 1984). Incontinence due to disease or trauma that impairs the anal sphincter muscles is treated surgically (Corman, 1983; Parks, 1984).

Fecal Impaction. The most common underlying cause of fecal incontinence in the elderly is fecal impaction. Fecal impaction is attributed to long-standing constipation resulting from immobility or decreased activity, dietary intake low in residue, inadequate fluid intake, and drugs, especially chronic laxative use, anticholinergics, and narcotic analgesics (Cefalu, McKnight, & Pike, 1981; Winograd & Jarvik, 1986). The older person with fecal incontinence due to impaction with overflow has frequent staining of liquid or semiformed stools (Klein, 1982; Winograd & Jarvik, 1986). A digital examination often reveals the problem, since 98% of cases of fecal impaction are restricted to the rectum (Klein, 1982; Smith, 1983; Wald, 1986).

The basic approach to treating the problem is to remove the impaction and initiate a bowel regimen to maintain normal bowel function (Smith, 1983; Tobin & Brocklehurst, 1986; Turner, 1987; Winograd & Jarvik, 1986). Clearance of the lower bowel is accomplished with a course of small bulk enemas. The enemas are discontinued when there is no return, which usually occurs within a period of 7 to

Table 10–4. TREATMENT OF FECAL INCONTINENCE

Gastrointestinal Disorders
1. Recognize change in bowel function as the presenting sign of a number of disorders.
2. Diagnose disorder.
3. Treat underlying cause, e.g., antibiotics, surgery, biofeedback, diet modification.

Fecal Impaction
1. Clear lower bowel:
   Course of small bulk enemas (7–10 days)
   Nightly or morning insertion of suppository
   In resistant cases, perform manual disimpaction or total gut irrigation.
2. Prevent recurrence of constipation:
   Bowel program
   Adequate dietary fiber
   Two liters of fluids daily
   Activity and exercise
   Encourage timely response to the urge to defecate.
   Add if indicated:
   Bulk laxatives
   Stool softeners
3. For long term therapy:
   Bowel program
   Daily to twice weekly suppositories.
4. For cognitively impaired:
   Bowel program
   Habit training
   (See under neurogenic disorders.)

Neurogenic Disorders
1. Initiate bowel program.
   Adequate dietary fiber
   Two liters of fluids daily
   Activity and exercise
   Consistent toileting time

2. Introduce habit training.
   Increase awareness of the urge to defecate
   Note elimination pattern. Plan scheduled toileting based on identified pattern or regular toileting after breakfast taking advantage of the gastrocolic reflex.
   Temporary use of suppositories to heighten rectal sensations and increase awareness of the defecation reflex
   Stool softeners as needed
   Suppositories or enemas to stimulate bowel movement if one does not occur for two consecutive days
3. Induce constipation with planned periodic evacuation.
4. Consider biofeedback for selected patients.

Environmental or Iatrogenic Factors
1. Identify cause and take necessary measures to correct the situation.
2. Initiate bowel program:
   Adequate dietary fiber
   Two liters of fluids
   Activity and exercise
   Avoid prolonged bedrest, immobility.
   Encourage timely response to urge to defecate.
3. Check medications:
   Note time of administration
   Monitor medications
   Sedatives, hypnotics
   Laxatives
   Narcotics
   Antacids
   Muscle relaxants
4. Monitor environmental factors:
   Timely response to call light
   Accessible toilet (commode, bedpan)
   Comfortable room temperature
   Privacy
   Unhurried, relaxed atmosphere
5. Use other measures:
   Select clothing that is easy to manipulate.
   Avoid restraints and siderails

(Data from Dodge, Backman, & Silverman, 1988; Cannon, 1981; Smith, 1983; Tobin & Brocklehurst, 1986; Winograd & Jarvik, 1986.)

10 days (Brocklehurst, 1985). Some treatment programs include purgatives using such methods as nightly or morning insertion of a suppository to set a planned time for elimination (Tobin & Brocklehurst, 1986). Concurrently, measures are taken to prevent the recurrence of constipation. These measures include advocating adequate dietary fiber, a minimum of 1.5 to 2 liters of fluids per day, exercise, and timely response to the urge to defecate (Winograd & Jarvik, 1986). Stool softeners or bulk laxative preparations may be required to ob-

tain the right consistency of stool, that is, a soft, moist, formed stool. Lactulose (15 to 30 mg) has been found to be effective in relieving constipation and can be given if necesary (Sanders, 1978; Winograd & Jarvik, 1986).

If long-term therapy is required, the bowel program consists of adequate intake of dietary fiber, adequate intake of fluids, activity and exercise, the administration of stool softeners, and twice weekly to daily suppositories (Smith, 1983; Tobin & Brocklehurst, 1986; Winograd & Jarvik, 1986).

Habit training is also an effective approach to manage overflow fecal incontinence secondary to fecal retention (McCormick & Burgio, 1984). Regular toileting is achieved by using the gastrocolic reflex that occurs after meals, usually following breakfast. The patient is instructed to attempt a bowel movement immediately after breakfast every day. An enema is administered to stimulate a bowel movement if one does not occur for 2 consecutive days (McCormick & Burgio, 1984).

In resistant cases of fecal impaction, manual disimpaction or total gut irrigation may be required (Brocklehurst, 1985; Smith, 1983). Manual removal of the impaction may be necessary to prevent mucosal necrosis or ulcer caused by the hardened fecal mass (Mager-O'Conner, 1984). This procedure should be used as a last resort, since irritation to the anus and rectum or damage to the anal sphincter can occur (Bergstrom, 1968). Removal starts with softening of the intestinal contents. Enemas with 30 to 60 ml of full-strength hydrogen peroxide or 115 ml of warm mineral oil will break the impaction or soften the stool (Mager-O'Conner, 1984; Wald, 1986).

Careful explanations as to the purpose of the treatment and the steps of the procedure and brief, clear instructions for the patient are essential. A topical anesthetic such as lidocaine ointment, 5%, may be applied 5 to 10 minutes prior to the impaction removal. The topical anesthesia lubricates the anorectal tissue and decreases the discomfort caused by the manual removal of hard stool (Mager-O'Conner, 1984). For disimpaction, a well lubricated, gloved index finger is gently inserted. Extreme care is used to break up the impaction in the rectum and remove the stool. Disimpaction should be completed in stages. Sudden evacuation of the large bulk of stool will lower intraabdominal pressure and may cause transient hypotension and dizziness. In the final step, a small retention enema or a suppository is administered to complete the evacuation (Bergstrom, 1968; Mager-O'Conner, 1984).

Whole gut irrigation to clear impaction has been described as a successful treatment approach in the British literature (Brocklehurst, 1985; Smith, 1983). While this drastic approach has not been used in the United States, it is included in this chapter as an alternative treatment in severe situations. To prepare the patient, a softening agent is given for 5 days prior to the procedure. Intravenous injections, one of furosemide, 40 mg, and the other of metoclopramide, 10 mg, are given. A nasogastric tube is inserted, and isotonic saline, warmed to body temperature, is infused at a rate of 2.5 to 3 liters per hour until the effluent begins to clear. An average of 8 liters of irrigant is required. This procedure is reported to produce minimal untoward effects on older persons.

Neurogenic Fecal Incontinence. Neurologic disorders, primarily central nervous system diseases such as strokes and Alzheimer's disease, are a major cause of fecal incontinence. Other conditions include spinal cord compression, tabes dorsalis, multiple sclerosis, peripheral neuropathy, and autonomic neuropathy as seen in diabetes mellitus (Schiller, 1986). The most common neurogenic type of fecal incontinence in the elderly is the uninhibited type. Moderate to severe mental impairment is seen in persons with this type of incontinence (Sowry, 1984; Winograd & Jarvik, 1986). With the loss of central inhibition to the defecation reflex, the older person is unable to inhibit the rectal contraction when there is distention in the rectum, and evacuation occurs (Smith, 1983). The person senses a feeling of urgency before the involuntary elimination occurs (Cannon, 1981). Patients with uninhibited neurogenic incontinence will pass a formed stool once or twice a day into the bed or clothing. This passage frequently follows the gastrocolic reflex (Smith, 1983).

The bowel program for the person with neurogenic fecal incontinence consists of steps to promote bowel regularity. The steps include physical exercise, high fluid intake, a diet that includes high fiber foods, and consistent toileting. Habit training is initiated. Measures are taken to increase the person's level of awareness of the urge to defecate. The time of elimination is noted and toileting is scheduled according to the pattern that is observed.

In settings where many patients must be cared for, it may be difficult to provide optimal scheduling routines. More staff time is required by the habit training approach, and there is a tendency on the part of the patient to rely on staff unless self-toileting is rewarded (McCormick & Burgio, 1984).

Another approach in habit training is to toilet the patient 30 minutes after each meal, when there is likely to be a response. Rectal suppositories are used to establish a consistent toileting time by increasing the rectal sensation and awareness of the urge to eliminate (Cannon, 1981). The use of suppositories is temporary and should be gradually discontinued as regularity is established by exercise, diet, and regular toileting (Cannon, 1981; Turner, 1987).

Neurogenic incontinence in the severely demented older person is treated by inducing constipation and planning periodic evacuation (Kane, Ouslander, & Abrass, 1984; Tobin & Brocklehurst, 1986; Winograd & Jarvik, 1986). Jarratt and Exton-Smith (1960) used kaolin and morphine in the morning and Senokot in the evening. Winograd and Jarvik (1986) recommended attempting a planned evacuation program employing a phosphate enema in the morning, two or three days per week, alternating with a constipating agent such as Lomotil on the other days. Brocklehurst's approach includes a program of constipating drugs given two or three times a day and enemas or suppositories for a planned evacuation on the fifth, sixth, and seventh days. For home care, an enema may be given first, followed by the administration of a bisacodyl suppository to produce further results 1 to 1½ hours later (Brocklehurst, 1985).

Electronic stimulators have been used to treat incontinence caused by some loss in nervous system control of the anal sphincter or the supporting pelvic musculature (Brocklehurst, 1985; MacLeod, 1987). An intraanal plug with electrodes is held in place by the contraction of anal muscles around the plug. The contraction is maintained by a constant tetanic current from a battery held in an apparatus worn over the implanted system. The success rate is low due to the low level of patient acceptance and the few patients available for long-term electric treatment (Brockle-

hurst, 1985). Good results were reported when the treatment was combined with pelvic floor exercises (Matheson & Keighley, 1981).

Persons with fecal incontinence due to peripheral and autonomic neuropathies, as well as those with anal sphincter surgery, trauma, and idiopathic fecal incontinence, may respond to biofeedback therapy (Kane, Ouslander, & Abrass, 1984; Wald, 1986). Studies that included older persons in the sample reported a success rate of 63% and higher (MacLeod, 1987; Whitehead, Burgio, & Engle, 1985). Biofeedback is appropriate for persons who are motivated, cognitively intact, and have rectal sensation and the ability to contract their external sphincter (Schiller, 1986; Wald, 1986). One method uses an intraanal plug containing two electrodes that are connected to an electromyometer or computer. The electrical impulses generated by the contracting sphincter may be audible and/or visible to the patient on the computer monitor. The older person is instructed in sphincter contraction (MacLeod, 1987). Another method is to create rectal distention by administering a small volume of air in a rectal balloon until the patient senses distention. Subsequently, smaller volumes of air are administered until the patient shows no further improvement in response (Wald, 1986). This biofeedback method uses operant conditioning to improve the older person's conscious threshold for sensation of rectal distention and increased control of internal anal sphincter contraction (Schiller, 1986). The advantages of the biofeedback approach are that it is simple and inexpensive and can be carried out in either the office or hospital (MacLeod, 1987).

Environmental and Iatrogenic Factors. A number of environmental and iatrogenic factors are responsible for what can be considered a temporary type of fecal incontinence. Once the underlying cause is identified and modifications are made or corrective actions taken, the incontinence problem is resolved. Illness and admission to a hospital or nursing home often mean an interruption in the older person's usual level of exercise and activity due to bedrest or immobility, a decrease in dietary and fluid intake, and a change in the usual manner and time of toileting. An older person who is in an unfamiliar environment may not be able to locate a toilet when one is needed. Accessibility becomes a problem when a toilet is shared or when the toilet is some distance from the older person's room. A call light not answered promptly, the unavailability of assistance when needed, a bedpan out of reach, restraints, and raised siderails are other reasons for the older person to become temporarily incontinent.

Several other environmental and iatrogenic factors need to be considered. Large doses and poor timing in the administration of laxatives and antacids often cause a loss of bowel control and incontinence. Sedatives, hypnotics, narcotics, and muscle relaxants decrease the older person's awareness of the urge to defecate and ability to get to the toilet on time. Toileting is best carried out in a warm, comfortable, relaxed, unhurried and private environment. These factors are often overlooked or are difficult to accommodate in hospitals and nursing homes. Multiple layers of clothing, buttons, snaps, and hooks are often difficult to manipulate for the older person with arthritis, stroke, or dementia. Clothing that is easy to manipulate and remove, such as pants with Velcro fasteners, allows the older person maximal independence in toileting and may prevent incontinence.

exceed 1 week (McEvoy, 1987). The type of elimination problem determines which laxative is used. For example, bulk-forming laxatives are indicated for the initial treatment of simple constipation, and stool softeners are used when straining at defecation is to be avoided or when the stools are hard and dry. The time of administration is determined by the time planned for the evacuation. When a bowel movement is planned in the morning, the laxative should be given in the evening. For the person who is on a bowel program with the bowel movement planned for the evening, the laxative is taken in the morning (McEvoy, 1987).

If laxatives are used for 1 week or less and the appropriate dosages are administered, the incidence of adverse side effects, such as diarrhea and fluid and electrolyte depletion, is rare. Stimulant laxatives are likely to be the most problematic. Caution is required when using preparations containing magnesium, sodium, or potassium in patients with decreased renal function. Judicious use is indicated with sodium-containing laxatives for patients on sodium-restricted diets and with preparations containing large amounts of sugar for diabetic patients (McEvoy, 1987). See Table 10–2 for a summary of the available oral laxative preparations, their actions, dose, precautions and side effects.

PHARMACEUTICAL PREPARATIONS

Laxatives

Laxatives are often self-prescribed and overused. They are also one of the most frequently prescribed medications in long-term care facilities (Lamy & Krug, 1978). Preventing constipation with proper diet, adequate fluid intake, exercise, and timely response to the defecation reflex is the preferred approach to establish and maintain normal bowel function. Laxatives should be used infrequently. When laxatives are indicated, the mildest oral laxative is the best choice for treatment. The lowest effective dose is given for a duration not to

Suppositories and Enemas

Suppositories and enemas are indicated when oral preparations are ineffective and when prompt and thorough bowel evacuation is desired. To treat constipation and fecal incontinence due to impaction, the recommended sequence for pharmaceutical preparations is as follows: suppositories, microenemas, phosphate enemas, and high soap enemas using a rectal tube (Turner, 1987).

Suppositories initiate the reflexes that stimulate peristalsis of the lower colon and rectum, resulting in relaxation of the external anal sphincter. They are helpful in the initial phase of a bowel management program and should be stopped once a regular pattern has been established. Most suppositories work in 30 minutes, so they should be inserted 30 minutes before results are desired. Proper insertion is important if the suppository is to be effective. Suppositories should be inserted beyond the internal and external sphincters and placed against the rectal wall. They are ineffective if inserted into the stool (Bergstrom, 1968).

Enemas are indicated when several days have passed since the last bowel movement or when there is an impaction. A small amount of tap water, 2 to 3 ounces given with a rubber syringe, is often enough to promote bowel response. If the stool is firm, sodium phosphate and biphosphate or an oil retention enema should be administered. In patients who lack anal sphincter tone, a Foley catheter with a large-sized bulb may be used to hold the fluid in the rectum (Bergstrom, 1968).

Large-volume enemas are avoided in bowel management programs, since total cleansing results in too little stool for defecation. Several days are then required for accumulation of stool to stimulate elimination (Bergstrom, 1968). Large-bulk soap and tap water enemas are not generally indicated for the older patient, since small-bulk enemas have been found to be as effective (Brocklehurst, 1985). It is recommended that no more than 1 pint of fluid be infused at a time (Rousseau, 1988a). Soapsuds or large-volume enemas cause discomfort, disrupt homeostasis, and may possibly lead to shock (Resnick, 1985). Acute colitis is another serious adverse effect of soapsuds enemas. Although the exact cause of colonic mucosal injury is not known, long-chain fatty acids have been implicated. Hard and soft soaps contain sodium and potassium salts of long-chain fatty acids (Rousseau, 1988b).

Table 10–3 lists the suppository and enema preparations used in treatment of constipation and fecal incontinence. The action, dose, precautions, and side effects of each preparation are also outlined.

SUMMARY

Constipation and fecal incontinence, for the most part, can be prevented. When they occur, they can be controlled, managed, or cured. Effective measures are available for these distressing conditions to make the patient more comfortable, prevent complications, make life easier for the caregivers, and lower the expense involved in care.

Normal bowel function can be established and maintained by a minimum daily fluid intake of 1500 to 2000 ml, a balanced diet including high fiber foods, exercise and activity, and timely response to the defecation urge. Constipation can be prevented with the same measures to ensure normal bowel function. Treatment of constipation includes an assessment to determine the cause of the problem, measures to eliminate the cause, appropriate treatment methods to relieve the constipation, and an individualized bowel regimen to prevent future occurrences. In the elderly, the common underlying causes of fecal incontinence are gastrointestinal disease, fecal impaction, neurogenic disorders, and environmental and iatrogenic factors. Specific interventions for each type of fecal incontinence have been presented in this chapter. A discussion on equipment and supportive measures has also been included.

Successful treatment of constipation and fecal incontinence is dependent on the knowledge that bowel dysfunction is not a way of life for the elderly, the belief that treatment is indicated and worthwhile, and the effort and commitment of the older incontinent person and all who are involved in the treatment program.

References

Alterescu, V (1986): Theoretical foundations for an approach to fecal incontinence. *J Enterost Ther*, 13:44–48.

Battle, EH, & Hanna, CE (1980): Evaluation of a dietary regimen for chronic constipation. *J Gerontol Nurs*, 6:527–532.

Behm, RM (1985): A special recipe to banish constipation. *Geriatr Nurs*, 6:216–217.

Benson, JA (1975): Simple chronic constipation. *Postgrad Med*, 57:55–60.

Bergstrom, DA (1968): *Care of Patients with Bowel and Bladder Problems: A Nursing Guide*. Minneapolis, American Rehabilitation Foundation.

Borgman, RF (1981): Dietary fiber and the aging process.

In Hsu, JM, & Davis, RL (eds): *Handbook of Geriatric Nutrition*. Park Ridge, NJ, Noyes Publications, 279–295.

Brocklehurst, JC (1985): The large bowel. *In* Brocklehurst, JC (ed): *Textbook of Geriatric Medicine and Gerontology* (ed 3). Edinburgh, Churchill Livingstone, 534–556.

Burkitt, DP (1982): Dietary fiber: Is it really helpful? *Geriatrics*, 37:119–126.

Burkitt, DP, & Meisner, P (1979): How to manage constipation with high-fiber diet. *Geriatrics*, 34:33–35, 38.

Cannon, B (1981): Bowel function. *In* Martin, N, Holt, NB, & Hicks, D (eds): *Comprehensive Rehabilitation Nursing*. New York, McGraw-Hill.

Cefalu, CA, McKnight GT, & Pike, JI (1981): Treating impaction: A practical approach to an unpleasant problem. *Geriatrics*, 36:143–146.

Corman, ML (1983): The management of anal incontinence. *Surg Clin North Am*, 63:177–191.

Davies, GJ, Crowder, M, Reid, B, et al. (1986): Bowel function measurement of individuals with different eating patterns. *Gut*, 27:164–169.

Davis, A, Nagelhout, MJ, Hoban, M, et al. (1986): Bowel management: A quality assurance approach to upgrading programs. *J Gerontol Nurs*, 12:13–17.

Dodge, J, Backman, C, & Silverman, H (1988): Fecal incontinence in elderly patients. *Postgrad Med*, 83:258–260, 263–264, 269–270.

Dudas, D (1986): Nursing diagnosis and interventions for the rehabilitation of the stroke patient. *Nurs Clin North Am*, 21:345–357.

Eastwood, MA, Fisher, N, Greenwood, CT, et al. (1974): Perspectives on the bran hypothesis. *Lancet*, 1:1029–1032.

Edgington, A, Shepherd, A, & Bainton, D (1983): Management of incontinence. *Health Soc Serv J*, 93:50–51.

Ellickson, EB (1988): Bowel management plan for the homebound elderly. *J Gerontol Nurs*, 14:16–19.

Friesen, AJ (1983): Adverse drug reactions in the geriatric client. *In* Pagliaro, LA, & Pagliaro, AM (eds): *Pharmacologic Aspects of Aging*. St. Louis, CV Mosby, 257–293.

Gorbien, MJ (1988): Constipation in the elderly: The Sepulveda GRECC method. *Geriatr Med Today*, 7:53–63.

Irvine, RE (1986): Faecal incontinence is not inevitable. *Br Med J*, 292:1618–1619.

Jarratt, AS, & Exton-Smith, AN (1960): Treatment of faecal incontinence. *Lancet*, 1:925.

Kane, RL, Ouslander, JG, & Abrass, IB (1984): *Essentials of Clinical Geriatrics*. New York, McGraw-Hill, 107–135.

Klein, H (1982): Constipation and fecal incontinence. *Med Clin North Am*, 66:1135–1141.

Lamy, PP, & Krug, BH (1978): Review of laxative utilization in a skilled nursing facility. *J Am Geriatr Soc*, 26:544–549.

Leigh, RJ, & Turnberg, LA (1982): Faecal incontinence: The unvoiced symptom. *Lancet*, 1:1349–1351.

MacLeod, JH (1987): Management of anal incontinence by biofeedback. *Gastroenterology*, 93:291–294.

Mager-O'Conner, E (1984): How to identify and remove fecal impactions. *Geriatr Nurs*, 5:158–161.

Matheson, DM, & Keighley, MRB (1981): Manometric evaluation of rectal prolapse and faecal incontinence. *Gut*, 22:126–129.

McCormick, KA, & Burgio, KL (1984): Incontinence: An update on nursing care measures. *J Gerontol Nurs*, 10:16–23.

McEvoy, GK (ed.) (1987): *Drug Information 87*. Bethesda, MD, American Society of Hospital Pharmacists.

Miller, J (1985): Helping the aged manage bowel function. *J Gerontol Nurs*, 11:37–41.

Moore, J (1984): Promoting continence: Confusion, ignorance, inconsistency. *Nurs Times*, 80:38–42.

Mowlam, V, North, K, & Myers, C (1986): Managing faecal incontinence. *Nurs Times*, 82:55–59.

Noekler, LS (1987): Incontinence in elderly cared for by family. *Gerontologist*, 27:194–200.

Okamoto, GA (1984): *Physical Medicine and Rehabilitation*. Philadelphia, WB Saunders.

Parks, AG (1984): Faecal incontinence. *In* Mandelstam, D (ed): *Incontinence and Its Management*. London, Croom Helm, 77–93.

Pattee, JJ, & West, MS (1988): Clinical aspects of a fiber supplementation program in a nursing home population. *Curr Ther Res*, 43:1150–1157.

Peto, JJ, & Skelton, D (1983): Drug selection and dosage in the elderly. *In* Pagliaro, LA, & Pagliaro, AM, (eds): *Pharmacologic Aspects of Aging*. St. Louis, CV Mosby, 294–336.

Resnick, B (1985): Constipation, common but preventable. *Geriatr Nurs*, 6:213–215.

Robinson, CH, Lawler, MR, Chenoweth, WL, et al. (1986): *Normal and Therapeutic Nutrition* (ed 17). New York, Macmillan.

Rousseau, P (1988a): Treatment of constipation. *Postgrad Med*, 83:339–345, 349.

Rousseau, P (1988b): No soapsuds enemas! *Postgrad Med*, 83:352–353.

Sanders, JF (1978): Lactulose syrup assessed in a double-blind study of elderly constipated patients. *J Am Geriatr Soc*, 26:236–239.

Sandman, PO, Adolfsson, R, Hallmans, G, et al. (1983): Treatment of constipation with high-bran bread in long-term care of severely demented elderly patients. *J Am Geriatr Soc*, 31:290–293.

Schiller, LR (1986): Faecal incontinence. *Clin Gastroenterol*, 15:687–704.

Shane, RE, & McLane, AM (1988): Constipation: Impact on etiological factors. *J Gerontol Nurs*, 14:31–33.

Sklar, M (1986): Gastrointestinal diseases. *In* Calkins, E, Davis, J, Ford, AB (eds): *The Practice of Geriatrics*. Philadelphia, WB Saunders, 555–575.

Smith, RG (1983): Fecal incontinence. *J Am Geriatr Soc*, 31:694–697.

Sowry, GSC (1984): Incontinence in general medical patients. *In* Mandelstam, D (ed): *Incontinence and Its Management*. London, Croom Helm, 94–102.

Stryker, R (1977): *Rehabilitive Aspects of Acute and Chronic Nursing Care*. Philadelphia, WB Saunders.

Thompson, WG (1980): Laxatives: Clinical pharmacology and rational use. *Drugs*, 19:49–58.

Tobin, GW, & Brocklehurst, JC (1986): Faecal incontinence in residential homes for the elderly. *Age Ageing*, 15:41–46.

Turner, A (1987): Constipation and faecal incontinence. *Professional Nurse*, 2:256–258.

Wald, A (1986): Fecal incontinence: Effective nonsurgical treatments. *Postgrad Med*, 80:123–130.

Whitehead, WE, Burgio, KL, & Engel, BT (1985): Biofeedback treatment of fecal incontinence in geriatric patients. *J Am Geriatr Soc*, 33:320–324.

Williams, SR (1984): *Basic Nutrition and Diet Therapy* (ed 7). St. Louis, Times Mirror/Mosby College Publishing.

Winograd, CH, & Jarvik, LF (1986): Physician management of the demented patient. *J Am Geriatr Soc*, 34:295–308.

CHAPTER
11

Immobility and Functional Mobility in the Elderly

DEBORAH MONICKEN, R.N., M.S.

This chapter focuses on immobility, including the cause of immobility and its conse-quences on the older client. Assessment and interventions toward functional mobility are presented to assist nurses in decreasing the negative consequences of immobility and in-creasing clients' functional mobility.

IMMOBILITY

Definition

The term "immobility" is used in a variety of ways. Immobility is an imposed restriction on the entire body. The term "disuse" refers to the lack of activity in a particular body part. These definitions do not provide a measure of impact on the individual person. Kottke (1966) stated that the impact of immobility is propor-tional to the duration, degree, and type of limitation. Focusing on immobility from this perspective will help the clinician determine the probable impact to body systems. Kottke also divided the causes of decreased activity into four areas: (1) neuromusculoskeletal re-strictions, (2) physical immobility, (3) pro-longed positions of the body in relation to gravity, and (4) decreased stimulation. Knowl-edge of the cause of the immobility will help the clinician understand the patient's limits. This knowledge can also help in the selection of interventions most practical to correct or modify the underlying cause.

Consequences

Physiologic Effects. Depending on the extent and time of immobilization, several body systems can be affected. As one system weakens, it creates vulnerability in others. For example, with loss of calcium from bone, hypercalcemia can develop and can lead to hypercalciuria and even encephalopathy. Immobility can lead to many physiologic changes (Miller, 1975). These changes are presented in Table 11–1.

Psychosocial Effects. There are psychosocial consequences of immobility. In the elderly these consequences have been identified as depression, fear and panic, and exacerbation of preexisting paranoia and organic brain syndrome, regressive behavior, social withdrawal, apathy, and even stupor, often simulating a semicomatose state (Miller, 1975). Oster (1976) describes loss of financial and personal independence and a lack of meaningful existence.

Causes

Rest. Rest has been used to provide optimal conditions for healing. Rest can be categorized in four forms: sleep, immobilization, diversion, and relaxation or leisure (Goldman, 1977). To be rested, one does not have to be immobile and, conversely, to be immobile does not imply rest.

Restraints. Misprescriptions for restraints in the name of safety may result in immobility. Patients who are believed to be in danger of falls are often restrained. Frengley and Mion (1986) monitored the use of physical restraints on patients on medical wards of an acute-care metropolitan hospital for a period of 15 weeks. They found that patients 70 years of age or older were more likely to be restrained, and for a longer period, than younger patients. Restrained patients had a hospital stay twice as long as unrestrained patients. When two long-term care Canadian hospitals were compared, the one that used fewer restraints had one-half the accident rate of the other. Bedrails are another form of restraint used to prevent falls. However, bedrails have not been dem-

Table 11–1. CONSEQUENCES OF IMMOBILITY ON BODY SYSTEMS

Body System	Consequences
Musculoskeletal	Thickening of joint capsule; loss of smoothness of cartilage surface; decreased flexibility of connective tissues; changes similar to osteoarthritis—joint contractures, demineralization of bone, bone loss; atrophy and shortening of muscle; decrease in muscle strength; decreased muscle oxidative capacity; decline in aerobic capacity
Pulmonary	Arterial oxygen desaturation; increased hypostatic pooling; increased risk of atelectasis and infection
Cardiovascular	Decreased cardiac output and stroke volume; increased peripheral resistance; net loss of total body water and total blood volume
Integumentary	Pressure sores
Gastrointestinal	General weakening of muscles, causing altered colonic motility, constipation
Urinary	Increased nitrogen, phosphorus, total sulfur, sodium, potassium, and calcium excretion; renal insufficiency; decreased glomerular filtration rate; loss of ability to concentrate urine; lower creatinine tolerance
Metabolic	Decreased basal metabolic rate; increased storage of fat or carbohydrate; negative nitrogen and calcium metabolic balance due to decreased absorption of protein and calcium intake; decreased glucose tolerance; metabolic alkalosis
Sensory	Decreased sensory stimulation (kinesthetic, visual, auditory, tactile); decreased social interaction; changes in affect, cognition, and perception

(Data from Harper & Lyles, 1988; Milde, 1988; Miller, 1975.)

onstrated to prevent falls; rather, they increase the height of the fall (Frengley & Mion, 1986).

Aging. Often the same changes that occur with immobility also occur in aging. Several studies agreed that aging affected the type II (fast-acting) muscle fibers (Grimby, Banneskiold-Samste, Hvid, et al., 1982; Larsson, Sjodin, & Karlssen, 1978; Tomonaga, 1977). Tomonaga (1977) noted that neuropathic changes were the most prominent cause of muscle change in people ages 60 to 69 years and 70 to 79 years. Atrophy of the type II muscle fibers was the next cause. In the 80 to 89 year age group, type II muscle fiber atrophy was the most prominent change. The changes occurred in the distal muscles of the lower extremity when caused by neuropathy, whereas type II muscle fiber atrophy was the cause in proximal muscles. Age-related changes in body systems essential to mobility are presented in Table 11–2.

Loss of flexibility and strength, changes in posture and gait, and pain increase the vulnerability of the elderly to immobility (Lewis, 1985). Increased stiffening of collagen decreases flexibility. Also, aging changes can be attributed to an alteration in muscle fibers, inability of the cardiovascular system to provide an adequate supply of blood, alteration in the muscle's chemical composition (that is, decreased potassium), and a decrease in the glycoproteins that maintain fluid content in muscle (Lewis, 1985). There is a loss of strength in antigravity muscles used in daily activities: quadriceps, hip extensors, ankle dorsiflexors, latissimus dorsi, and triceps (Browse, 1965). An increase in activity may be needed to maintain their strength (Browse, 1965). Lewis (1985) noted decreased flexibility and strength and changes in the intervertebral disc affect posture. When standing, the vertical axis should run down an imaginary line through the ear, acromion, greater trochanter, posterior patella, and lateral malleolus. However, in the elderly, the vertical axis changes such that the position of the head is forward, shoulders rounded, slight kyphosis of the upper back, flattening or accentuation of the lumbar curve particularly with frequent sitting, and slight flexion of the hips and knees. Changes in gait are due to an alteration in balance, strength, and flexibility. Chemical and circulatory deficiencies cause a shuffling gait and a decreased heel-to-floor angle, increasing the potential for falls (Lewis, 1985).

Pain may be a problem related to mobility in the elderly. Pain due to decreased production and liberation of enkephalins (a natural analgesic) may be a secondary effect of aging (Lewis, 1985). In addition, a tendency toward decreased activity or hypokinesis resulting in

Table 11–2. BODY SYSTEM CHANGES ASSOCIATED WITH AGING

Body System	Changes
Musculoskeletal	Changes in joint surface, ligaments, tendons and connective tissues; decreased bone density increasing vulnerability for fracture; loss of both number and size of muscle fibers; atrophy with fibrous tissues replacing muscle; increased atrophy of proximal muscles of lower extremity with neuropathic changes of distal leg; decline in muscle strength (10% to 25% less than that of a 25-year-old)
Pulmonary	Loss of elastic recoil of the lungs with increase in airway resistance; reduced vital capacity; decrease in chest wall compliance; 50% reduction in maximal voluntary ventilation and decreased gas exchange
Cardiovascular	Increase in blood pressure; decrease in stroke volume; decreased cardiac reserve and decreased perspiration capability leading to a decline in compensatory response to physical and emotional stress (i.e., exercise, heat)
Integumentary	Decreased subcutaneous adipose tissue; decreased elasticity of connective tissue; loss of sweat and sebaceous glands
Nervous	Central nervous system changes including a decrease in weight of brain resulting from postmitotic cells and probable decrease in neural cell size; decrease in cerebral blood flow; reduction of nerve conduction velocity; decrease in rate and magnitude of the reflex response; increase in arousal threshold; decrease in alpha waves/second; decrease in sensory activity; decline in perceptual motor response; decreased myoneural transmission; decreased speed of muscle contraction and increase in postural sway, resulting in loss of balance

(Data from Harper & Lyles, 1988; Payton & Poland, 1984.)

long-term sitting accounts for the tightness of the flexor muscles. There are also secondary aging changes that are due to environmental influences, such as poor nutrition, injury, disease, and hypokinesis leading to a posture the elderly person may finally assume (Kaufman, 1987). Arthritis, osteoporosis, polymyalgia, and neurologic disorders commonly occur in the aged, causing further restrictions in mobility.

With aging, several reasons for falls have been suggested: postural sway (Overstall, Johnson, & Exton-Smith, 1978), visual-perceptual disturbance (Tobis, Nayak, & Hoehler, 1981), or a combination of musculoskeletal, visual, and vestibular factors (Tobis, et al., 1981). If falls become a part of the older person's history, fear and ultimately decreased mobility can occur. (See Chapters 14 and 15 on falls.)

MOBILITY ASSESSMENT

In the assessment of mobility, there are four areas to be considered: range of motion, strength, coordination/balance, and tolerance.

Range of Motion

Range of motion (ROM) is measured with the body in a vertical or supine anatomic position with the legs and arms at the sides, which represents neutral or zero degrees of motion (Figure 11–1).

As the extremity moves toward the head, the degrees of motion increase. Exceptions to this measurement occur with the trunk and neck movements, shoulder rotation, elbow pronation and supination, and hip rotation.

For the trunk and neck the degrees of motion increase as the trunk or head moves toward the feet (Figure 11–2). External and internal rotation of the shoulder is assessed with the humerus abducted to 90°. This is zero position for measuring external and internal shoulder rotation, with the degrees of motion increasing when the shoulder is externally or internally rotated (Figure 11–3). For supination and pronation, the elbow is flexed at 90°, with the thumb facing up (zero degrees of motion). The degrees of motion increase as the arm is supinated or pronated (Figures 11–4 and 11–5). Hip rotation is assessed with the hip and

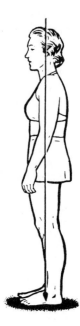

Normal

Figure 11–1. Note the central axis when the body is in anatomic position. (From Daniels, L, and Worthingham, C.: *Therapeutic Exercise for Body Alignment and Function.* Philadelphia, WB Saunders, 1977, p 12. Reprinted with permission.)

knee in 90° of flexion (zero degrees of motion), the degrees of motion increasing when the leg is rotated externally or internally (Figure 11–6). See Table 11–3 for maximum range of motion for specific joints.

Reaching maximal ROM is not essential for a person to be functional. However, certain degrees of motion are essential to accomplishing certain skills. It is important to determine the necessary movements to perform an action or activity. If the activity is necessary but the movement is not possible, alternatives are needed to accomplish the desired activity. Equipment modifications and caregiver education can help provide the adaptations necessary to accomplish the task.

Strength

Adequate ROM does not assist the person to accomplish an activity without adequate

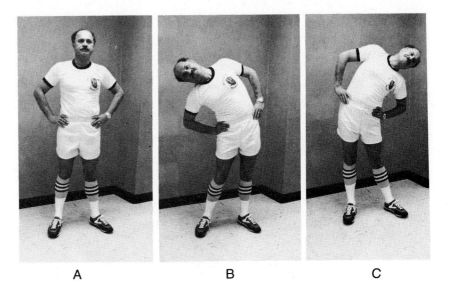

Figure 11–2. *(A, B, C)* Movement away from the central axis. (From Pollock, ML, Wilmore, JH, and Fox, SM III: Exercise in Health and Disease. Philadelphia, WB Saunders, 1984, p 328. Reprinted with permission.)

A   B   C

strength. Brown (1987) discriminates between strength and power. Strength is the maximal tension or force developed in a muscle, and power is the amount of tension developed within a period of time. Both strength and power decrease with age, which is one reason for the more limited skills of the elderly athlete. "Strength," as used here, will serve as the general representation of strength and power. Strength assessment, though subjective, is reported with numbers (i.e., 5, 4, etc.) or words (excellent, very good, etc.) to define

the levels of strength. Strength is assessed by comparing both sides of the patient and determining how well the patient can maintain a position against the resistance of the examiner. In the lowest strength levels of 1 and 2, the muscle itself must be palpated to check for contraction and the limb must be cradled to prevent its weight from interfering with movement. The person who has minimal or no strength potentials (i.e., one judged as 0, 1, or 2) is classified as weak and presents a challenge to nurses. However, the nurse must consider what level of strength a person needs

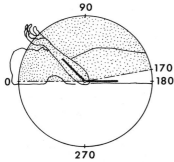

Figure 11–3. Shoulder: external and internal rotation. (From Cole, TM and Tobis, JS: Measurement of musculoskeletal function. *In* Kottke, FJ, Stillwell, GK, and Lehmann, JF (eds). Krusen's Handbook of Physical Medicine and Rehabilitation, ed 3. Philadelphia, WB Saunders, 1982, p 25. Reprinted with permission.)

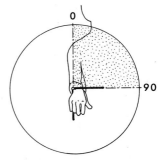

Figure 11–4. Radioulnar joint: pronation. (From Cole, TM, and Tobis, JS: Measurement of musculoskeletal function. *In* Kottke FJ, Stillwell, GK, and Lehmann, JF (eds): Krusen's Handbook of Physical Medicine and Rehabilitation, ed 3. Philadelphia, WB Saunders, 1982, p 26. Reprinted with permission.)

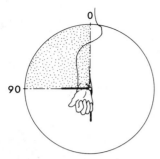

Figure 11–5. Radioulnar joint: supination. (From Cole, TM, and Tobis, JS: Measurement of musculoskeletal function. *In* Kottke, FJ, Stillwell, GK, and Lehmann, JF (eds): Krusen's Handbook of Physical Medicine and Rehabilitation, ed 3. Philadelphia, WB Saunders, 1982, p 26. Reprinted with permission.)

to function in his/her environment. For example, Mr. G. is in generally good health with a strength of 3 in his upper extremities, which is adequate for him to get himself around the home. However, this strength level is not adequate for future needs when ambulation on crutches or a walker is required. Strengthening exercises should begin immediately.

An area of strength assessment where health care providers are frequently fooled is in gauging an imbalance in opposing muscles, that is, flexors versus extensors. For instance, a person appears to be functional with full ROM—that is, drinking from a cup or bending

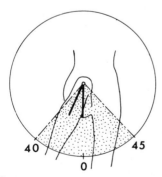

Figure 11–6. Hip: external-internal rotation of the hip (flexed position). (From Cole, TM, and Tobis, JS: Measurement of musculoskeletal function. *In* Kottke, FJ, Stillwell, GK, and Lehmann, JF (eds). Krusen's Handbook of Physical Medicine and Rehabilitation, ed. 3. Philadelphia, WB Saunders, 1982, p 30. Reprinted with permission.)

Table 11–3. MAXIMUM RANGE OF MOTION

Joint	Direction/Degrees
Neck	Flexion/45°
	Extension/55°
	Lateral bending/40°
	Rotation/70°
Back	Flexion/75°
	Extension/30°
	Lateral bending/35°
	Rotation/30°
Shoulder	Flexion/180°
	Extension/50°
	External rotation/90°
	Internal rotation/90°
	Abduction/180°
	Adduction/50°
Elbow	Flexion/160°
	Supination/90°
	Pronation/90°
Wrist	Extension/70°
	Flexion/90°
	Radial deviation/20°
	Ulnar deviation/20°
Fingers	Metacarpophalangeal hyperextension/30°
	Flexion/90°
	Proximal interphalangeal flexion/120°
	Distal interphalangeal flexion/80°
Hip	Flexion/90° (with knee at 120°)
	Hyperextension/15°
	Abduction/45°
	Internal rotation/40°
	External rotation/80°
Knee	Hyperextension/15°
	Flexion/130°
Ankle	Dorsiflexion/20°
	Plantar flexion/45°
	Inversion/30°
	Eversion/20°

(Data from Cole & Tobis, 1982; Swartz, 1989.)

the arm all the way up. But this person may not be able to achieve full ROM in the opposite direction—that is, extending the elbow. This is particularly deceiving when the weaker muscle is being pulled by gravity so that it appears strong; on close assessment, full ROM is not achieved. Contractures can rapidly develop with a shortening of the stronger muscle. Commonly, this is seen in flexion positions due somewhat to the nature of the injury and splinting of the injured joint. However, another cause is maintaining patients in positions that foster flexion patterns. While it is normal for some ROM to be lost in the shoulders and hips, frequently the hip and knee flexors and the hip rotators lose ROM due to long periods of sitting and decreased use of these muscles in activities (Lewis, 1985).

Coordination and Balance

Coordination and balance assessment determines the degree of physical control and independent movement that a person requires to hold a posture or perform an action. When dizziness, fainting, or falls trouble the older person, definitive testing should be done (Venna, 1986).

For a simple test of imbalance, Mathias, Nayak, and Isaacs (1986) found good correlation between their "get up and go" test and the more sophisticated laboratory tests of gait and imbalance. Mathias and associates had elderly people get up from a chair, walk to the wall, turn without touching the wall, walk back to the chair, turn around, and sit down. This activity was then scored with numbers from 1 (normal) to 5 (severely abnormal). Elderly persons with a score of 3 or more were considered at risk of falling. (See Chapter 15 for an explanation of this test.)

Tolerance

Tolerance is both physical and psychological. Assessment of physical tolerance includes cardiovascular and respiratory response, fatigue, and pain response. Assessment of psychological tolerance includes factors such as motivation and depression. The elderly person's blood pressure, pulse, respirations, pain/discomfort, and attentiveness should be assessed before, during, and after a test exercise. Allan (1985) advises obtaining a health history before an exercise program is started. The history includes a current health status, medications, coronary disease history and risk factors, activity-limiting disease, and personal social history. Personal social history includes previous coping and current environment. Knowledge of the individual's prognosis/progression, determined by the state of health or

presence of disease, helps the nurse to determine realistic goals and select nursing interventions that will achieve those goals within a given time frame.

Factors That Affect Mobility

Cognition, social support, patient's preference, and environment all affect mobility. For example, if cognition is impaired, the degree of independence will be limited. The patient with Alzheimer's disease is an example of the impact of cognition on a person's functional ability. Though this person might score very well on the physical assessment areas, cognitive deficits require that most activities be supervised and the selection of skills be safety-dependent.

In assessing social support, the nurse evaluates the physical, intellectual, and emotional capabilities of the caregiver. Also, the larger social support circle of the caregiver and elderly patient is assessed in terms of its ability to provide caregiver relief, support, and socialization. The nurse proceeds with caution in making interventions with the caregiver. When the social support is limited or the physical and emotional care demands are high, the caregiver may decide to set priorities that limit, modify, or eliminate certain types of care. These decisions may be detrimental to the elderly patient. In settings involving caregivers the nurse can provide guidance to the caregiver concerning optimal, realistic goals for the patient.

Personal preference determines how much an individual will change or alter his or her behavior. Given the many adjustments that aging requires, a willingness to change yet another sphere of life may be too great a demand. Where possible, options that limit change and keep the person's lifestyle or belief system consistent should be considered.

Variations in environments can enhance or limit a person's independence. It is important to know the planned discharge environment to determine the activities and actions an individual will need to function.

FUNCTIONAL MOBILITY

Function

"Functional" refers to that which the patient needs in a given setting. This is an important concept to embrace. It demands that the practitioner focus on what each individual patient needs, rather than on what the practitioner thinks the patient needs or what other patients have done. Patients may be alike in physical capabilities, but *function* depends on other elements, including caregiver involvement and environment. The nurse must always consider how the patient and caregiver will cope and which approaches they will use to achieve their goals. For example, a nurse was helping a stroke patient practice dressing when the patient remarked, "My wife always does this for me." "Well," declared the nurse, "you should learn to do this yourself." The patient responded, "I do most things for myself but my wife likes to dress me because it's faster, you know." After many hours of therapy and nurse teaching, the patient was discharged. On a subsequent clinic visit, the patient and wife declared that all was well, the wife stating that the only thing she did for the patient was dress him. "It's faster, you know."

Mobility

"Mobility" refers to actions or activities a person performs, which should be described in definitive, measurable terms, for example, independent ambulation at home for a functional distance of 50 feet or being able to perform basic activities of daily living with supervision. Determining mobility requires that the patient be considered in day-to-day, event-to-event, week-to-month activities. This will help to include all important functions.

Goal Setting

In order to achieve functional mobility, goals must be set. The goal should reflect the patient's condition, prognosis, and time con-

straints for care. Also, the goal should be measurable and realistic. Goals should have a "long life" in servicing the patient's needs. For instance, a partially paralyzed patient may be able to do a stand pivot transfer at present but spasms are noted to be developing in the lower extremities. This transfer may become impossible, unsafe, or unworkable in the near future. Therefore, it might be better to train the patient to perform another type of transfer, such as a slide-over transfer (Figure 11–7).

When goals are written in descriptive, measurable terms, their achievement by the person is observable. Most mobility goals reflect a developmental progression (growth) of skill. To attain a goal, short-term goals (STGs) should be listed in a priority sequence that fosters a person's motor or skill development. A method to determine STGs and their priority placement is to reduce a goal to specific activities, look logically at which activity must precede the next, and then determine the priority or developmental progression. For example, a recovering stroke patient is lying in bed. Given the assessment data, the goal is for the patient to do an independent stand pivot transfer at home. Breaking down that goal, the patient would have to demonstrate

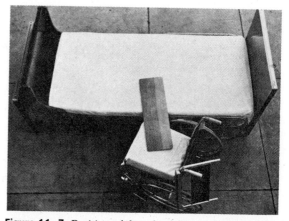

Figure 11–7. Position of the wheelchair and sliding board for a lateral sliding transfer. (From Ellwood, PM, Jr: Transfers—Method, equipment, and preparation. *In* Kottke, FJ, Stillwell, GK, and Lehmann, JF (eds). Krusen's Handbook of Physical Medicine and Rehabilitation, ed 3. Philadelphia, WB Saunders, 1982, p 483. Reprinted with permission.)

the following physical activities: rolling side-to-side in bed, sitting up in bed, balanced sitting on the side of the bed, standing, pivoting, and sitting down. Since the goal includes independence at home, these activities require that the patient have the strength, cognition, and judgment to safely do the transfer alone and that the transfer can be done in several settings in the home (e.g., toilet and tub). Setting priorities means that a person must be able to sit before standing and stand before pivoting and that he or she must be able to do both dependently before being able to do them independently.

In another example, the stated goal was for the patient to be "independent in all of personal care in order to live alone at home." This includes not only the basic activities of daily living but also the instrumental activities of daily living, such as selecting appropriate clothing for weather conditions, shopping, and doing laundry. These skills are necessary for patients living alone without support systems.

PROMOTING FUNCTIONAL MOBILITY AND HEALTH

Exercise

There are many aspects and parameters to evaluate when considering therapeutic mobility and aggressive exercise programs for the elderly. In mobility prescription, the approach to treatment must often be uniquely tailored and not always conventional. Given the need to balance the individual's present chronic disorders, stamina, and environments, all aspects of the individual must be addressed or decisions may be made that actually impede the person's mobility.

The effects of activity in reducing, preventing, or improving body changes are well documented. Parent and Whall (1984) showed a strong positive correlation between increased activity and improved self-esteem and a strong negative correlation between high self-esteem and depression. Simpson (1986) described the

following positive health effects from exercise: increased energy, improved sleeping and eating, decreased aches and pains, decreased stress, and decreased smoking and alcohol use. Simpson noted benefits to the cardiovascular, respiratory, and musculoskeletal systems with improved oxygen transport, decreased blood pressure, heart rate, and blood lactate, increased lung vital capacity, decreased body fat, increased lean body mass, and increased muscle strength and joint flexibility. The positive psychological changes occur sooner in the elderly than in the young (Simpson, 1986).

To guide in the prescription of exercise, stress tests are advised for anyone with a positive cardiovascular history or physical findings. People who require special monitoring are those who are on the following medications: beta blockers because they cause a decreased heart rate, antihypertensives because their effect may be magnified by exercise, and antidepressants and neuroleptics, which can produce postural blood pressure changes particularly with exercise (Simpson, 1986). Eiserman (1986) reported dizziness from loss of potassium with diuretics, impaired heat dissipation with phenothiazines, and increased risk of heat stroke with amphetamines, barbiturates, and alcohol. In a discussion of the use of medication in conjunction with exercise, Chapron and Besdine (1986) noted the need to monitor the following side effects: postural hypotension, fatigue, weakness, depression, confusion, involuntary movements, dizziness, vertigo, ataxia, and urinary incontinence.

Regardless of functional potential, few patients should be eliminated from rehabilitation programs. Any goals, no matter how limited, that can possibly enhance a patient's discharge status, quality of life, or level of independence should be given at least a short-term trial. Schuman and associates (1981) demonstrated positive effects on certain levels of demented patients when specialized programs were used, though the authors note that this program exceeds standard rehabilitation components. Whatever the exercise, the elderly person needs to be aware of the problems with thermoregulation and hydration due to age-related body changes. Eiserman (1986) noted that with exercise, the body core temperature increases. This increase is relieved by increased cutaneous blood flow, increased cardiac output, and cooling by evaporation of perspiration. In the elderly, there is a decreased cutaneous vasculature and cardiac output response. In addition, the elderly have a decreased fluid volume and the kidneys retain less fluid. These physical changes make the elderly person less adaptable to exercise. In warm, humid weather there is an increased risk of heat stress, heat cramps, heat exhaustion, and heat stroke (i.e., hyperthermia, a body temperature in excess of 40°C). Thirst in the elderly is not a good indicator of fluid needs since thirst symptoms lag 2 to 3 days behind actual needs. With changes in climate, the elderly should decrease or slowly work into activity. With heat at or above 27°C or humidity at or above 80%, exercise should be decreased. It is also recommended that the elderly drink extra water before exercise, drink up to 6 to 8 ounces every 15 minutes during exercise, avoid alcohol and excess protein, and wear loose, porous, light clothing and a hat (Eiserman, 1986). Simpson (1986) suggests that exercise not be done for 30 minutes to 1 hour after eating, that it begin with gentle flexing and stretching, that the exercise period be tapered off slowly, not abruptly, and that the person gradually work up activity.

Good cardiovascular exercises such as some aerobic exercises may be contraindicated given a preexisting condition. In these situations, specialized programs or exercises like jarming (jogging with arms, like conducting an orchestra), swimming, and walking may be considered (Simpson, 1986). Motivators to exercise include ready access to the exercise facility, freedom from injury, and spousal support or participation in the program. Education, daily schedule, and group/partner exercise are also considered important (Simpson, 1986).

Most nurses are familiar with providing passive range of motion (PROM) or ambulation for patients. However, many nurses do not always understand the activity needs of patients between these two extremes. A person's joint elasticity may be maintained with PROM, but to decrease muscle atrophy and improve muscle strength activities must be used that require the person to contract the muscle. PROM should be prescribed only when there is no indication of voluntary muscle motion. The nurse should continually assess the patient for possible muscle movement in order to advance the patient to the next level of exercise, such as active assisted range of motion (AAROM), active range of motion (AROM), or active resistive range of motion (ARROM) (Table 11–4).

In conjunction with exercise, positioning also helps to maintain or increase the desired ROM in patients with diminished mobility. The art of positioning patients comfortably in extension positions—side-lying with extremities in extension, three-quarters prone and prone—can provide the slow stretch needed to help prevent atrophy and contractures. Semi-Fowler's is a commonly used position. However, it can accentuate problems with posture (flexion) and skin condition (shearing) (Figure 11–8).

To exercise a patient with a strength rating of 1 or 2, the nurse does AAROM. At a strength of 1, the nurse should support the limb while having the patient contract the muscle. While moving the limb, the nurse should palpate to assess if the muscle is contracting. At a strength of 2, the patient's limb should be cradled to help eliminate the patient

Table 11–4. STRENGTH ASSESSMENT

Strength Rating	Description	Exercise*
5	Able to oppose against maximal resistance	ARROM
4	Able to oppose against moderate resistance	ARROM
3	Able to move the weight of limb against gravity	AROM
2	Able to move limb if gravity removed	AAROM
1	Able to contract muscle	AAROM
0	None	PROM

(Data from Brown, 1987; Swartz, 1989.)
*ARROM—active resistive range of motion; AROM—active range of motion; AAROM—active assisted range of motion; PROM—passive range of motion.

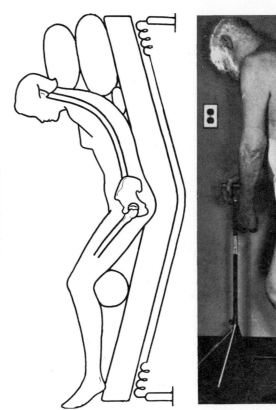

Figure 11–8. The prolonged bedfast position without maintenance of the normal range of motion results in a kyphosis of the spine and flexion contractures of the hips, knees, and ankles. (From Kottke, FJ: Therapeutic exercise to maintain mobility. In Kottke, FJ, Stillwell, GK, and Lehmann, JF (eds). Krusen's Handbook of Physical Medicine and Rehabilitation, ed. 3. Philadelphia, WB Saunders, 1982, p 397. Reprinted with permission.)

having to lift the weight of the limb against gravity. The patient should be moved through the full ROM. Patients doing their own exercise should be checked to ensure that full ROM is accomplished and that an imbalance in strengths of opposing muscle is not present. As voluntary function returns, Steinberg (1986) points out that agonist and antagonist (opposing muscle groups) should be simultaneously exercised. If one group is stronger, it should not be overexercised. Isometric exercise can be helpful, provided the patient is well instructed in breathing and in the execution of the exercise.

To maintain or enhance strength at a 3, 4, or 5 rating, some type of resistance such as a weight must be used. At a strength of 3, the patient's own body weight is often adequate for resistance. In a bed or wheelchair, the patient can do resistive exercise by using a trapeze for chin-ups, doing wheelchair propulsion or wheelchair push-ups for the arms, or even doing sit-ups in bed.

With any exercise, the physician must be made aware of the exercise; also, the patient must be assessed for ability and tolerance. When exercising to strengthen a muscle group, it must be known which exercise works which muscle and which muscle will be needed for a task. Physical and occupational therapists are important resources, especially where exercise routines are not established. All levels of nursing staff must work toward practicing rehabilitative rather than custodial care (Heller, Bausell, & Ninos, 1984).

Mobility Aids

Controversies exist over which mobility aids are most effective. For example, many arguments have been generated about whether to focus on ambulation or to advance straight to wheelchair adaptation. "He'll just sit in that chair and lose strength," argues one health practitioner, and another retorts, "He's not that good at ambulation. He'll be confined to a distance of 50 feet." Who is right? Either professional may be right. In fact, until recently, there was little research to substantiate the benefits of one approach over another. In reality, a balance of clinical data and individual patient needs provides the best direction.

Some research has been conducted regarding the physiologic impact of various mobility-assisted approaches. Wheelchair propulsion has always been thought to cause greater exhaustion to the patient than ambulation, even when prosthesis was necessary. In a study by Fisher and Patterson (1981) comparing two types of crutch walking with healthy adults on flat and step-up terrain, there was a high energy cost with crutch ambulation. Based on these results, the authors suggested very careful evaluation of cardiovascular patients for crutch walking. Upper extremity endurance aerobic exercise may be indicated in preparation of the patient for crutch walking. This study also noted that for both normal and crutch-walking ambulation, stair-climbing costs less energy than ramps per amount of vertical rise if horizontal distance is not included. Therefore, in some cases, it might be easier for a patient to walk the stairs than take a ramp, depending on distance and degree of incline. The surface of a terrain should also be considered. It is easier to move a wheelchair on a hard surface than on a soft one (i.e., plush carpet), and there is a big difference in ambulation on grass as compared to a tiled floor. When a mobility program is prescribed, it should be tested on appropriate terrains.

Much effort has been invested in preparing lower extremity amputees and even bilateral amputees to walk with prostheses. In practice, many amputees have discarded their prostheses for wheelchairs. This is seen more often with persons of advanced age, poor tolerance, bilateral amputation, or above-the-knee amputation. In a study by DuBow and associates (1983) on bilateral lower extremity amputees, the velocity with which a patient moved did not vary whether a wheelchair or ambulation was used. However, heart rate and oxygen consumption increased significantly with ambulation, whereas the amputee did not experience any more changes than the normal subject when using a wheelchair at his or her own pace.

EVALUATION

With any prescribed activity, an evaluation of its impact on the person should be made. Parameters including vital signs, skin condition, and tolerance should be routinely checked. In many cases, ongoing followup is also essential. With chronic progressing disorders (i.e., multiple sclerosis, Parkinson's, organic brain syndromes) where the patient's condition deteriorates with the disease process, adaptation in equipment, environment, and exercise is often needed. Early recognition of changes can help to prevent muscular deterioration, contractures, injuries, and many other problems. In areas where respite care is available, updates on care protocols can be made. Through clinics, routine review of activity regimens should be as common as monitors of blood pressure or weight. With early prevention and restoration, happier, healthier years of life may be available to the elderly.

SUMMARY

In this chapter, functional mobility was presented as a broad concept that includes both mobility and function. The physical and psychosocial effects of immobility on the elderly were delineated. Assessment of the patient's mobility status is essential to plan for functional mobility. Through careful planning and attention to special qualities of each patient, complications and restrictions can be prevented. Exercise maintains functional mobility.

References

Allan, JD (1985). Exercise program. *In* Bulechek, GM, & McCloskey, JC (eds): *Nursing Interventions: Treatment for Nursing Diagnosis*. Philadelphia, WB Saunders, 198–219.

Brown, M (1987): Selected physical performance changes with aging. *Top Geriatr Rehab*, 2:68–76.

Browse, N (1965): *The Physiology and Pathology of Bed Rest*. Springfield, IL, Charles C Thomas.

Chapron, D, & Besdine, R (1987): Drugs as an obstacle to rehabilitation: A primer for therapists. *Top Geriatr Rehab*, 2:63–81.

Cole, TM, & Tobis, JS (1982): Measurement of musculoskeletal function. *In* Kottke, FJ, Stillwell, GK, & Lehmann, JF (eds): *Krusen's Handbook of Physical Medicine and Rehabilitation* (ed 3). Philadelphia, WB Saunders, 19–55.

Daniels, L, & Worthingham, C (1977): *Therapeutic Exercise for Body Alignment and Function*. Philadelphia, WB Saunders.

DuBow, L, Witt, O, Kadaba, M, et al. (1983): Oxygen consumption of elderly persons with bilateral below knee amputation: Ambulation vs. wheelchair propulsion. *Arch Phys Med Rehabil*, 64:255–259.

Eiserman, PL (1986): Hot weather, exercise, old age, and the kidneys. *Geriatrics*, 41(5):108–114.

Ellwood, PM (1982a): Bed positioning. *In* Kottke, FJ, Stillwell, GK, & Lehmann, JF (eds): *Krusen's Handbook of Physical Medicine and Rehabilitation* (ed 3). Philadelphia, WB Saunders, 465–472.

Ellwood, PM (1982b): Transfers—Methods, equipment, and preparation. *In* Kottke, FJ, Stillwell, GK, & Lehmann, JF (eds): *Krusen's Handbook of Physical Medicine and Rehabilitation* (ed 3). Philadelphia, WB Saunders, 473–491.

Fisher, SV, & Patterson, RP (1981): Energy cost of ambulation with crutches. *Arch Phys Med Rehabil*, 62:250–256.

Frengley, JD, & Mion, LC (1986): Incidence of physical restraints on acute general medical wards. *J Am Geriatr Soc*, 34:565–568.

Goldman, R (1977): Rest: Its use and abuse in the aged. *J Am Geriatr Soc*, 25:433–438.

Grimby, G, Banneskiold-Samste, B, Hvid, K, et al. (1982): Morphology and enzymatic capacity in arm and leg muscles in 78–81 year old men and women. *Acta Physiol Scand*, 115:125–134.

Harper, CM, & Lyles, YM (1988): Physiology and complications of bed rest. *J Am Geriatr Soc*, 36:1047–1054.

Heller, B, Bausell, R, & Ninos, M (1984): Nurses' perceptions of rehabilitation potential of institutionalized aged. *J Gerontol Nurs*, 10:(7):22–26.

Kaufman, T (1987): Posture and age. *Top Geriatr Rehab*, 2:13–28.

Kottke, FJ (1966): The effects of limitation of activity upon the human body. *JAMA*, 196:117–122.

Kottke, FJ (1982): Therapeutic exercise to maintain mobility. *In* Kottke, FJ, Stillwell, GK, & Lehmann, JF (eds): *Krusen's Handbook of Physical Medicine and Rehabilitation* (ed 3). Philadelphia, WB Saunders, 398–402.

Larsson, L, Sjodin, B, & Karlssen, J (1978): Histochemical and biochemical changes in human skeletal muscle with age in sedentary males, age 22–65. *Acta Physiol Scand*, 103:31–39.

Leslie, LR (1982): Training for functional independence. *In* Kottke, FJ, Stillwell, GK, & Lehmann, JF (eds): *Krusen's Handbook of Physical Medicine and Rehabilitation* (ed 3). Philadelphia, WB Saunders, 501–507.

Lewis, C (1985): Clinical implications of musculoskeletal changes with age. *In* Lewis, C (ed): *Aging: The Health Care Challenge*. Philadelphia, FA Davis, 117–140.

Mathias, S, Nayak, U, & Isaacs, B (1986): Balance in elderly patients: The "get-up-and-go" test. *Arch Phys Med Rehabil*, 67:387–389.

Milde, FK (1988): Impaired physical mobility. *J Gerontol Nurs*, 14(3):20–24.

Miller, MB (1975): Iatrogenic and nursigenic effects of prolonged immobilization of the ill aged. *J Am Geriatr Soc*, 23:360–369.

Oster, C (1976): Sensory deprivation in geriatric patients. *J Am Geriatr Soc*, 24:461–464.

Overstall, P, Johnson, A, & Exton-Smith, A (1978): Instability and falls in the elderly. *Age Ageing*, 7:92–96.

Palmore, WB (1986): Trends in the health of the aged. *Gerontologist*, 26:298–302.

Parent, CJ, & Whall, AL (1984): Are physical activity, self-esteem and depression related? *J Gerontol Nurs*, 10(9):8–11.

Payton, OD, & Poland JL (1984): Aging process. Implications for clinical practice. *Phys Ther*, 63:41–48.

Pollock, ML, Wilmore, JH, & Fox, SM, (1984): *Exercise in Health and Disease*. Philadelphia, WB Saunders.

Schuman, JE, Beattie EJ, Steed, DA, et al. (1981): Geriatric patients with and without intellectual dysfunction: Effectiveness of a standard rehabilitation program. *Arch Phys Med Rehabil*, 62:612–618.

Simpson, WM (1986): Exercise: Prescriptions for the elderly. *Geriatrics*, 41(1):95–100.

Steinberg, F (1986): Rehabilitating the older stroke patient: What's possible. *Geriatrics*, 41(3):85–97.

Swartz, MH (1989): *Textbook of Physical Diagnosis*. Philadelphia, WB Saunders.

Tobis, JL, Nayak, L, & Hoehler, F (1981): Visual perception of verticality and horizontality among elderly fallers. *Arch Phys Med Rehab*, 62:619–622.

Tomonaga, M (1977): Histochemical and ultrastructural changes in senile human muscle. *J Am Geriatr Soc*, 3:125–131.

Venna, N (1986): Dizziness, falling and fainting: Differential diagnosis in the aged. *Geriatrics*, 41(6):30–42.

CHAPTER
12

Pressure Sores

JOYCE TAKANO STONE, R.N.C., M.S.

INTRODUCTION

This chapter presents current theories on the etiology and pathophysiology of pressure sores. Implications for nursing care with assessment, prevention, and management approaches are discussed. Areas in need of further exploration and study are identified.

Terminology

"Bedsores," "decubitus ulcers," "pressure ulcers," and "pressure sores" are terms used interchangeably. The term "decubitus" was derived from Latin and means "lying down" (Berecek, 1975a). For many years, the terms "bedsores" and "decubitus ulcers" were appropriate and popular, since the condition occurred most frequently in bedridden, recumbent patients. The term "pressure sore" will be used in this chapter, in concert with current knowledge and understanding that the condition is primarily the result of pressure from a number of surfaces, such as bed, chair, floor, and brace, and from positions other than the recumbent one.

Background and Significance

The pressure sore is a familiar problem recognized since antiquity (Parish, Witkowski, & Crissey, 1983). In modern times, pressure sores continue to be a serious health hazard. An estimated 1.5 to 3 million persons in the United States have pressure sores (Cowart, 1987). The impact of pressure sores on morbidity, mortality, and cost of health care is tremendous (Cooney & Reuler, 1984). The prevalence rate of pressure sores in the general hospital population is estimated to be 3 to 5% (Constantian, 1980; Horsley, 1981; Reuler & Cooney, 1984). An estimated 15 to 30% of nursing home residents develop pressure sores (Fowler, 1982; Michocki & Lamy, 1976b). In a study on 5,000 new admissions to a nursing home, the investigators found that 20% of the new residents had at least one pressure sore (Spector, Kapp, Tucker, et al., 1988). The highest incidence of pressure sores is among the elderly (Barbenel, Jordan, & Nicol, 1977; David, 1984; Horsley, 1981).

There is evidence of an increase in the incidence of pressure sores (Exton-Smith, 1987; Norton, McLaren, & Exton-Smith, 1962). This increase is attributed to the growing number of elderly and advances made in medical science that prolong life. With the extension of life, pressure sores have become the hallmark of the debilitated and those suffering from chronic illness and long-term disabilities (Berecek, 1975a).

A high mortality rate, approximately 60,000 deaths per year, is associated with complications of pressure sores (Bryan, Dew, & Reynolds, 1983; Maklebust, 1987). From 7 to 8% of the deaths in the spinal cord injured population are attributed to pressure sores (Cooney & Reuler, 1984; Dinsdale, 1974). Among the elderly in nursing homes, the presence of pressure sores is a poor prognostic sign. The mortality rate in this group exceeds 66% (Michocki & Lamy, 1976b; Vasile & Chaitin, 1972).

Treatment costs for each pressure sore range from 14 to 25 thousand dollars, with a total cost estimate in the range of 3.5 to 7 billion dollars annually (Maklebust, Mondoux, & Sieggreen, 1986). Allman and associates (1986) reported that hospitalized patients with pressure sores had a median total length of hospitalization of 46 days as compared to the 11 days median stay for all patients. The median total charge for patients with pressure sores was 27 thousand dollars; the median charge for all patients was 7 thousand dollars. Labor intensive effort is required to treat a slow-healing pressure sore. It is estimated that once a pressure sore develops, a patient requires 50% more nursing care (Agate, 1985a).

The importance of the pressure sore problem in nursing was shown in a recent survey conducted by Brower and Crist (1985) examining research priorities in gerontologic nursing and long-term care. The study of the prevention, formation, and treatment of pressure sores was rated as one of the top priorities for research by nurses in nursing homes and home health agencies. This research was identified as being extremely important for patient welfare, nursing education, and nursing practice (Brower & Crist, 1985). While there is the recognized need for continued research regarding pressure sores, the current level of clinical practice does not reflect the advances in the prevention and treatment of pressure sores generated by research. There is failure and time lag in the implementation of research findings in clinical practice (Gould, 1986).

ETIOLOGY

The exact mechanism and processes involved in pressure sore development have not been defined. However, several extrinsic and intrinsic factors have been implicated as having major contributing roles in the pathophysiologic events leading to the development of the pressure sore (Table 12–1).

Table 12–1. PREDISPOSING FACTORS FOR PRESSURE SORE DEVELOPMENT

Extrinsic Factors
 Pressure
 Friction
 Moisture
 Shear
Intrinsic Factors
 Limited mobility
 Old age
 Poor nutritional status
 Specific clinical diagnosis or condition of patient
  Cardiovascular disease
  Fractures
  Diabetes
  Neurologic disorders
  Altered mental status
  Rheumatologic disease
  Spasms and contractures
  Incontinence

Extrinsic Factors

The extrinsic (mechanical) factors that contribute to the development of pressure sores are pressure, friction, shearing force, and moisture.

Pressure. Pressure is the essential element in the development of pressure sores. It is defined as the force exerted on a unit area (Reuler & Cooney, 1981). Pressure sores develop when there is an inadequate blood supply to the tissues, with resultant compromise of nutrition and oxygenation of the tissues. Normally the capillary arteriolar limb pressure is 32 mm Hg, the midcapillary pressure is 20 mm Hg, and the venous limb pressure is 12 mm Hg (Reuler & Cooney, 1984). The pressure is not evenly distributed in humans but is concentrated in specific areas, such as over the bony prominences. Pressure of sufficient intensity and duration over bony prominences results in tissue damage. When pressure exceeds 70 mm Hg over an area for more than 2 hours, there may be irreversible tissue damage (Dinsdale, 1974; Kosiak, 1961). However, if pressure is altered every 5 minutes, few changes occur (Kosiak, 1961). By removing the excessive pressure before the critical time of 1 to 2 hours expires, there is compensation for compromised circulation through the mechanism of reactive hyperemia. This mechanism restores adequate tissue nutrition by flooding the deprived area with blood, and it prevents the irreversible pathologic changes (Berecek, 1975a).

Over 30 years ago, Husain's work (1953) indicated that the duration of pressure was more important than its intensity; that is, high pressure for a short time was safer than lower pressure for a prolonged time. More recently, Daniel, Priest, and Wheatley (1981) found that muscle damage occurred at high pressure of short duration and skin damage occurred at high pressure of long duration. Their work suggests that the threshold for the development of pressure sores is lowered by changes in soft tissue coverage.

The compression of soft tissue between a bony prominence and a contact surface under a person results in a cone-shaped pressure gradient area. A cone of tissue destruction occurs from the skin through each layer of tissue to the bony prominence (Agris & Spira, 1979). The tip of the cone, like the tip of an iceberg, is visible on the skin surface, while the other 70%, or the base of the cone, forms a larger undermined area overlying the bone (Figure 12–1) (Agris & Spira, 1979; Reuler & Cooney, 1984; Shea, 1975). As noted by Daniel and associates (1981), fat and muscle resist pressure injury less well than skin. With fat and muscle being closer to bony prominences than the skin, pressure is concentrated in smaller areas in these deeper tissues. This may explain why small cutaneous ulcers overlay much larger areas of fat and muscle destruction (Constantian, 1980). Guyton, Granger, and Taylor (1971) provided a description of the physiologic effect of the pressure gradient. Normally a negative interstitial fluid pressure exists, balanced by a positive solid tissue pressure, resulting in a total tissue pressure of zero. External pressure causes an increase in interstitial fluid pressure. When the pressure exceeds 12 mm Hg in the venous limb, it creates an increase in total tissue pressure, leading to increased capillary arteriolar pressure, filtration of fluid from capillaries, edema, and autolysis. The pressure gradient also causes occlusion of the lymphatic vessels (Reuler & Cooney, 1981). The pressure impairs the

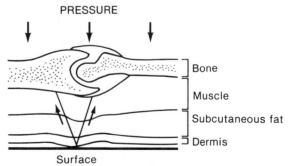

Figure 12–1. Pressure gradient. A cone-shaped pressure gradient is formed when there is compression of soft tissue between the bony prominence and the surface under the person. (Redrawn from Reuler, JB and Cooney, TG: The pressure sore: Pathophysiology and principles of management. Ann Intern Med, *94*:662, 1981. Reprinted with permission from the American College of Physicians.)

function of active contractility of lymphatics. In combination with changes in the blood microvascular system, tissue necrosis occurs as anaerobic metabolic waste products accumulate.

Shearing Force. The shearing phenomenon occurs when the head of the bed is raised, causing the torso to slide down, transmitting pressure to the sacrum and deep fascia (Figure 12–2). The loosely attached superficial sacral fascia slides over the firmly attached deep fascia, where the blood vessels pass to the skin. This causes stretching, angulation, obliteration, or rupture of the vessels, leading to platelet thrombosis and resulting in tissue necrosis from the deprivation of blood supply (Reichel, 1958). The shearing force is further accentuated because subcutaneous fat, lacking tensile strength, is particularly vulnerable to injury from mechanical forces (Reuler & Cooney, 1981). The tissue necrosis that results differs from the type due to direct compression in that the ulcer is widely undermined at its base (Constantian, 1980). Shearing forces are the probable cause of sores on the heels or on the anterior tibial region. Blisters or abrasions precede the formation of ulcers (Constantian, 1980; Exton-Smith, 1976). In the presence of a sufficiently high level of shearing force, half the amount of pressure is necessary to produce vascular occlusion as when shearing force is absent. The combination of the two forms of

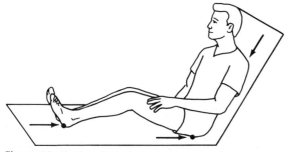

Figure 12–2. Shearing phenomenon. The shearing phenomenon occurs when the torso slides downward on a surface, transmitting pressure to the sacrum and deep fascia. (Redrawn from Longe, RL: Current concepts in clinical therapeutics: Pressure sores. Clin Pharm, 5:674, 1986. All rights reserved. Adapted with permission from the American Society of Hospital Pharmacists.)

stress, shear and pressure, is believed to cause damage to soft tissue (Bennett & Lee, 1985; 1988).

Friction. Friction is caused when two contact surfaces move across each other, such as skin across bed sheets. The resulting damage is removal of the outer protective stratum corneum, accelerating the onset of ulceration (Reuler & Cooney, 1981).

Moisture. In the presence of moisture created by perspiration or fecal or urinary soilage, there is a fivefold increase in the risk of pressure sore formation over the sacrum and buttocks (Agate, 1985b; Reuler & Cooney, 1981). With dampnesss at the contact surface, there is an increase in static friction between the surface and the skin. This can fix a frail, weak patient in one position (Lowthian, 1977). Moisture also causes maceration of the skin, which weakens it and makes it more susceptible to infection (Lowthian, 1977).

Intrinsic Factors

There are several intrinsic factors implicated in the pathogenesis of pressure sores. The presence of one or more of these factors, in conjunction with the previously discussed four extrinsic factors, is thought to increase a person's susceptibility to the development of pressure sores. These risk factors include limited mobility, advanced age, poor nutritional status, incontinence, and specific clinical diagnoses or conditions.

Limited Mobility. The protective mechanism of spontaneous movement occurs during sleep and at various times throughout the day, causing a person to move and shift weight when the pressure tolerance of the tissue has been reached. This protective mechanism can become impaired under several conditions: (1) if there is a loss of sensitivity in local tissues such as that experienced by paraplegics; (2) if there is decreased central nervous system response to the sense of discomfort due to anesthesia, heavy use of sedative/hypnotics, or severe mental deterioration; or (3) if there is a physical disability preventing movement (Agate, 1985a; Ek & Boman, 1982; Exton-Smith

& Sherwin, 1961; Norton, 1975). Movement may also be restricted by various types of apparatus and restraints. A person experiencing severe pain may intentionally restrict or limit movements.

Advanced Age. Several studies support the clinical observation that the elderly are especially vulnerable and susceptible to developing pressure sores. Norton, McLaren, and Exton-Smith (1962) reported that, in their study of 250 patients with pressure sores, the average age of the patients who developed pressure sores was 79.9 years. They found that nearly twice as many patients over 85 years of age developed pressure sores as compared to those under 75 years of age. Barbenel and associates (1977) noted that 70% of all patients with pressure sores were over 70 years of age. In her study of 885 patients with pressure sores, David (1984) found that 85% were over 65 years of age and 37% were older than 80 years.

Several age-related changes in the skin increase the elderly's risk for pressure sores. These changes include epidermal atrophy, a decreased turnover rate of cells in the stratum corneum, stiffening of dermal collagen, and a decrease in dermal blood vessels (Boss & Seegmiller, 1981).

Poor Nutritional Status. General malnutrition and deficiencies in zinc, iron, acorbic acid, and protein contribute to pressure sore development (Agate, 1985b). A study by Pinchcofsky-Devin and Kaminiski (1986) on 232 nursing home patients showed a definite correlation between pressure sore development and deteriorating nutritional status. All patients who had a pressure sore on admission or developed a pressure sore later were severely malnourished. The more severe the pressure sore, the greater the malnutrition. The researchers recommended nutritional intervention when the serum albumin level is below 3.3 gm% and the total lymphocytic count (TLC) drops below 1220.

With marked loss of weight and muscular atrophy, a person loses the natural protective padding of subcutaneous tissue and muscle bulk. With less padding over bony prominences, vulnerability increases for pressure

sores due to the sharper gradients and higher peaks of pressure on an area (Lindan, Greenway, & Piazza, 1965). Allman and associates (1986) also reported a relationship between low serum albumin levels and pressure sores. They indicated a threefold increase in the risk of developing a pressure sore with every gram decrease in the serum albumin level. An inadequate amount of protein results in a negative nitrogen balance, leading to edema of the dependent parts of the body. Edema causes decreased elasticity, resiliency, and vitality of the skin, making it more susceptible to damage. Edema also results in a slower rate of diffusion of oxygen and metabolites from the capillaries to the cells (Berecek, 1975). Research has shown that healing does not occur when a patient is in negative nitrogen balance. Also, ascorbic acid is necessary to prevent pressure sores (Berecek, 1975).

Specific Clinical Diagnoses or Conditions. Several conditions place the older person at greater risk for pressure sore development. Cardiovascular disease may interfere with adequate perfusion of the skin's capillary bed. Edema, anemia, and hypotension reduce the efficiency or level of oxygen delivery (Agate, 1985b; Tepperman, DeZwirek, Chiarcossi, et al., 1977). Fractures, diabetes, and neurologic and rheumatologic diseases may predispose patients to pressure sore development because of compromised mobility or motor or sensory deficits (Tepperman, et al., 1977). Confused, demented, and depressed patients may be at risk for pressure sores if they do not understand and cooperate with the treatment plan and fail to change position or eat an adequate diet. Emotional stress has been identified as a contributing factor to pressure sore risk. When a person is stressed, there is a greater likelihood of tissue breakdown due to increased glucocorticoid production by the adrenal glands causing inhibition of collagen formation (Maklebust, 1987).

Spasms—involuntary, uncontrollable muscle contractions—cause repeated internal abrasions of the fascia and subcutaneous tissues, placing the patient at greater risk for pressure sores (Roaf, 1976). The administration of medications such as diazepam and dantrolene sodium may be indicated to help control short, sudden movements. If the condition is severe and unresponsive to medications, other measures may be considered, such as anterior rhizotomy or alcohol injections (Agris & Spira, 1979; Garrigues, 1987).

Contractures create problems in positioning, moving, and maintaining daily hygiene. They place the older person at greater risk for pressure sores (Agris & Spira, 1979). Flexion contractures can occur rapidly and can be prevented by placing the patient in the prone position and instituting range of motion exercises at least twice a day.

In patients admitted with acute illnesses, unconsciousness, dehydration, and paralysis were the three factors that placed them at risk for pressure sore development (Andersen, Jensen, Kvorning, et al., 1982). Data from almost 5,000 nursing home residents showed that certain characteristics were associated with persons having pressure sores on admission: older age, male, nonwhite, coming from a hospital, unable to perform activities of daily living of bathing and transferring, being bed- or chairfast, requiring catheterization, experiencing fecal incontinence, and having no rehabilitation potential (Spector, Kapp, Tucker, et al., 1988).

Incontinence. Incontinence was identified by Norton and associates (1962) as the single most reliable predictor of pressure sore development. Incontinence causes maceration of the skin, increasing the risk of pressure sores. The moisture from incontinence is taken up by the stratum corneum. The outcome is bacterial contamination and lowered resistance of the epidermis to shearing forces (Parish, et al., 1983).

CLINICAL PRESENTATION

Location

At greatest risk for pressure sore formation are areas where a high proportion of the body weight is brought to bear upon a small area and where a bony prominence lies close beneath the skin (Agate, 1985a). More than 90%

of pressure sores are located on the lower part of the body (Reuler & Cooney, 1984; Seiler & Stahelin, 1986). The sacral and coccygeal areas, the greater trochanter, the heel, and the ischial tuberosities are the most common sites for pressure sore formation (Agate, 1985a; Reuler & Cooney, 1981).

For the patient in the supine position, potential sites for pressure sores include the occiput, scapula, spinous processes, elbow, sacrum, posterior calf, and heels. For those maintaining a prone position, pressure areas include the cheek and ear, acromion process, anterior chest, iliac crest, thigh, knees, and dorsum of the feet and ankle. In the lateral position, the ear and side of the head, the acromion process, ribs, greater trochanter, medial and lateral surface of the knee, and the external malleolus are the vulnerable areas. In the sitting position, the scapula, ischial tuberosities, sacrum, coccyx, popliteal areas, heels, and plantar surface of the foot are susceptible for pressure sores (Figure 12–3) (Gosnell, 1987; Parish, et al., 1983; Reuler & Cooney, 1981).

Classification

There are several systems for classification of pressure sores, with the grade or stage being determined by the amount of tissue damaged (Parish, et al., 1983; Shea, 1975). It is helpful to use the stages to describe, document, and evaluate the progression or healing of the wound. However, no one classification system is universally accepted (Maklebust, 1987). In 1989, a national conference was convened by the National Pressure Ulcer Advisory Panel. This consensus conference put forth a classification system that combined several of the most commonly used pressure sore staging systems. The proposed system is viewed as a step in the evolution of a classification system that would eventually be universally accepted (National Pressure Advisory Panel, 1989). This new system will be used in this chaper (Figure 12–4).

Pre-pressure Sore Stage. In the pre-pressure sore stage, blanchable erythema is an important sign. It appears as ill-defined reactive

Supine

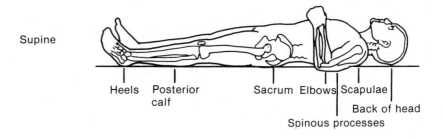

Heels   Posterior   Sacrum Elbows Scapulae
         calf
                                                    Back of head
                             Spinous processes

Prone

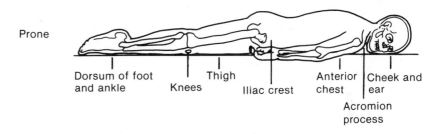

Dorsum of foot   Thigh   Anterior   Cheek and
and ankle   Knees   Iliac crest   chest   ear
                                   Acromion
                                   process

Figure 12–3. Common locations of pressure sores. (Redrawn from Gosnell, DJ: Assessment and evaluation of pressure sores. Nurs Clin North Am, 22:403, 1987; and Maklebust, J: Pressure ulcers: Etiology and prevention. Nurs Clin North Am, 22:364, 1987. Adapted with permission from WB Saunders Company.)

Lateral

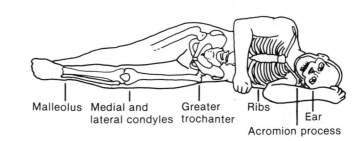

Malleolus   Medial and   Greater   Ribs
         lateral condyles   trochanter   Ear
                               Acromion process

Sitting

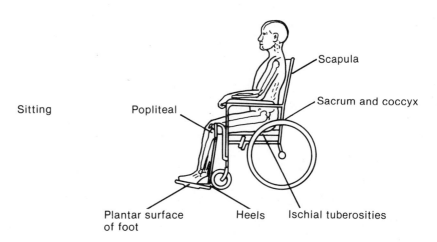

                                   Scapula

                                   Sacrum and coccyx

Popliteal

Plantar surface   Heels   Ischial tuberosities
of foot

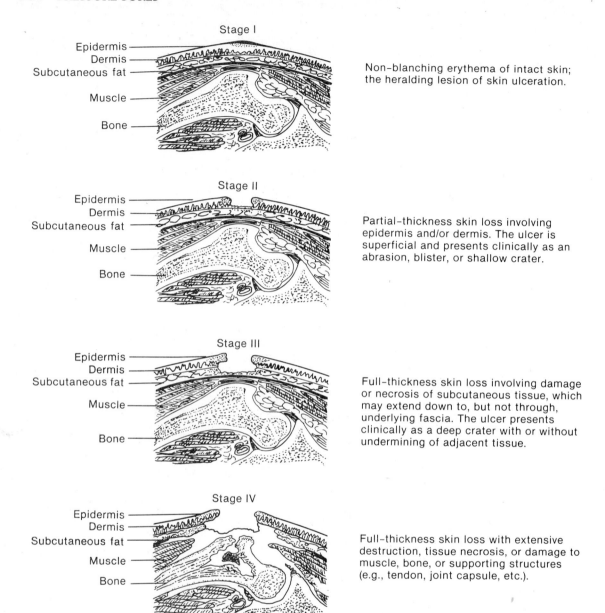

Stage I

Epidermis
Dermis
Subcutaneous fat
Muscle
Bone

Non-blanching erythema of intact skin; the heralding lesion of skin ulceration.

Stage II

Epidermis
Dermis
Subcutaneous fat
Muscle
Bone

Partial-thickness skin loss involving epidermis and/or dermis. The ulcer is superficial and presents clinically as an abrasion, blister, or shallow crater.

Stage III

Epidermis
Dermis
Subcutaneous fat
Muscle
Bone

Full-thickness skin loss involving damage or necrosis of subcutaneous tissue, which may extend down to, but not through, underlying fascia. The ulcer presents clinically as a deep crater with or without undermining of adjacent tissue.

Stage IV

Epidermis
Dermis
Subcutaneous fat
Muscle
Bone

Full-thickness skin loss with extensive destruction, tissue necrosis, or damage to muscle, bone, or supporting structures (e.g., tendon, joint capsule, etc.).

Figure 12—4. Classification of pressure sores. (Based on the National Pressure Ulcer Advisory Panel, 1989.)

erythema, ranging in hue from pale to bright red. Digital compression on the area produces blanching, with the erythema returning with the removal of the finger. A slight edematous area may be noted, as well as an elevation of temperature felt by the back of the examiner's hand. These signs are especially important in detecting blanchable erythema in dark-skinned individuals (Feustel, 1982; Parish, et al., 1983). If pressure is removed, the skin will return to normal, usually within 24 hours (Parish, et al., 1983).

Stage I. The initial sign of this stage is nonblanchable erythema, wherein the redness does not fade when digital compression is applied and then removed (National Pressure Ulcer Advisory Panel, 1989). The color range is from red to dusky cyanosis. The area of pressure is irregular and ill-defined and reflects the shape of the object creating the pressure or the bony prominence underlying the skin. Tenderness and pain are present if sensory innervation is intact. The acute inflammatory response involves all soft tissue layers. There is swelling and induration with associated heat (Parish, et al., 1983; Shea, 1975). If not arrested at this stage, the pressure sore will progress to stage II.

Stage II. In stage II, there is extension of the acute inflammatory response leading to a fibroblastic response in all layers. Partial-thickness skin loss involves the epidermis or epidermis and dermis (National Pressure Ulcer Advisory Panel, 1989). The ulcer is shallow and surrounded by a broad, indistinct area of heat, erythema, and induration (Shea, 1975). The patient complains of pain and tenderness if the neurologic system is intact. Healing at this stage usually requires 2 to 3 weeks (Parish, et al., 1983).

Stage III. There is extension through the dermis into the subcutaneous fat in the stage III pressure sore. Stage III presents the classic appearance of a pressure ulcer with a full-thickness defect extending into the subcutaneous fat, which may extend down to, but not through, underlying fascia (National Pressure Ulcer Advisory Panel, 1989). A distinct ulcer margin is formed as the epidermis thickens and rolls over the edge toward the ulcer base. There is intensive reactive fibrosis, inflammation, and retraction in the dermis and subcutaneous fat. The loss of fluid and protein from these open, draining wounds is significant. Clinically, the patient has fever, dehydration, anemia, and leukocytosis (Shea, 1975).

Stage IV. The skin surrounding the pressure sore is erythematous, warm, and indurated. The size of the ulcerated area may be deceiving, with a small lesion opening to a much larger necrotic area beneath. There is full-thickness skin loss with extensive destruction, tissue necrosis, or damage to muscle, supporting structures such as tendon and joint capsule, and bone (National Pressure Ulcer Advisory Panel, 1989). Infection is present with exudation, foul odor, purulent drainage, and surrounding cellulitis. This is considered a toxic state, and requires aggressive life-saving measures and extensive surgery to resect all necrotic tissues (Parish, et al, 1983; Shea, 1975).

Other Types of Pressure Sores

A fairly common type of pressure sore is one that is covered by a black membrane. The black eschar is a sharply defined, tough, membranous form of dry gangrene that adheres to the site where full-thickness (skin to muscle or bone) tissue death has occurred within a relatively short period of time. Coagulation necrosis is the end of a process that starts with a shearing force against a skin surface, causing the stretching and tearing of the large blood vessels at the level of the subcutaneous fat and superficial fascia. The subcutaneous fat lacks the tensile strength to withstand distortion, and necrosis results from vascular occlusion and lack of reperfusion to the tissues (Parish, et al., 1983). The eschar is usually surrounded by nonblanchable erythema. Unless surgically debrided, it will persist for weeks without healing and without ulcerating to an open lesion (Agate, 1985a; Parish, et al., 1983).

Some large pressure sores appear to develop within a very short period of time. These pressure sores are usually the result of some event that took place previously, such as during a long surgical procedure or as a result of a "long lie" when a person who fell at home lies on a hard linoleum floor or in a bathtub for a period of time before being discovered. In these patients, the skin is initially intact but the deeper muscle tissue, being especially susceptible to pressure, has undergone necrosis. This hidden necrosis tends to burst through like an abscess, leaving a deep cavity. The prognosis for healing is poor, and the injury can result in death (Agate, 1985a).

A very serious but rare type of pressure sore results from a thrombosis of the inferior vena cava. The sore seemingly develops overnight, appearing as a huge area of total tissue infarction, 10 to 20 cm in size, over the buttocks and sacrum. The prognosis for survival is very poor (Agate, 1985a).

PREVENTION AND MANAGEMENT

Prevention

While controversies and conflicting opinions prevail about pressure sore treatment, there is total agreement that prevention of pressure sores is of utmost importance and that quality nursing care is the critical element in prevention. Mechanical devices, materials, and pharmaceutical preparations are only adjuncts to nursing care. It is the identification of the patient at risk and the careful daily observation of patients for early indications of pressure sores that form the basis of a prevention protocol (Agris & Spira, 1979; Bliss & McLaren, 1967). Nurses must continuously observe, assess, initiate appropriate measures to prevent and treat pressure sores, and evaluate the outcome of their interventions. Danger lies in a false sense of security and reliance on the adjuncts to nursing care (Tepperman, et al., 1977).

Preventive measures consist of identifying the patient at risk for pressure sore development and taking the necessary steps to eliminate the causative factors of pressure, shearing, friction, and moisture.

Identifying the Patient at Risk. Assessment is the first step in the prevention of pressure sores. By identifying the patient at risk and quickly acting on the potential problem, pressure sores can be prevented in most patients.

Assessment Tools. Assessment tools have been developed that take into consideration several important predisposing factors. One of the most widely used tools was developed by Norton in 1962. Norton identified physical condition, mental condition, activity, mobility, and incontinence as critical risk factors to assess (Norton, et al., 1962; Norton, 1975). The

Norton Scale frequently serves as the basis for newer tools that have been designed. It remains widely used because it is a good screening tool to identify those at risk and is easy for staff to use in any setting.

Isler (1972) designed a scale similar to Norton's, specifying nutrition under general condition and adding surgery as an important variable for consideration. Williams (1972) studied 20 variables associated with pressure sores. Factors found to be important were thinness of patient, infection other than genitourinary, elevated temperature, and taking corticosteroids. The Gosnell Scale included the categories found in the Norton Scale and in Williams' work. Nutrition was substituted for the physical condition category, and vital signs, skin appearance, tone, sensation, and medications were added to areas for assessment (Gosnell, 1973). Resio and Verhonick (1973) studied a large number of variables and confirmed Williams' finding that thinness of patient played a significant role in pressure sore development. Their study did not uphold some of the other variables studied by Williams, such as sex, mental status, and skin condition. Utilizing experts on pressure sores and available information, Abruzzese (1985) developed the Assessment of Decubitus Ulcer Potential Scale, which includes forms to record treatment of the pressure sore and the healing process, to chart position changes and pressure areas to avoid, and to identify and alert others to potential problem areas.

A new tool, the Braden Scale, shows promise as a clinical tool for predicting pressure sore risk (Taylor, 1988). The tool consists of six subscales—sensory perception, activity, mobility, moisture, friction, and nutrition. Levels are described for each subscale. Sensitivity and specificity of the Braden Scale are high (Bergstrom, Braden, Laguzza, et al., 1987).

These assessment scales have been helpful in identifying the patient at risk for pressure sore development. An assessment at the time of admission, periodically during the hospital stay, and again during the continuum of care (e.g., at home, in nursing home or clinic) will provide sufficient vigilance to prevent pressure sores. To assess and identify the patient at risk, the existing assessment tools may be modified and adapted by nurses to meet their specific needs.

Instrumental Methods. Several sophisticated instruments have been developed to detect potential areas for skin breakdown. It has been known that death of skin precedes actual breakdown to open sores. During this early stage, it has been found that the temperature may be low at the site of dead skin but higher in the surrounding area (Agate, 1985a). Skin thermography and radiometric methods were developed to precisely define cold areas and predict where pressure sores might occur. Use of the instrumental methods is not widespread because of high cost, the difficulties in interpretation of results, and the need for specially trained personnel. In addition, the information obtained may not alter current treatment and management (Agate, 1985a).

Preventive Measures. *Pressure, Shearing, Friction, and Moisture.* The relief of pressure leads to recirculation and oxygenation in the microvessels of the skin (Seiler & Stahelin, 1985). Keeping a person active and moving is the best method to prevent pressure sores. However, for those with limited mobility, frequent positional change is one of the most effective preventive measures. A full 180° turn is not required for pressure relief; a 20° to 30° turn is adequate (Shea, 1985), as are small shifts in body weight (Horsley, 1981). Designing a turning schedule and, where possible, grouping patients who require frequent turning may help to ensure that a scheduled change in position is carried out (Patterson & Fisher, 1986).

Patients can be taught to protect themselves from pressure by shifting weight, changing positions, and carefully monitoring pressure points. Patients may not be aware of their role in the overall prevention program and the importance of these simple preventive measures. Families can assist in reminding older persons to move and in helping them move and change position. Setting an alarm clock or timing device can serve to remind patients to turn (Seiler & Stahelin, 1985).

The magnitude of pressure is determined by the hardness of the supporting surface; measures should be taken to reduce excessive pressure. A number of pressure-relieving devices are available (see Table 12–2).

Proper technique must be used in turning, positioning, and moving a patient in bed, in transferring to a chair or gurney, and in placing a patient on and off a bedpan. Using proper technique will reduce trauma to the skin resulting from pressure, friction, and shearing. As the patient is turned and positioned, pillows and towel rolls are used to support the position and alignment of the spine. A pillow between the legs in the side-lying position prevents pressure from the weight of one extremity on another and prevents moisture from skin touching skin. The prone position, with soft pillows supporting the bony prominences or a soft mattress, provides the most even distribution of weight (Feustel, 1982; Seiler & Stahelin, 1985).

There is evidence that pressure over the ischial tuberosities is significantly higher when persons sit with the feet supported rather than hanging free. The weight is shifted back to a smaller, more concentrated area directly over the ischial tuberosities when the feet are supported (Lindan, Greenway, & Piazza, 1965). Using protective cushions on the chair and limiting time in the sitting position will help to reduce pressure.

Rubber rings and doughnut-shaped cushions should be avoided, since they tend to cause occlusion of circulation and poor distribution of pressure, with higher points of pressure falling along the inner and outer borders (Tepperman, et al., 1977).

Heavy blankets add to the pressure exerted on vulnerable areas. This pressure can be avoided by leaving some slack in the linen and blankets over the feet. Tucking linen in tightly restricts movement, prevents air flow, and adds pressure on the extremities. Lightweight blankets and devices such as bed cradles and footboards help to relieve some of the pressure.

Tubing (intravenous, oxygen, nasogastric, drainage catheters) has to be positioned so that the patient is not lying on it. Care must be taken to keep the patient's bed free of food crumbs, hairpins, and plastic packaging for medical equipment.

The linen should be clean, dry, and wrinkle-free. Damp, wrinkled linen and incontinence pads can produce ridges of concentrated pressure and can be abrasive and irritating. Dampness results in static friction between the surface and the skin (Lowthian, 1977). The use of socks has been found to help decrease friction over the heels. Either special socks manufactured with a foam lining or regular socks may be used (Bliss & McLaren, 1967; Lowthian, 1977).

To prevent friction, movement in bed is achieved by lowering the head of the bed, removing the pillow, and lifting the patient on a turning sheet, rather than by dragging the patient or pulling up on the shoulders. A trapeze is used so that the patient can bend the knees and help shift upward in bed.

Shearing can be avoided by keeping the bed elevated no more than 30°; the person should not be placed in a reclining sitting posture (Lowthian, 1977). Footboards, elevated knee gatches, and properly adjusted foot/leg supports on wheelchairs will alleviate shearing. Attention must be given to proper position when the older person is sitting in a chair. Allowing the patient to slide and slouch in a chair causes shearing and friction of the sacral area.

Nutrition. Nutritional intake should be adequate to meet the general daily requirements plus the additional demands resulting from illness or surgery. Nutrition repletion is necessary to reverse protein catabolism, to replace fluid and protein losses, and to correct anemia or edema (Reuler & Cooney, 1981). Dietary consultation is helpful to determine the patient's caloric and protein requirements and to tailor a diet regimen to meet the requirements.

Skin Care. A major preventive measure is to protect the skin to avert early skin breakdown. Avoidance of harsh soaps, perfumed powders, and alcohol and carefully rinsing off soap during patient bathing have been suggested to prevent drying and irritation of the skin. Avoiding plastic-lined materials next to the skin will help maintain low humidity interface. A sheepskin is soft and resilient, provides a smooth surface, distributes pressure, and is effective in absorbing moisture (Michocki & Lamy, 1976a; Reuler & Cooney, 1984). However, sheepskins create a relatively high static friction against the skin and are not suitable for incontinent patients (Lowthian, 1977).

In the past, massage had been advocated to stimulate the local skin blood flow and reduce ischemic injury. Current practice is to avoid massage when there is nonblanchable erythema. Vigorous massage is thought to cause additional damage (Ek, Gustavsson, & Lewis, 1985).

Incontinence. Incontinence can be controlled in most situations (see Chapters 9 and 10). When the patient is incontinent, special skin care is indicated to keep the skin clean, dry, and protected from feces and urine. Timely skin care with thorough washing and rinsing, gentle drying, and application of light talc or protective cream or ointment helps to prevent skin irritation and maceration (Norton, 1975). While taking measures to find the cause and control incontinence, the use of highly absorbent disposable adult briefs, external catheters, and fecal incontinence bags may be helpful to prevent skin irritation and breakdown.

Management and Staged Treatment of Pressure Sores

Preventive measures are continued in the treatment phase in order to prevent the development of additional pressure sores and to avoid further trauma and damage in the affected area. The goal of staged treatment is to promote wound healing. General care is focused on maintaining optimal physiologic function and correcting the underlying medical disease.

Several comprehensive articles are available to describe the many approaches to pressure sore treatment; the reader is referred to them for extensive review (Berecek, 1975b; David, 1982; Doughty, 1988; Longe, 1986; Lowthian, 1977; Maklebust, et al., 1986; Melcher, Longe, & Gelbart, 1988; Michocki & Lamy, 1976a; Mikulic, 1980; Morgan, 1975; Nierman, 1978).

Much confusion and mixed opinions exist

about the "ingredients" for a recipe to cure pressure sores. A multitude of ointments, solutions, sprays, dressings, and supportive devices are available for treatment (Table 12–2). Some of the available treatment methods are not recommended, based on current research findings. However, the research to date on the treatment of pressure sores has provided limited information for the clinician. The studies have tended to consist of small samples, to test a limited number of variables, and to have inadequate controls (David, 1984). At the present time, further study is needed on most therapeutic measures to prove their effectiveness (Ek, 1987), and no standard treatment regimen can be prescribed (David, 1982). The

Table 12–2. PARTIAL LISTING OF PRESSURE SORE TREATMENT METHODS*

Physical Agents

Air	Infrared	Ultrasound
Cold	Massage	Ultraviolet
Heat	Oxygen	Vibration
Heat lamp	Sunlight	Whirlpool (hydrotherapy)
Hyperbaric oxygen		

Special Beds, Mattresses, Cushions, Appliances for Pressure Relief

Air	Gel	Trapeze bar
Alternating air	Sand	Sheepskin
Low air	Turning beds	Foot cradle
Fluidized air	Water	
Foam		

Topical Agents

Acetic acid	Gentian violet
Alcohol	Hexachlorophene
Antacids	Honey paste
Antibiotics	Hydrogen peroxide
Gentamicin	Hypochlorite solutions
Penicillin	Iodoform
Sulfathiazole	Karaya gum
Nitrofurazone	Linseed oil
Balsam Peru	Maggots
Benzoin, tincture	Pectin paste
Boric acid	Povidone iodine
Cornstarch	Ringer's solution
Eggwhite	Saline
Enzymes	Silicone spray
Collagenase	Silvadene (silver sulfadiazine)
Fibrinolysin + desoxyribonuclease	Stilbestrol
Trypsin	Sugar
	Disaccharide
	Monosaccharide
	Titanium
	Zinc

Dressings

Dry	Transparent polyurethane	Hydrogel, nonadhering
Wet-to-dry	Hydrocolloid	Polyurethane foam, nonadhering
Wet	Absorptive	
Periodically wet	Gauze	
	Powder	
	Beads	
	Starches	

(Data from Berecek, 1975b; David, 1982; Doughty, 1988; Longe, 1976; Lowthian, 1977; Maklebust, et al., 1986; Melcher, Longe, & Gelbart, 1988; Michocki & Lamy, 1976a; Mikulic, 1980; Morgan, 1975; Nierman, 1978.)
*This table illustrates the variety of treatment approaches available for pressure sores. Inclusion of products in the list does not imply recommendation.

decision on what to use is often based on personal preference.

Each patient who presents a problem of skin integrity needs careful assessment. The nurse must then determine a plan of care based on sound scientific information on the etiology and pathophysiology of pressure sores and the alternative approaches to treatment available in the clinical setting. Once a plan of care has been determined, consistency and continuity of a planned approach are essential for effective treatment (Ameis, Chiarcossi, & Jimenez, 1980; Tooman & Patterson, 1984).

In this chapter, basic principles and goals for treatment are delineated for the staged treatment of pressure sores. The selection of devices, materials, and pharmaceutical preparations is left to the clinician. Several factors enter into decisions for prevention and treatment. Factors to be considered include space, cost, time, the qualifications and number of staff or care providers, and the ease in handling, storing, maintaining, and using equipment and materials. The cost of suitable and effective equipment is not always prohibitive. The use of specialized equipment in the prevention of pressure sores in selected high-risk patients may prove less expensive than the treatment of pressure sores (Exton-Smith, 1987).

Stages I and II. Superficial ulcers are sufficiently vascularized, and are clean, granulating, and oxygenated (Seiler & Stahelin, 1985). Seventy to 80% of pressure sores are superficial and can be managed with conservative treatment (Coodley, Lincer, Parham, et al. 1983; Reuler & Cooney, 1981).

The treatment of stage I pressure sores consists of (1) relief of pressure and (2) general supportive measures to maintain skin integrity (Melcher, et al., 1988; Reuler & Cooney, 1981; Shea, 1975).

With stage II pressure sores, the goal of treatment is to prevent further insult and trauma by (1) relieving pressure and (2) permitting the normally well-vascularized skin to heal through local wound cleansing (Shea, 1975).

Pressure relief has been discussed under preventive measures; it cannot be overempha-

sized in any program for the prevention and treatment of pressure sores. The patient should not lie on the pressure sore even for brief periods. Without pressure relief, all other therapeutic measures are ineffective (Seiler & Stahelin, 1986). A frequently used quotation is that of Dr. Vilan of Paris: "You can put anything you like on a pressure sore except the patient" (Guttman, 1976). There is sophisticated, costly pressure relieving equipment on the market to use for treating skin breakdown and preventing progression of the condition. However, efforts to prevent moisture, friction, and shearing must be carried out concurrently.

The purpose of local wound care is to control bacterial contamination and promote healing. A number of substances and products are available for wound care (Table 12–2). The efficacy of most has not been carefully studied and critically evaluated (Coodley, et al., 1983; Cooley & Reuler, 1981; David, 1982). In an extensive review of the English literature covering the period 1900 to 1974, Morgan (1975) concluded that most studies on topical agents had either no control groups or inadequate ones, small sample population or a single patient history, and mixed types of ulcers included in the study. Healing of pressure sores was asserted in some studies but not supported by objective data. There was no followup data available, and the rate of healing with topical agents was not compared with various surgical approaches.

Surface application of pastes, ointments, powders, and creams is thought to be ineffective and may retard healing (Melcher, et al., 1988). For example, topical antibiotics are not effective because they are neither absorbed into the wound nor effective against bacterial growth in granulation tissue (Agris & Spira, 1979; Melcher, et al., 1988). The efforts to improve blood supply in the already inflamed wound by physical, chemical, and pharmacologic means are of questionable value and may actually retard healing (Longe, 1986; Shea, 1975). The use of a heat lamp is contraindicated; a rise in temperature increases the metabolic demands of the skin and places additional stress on a compromised area (Maklebust, 1987). Studies have shown that massaging did not have any long-term effect on local skin blood flow and actually reduced blood flow in persons with nonblanchable erythema (Ek, et al., 1985). Systemic application of vasodilators is contraindicated. By opening arteriovenous anastomoses, they may effect a decrease in blood flow through the affected area (Seiler & Stahelin, 1986). Adhering ointments, powders, and pastes are to be avoided (Seiler & Stahelin, 1985). Pastes and ointments on pressure sores may promote bacterial growth and impede the reepithelialization process (Michocki & Lamy, 1976a). Other substances to avoid are potentially allergenic agents, such as dyes, and antibiotics and cytotoxic agents, such as local disinfectants and acidifying agents (Seiler & Stahelin, 1985). For example, alcohol may remove the essential fatty constituents from the skin; rubbing with alcohol can cause skin dryness, irritation, and abrasion (Michocki & Lamy, 1976a). While antiseptics such as 1% providone iodine, 0.25% acetic acid, 3% hydrogen peroxide, and 0.5% sodium hypochlorite are known to be effective bactericidal agents, a recent study found that acetic acid and hydrogen peroxide are not useful adjuncts in wound care since bactericidal concentrations are toxic to fibroblasts (Lineaweaver, Howard, Soucy, et al., 1985). Mild soap and water and normal saline are considered safe and are recommended for treating stage I and II pressure sores (Dimant & Francis, 1988; Garrigues, 1987).

The role of the dressing is to protect the open area from contamination and the new granulating tissue from trauma (Seiler & Stahelin, 1985; Sieggreen, 1987). Several factors should be taken into consideration in selecting a dressing. The material should not cause further trauma to the healing tissues during dressing change (Neuberger, 1987). All wound covers should be permeable to allow the tissues adequate oxygen access. Wound healing is enhanced when the pressure sore and surrounding tissues can freely take up oxygen and expel carbon dioxide. Nonpermeable materials such as plastics and aluminum, silver, and gold foils, should not be used. A dressing

that provides a moist microenvironment and maintains a temperature close to body temperature promotes wound healing. Under these conditions, epithelial cells migrate and achieve optimal miotic activity (Seiler & Stahelin, 1985). An advantage of most of the occlusive and semiocclusive dressings is that they provide a moist microenvironment and can be left in place for several days (Garrigues, 1987). A shorter interval between dressing changes is associated with a poorer response to therapy (Yarkoney, Kramer, King, et al., 1984).

Stages III and IV. Stage III and IV pressure sores require a broader, more comprehensive approach to care. Supportive care to treat anemia, dehydration, protein depletion, and infection is essential to promote wound healing (Shea, 1975). Delayed wound healing and depression of cellular immunity are both associated with malnutrition (Agarwal, Del Guercio, & Lee, 1985). Nutritional intervention includes oral supplements such as canned polymeric diets. If oral intake is not sufficient to improve the nutritional status of the older person, nasogastric feedings or parenteral nutrition may be required to provide the additional nutrients necessary for healing (Pinchcofsky-Devin & Kaminski, 1986). Wound care consists of debridement to remove the devitalized, necrotic tissue that promotes infection, delays granulation, and impedes healing (Melcher, et al., 1988; Reuler & Cooney, 1981). Debridement is achieved with topical methods using dressings and various pharmacologic preparations, hydrotherapy, or surgery (Melcher, et al., 1988; Parish, et al., 1983). When a small amount of debridement is required, a common treatment modality is the application of wet to dry dressings. The gauze pads are opened, fluffed, and dampened with normal saline solution (Garrigues, 1987). Care should be used to place the moistened dressing in the wound and not on healthy tissue, and to change the dressing before it is dry. It is essential to stop this treatment when the wound begins to epithelialize, since the dry phase removes new epithelial cells from the wound, delaying the healing process (Constantian & Jackson, 1980). Enzymatic agents may be prescribed to debride necrotic tissue. These agents do not penetrate eschar and are not effective if there is a large amount of necrotic tissue (Melcher, et al., 1988).

Surgery is often the preferred method to treat pressure sores in the advanced stages. The surgical approach includes excision of the ulcer, scar tissue, and usually the bony prominence, followed by closure of the defect (Agris & Spira, 1979; Garrigues, 1987). The reader is referred to Agris and Spira and Garrigues for detailed discussion and diagrams of the surgical procedures used for treating pressure sores.

Primary closure is used, with skin grafts, skin flaps, or skin flaps plus muscle interposition when there is adequate skin, subcutaneous tissue, and muscle in the adjacent area. If there have been multiple breakdowns and adequate tissue is not available, secondary procedures are necessary. These include the use of musculocutaneous flaps plus skin grafts and muscle interposition and skin grafts. The tertiary procedures are used if primary and secondary procedures have not been successful. Amputation and fillet of the lower extremity, removal of bone and use of muscle and subcutaneous tissue to cover the defect, is the most common tertiary method in treating recurrent, extensive ulcers. Large tissue flaps, obtained from a distant site, may also be used to cover extensive ulcers.

An average healing period of 4 to 6 weeks is to be expected with close followup required after discharge from the hospital (Agris & Spira, 1979; Coodley, et al., 1983). Even after weeks, healing by secondary intention often results in a poorly epithelialized area over the bony prominence, leaving the area vulnerable to further breakdown (Agris & Spira, 1979).

As with general postoperative care, special attention is paid to maintain adequate nutrient and fluid intake, to control pain, and to maintain bowel and bladder function. The surgical site is observed for drainage and infection. Special attention is given to prevent localized pressure areas by careful positioning with padding under bony prominences. There are frequently specific written instructions provided for when and how the patient may be turned.

A bed cradle is used to keep pressure off the surgical site, and a trapeze is used to help move the patient. Drains are often placed in the wound under the flap and kept in place until the drainage is less than 15 ml in 24 hours (Agris & Spira, 1979). The type of dressing and the frequency of dressing change are specified by the surgeons. Activity is gradually increased from bedrest to chair to full ambulation.

Treatment Methods of the Future

Current research may lead to new treatment approaches to heal pressure sores more rapidly and effectively. Some of the modalities being studied include (1) an injectable preparation of collagen to augment soft tissue; (2) dressings that protect the wound, improve the wound environment, and deliver timed-release medications for wound repair; (3) electrical stimulation to accelerate wound healing; and (4) topical application of growth factors to stimulate granulation tissue formation and accelerate epithelialization (Mulder & LaPan, 1988).

COMPLICATIONS

Life-threatening complications occur with pressure sores. Infections are common and should be considered when a pressure sore does not heal after the removal of pressure (Sugarman, 1985). Systemic infections carry a high mortality rate in elderly patients (Bryan, Dew, & Reynolds, 1983; Galpin, Chow, Bayer, et al., 1976). The most common sources of infectious complications are gram-negative enteric organisms and anaerobic organisms (Cooney & Reuler, 1984).

Osteomyelitis is a complication in the advanced stages of pressure sores (Parish, et al., 1983; Shea, 1975). Diagnostic procedures used to determine the presence of osteomyelitis include plain radiography, technetium 99m bone scan, and computed tomography (CT), with bone biopsy and culture to confirm if the results of the previous procedures are positive (Cooney & Reuler, 1984).

Other serious but rare complications include pyarthrosis with extension to deep structures such as bowel and bladder, tetanus, and amyloidosis. Although the pressure sore may appear superficial, deep sinus tracts may extend to the joint space. Sinography helps to delineate the area requiring surgical debridement. Tetanus toxoid is indicated for patients with deep pressure sores whose immunization status is questionable (Reuler & Cooney, 1981).

SUMMARY

Pressure sores are a major concern in geriatric care. They are costly and debilitating. Prevention of pressure sores is critical; once a pressure sore develops, additional hospitalization time and nursing care are required. Much controversy surrounds the treatment of pressure sores. While there are many approaches to treatment, basic treatment includes relief of pressure, promotion of wound healing, and prevention of complications.

References

Abruzzese, RS (1985): Early assessment and prevention of pressure sores. *In* Lee, BY (ed): *Chronic Ulcers of the Skin*. New York, McGraw-Hill, 1–19.

Agarwal, N, Del Guercio, LRM, & Lee, BY (1985): *In* Lee, BY (ed): *Chronic Ulcers of the Skin*. New York, McGraw-Hill, 133–145.

Agate, JN (1985a); Aging and the skin—pressure sores. *In* Brocklehurst, JC (ed): *Textbook of Geriatric Medicine and Gerontology* (ed 3). Edinburgh, Churchill Livingstone, 915–934.

Agate, JN (1985b): Pressure sores. *In* Pathy, MS (ed): *Principles and Practice of Geriatric Medicine*. New York, John Wiley & Sons, 899–906.

Agris, J, & Spira, M (1979): Pressure ulcers: Prevention and treatment. *Clin Symp* 31:2–32.

Allman, RM, Laprade, CA, Noel, LB, et al. (1986): Pressure sores among hospitalized patients. *Ann Intern Med*, 105:337–342.

Ameis, A, Chiarcossi, A, & Jimenez, J (1980): Management of pressure sores. Comparative study in medical and surgical patients. *Postgrad Med*, 87:177–182.

Andersen, KE, Jensen, O, Kvorning, SA, et al. (1982): Prevention of pressure sores by identifying patients at risk. *Br Med J*, 284:1370–1371.

Barbenel, JC, Jordan, MM, & Nicol, SM (1977): Incidence of pressure sores in the greater Glasgow Health Board Area. *Lancet*, 2:548–550.

Bennett, L, & Lee, BY (1985): Pressure versus shear in pressure sore causation. *In* Lee, BY (ed): *Chronic Ulcers of the Skin*. New York, McGraw-Hill, 39–56.

Bennett, L, & Lee, BY (1988): Vertical shear existence in animal pressure threshold experiments. *Decubitus*, 1:18–24.

Berecek, KH (1975a): Etiology of decubitus ulcers. *Nurs Clin North Am*, 10:157–170.

Berecek, KH (1975b): Treatment of decubitus ulcers. *Nurs Clin North Am*, 10:171–210.

Bergstrom, N, Braden, BJ, Laguzza, A, et al. (1987): The Braden Scale for predicting pressure sore risk. *Nurs Res*, 36:205–210.

Bliss, MR, & McLaren, R (1967): Preventing pressure sores in geriatric patients. *Nursing Mirror*, 123:(19):434–437, 444.

Boss, GR, & Seegmiller, JE (1981): Age-related physiological changes and their clinical significance. *West J Med*, 135:434–440.

Brower, HT, & Crist, MA (1985): Research priorities in gerontological nursing for long-term care. *Image*, 17(1):22–27.

Bryan, CS, Dew, CE, & Reynolds, KL (1983): Bacteremia associated with decubitus ulcers. *Arch Intern Med* 143:2093–2095.

Cooney, TG, & Reuler, JB (1984): Pressure sores. *West J Med*, 140:622–624.

Constantian, MB (ed) (1980): *Pressure Ulcers: Principles and Techniques of Management*. Boston, Little, Brown.

Constantian, MB, & Jackson, HS (1980): Biology and care of the pressure ulcer wound. *In* Constantian, MB (ed): *Pressure Ulcers: Principles and Techniques of Management*. Boston, Little, Brown, 69–100.

Coodley, E, Lincer, F, Parham, A, et al. (1983): Management of decubitus ulcers. *Comp Ther*, 9:61–66.

Cowart, V (1987): Pressure ulcers preventable, say many clinicians. *JAMA*, 257:589–590.

Daniel, RK, Priest, DL, & Wheatley, DC (1981): Etiologic factors in pressure sores: An experimental model. *Arch Phys Med Rehabil*, 62:492–498.

David, JA (1982): Pressure sore treatment: A literature review. *Int J Nurs Stud*, 19:183–191.

David, JA (1984): Tissue breakdown. *Nursing Mirror*, 158(10):i–x.

Dimant, J, & Francis, ME (1988): Pressure sore prevention and management. *J Gerontol Nurs*, 14:18–25.

Dinsdale, SM (1974): Decubitus ulcers: Role of pressure and friction in causation. *Arch Phys Med Rehabil*, 55:147–152.

Doughty, D (1988): Management of pressure sores. *J Enterost Ther*, 15:39–44.

Ek, AC (1987): Prevention, treatment and healing of pressure sores in long term care patients. *Scand J Caring Sci*, 1:7–13.

Ek, AC, & Bowman, G (1982): A descriptive study of pressure sores: The prevalence of pressure sores and the characteristics of patients. *J Adv Nurs*, 7:51–57.

Ek, AC, Gustavsson, G, & Lewis, OH (1985): The local

skin blood flow in areas at risk for pressure sores treated with massage. *Scand J Rehab Med, 17*:(2):81–86.

Exton-Smith, AN (1976): Prevention of pressure sores: Monitoring mobility and assessment of clinical condition. *In* Kenedi, RM, Cowden, JM, & Scales, JT (eds): *Bedsore Biomechanics.* Baltimore, University Park Press, 133–130.

Exton-Smith, AN (1987): The patient's not for turning. *Nursing Times, 83*:(42):42–44.

Exton-Smith, AN, & Sherwin, RW (1961): The prevention of pressure sores: Significance of spontaneous bodily movements. *Lancet, 2*:1124–1126.

Feustel, DE (1982): Pressure sore prevention. *Nursing '82, 12*(4):78–83.

Fowler, E (1982): Pressure sores: A deadly nuisance. *J Gerontol Nurs, 8*:680–685.

Galpin, JE, Chow, AW, Bayer, AS, et al. (1976): Sepsis associated with decubitus ulcers. *Am J Med, 61*:346–350.

Garrigues, NW (Spring, 1987): Pressure ulcers. *Curr Conc Wound Care, 10*:4–10.

Gosnell, DJ (1973): An assessment tool to identify pressure sores. *Nurs Res, 22*:55–59.

Gosnell, DJ (1987): Assessment and evaluation of pressure sores. *Nurs Clin North Am, 22*:399–415.

Gould, D (1986): Pressure sore prevention and treatment: An example of nurses' failure to implement research findings. *J Adv Nurs, 11*:389–394.

Guttman, L (1976): The prevention and treatment of pressure sores. *In* Kenedi, RM, Cowden, J, & Scales, JT (eds): *Bedsore Biomechanics.* Baltimore, University Park Press, 153–159.

Guyton, AC, Granger, HJ, & Taylor, AE (1971): Interstitial fluid pressure. *Physiol Rev, 51*:527–563.

Horsley, JA (1981): *Preventing Decubitus Ulcers* (CURN Project). New York, Grune & Stratton.

Husain, T (1953): An experimental study of some pressure effects in tissues with reference to the bedsore problem. *J Pathol Bacteriol, 66*:347–358.

Isler, C (1972): Decubitus: Old truths, and some new ideas *RN, 39*(7):42–45.

Kosiak, M (1961): Etiology of decubitus ulcers. *Arch Phys Med Rehabil, 42*:19–29.

Lindan, O, Greenway, RM, & Piazza, JM (1965): Pressure distribution on the surface of the human body: I. Evaluation in lying and sitting positions using a "bed of springs and nails." *Arch Phys Med Rehabil, 46*:378–385.

Lineaweaver, W, Howard, R, Soucy, D, et al. (1985): Topical antimicrobial toxicity. *Arch Surg, 120*:267–270.

Longe, RL (1986): Current concepts in clinical therapeutics: Pressure sores. *Clin Pharm, 5*:669–681.

Lowthian, PT (1977): A review of pressure sore prophylaxis. *Nursing Mirror, 144*(10):vii–xv.

Maklebust, J (1987): Pressure ulcers: Etiology and prevention. *Nurs Clin North Am, 11*:359–377.

Maklebust, J, Mondoux, L, & Sieggreen, M (1986): Pressure relief characteristics of various support surfaces used in prevention and treatment of pressure ulcers. *J Enterost Ther, 13*:85–89.

Melcher, RE, Longe, RL, & Gelbart, AO (1988): Pressure sores in the elderly. *Postgrad Med, 83*:299–308.

Michocki, RJ, & Lamy, PP (1976a): The care of decubitus ulcers. *J Am Geriatr Soc, 24*:217–224.

Michocki, RJ, & Lamy, PP (1976b): The problem of pressure sores in a nursing home population: Statistical data. *J Am Geriatr Soc, 24*:323–328.

Mikulic, MA (1980): Treatment of pressure ulcers. *Am J Nurs, 80*:1125–1128.

Morgan, JE (1975): Topical therapy of pressure ulcers. *Surg Gynecol Obstetr, 141*:945–947.

Mulder, GD, & LaPan, M (1988): Decubitus ulcers: Update on new approaches to treatment. *Geriatrics, 43*:37–50.

National Pressure Ulcer Advisory Panel (1989): *Consensus Development Conference Statement.* West Seneca, NY.

Neuberger, GB (1987): Wound care. *Nursing '87, 17*(2):34–37.

Nierman, MM (1978): Treatment of dermal and decubitus ulcers. *Drugs, 15*:226–230.

Norton, D (1975): Research and the problem of pressure sores. *Nursing Mirror, 140*(7):65–67.

Norton, D, McLaren, R, & Exton-Smith, AN (1962): *An Investigation of Geriatric Nursing Problems in Hospitals.* London, The National Corporation for the Care of Old People.

Parish, LC, Witkowski, JA, & Crissey, JT (1983): *The Decubitus Ulcer.* New York, Masson.

Patterson, RP, & Fisher, SV (1986): Sitting pressure-time patterns in patients with quadriplegia. *Arch Phys Med Rehabil, 67*:812–814.

Pinchcofsky-Devin, GD, & Kaminski, MV, Jr (1986): Correlation of pressure sores and nutritional status. *J Am Geriatr Soc, 34*:435–440.

Reichel, SM (1958): Shearing force as a factor in decubitus ulcers in paraplegics. *JAMA, 160*:762–763.

Resio, DT, & Verhonick, PJ (1973): On the measurement and analysis of clinical data in nursing. *Nurs Res, 22*:388–393.

Reuler, JB, & Cooney, TG (1981): The pressure sore: Pathophysiology and principles of management. *Ann Intern Med, 94*:661–666.

Reuler, JB, & Cooney, TG (1984): Pressure sores. *In* Cassel, CK, & Walsh, JR (eds): *Geriatric Medicine, Vol I.* New York, Springer-Verlag, 508–516.

Roaf, R (1976): The causation and prevention of bedsores. *In* Kenedi, RM, Cowden, JM, & Scales, JT (eds): *Bedsore Biomechanics.* Baltimore, University Park Press, 5–9.

Seiler, WO, & Stahelin, HB (1985): Decubitus ulcers: Treatment through five therapeutic principles. *Geriatrics, 40*:30–36, 39–42, 44.

Seiler, WO, & Stahelin, HB (1986): Recent findings on decubitus ulcer pathology: Implications for care. *Geriatrics, 41*:47–50, 53–60.

Shea, JD (1975): Pressure sores—classification and management. *Clin Orthop Rel Res, 112*:90–100.

Sieggreen, MY (1987): Healing of physical wounds. *Nurs Clin North Am, 22*:439–447.

Spector, WD, Kapp, MC, Tucker, RJ, et al. (1988): Factors associated with presence of decubitus ulcers at admission to nursing homes. *Gerontologist, 28*:830–834.

Sugarman, B (1985): Infection and pressure sores. *Arch Phys Med Rehabil, 66*:177–179.

Taylor, KJ (1988): Assessment tools for the identification of patients at risk for the development of pressure sores. *J Enterost Ther, 15*:201–205.

Tepperman, PS, DeZwireck, CS, Chiarcossi, AL, et al.

(1977): Pressure sores: Prevention and step up management. *Postgrad Med*, 62:83–89.

Tooman, T, & Patterson, J (1984): Decubitus ulcer warfare: Products vs process. *Geriatr Nurs*, 5:166–167.

Vasile, J, & Chaitin, H (1972): Prognostic factors in decubitus ulcers of the aged. *Geriatrics*, 27:126–129.

Williams, A (1972): A study of factors contributing to skin breakdown. *Nurs Res*, 21:238–243.

Yarkony, GM, Kramer, E, King, R, et al. (1984): Pressure sore management: Efficacy of a moisture reactive occlusive dressing. Arch Phys Med Rehabil, 65:597–600.

CHAPTER
13

A Protocol for the Management of Patients at High Risk for Pressure Sores

BARBARA L. SATER, R.N.C., M.S.N.
JUDY R. HENSLEY, R.N.C.
JOYCE TAKANO STONE, R.N.C., M.S.

INTRODUCTION

Despite the expansion of knowledge in areas of cause, prevention, and treatment, pressure sores continue to be problematic. Nurses have observed that the problems lie in four areas: (1) lack of a system to accurately determine risk status; (2) inability to differentiate between low-risk (or at-risk) from high-risk patients; (3) inadequate methods to target prevention and treatment interventions, which at present are indiscriminately applied; and (4) inconsistent application of treatments for pressure sores. The following description illustrates a common scenario in the inconsistent management of pressure sores:

Nurse 7:00 am–3:00 pm: Treats the patient's granulating wound with moist dressing; uses Stomahesive around the wound; puts dressing on the wound, pours saline irrigant on the 4 × 4s and tapes the dressings to the Stomahesive edges. *Reasonable, therapeutic method of treatment.*
Nurse 3:00 pm–11:00 pm: Removes the dressing and decides to use Duoderm, which acts as an absorptive agent and a cover; removes the Stomahesive, irrigates the wound, pats the surrounding healthy skin dry, applies the Duoderm, and secures the dressing. *Good, reasonable, therapeutic method of treatment.*
Nurse 11:00 pm–7:00 am: Is upset because she cannot see the wound bed and would like to chart her findings; removes the tape and lifts the Duoderm away from the wound; irrigates with

Ringer's lactate. Her preference is a selectively permeable membrane by Johnson & Johnson. She selects a size that will overlap the wound edges, applies the dressing, and secures the edges with tape. *Reasonable, therapeutic method of treatment.*

Nurse 7:00 am–3:00 pm (24 hours have elapsed): Becomes alarmed when she sees the yellow-brown colored liquid under the membrane; removes the membrane and is content that there is no odor. She irrigates the wound, sees that it is clean, and decides to use an absorptive powder (manufactured by Bard). She places it in the wound, puts two 4 × 4s over the wound, and secures the edges with tape. *Good, reasonable method of treatment.*

Anonymous

Although treatment interventions are appropriate, they are inconsistently applied in the above scene. This results in disruption and delay in wound healing, as well as wasted nursing time.

In this chapter, a protocol for pressure sore management in an acute-care setting is presented. The protocol is based upon the results of a multiphase study conducted in an acute-care hospital over a period of several years. The pressure sore management program includes three components: identification of patients at risk for pressure sores, preventive measures, and treatment of pressure sores. Each component of the management program (identification, prevention, and treatment) will be discussed within the context of the pressure sore study. The process of determining risk status for patients will be reviewed, followed by our protocol for the prevention and treatment of pressure sores. A compilation of studies on the prevention and treatment of pressure sores is included. Products and equipment that were selected for the protocol are described. This program may be implemented in acute- or long-term care facilities and provides the nurse with a practical and effective approach to an age-old problem.

IDENTIFICATION OF RISK STATUS

The identification of factors or combinations of factors that lead to pressure sore develop-

ment and control of these factors have been the focus of pressure sore treatment and research. A constellation of related factors that predispose and contribute to pressure sores is identified and discussed in Chapter 12.

Profiles that are composites of factors have been developed to predict risk for pressure sore development. The Norton Scale, the first profile designed (Norton, McLaren, & Exton-Smith, 1975), continues to serve as a prototype (Andrews, Jensen, Korning, et al., 1982; Gosnell, 1973; Meissner, 1980; Taylor, 1980) (Table 13–1). The Norton Scale was chosen as the assessment tool for the Pressure Sore Management Protocol because it is a screening device that can be used to rapidly assess the patient's risk for pressure sore development. Nurses can complete the Norton Scale assessment in approximately 1 to 2 minutes per patient (Gaston, unpublished, 1983; Norton, et al., 1975). The Norton Scale is also a reliable and practical clinical tool. One disadvantage of the Norton Scale was discovered when Goldstone and Goldstone (1982) examined its predictive ability by using it to assess 40 subjects in two matched samples in a general hospital. Specific components of the Norton Scale were tested against the total score to determine predictive power. The investigators concluded that the Norton Scale, with all the components, was reliable but tended to overpredict pressure sores. In order to improve the predictive power of the Norton Scale, additional information is needed to more closely identify those patients at risk.

INSTRUMENT TO DIFFERENTIATE RISK STATUS

Factors in Pressure Sore Development (FPSD) is an instrument designed to collect data concurrently on specific events, patient characteristics, and conditions during hospitalization (Table 13–2). The authors of this chapter conducted a medical record review using the FPSD that yielded a subgroup of patients who were considered at *high risk* for pressure sore development. Risk factors that were present during the patients' hospitaliza-

Table 13–1. NORTON SCALE AND NORTON PLUS SCALE

Norton Scale

A Physical Condition	B Mental State	C Activity	D Mobility	E Incontinence	Total Score
4 Good	4 Alert	4 Ambulant	4 Full	4 Not	_____
3 Fair	3 Apathetic	3 Walks with help	3 Slightly limited	3 Occasional	
2 Poor	2 Confused	2 Chairbound	2 Very limited	2 Usually urine	
1 Bad	1 Stupor	1 Bedrest	1 Immobile	1 Double Incontinence	

Norton Plus Scale
(For determining high risk for pressure sores)

Check ONLY if YES	*YES*
Diagnosis of diabetes	_____
Diagnosis of hypertension	_____
Hematocrit (M) <41%	_____
(F) <36%	_____
Hemoglobin (M) <14 g/dl	_____
(F) < 12 g/dl	_____
Albumin level <3.3 g/dl	_____
Febrile >99.6°F	_____
5 or more medications	_____
Changes in mental status to confused, lethargic within 24 hours	_____
TOTAL Number of Checkmarks	
Norton Scale Score	_____
Minus total from above	_____
Norton Plus Score	_____

(From Norton, D, McLaren, R, & Exton-Smith, AN: An Investigation of Geriatric Nursing Problems in Hospital. Edinburgh, Churchill-Livingstone, 1975, 225. Reprinted with permission.)

tions were analyzed. Factors that were common to the high-risk group were a diagnosis of diabetes or hypertension; fever; urinary incontinence; mental status changes; bedrest; poor nutrition; low hemoglobin, hematocrit, and albumin; edema; taking five or more medications; and decreased sensation in a body part. Excluding the risk factors that were already on the original Norton Scale, the factors seen in 60% or more of the subgroup patients were used to compose the Norton Plus Scale (NPS) (see Table 13–1). Items on the NPS are diagnosis of diabetes or hypertension; low hemoglobin, hematocrit, and albumin; fever; taking five or more medications; and change in mental status to lethargy or confusion within 24 hours. Each item is given a score of one; the sum of these is subtracted from the Norton Score. A Norton Plus Score of 10 or below indicates that the patient is at high risk for pressure sore development. Hospitalized patients who are deemed at risk for pressure

sores by the Norton Scale may be assessed with the NPS to determine if they are at high risk. Patients who are at high risk may then receive high-risk prevention measures.

The FPSD provides a more comprehensive profile of pressure sore vulnerability, and it may be used to differentiate risk status, that is, those at risk from those at high risk. While the FPSD is a lengthy instrument at present, further research on the FPSD with a larger patient population is required to revise the instrument for practical, clinical application.

PREVENTION AND TREATMENT: A REVIEW OF PRESSURE SORE MANAGEMENT PROGRAMS

Effective pressure sore management relies on a systematic approach for prevention and treatment. A systematic approach includes a method for identifying risk status, preventive

Table 13–2. FACTORS IN PRESSURE SORE DEVELOPMENT (FPSD) OUTLINE

I. A. Sociodemographics
    B. Past medical history
II.   Pressure sore history, description, treatment
III. A. Patient profile during hospitalization/flow sheet
        1. Weight, incontinence, temperature
        2. Mental status and behavior
        3. Methods of feeding
        4. Specialized skin care equipment
        5. Activity
        6. Medications
        7. Surgical procedure
        8. Diagnostic procedure
        9. Special treatments
       10. Lab findings
       11. Compromised positions
       12. Decreased sensation/edema
       13. Nutritional state
       14. Smoker/nonsmoker
     B. Discharge status

measures for at-risk and high-risk patients, and treatments for pressure sores based on the degree of tissue involvement. Success of such an approach has been reported in several studies. Ameis, Chiarcossi, and Jiminez (1980) reported the results of a 5-month study in which patients on medical and surgical units in a general hospital were assessed for pressure sores. A team approach was used to maintain a consistent pattern of assessment and management. Treatment protocols were implemented according to stages of pressure sores. Preventive measures included proper positioning, enforced turning schedules, and use of pressure relief mattresses and pads. Aids used to decrease external forces included sheepskin boots, sheepskin sheets, foam cushions (Temper foam), gel cushions, and elbow pads. Topical treatments included brown soap, benzoyl peroxide (Benoxyl), fibrinolysin with desoxyribonuclease (Elase), ultraviolet light, and ventilation by fan. The incidence of pressure sores per week decreased from 12% on the surgical unit and 29% on the medical unit to zero using this approach. Ameis and associates attributed their results to control of causal factors and the application of a systematic approach for the prevention and treatment of pressure sores in the early stages.

Khun and Wygonoski (1984) described a prevention and treatment protocol that was implemented in a nursing home by a multidisciplinary team. Patients were assessed for pressure sore risk using a decubitus ulcer evaluation tool. The prevention protocol included instructions for skin care, turning, diet, vitamins, physical therapy, protective pads, bowel and bladder regimens, and psychological assessment. Treatment of patients with pressure sores was evaluated by measuring the pressure sore, recording observations of the wound, photographing the wound, and obtaining a wound culture if necessary. The authors concluded that an orderly approach improved the care of patients with pressure sores by providing the health care workers with a system for classifying pressure sores and a method for evaluating healing rates for each stage.

Fowler (1982) described guidelines for a systematic approach for preventing and treating pressure sores. Patients at risk for pressure sore development were entered into a five-step protocol. The steps included (1) pressure relief with devices such as foam pads, gel pads, water mattresses, alternating pressure pads, air-fluidized beds, and heel and elbow protectors; (2) skin care with moisturizing topical agents and protective film barriers; (3) patient movement with turning and positioning schedules and trapeze bars; (4) nutritional care with a dietitian consultation; and (5) patient teaching for patient and care providers. Chemical enzymatic agents and granulation aids for wound debridement and absorption were recommended in the protocol. The guidelines were offered to assist clinicians in the development of a systematic approach to pressure sore management. The products recommended in the protocol were found useful by the author, but they require controlled clinical trials to validate their effectiveness. In our study of pressure sore prevention on a medical unit in an acute-care hospital, a systematic approach to pressure sore prevention was utilized. The incidence of pressure sores was reduced to 1.5%, while on comparison units the incidence was 4% (Takano-Stone & Sater, 1982). The protocol for this study is described later in this chapter.

Pressure sore treatment protocols reported above included interventions for all stages of pressure sores—stages I through IV. Generally speaking, prevention of pressure sores and treatment of pressure sores in stages I and II are the domain of nursing practice. In later pressure sore stages, stages III and IV, treatment includes specialized equipment, medication, and surgery. These stages are the domain of medical practice. Therefore, in the protocol described in this chapter, the prevention and treatment for patients with stages I and II have been emphasized, and treatment in advanced stages has been excluded.

DEVELOPMENT OF A PRESSURE SORE MANAGEMENT PROTOCOL

The following section describes the authors' preliminary work on pressure sores, which began in 1981 and led to the current protocol (Sater, Takano-Stone, Umeh, et al., 1987).

Study 1: Prevention of Pressure Sores

The purpose of the original study, Descriptive Study of Critical Factors in Pressure Sore Development, was to examine the effect of a systematic approach to prevention and treatment on the incidence of pressure sores. For 7 months each patient admitted to the 30-bed medical unit in an acute-care hospital was assessed on admission and again biweekly for pressure sore risk, using the Norton Scale.

Of the 522 patients who were evaluated with the Norton Scale, 457 (87.5%) scored 12 or above and were considered at low risk for pressure sores. Sixty-five (12.5%) scored 12 or below and were considered at risk for pressure sore development. These patients were provided with the protocol for prevention. Of the 65 patients at risk, eight patients (12.3%) developed pressure sores. In addition, one patient with a score of 15 developed a pressure sore.

In this study, the Norton Scale did not differentiate in 12.5% of the low-scoring patients those who developed pressure sores from those who did not. In addition, the Norton Scale provided limited information to describe the patients at risk. Since a large number (12.5%) of the total population was at risk, there was a need to further differentiate those at risk (those having low scores) from those at high risk, that is, those who developed pressure sores in spite of a prevention protocol. It was postulated that interventions could be targeted according to the level of risk.

During this study an additional measurement problem emerged, namely, the need to objectively measure pressure sores. A rating system was needed that included both an inter-rater reliability measure in the staging procedure for pressure sores for both initial and ongoing assessments and an objective measure to determine circumference, width, and depth of the pressure sore. In our proposed study, this problem is addressed, and the procedure for the initial and ongoing assessment of pressure sores will use a panel of clinicians reviewing both photographs for rating stages and healing and measurements with various devices to determine the rate of healing. In addition, the rater's judgment will be compared with measurements using devices such as the Kundin wound gauge instrument (Figure 13–1) to provide a precise description of the wound. With the Kundin wound gauge instrument, the area of surface (flat) lesions and the volume of crater wounds can be calculated using the formulas accompanying the instrument package.

Study 2: Determining Risk Status

The second study was conducted from 1983 to 1985. The specific aims of this study were (1) to differentiate between patients simply at risk and those at high risk for the development of pressure sores and (2) to delineate those factors that are critical in pressure sore development in both groups. In the study hospital, an instrument was developed by Carpendale (1980) for an epidemiologic study on pressure sores. The original instrument included sociodemographic data, past medical and pres-

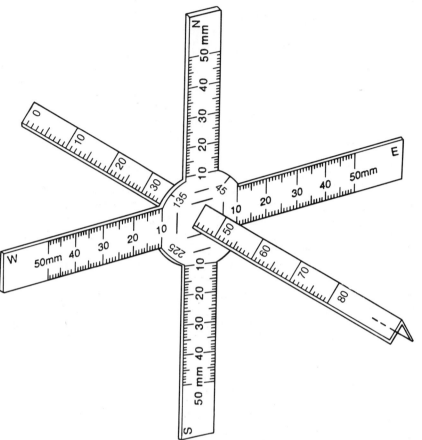

Figure 13–1. Kundin wound gauge. (Courtesy of Jane Kundin, San Mateo, CA. Used with permission.)

sure sore history, and the number, stage, and location of pressure sores developed during hospitalization. This instrument was revised to include a list of factors associated with pressure sore development, such as changes in a patient's condition, treatments, transfers within the hospital, and dietary restrictions. Nursing interventions aimed at the treatment of pressure sores were also documented. In the revised instrument, Factors in Pressure Sore Development (FPSD), flow charts were included to allow data to be collected prospectively during hospitalization. The instrument provided a method for recording the natural history of pressure sore formation and its resolution.

In the second study, a retrospective medical record review using the FPSD was conducted on those patients who had developed pressure sores during study 1. The aim of the review was to find common factors in the high-risk group differentiating them from those at risk. Factors common to this group were a diagnosis of diabetes or hypertension; mental status described as lethargic, confused, or depressed; taking five or more medications; below normal hematocrit and hemoglobin; febrile state; urinary incontinence; and bedrest. In our proposed study, the use of the FPSD concurrently throughout the hospital stay on patients at risk for pressure sores will enable us to collect data on medical diagnoses and other potential contributing factors.

Problems with study 2 were the small sample size and incomplete data in the medical records. The review of the literature and our previous work pointed out several critical issues that were considered in the proposed study.

First, there was no standard protocol for the prevention and treatment of pressure sores. Each clinician or unit determined its own protocols, and thus treatment protocols changed as often as work shifts in a hospital. A wide array of equipment, materials, and pharmaceuticals are available for the prevention and treatment of pressure sores. New products are constantly being introduced, while old products are being modified and improved. The clinician has many choices.

A review of literature (1978–1988) on the prevention and treatment of pressure sores revealed descriptive and comparative studies on products and treatment approaches and commentaries based on personal experiences. A summary of the studies found in the review and a small number found in the preceding 4 years can be found in Table 13–3. The studies on products represented only a small number of brand names. The studies did not compare similar product types, such as Restore, Duoderm, and Tegasorb occlusive dressings. It was difficult to find conclusive documentation that would help the clinician decide which product would be most effective in the prevention or treatment of pressure sores. The treatment studies did not compare a variety of treatment approaches but generally compared only two approaches. No single treatment has been proved to be superior (Tooman & Patterson, 1984), and therefore none is recommended.

The other problems noted with the studies include (1) insufficient number of subjects, (2) inadequate description of the study population, (3) insufficiently indicated or unmatched stage of pressure sore, (4) inadequate control of variables, (5) insufficient consideration of multiple variables, and (6) insufficient details about the treatment approach being studied. The overall lack of negative findings may lend support for the long-held clinical belief that pressure sores can be prevented and treated effectively if the problem is attended to and if there is consistency in the treatment used. The method used is not necessarily important.

Second, pressure sores are treated according to stages. Stages are determined by the degree of tissue involvement, and they range from stages I to IV. Stages I and II are the early stages and are usually treated by employing nursing interventions. These interventions do not include treatment technologies customarily reserved for the advanced stages, such as special beds. There were few studies on the effects of a treatment protocol using a systematic prevention and treatment approach in a general hospital. There were no studies comparing systematic treatment with standard nursing care on the rate of healing of pressure sores.

Third, a major problem with studies of pressure sore prevention and treatment has been the lack of an instrument to objectively measure the pressure sore and to evaluate the rate of healing with different treatments. Rate of healing is the primary method to determine the effectiveness of pressure sore treatment. Yet, studies have relied on descriptive methods or two-dimensional measurements to assess healing. For example, in a study comparing two pressure sore dressings, Sebern (1986) examined the effectiveness of the interventions by measuring width and length of the pressure sore. The area was then calculated by assuming an elliptical shape. Since the shape of pressure sores is seldom symmetrical, the area of the pressure sore was obtained using a formula to calculate an elliptical shape, i.e., $\frac{1}{2}$ length $\times$ $\frac{1}{2}$ width $\times$ π (Sebern, 1986). Roesler (1983) studied the rate of pressure sore healing with an instrument that measured the volume, depth, and circumference of the wounds. Wound measurement was performed periodically, and it objectively demonstrated the rate of healing. Unlike previous studies, Roesler used a three-dimensional measure, the Kundin wound gauge, to determine rate of healing of pressure sores. Since this technique is relatively new, there have been few studies that utilize this measurement to assess rate of healing. Measuring pressure sore volume from a mold made of Jeltrate (used for dental impressions) has been described by Resch, Kerner, Robson, and associates (1988). Another method of measuring sores has been

Text continued on page 282

Table 13–3. SUMMARY OF PRESSURE SORE PREVENTION
AND TREATMENT STUDIES (1978–1988)

			Mattresses		
Author	*Title of Study*	*Year*	*Subjects*	*Product*	*Findings*
Exton-Smith Overstall Wedgwood Wallace	Use of the "Air Wave System" to Prevent Pressure Sores in Hospital (Descriptive)	1982	31 matched pairs of patients at high risk for pressure sores	Air wave system— two layers of air cells	In comparison to the conventional large-cell ripple mattress, the airwave system was significantly more effective in preventing and reducing the severity of pressure sores and in promoting recovery from existing sores. It was more reliable and free from mechanical breakdown.
Maklebust Mondoux Sieggreen	Pressure Relief Characteristics of Various Support Surfaces Used in Prevention and Treatment of Pressure Ulcers (Comparative)	1986	13 healthy volunteers (3 men, 10 women) with various body characteristics Weight: 120–248 lb. Height: 5'2"–6'2" Age: 23–55 years	Conventional hospital mattress 2" convoluted foam pad Biogard Critical Care flotation unit Sof-Care bed cushion	The mean sacral pressures for all support surfaces were below 32 mm Hg. The trochanteric reading showed only Sof-Care reduced pressure significantly from that of regular hospital mattress. All support surfaces reduced pressure on the heel significantly more than the hospital mattress.
Seiler Allen Stahelin	Decubitus Ulcer Prevention: A New Investigative Method Using Transcutaneous Oxygen Tension Measurement (Comparative)	1983	10 healthy subjects, age 18–50 years	Hospital mattress Exam table Super-soft mattress (latex foam, 20 cm thick)	Sacral skin oxygen remained in the normal range when on super-soft mattress or in the 30° lateral position. Lying dorsally on hard table and normal mattress deoxygenated the sacral skin area.
Stoneberg Pitcock Myton	Pressure Sores in the Homebound: One Solution (Comparative)	1986	127 homebound patients age 40–94 years bedfast for at least 1 week, 64 on foam, 22 on regular mattress, 41 on alternating pressure pads	Alternating pressure pads (APP) Foam mattress Regular mattress	Patients on APP had fewer pressure sores; 43 of 64 on foam developed a new pressure sore; 4 of 22 on a regular mattress developed a new pressure sore; 1 of 41 on APP developed a pressure sore.

			Air-fluidized Bed		
Author	*Title of Study*	*Year*	*Subjects*	*Product*	*Findings*
Barnes Rutland	Air-fluidized Therapy as a Cost-Effective Treatment for a "Worst Case" Pressure Necrosis (Descriptive)	1986	One patient, 63-year-old paraplegic with extensive stage IV sacral pressure sore	Clinitron bed	Cost effective. Total daily charges substantially less with air-fluidized bed. Nursing time saved = 195 minutes per day. Stage IV ulcer improved to stage III and patient could be discharged to nursing home.

Table 13–3. SUMMARY OF PRESSURE SORE PREVENTION
AND TREATMENT STUDIES (1978–1988) *Continued*

	Air-fluidized Bed *Continued*				
Author	*Title of Study*	*Year*	*Subjects*	*Product*	*Findings*
Dolezal Cohen Schultz	The Use of Clinitron Therapy Unit in the Immediate Postoperative Care of Pressure Ulcers (Descriptive)	1985	16 patients, majority with spinal cord injuries	Clinitron bed	All patients except one healed in 2 weeks. Clinitron bed increased patient comfort and simplified nursing care. Additional cost of bed represented only 4% to 6% of total hospital bill.
Allman Walker Hart Laprade Noel Smith	Air-fluidized beds or Conventional Therapy for Pressure Sores (Comparative)	1987	65 patients completed the study. Topical therapy was standardized for both groups. Mean age was 65 and 67 years in experimental and control groups, respectively.	Clinitron bed Conventional therapy (Lapidus air mattress)	Clinitron bed group showed decrease in ulcer surface area, especially effective in larger sores, and increased patient comfort. Improvement characteristics: higher protein nitrogen and small sore. Failure to improve: high leukocyte count or creatinine level and history of flap, amputation, undermining of sore, oliguria. Outcome was not associated with medical conditions, age, sex, race, usual blood chemistries, or pressure sore characteristics.

	Wound Dressing: Hydrocolloid				
Author	*Title of Study*	*Year*	*Subjects*	*Product*	*Findings*
Fellin	Cost Savings by Substituting Hydrocolloid for Gauze Dressings (Descriptive)	1984	4 debilitated patients with chronic wounds	Hydrocolloid dressing (Duoderm)	Substantial cost savings on a day-to-day basis using a hydrocolloid dressing.
Mulder Albert Grimwood	Clinical Evaluation of a New Occlusive Hydrocolloid Dressing (Descriptive)	1985	18 patients, 24 ulcers induced by venous stasis, pressure, ischemia, neurotrophy, surgery Two case reports and other descriptive data	Duoderm	Reduced healing time when other treatments had failed. Difficulty in securing dressing to weight bearing areas. Lesions recurred in 4 patients within 3 months of discontinuing use of dressing.
Taylor	Duoderm Wafers (Descriptive)	1985	13 patients in two geriatric hospital wards; 18 sores	Duoderm	Duoderm saved nursing time, cost less, increased patient comfort, had excellent adhesion, and increased rate of healing. Difficult to apply on certain areas, heel or sacral cleft.

Table continued on following page

Table 13–3. SUMMARY OF PRESSURE SORE PREVENTION
AND TREATMENT STUDIES (1978–1988) *Continued*

			Wound Dressing: Hydrocolloid *Continued*		
Author	*Title of Study*	*Year*	*Subjects*	*Product*	*Findings*
Tudhope	Management of Pressures Ulcers with a Hydrocolloid Occlusive Dressing: Results in 23 Patients (Descriptive)	1984	23 patients from 50–97 years of age; 30 pressure ulcers	Duoderm Sores irrigated with hydrogen peroxide and saline	14 (47%) of the ulcers healed, 12 (40%) moderate to marked improvement, 3 (10%) mild improvement, 1 (3%) deteriorated. Less painful in 43%. Little correlation between patient condition and initial ulcer status and time of healing.
Yarkony Kramer King Lukane Carle	Pressure Sore Management: Efficacy of a Moisture Reactive Occlusive Dressing (Descriptive)	1984	21 patients from 16–61 years of age, mean 32; 25 pressure sores that had received previous treatment ranging from 2 weeks to 1 year, mean 2½ months	Duoderm compared to previous treatment	56% of the ulcers showed marked improvement or complete healing compared to 8% of the ulcers with previous treatment. Of the 16 ulcers that showed no improvement with previous treatment, 44% healed or demonstrated marked improvement.
Ryan	Treatment Using Stomahesive (Descriptive)	1976	10 patients with 19 pressure sores	Stomahesive	Stomahesive is successful in treating pressure sores.
Alvarez Mertz Eaglstein	The Effect of Occlusive Dressing on Collagen Synthesis and Re-epithelialization in Superficial Wounds (Comparative)	1983	Young Yorkshire pigs—2 animals treated with Duoderm; wet-to-dry gauze and air exposure treatment of 6 animals	Two different occlusive dressings: Op-Site and Duoderm and nonocclusive wet-to-dry dressing	Increased collagen synthesis and reepithelialization in wounds treated with occlusive dressings. Reepithelialization increased beneath both oxygen-impermeable and oxygen-permeable dressings. New epidermis was damaged with the removal of the wet-to-dry dressing and one of the occlusive dressings.
Boykin Winland-Brown	Pressure Sores: Nursing Management (Comparative)	1986	21 subjects, 15 females, 6 males living at home. Age range 67–96 years; average age 83 years; 11 had pressure sores, 10 were at risk on the Norton Scale, <14.	HCD-hydrocolloid dressing, povidone-iodine	HCD resulted in a decrease in the size of pressure sore approximately twice that of povidone-iodine. No improvement in risk factor following adherence to prevention guidelines.

Table 13–3. SUMMARY OF PRESSURE SORE PREVENTION
AND TREATMENT STUDIES (1978–1988) *Continued*

	Wound Dressing: Hydrocolloid *Continued*				
Author	*Title of Study*	*Year*	*Subjects*	*Product*	*Findings*
Brady	Management of Pressure Sores with Occlusive Dressings in a Select Population (Comparative)	1987	13 pressure sites in 7 patients age 57–87 years, mean age 71 years, median age, 74 years. All neurologic diagnoses; unconscious, stuporous, or confused	1—Duoderm 6—Duoderm and Duoderm granules 6—Op-Site Previous treatment: wet-to-dry dressing. Betadine collagenase and Neosporin powder were also previously used.	Within 3 weeks all pressure sores showed dramatic improvement. Showed less time involved with new dressings. Previous costs $26–$298; dropped to $5–$50. Average savings of $125.34 per patient per week.
Cherry Ryan	Enhanced Wound Angiogenesis with a New Hydrocolloid Dressing (Comparative)	1985	2 experimental models: (1) chick embryo chorioallantoic membrane (CAM), 23 eggs—disc of hydrocolloid dressing (HCD); 16 control; 17 with Silastic material same weight as HCD; (2) 7 pigs; full-thickness, circular wounds; half of wounds treated with hydrocolloid, half with nonadhesive gauze.	Hydrocolloid dressing versus dry dressing	Angiogenic response of a hydrocolloid dressing shown to enhance healing. Wounds treated with HCD exhibited an increase in vascularity and stimulus of angiogenesis found on CAM with oxygen-permeable hydrocolloid dressing.
Gorse Messner	Improved Pressure Sore Healing with Hydrocolloid Dressing	1987	Group I—27 patients with 76 pressure sores; Group II—25 patients with 52 pressure sores; 38% of the patients had severe nutritional depletion	Group I treated with hydrocolloid dressing (HCD); Group II treated with Dakin's solution, wet-to-dry dressing	In HCD group, 66 pressure sores (86.8%) improved as compared to 36 (69.2%) in the wet-to-dry group. Significantly more pressure sores that resolved or were healing were in patients receiving adequate nutritional support.
	Wound Dressing: Moisture Vapor-permeable				
Author	*Title of Study*	*Year*	*Subjects*	*Product*	*Findings*
Ahmed	Op-Site for Decubitus Care (Descriptive)	1982	65 patients with 109 pressure ulcers; age 38–95 years; average age 70 years.	Op-Site	Op-Site hastened healing. Dressing was well tolerated by patients. Decreased nursing time.

Table continued on following page

Table 13–3. SUMMARY OF PRESSURE SORE PREVENTION
AND TREATMENT STUDIES (1978–1988) *Continued*

	Wound Dressing: Moisture Vapor-permeable *Continued*				
Author	*Title of Study*	*Year*	*Subjects*	*Product*	*Findings*
Chrisp	New Treatment for Pressure Sores (Descriptive)	1977	8 patients, 3 case reports	Op-Site	Op-Site was effective in healing sores. Effective in preventing stage I sores from worsening. Increased patient comfort.
Hutchinson	Pressure Areas	1980	3 patients	Op-Site	Patient satisfaction based on dressing being comfortable, less frequent dressing changes, able to bathe and shower. Same difficulty in application. Expensive, but less nursing time required.
Lingner Rolstad Wetherill Danielson	Clinical Trial of a Moisture Vapor-Permeable Dressing on Superficial Pressure Sores (Descriptive)	1984	30 females, 40 males, average age 62 years; 100 pressure sores; other preventive sore care not controlled	Tegaderm	Grade I sores healed faster than grades III and IV. Healing rate for grades I and II was 90%.
Porreca Chagares	Op-Site: A Treatment for Pressure Sores in the Orthopaedic Patient Population (Descriptive)	1983	38 patients, average age 80 years; treated over 10-month period; 68 ulcers, no stage I or V	Op-Site	55% of stage II ulcers healed completely; 36% of stage III ulcers healed completely; 10% of stage IV ulcers healed completely.
Tooman Patterson	Decubitus Ulcer Warfare: Product vs Process (Descriptive)	1984	19 ulcers, majority of patients over age 65 years, frail, poor nutritional status; 20-day treatment program	Op-Site	Consistent treatment using Op-Site resulted in improvement in the original 19 ulcers. Success attributed to consistent treatment approach.
Alper Welch Ginsberg Bogaars Maguire	Moist Wound Healing Under a Vapor Permeable Membrane (Comparative)	1983	18 patients, 10 with unilateral ulcers, 8 with bilateral ulcers; ulcers include pressure, vascular, and diabetic ulcers.	Op-Site compared with benzoyl peroxide in bilateral group	Op-Site increased rate of healing when compared to control group.
Kurzuk-Howard Simpson Palmieri	Decubitus Ulcer Care: A Comparative Study (Comparative)	1985	43 patients age range 36–94 years; mean age 76 years; 5 subjects in Op-Site group and 6 in alternative treatment	Op-Site and standard nursing care (alternative treatment)	No difference in rate of improvement in Op-Site group and alternative treatment group. Op-Site required far less nursing time.

Table 13–3. SUMMARY OF PRESSURE SORE PREVENTION
AND TREATMENT STUDIES (1978–1988) *Continued*

Wound Dressing: Moisture Vapor-permeable *Continued*					
Author	*Title of Study*	*Year*	*Subjects*	*Product*	*Findings*
Mertz Marshall Eaglstein	Occlusive Wound Dressing to Prevent Bacterial Invasion and Wound Infection (Comparative)	1985	3 young Yorkshire pigs; partial-thickness wounds made; 2 animals, 12 wounds each; 1 animal, 24 wounds	Op-Site Vigilon Duoderm	Wounds challenged with *S. aureus* or *P. aeruginosa.* Bacterium isolated on 0% of Duoderm, 50% of Op-Site and Vigilon dressed wounds challenged with *S. aureus,* and 100% wounds challenged with *P. aeruginosa.*
Oleske Smith White Pottage Donovan	A Randomized Clinical Trial of Two Dressing Methods for the Treatment of Low-Grade Pressure Ulcers (Comparative)	1986	N = 16, age 52–93 years, mean age 69 years; standard deviation, 6; variety of underlying illnesses; most common was congestive heart failure. All ulcers were in gluteal or coccyx areas.	Two types of dressing: normal saline, polyurethane	Pressure sores treated with polyurethane occlusive dressing had a larger mean decrease in total surface area as compared to ulcers treated with saline. The two groups were not found to be significantly different in ulcer grade and largest wound diameter.
Sebern	Pressure ulcer Management in Home Health Care: Efficacy and Cost Effectiveness of Moisture Vapor Permeable Dressing (Comparative)	1986	77 ulcers excluding grades I and IV; average ages 72 years (gauze) and 76 years (Op-Site)	Op-Site and wet-to-dry gauze dressing	Op-Site improved the rate of healing and was more cost effective in treatment of grade II ulcers. No significant difference in healing rates or cost for grade III ulcers.
Topical					
Author	*Title of Study*	*Year*	*Subjects*	*Product*	*Findings*
Aronoff Friedman Doedens Lavell	Case Report: Increased Serum Iodide Concentration from Iodine Absorption through Wounds Treated Topically with Povidone-Iodine (Descriptive)	1980	N = 2	Povidone-iodine (Betadine)	Found increased serum iodide concentrations secondary to iodine absorption through wounds treated with povidone-iodine. Cardiovascular instability and renal failure occurred concurrently with systemic iodide accumulation.
DelaCruz Brown Leikin Franklin Hryhorczuk	Iodine Absorption After Topical Administration (Descriptive)	1987	One case study, elderly woman	Iodine dressing applied every 4 hours over 3–5 weeks.	Absorption of iodine after prolonged application of povidone-iodine to a relatively small surface area of denuded skin can result in considerable iodine absorption.

Table continued on following page

Table 13–3. SUMMARY OF PRESSURE SORE PREVENTION
AND TREATMENT STUDIES (1978–1988) *Continued*

			Topical *Continued*		
Author	**Title of Study**	**Year**	**Subjects**	**Product**	**Findings**
Gerber Van Ort	Topical Application of Insulin to Pressure Sores: A Questionable Therapy (Descriptive)	1981	14 subjects in pilot followed by 29 geriatric subjects randomly assigned to either an experimental or control group	Regular insulin	No statistically significant difference between subjects treated with topical insulin therapy and those in a comparative group (both pilot and study). Concluded efficacy of treatment not demonstrated and should not be used (questionable safety, insufficient scientific rationale, lack of sound research). Not FDA approved; old drug, new use. Limits of safe dose not known.
Lee Ambus	Collagenase Therapy for Decubitus Ulcers (Descriptive)	1975	11 patients, age 47–90 years; treatment for 4 weeks; 28 advanced dermal ulcers, 17 collagenase, 11 placebo	Collagenase ointment (Santyl)	14 of 17 treated with collagenase improved. None of the placebo patients showed improvement.
Rao Sane Georgiev	Collagenase in the Treatment of Dermal and Decubitus Ulcers (Descriptive)	1975	24 patients, age 41–91 years, average age 70.4 years; Decubitus ulcers, duration 1 month to 12 years; require debridement; treatment average 3 weeks	Collagenase ointment (Santyl)	Odor, pus, wound size, and degree of necrosis decreased. Granulation increased. Reduced incidence of hypertrophic scanning.
Parish Witkowski	Use of Dextranomer in Decubitus Ulcers (Descriptive)	1981	4 patients treated up to 3 months, 6 mm punches taken from a variety of pressure sores	Dextranomer	Minimal inflammatory response, no irritation in the presence of dextranomer left in wound. Dextranomer may be used for long periods without any tissue damage.
Shimamoto Shimamoto Fujihata Nakamura Matsuura	Topical Application of Sugar and Povidone-Iodine in the Management of Decubitus Ulcers in Aged Patients (Descriptive)	1986	15 elderly patients with 25 pressure ulcers; age 65–90 years; sacral area was site for most of the ulcers.	Mixture of granulated sugar, 310 g; povidone-iodine solution, 28 ml; and povidone-iodine gel, 90 g	Area remained unchanged in 12 of 25 ulcers; of the remaining 13 ulcers, 6 decreased in size while 7 increased. Mixture did not debride the wound of eschar.

Table 13–3. SUMMARY OF PRESSURE SORE PREVENTION
AND TREATMENT STUDIES (1978–1988) *Continued*

			Topical *Continued*		
Author	*Title of Study*	*Year*	*Subjects*	*Product*	*Findings*
Knutson Merbitz Creekmore Snipes	Use of Sugar and Povidone-Iodine to Enhance Wound Healing (Comparative)	1981	N = 759; 154 (20.3%) with standard therapy and 90 (11.9%) with sugar and povidone-iodine (PI) solution; 515 (67.8%) with compound mixture sugar, PI solution, and PI ointment; a variety of wounds, burns, and ulcers were treated.	Sugar Povidone-iodine (PI) solution Povidone-iodine (PI) ointment	All wounds, burns, and ulcers rapidly became clean.
Kucan Robson Heggers Ko	Comparison of Sulfadiazine, Povidone-Iodine and Physiologic Saline in the Treatment of Chronic Pressure Ulcers (Comparative)	1981	N = 40; 15 silver sulfadiazine cream, 14 saline, 11 povidone-iodine solution	Silver sulfadiazine cream Povidone-iodine solution	In preparing pressure ulcers for closure, found 100% of the patients treated with silver sulfadiazine cream had the necessary bacterial count (less than 10^5 per gram of tissue); 78.6% of those treated with saline and 63.6% of those treated povidone-iodine solution had suitable bacterial count.
Parish Collins	Decubitus Ulcers: A Comparative Study (Comparative)	1979	17 patients with 34 decubitus ulcers; all were moist ulcers, not dry	Dextranomer Collagenase	All 7 in the Dextranomer group and 2 of 5 in the collagenase group improved. None of the 5 patients on sugar and egg white improved. Dextranomer treatment was significantly more effective. No side effect from any treatment. Noted frequency of turning, diet, cleaning patients, and changing linen did not affect progress of healing.
Yucel Basmajian	Controlled Study of Healing Effect of Enzymatic Spray (Comparative)	1974	21 decubitus ulcers, ages 18–47 years; spinal cord injury with other conditions to complicate healing; 16 closely matched (size, location, depth) in 8 pairs	Granulex enzymatic spray, Routine treatment	Enzymatic spray-treated ulcers healed at 2.5 times faster rate than the routinely treated counterpart.

Table continued on following page

Table 13–3. SUMMARY OF PRESSURE SORE PREVENTION
AND TREATMENT STUDIES (1978–1988) *Continued*

			Miscellaneous		
Author	*Title of Study*	*Year*	*Subjects*	*Product*	*Findings*
Akers Gabrielson	Effect of High Voltage Galvanic Stimulation on Rate of Healing of decubitus ulcers (Comparative)	1984	14 spinal cord-injured patients	Nerve stimulation, whirlpool, and whirlpool nerve stimulation	Reduction in ulcer size no matter what treatment. Greatest rate of healing was with nerve stimulation alone, then combined whirlpool and nerve stimulation.
Kaada	Promoted Healing of Chronic Ulceration by Transcutaneous Nerve Stimulation (TNS) (Descriptive)	1983	10 patients, 5 females, 5 males; average age 66 years (range 53–77 years); ulcers included vascular, pressure, scleroderma, neuropathy	Nerve stimulation	Resistant ulcers treated for months or years healed completely in a few weeks or healed sufficiently to permit grafting.
Wills Anderson Beattie Scott	A Randomized Placebo-controlled Trial of Ultraviolet Light in the Treatment of Superficial Pressure Sores (Comparative)	1983	16 patients, mean ages 87 years (treatment) and 80 years (control)	Ultraviolet light and placebo	Increased the rate of healing by 2 weeks when compared to control group.

developed that uses photography and a microcomputer. This method shows a high level of repeatability and interobserver reliability (Anthony, 1985), but the cost for general clinical use may be prohibitive.

Finally, there is a belief among clinicians that more aggressive prevention will reduce the incidence of pressure sores. It is also believed that aggressive treatment in the early stages can reduce the progression of pressure sores to the later stages. However, this belief lacks empirical proof. These problems were considered in the design of the proposed study, which resulted in the development of the Pressure Sore Management Protocol (Table 13–4).

Pressure Sore Management Protocol

Assessment

1. At the time of admission to the medical/surgical unit and every Monday and Thursday all patients will be assessed by the nursing staff for pressure sore risk using the Norton Scale.

2. Patients who score 12 or lower on the Norton Scale will be identified as at risk for pressure sores.

3. Patients at risk for pressure sores will be assessed with the Norton Plus Scale to determine if they are at high risk. A Norton Plus Score of 10 or lower indicates high risk. Patients at high risk for pressure sores will be placed on the high-risk prevention protocol.

4. All patients at risk will be assessed using the Norton Plus Scale every Monday and Thursday thereafter.

5. Patients at risk for pressure sores will receive Protocol A. Patients at high risk will receive Protocol B.

Protocol A: Prevention for Patients at Risk. The Prevention Protocol consists of explaining to the subject the protocol and a rationale for the treatment. Measures outlined in the Prevention Protocol are aimed at providing metic-

Table 13–4. PRESSURE SORE MANAGEMENT PROTOCOL

Assessment: Identification of Risk Status

1. On admission, determine risk for pressure sore development using the Norton Scale.
2. Assess every Monday and Thursday during hospitalization using the Norton Scale.
3. Depending on Norton Scale Score:
   Norton score of 13 or above indicates no special procedure.
   Norton score of 12 or below, assess with Norton Plus Scale.
4. Norton Plus Score of 11 or above, place on Protocol A. Norton Plus Score of 10 or below, place on Protocol B.

Prevention Protocol

1. Explain each step of protocol and rationale to patient. Secure his/her cooperation.
2. Prevent pressure:
   a. Turn and position patient every 2 hours while in bed.
   b. Active/passive range of motion every shift.
   c. Up in chair at least once a day if not contraindicated. Use a 3–4″ foam cushion on chair.
   d. Advance activity as tolerated.
3. Meticulous skin care:
   a. Inspect pressure areas and gently massage bony prominences a minimum of once every shift. DO NOT massage if nonblanching erythema is present.
   b. Use skin care kit to keep skin clean and dry, applying skin cream to prevent excessive dryness and ointment to perineal area if incontinent.
   c. Avoid direct skin contact with plastic-lined bedpads.
4. Prevent shearing/friction:
   a. Avoid wrinkles in sheets.
   b. Teach patient use of overhead trapeze bar to move around in bed.
   c. Lift, do not pull patient across linen.
   d. Do not elevate head of bed more than 30°.
5. Nutrition:
   a. Monitor fluid and nutrient intake by measurement of intake and output and through calorie count.
   b. Obtain dietary consult for diet analysis.
   c. Record admission height and weight and weekly weight.
   d. Record albumin, hemoglobin, and hematocrit levels.
6. Control incontinence:
   a. Identify type of incontinence.
   b. Implement appropriate bowel or bladder regimens.
   c. Use external catheter for urinary incontinence, if necessary, or disposable briefs.
   d. Provide meticulous skin care.

Prevention Protocol A:

1. Includes use of Prevention Protocol.
2. Place air mattress on bed.

Prevention Protocol B:

1. Includes use of Prevention Protocol.
2. Place Vaperm on bed.

Protocol/Pressure Sore Stage I:

1. Continue with Prevention Protocol.
2. All patients are placed on the Vaperm mattress.
3. Apply occlusive dressing to reddened areas.
4. Change dressing every 7 days or as needed. Dressings that are pulling, wrinkled, or loosened or that have exudate require change.
   Exception: Atrophic skin
   a. Do not use any adhesive material on subjects with atrophic skin, e.g.:
      (1) Patients who have been on long-term steroid therapy.
      (2) Patients who have three or four senile purpura on arm.
   b. Protocol for patients with atrophic skin:
      (1) Continue with prevention protocols.
      (2) Use foam-lined molded boots (Spenco) to provide extra protection to heels/ankles if needed.
      (3) Use Granulex aerosol spray to protect reddened areas.

Table continued on following page

Table 13–4. PRESSURE SORE MANAGEMENT PROTOCOL *Continued*

Protocol/Pressure Sore Stage II:
1. Continue with Prevention Protocol.
2. All patients are placed on the Mediscus bed.
3. Apply occlusive dressing to pressure sore. For atrophic skin, use Granulex aerosol spray.
4. Change dressing and measure and care for pressure sore every Monday and Thursday, more frequently if leakage of exudate occurs or if signs of infection appear.

Pressure sore care:
   a. Check for infection—redness, edema surrounding dressing, increased skin warmth, purulent drainage.
      (1) If infection present, notify physician.
      (2) If no infection present, proceed with protocol.
   b. Cleanse area with saline, gently dry with 4 × 4.
   c. Apply a new occlusive dressing.

ulous skin care; preventing pressure by turning and range of motion schedules and advancement of activity as tolerated; preventing shearing and friction by proper transfer techniques and positioning; assuring adequate nutrition; and controlling incontinence. Specific equipment to be used includes air mattresses, cushions, and overhead trapeze bars on the beds of all patients at risk.

Protocol B: Prevention for Patients at High Risk. This protocol includes all of the treatment in protocol A. The Vaperm mattress is substituted for the air mattress in protocol A.

Staged Treatment

Treatment of Stage I Pressure Sores. Prior to treatment, the physician is notified and the protocol explained. Reports of the condition of the pressure sore and the treatment are documented on the patient's medical record. Prevention protocol B is used or continued at this level. Patients are placed on the Vaperm mattress. An occlusive dressing is applied and is changed as needed, but it may remain for 7 days.

Treatment of Stage II Pressure Sores. In stage II pressure sores, an occlusive dressing is also used. Assessment of the pressure sore and wound care is carried out every fourth day or more frequently if leakage occurs or if signs of infection appear. After 4 days the dressing is changed. If infection is present, the condition is reported to the physician for treatment. If no infection is present, the area is cleansed with saline and gently patted dry with a 4 × 4 gauze dressing. An occlusive dressing is then reapplied. Patients with a stage II pressure sore are placed on a low-pressure bed, such as the Mediscus Bed (Figure 13–2).

Patients who advance to pressure sore stage III or IV require medical intervention and will be referred to the physician.

PREVENTION AND TREATMENT EQUIPMENT

A description of prevention and treatment equipment used in the protocol is provided,

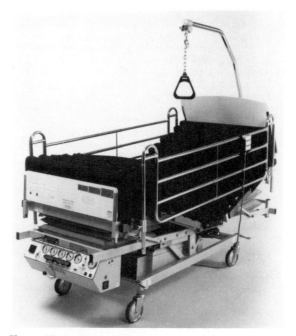

Figure 13–2. Air support therapy system in a low pressure bed. (Courtesy of Mediscus Products, Inc. Used with permission.)

along with advantages and disadvantages we found in using a particular product (Table 13–5). Equipment is grouped according to the following categories: (1) pressure relief devices, (2) protective skin care products, and (3) mobility equipment.

1. Relief of sustained pressure, which permits tissue reoxygenation, is the first and foremost principle in pressure sore prevention. An increase in oxygen tension is accomplished by mechanical decompression of the microvessels and never by massage or local applications (Berecek, 1975). A rapidly expanding technology in the area of super-soft pressure relief equipment has led to the availability of numerous devices for patients and health care providers.

2. The application of protective skin care items helps to maintain the integrity of the epidermis by keeping it lubricated (Skin Care Kit), covered (wound dressings), and dry (Wings disposable briefs).

3. A trapeze bar allows the patient to move independently and spontaneously when uncomfortable. Discomfort from compression of the skin and subcutaneous tissue prompts a

Table 13–5. PREVENTION AND TREATMENT EQUIPMENT AND MANUFACTURERS

Pressure Relief Devices
Air Mattresses:
  Sof-Care Mattress/Cushion (Gaymar Industries, Inc., Orchard Park, New York)
  Waffle Mattress/Cushion (EHOB, Inc., Indianapolis, Indiana)
Vaperm Mattress (Beauvale Medical, Derbyshire, England)
Sheepskin Protectors, Heel and Elbow
Spenco Boots (Orthopedic Systems, Inc., Hayward, California)
Mediscus Air Bed (Mediscus Products, Ltd., Derbyshire, England)
Protective Skin Care Products
  Wound Dressings:
    Restore (Hollister)
    Duoderm (Squibb)
    Tegasorb (3M)
  Granulex Aerosol (Dow B. Hickman, Inc.)
  Skin Care Kit (United, Division of Howmedica, Inc.)
  Disposable Briefs (Wings, Professional Medical Products)
Patient Mobility Equipment
  Trapeze Bars

---

change in position with consequent relief of pressure (Exton-Smith & Sherwin, 1961). A trapeze bar also assists in lifting and moving the patient to avoid sliding the patient against a stationary force. Sliding or pulling patients across the bed results in a shearing force. The skin over the sacrum tends to remain in the same position because of the friction between the skin and the bed (Norton, McLaren & Exton-Smith, 1975). The sacral tissue is vulnerable to shearing force also when the head of the bed is raised and the patient slides downward.

Pressure Relief Devices

Air Mattress/Cushion (Sof-care, Waffle). An air mattress/cushion provides comfort and protection for patients at risk for pressure sores. Heat, moisture, pressure, and shearing are reduced. The required amount of air varies according to the size of the patient and can be controlled by simple checking and inflating or deflating as needed. The mattress/cushion can be easily cleaned and is disposable after each patient use. Disadvantages are the need for air inflation and frequent checking to ensure an adequate amount of air. Special caution has to be taken when sharp objects or heat (lit cigarettes, heaters) come in contact with the product.

Vaperm Mattress. The Vaperm mattress and cover is a complete patient support system. The porous mattress and the water-vapor permeability of the waterproof covering increase the evaporation of water from the supported area. The mattress is made from open-cell, fatigue-resistant foams of varying density. Compliant top layers and firm bottom layers provide cushioning for the patient's bony prominences while conforming to the contour of the patient. The outer covering is a waterproof, water-vapor permeable stretch film cover. This cover eliminates the need for a draw sheet.

Sheepskin Heel and Elbow Protectors. The popularity of sheepskin pads has led to the development of elbow and heel pads made from wool or a synthetic. Advantageous characteristics of sheepskin protectors include (1) dry, resilient, dispersion of pressure over the body area; (2) frictionless contact when the skin surface rubs or slides over the sheepskin; (3) absorbency and drying through the natural properties of wool; and (4) washability and durability, especially if synthetic sheepskin is used. Disadvantageous characteristics of sheepskin include the following: (1) generates heat and perspiration; (2) it is impractical to change after frequent soiling; and (3) it is destructible with repeated laundering if natural wool is used (Berecek, 1975). In addition, the protectors must be checked periodically for slippage from the body part, heel, or elbow on which they are applied.

Spenco Boots. Spenco boots are very useful in the protection of the foot and ankle. There are two parts for each boot. The inner part is like a small eggcrate of 1 to 1½ inches of foam with indentations throughout. The outer shell is a formed, pliable foam with a waterproof coating. A Velcro strap secures the boot onto the patient's foot.

Mediscus Air Bed. The Mediscus bed is an air support system that uses 21 air sacks to support the patient. It is flexible, with a water vapor-permeable cover that is waterproof. The Mediscus bed is temperature controlled, which enables the nurse to find the most comfortable temperature for the patient. "The water vapor diffuses through the sac wall and is swept away by the filtered temperature controlled air, which flows through the bed at approximately 80 cubic feet per minute (140 m³/hr)" (Mediscus Low Air Loss System). The Mediscus bed does not dehydrate the bedridden patient. There are five groups of air sacks. Each group has its own pressure control valve and indicator so it can be adjusted to provide the correct support for each patient. Patient mobility and safety are improved because the air sacks can be adjusted to provide support and protection for sitting patients or for positioning bedridden patients. The ability to increase the pressures in all the air sacks gives the nurse a firm surface to move and position a patient with minimum lifting.

Protective Skin Care Products

Wound Dressings (Restore, Duoderm, Tegasorb). These are hydrocolloid dressings that form a protective gel over the wound bed to speed epithelialization. The dressing absorbs wound exudate, odor, and bacteria; reduces edema; and provides a barrier against infection. The dressings are designed to be left in place for up to 1 week, which eliminates frequent dressing changes.

Granulex Aerosol. Granulex has three ingredients: (1) trypsin, (2) balsam Peru, and (3) castor oil. Trypsin is an enzymatic debridement agent that helps in the promotion of normal healing. Balsam Peru increases circulation and has a mildly bactericidal property. Castor oil improves epithelialization by reducing premature epithelial desiccation and cornification. It also protects the wound, reducing the patient's pain and discomfort (Yucel, 1974). Aerosols have the advantage of eliminating all extraneous physical contact with the wound. These products are advantageous because they eliminate dressing changes for patients who have paper-thin skin due to steroid therapy.

Skin Care Kit. The Skin Care Kit consists of a skin cleanser, ointment, and protective moisturizer. The skin cleanser is a nonirritating, pH balanced solution that is sprayed onto the skin to remove residue and then is rinsed off with water. The cleanser is composed of water, lauramine oxide, and propylene glycol. The ointment is a petroleum salve to protect the skin. The protective moisturizer is a lanolin anhydrous product to restore moisture and oil to the skin and help maintain skin integrity. The moisturizer penetrates the skin sufficiently to leave it lubricated but not oily.

Disposable Briefs (Wings). The disposable brief is a layered, absorbent material that is contoured to fit the body. The deeper layers absorb most of the moisture, thus keeping the skin dry.

Mobility Equipment

A trapeze bar assists in the patient's mobility and the nurse's efforts in positioning the patient to avoid friction and shearing force. If the head of the bed must be elevated, the patient may use the trapeze bar to adjust positions and prevent pressure.

SUMMARY

The Pressure Sore Management Protocol was the outcome of a series of studies in pressure sore development that were conducted over a period of several years in an acute-care hospital. The studies were divided into phases: (1) identification of patients at risk for pressure sore development; (2) differentiation of levels of risk; and (3) development of prevention and treatment interventions. The protocol is designed to decrease the incidence of pressure sores and to offer guidelines to nurses in the care of early stage pressure sores.

The distinguishing features of the protocol are (1) providing a method to differentiate at-risk from high-risk patients; (2) differentiating treatment for at-risk and high-risk patients; and (3) intensifying care for beginning pressure sores (stages I and II) to prevent their progression to advanced stages III and IV. There is no single product or procedure that is definitive in the management of pressure sores. Rather, products selected for the protocol are generically grouped according to principles of skin and wound care. The protocol is based upon the concept of a systematic approach—one emphasizing consistent application of steps in the procedure. The principles of skin and wound care, together with a systematic approach, are supported by the literature.

The body of knowledge in pressure sore management is extensive, yet minimal impact has been made on clinical nursing practice (Gould, 1986). This is partially due to a lack of knowledge about pressure sore research findings and a failure in communicating current information to bridge theory and practice. The Pressure Sore Management Protocol, with its focus on patients at high risk, is based upon existing knowledge in pressure sore management, our research of several years in the management of pressure sores, and our experience as practicing nurses. The protocol is one component of a new study, A Controlled Clinical Study of Pressure Sore Treatment, which is underway. The study will test the effectiveness of a systematic approach on the incidence rate, rate of healing, length of hospital stay, and costs of early stage pressure sores in hospitalized patients. The study is intended to address some of the gaps in our present knowledge about pressure sore development and treatment.

References

Ahmed, MC (1982): Op-Site for decubitus care. *Am J Nurs,* 82:61–64.

Akers, TK, & Gabrielson, AL (1984): The effect of high voltage galvanic stimulation on the rate of healing of decubitus ulcers. *Biomed Sci Instrum,* 20:99–100.

Allman, RM, Walker, JM, Hart, MK, et al. (1987): Air-fluidized beds or conventional therapy for pressure sores. *Ann Intern Med,* 107:641–648.

Alper, JC, Welch, EA, Ginsberg, M, et al. (1983): Moist wound healing under a vapor permeable membrane. *J Am Acad Dermatol,* 8:347–353.

Alvarez, DM, Mertz, PM, & Eaglstein, WH (1983): The effect of occlusive dressing on collagen synthesis and re-epithelialization in superficial wounds. *J Surg Res,* 35:142–148.

Ameis, A, Chiarcossi, A, & Jiminez, J (1980): Management of pressure sores. *Postgrad Med,* 67:177–184.

Andrews, KE, Jensen, O, Korning, SA, et al. (1982): Prevention of pressure sores by identifying patients at risk. *Br Med J,* 284:1370–1371.

Anthony, D (1985): Measuring pressure sores. *Nurs Times,* 81:57–61.

Aronoff, GR, Friedman, SJ, Doedens, DJ, et al. (1980): Case report. Increased serum iodide concentration from iodine absorption through wounds treated topically with povidone-iodine. *Am J Med Sci,* 279:173–176.

Barnes, S, & Rutland, BS (1986): Air-fluidized therapy as a cost-effective treatment for a "worst-case" pressure necrosis. *J Enterost Ther,* 13:27–29.

Berecek, KH (1975): Treatment of decubitus ulcers. *Nurs Clin North Am,* 10:171–210.

Boykin, A, & Winland-Brown, J (1986): Pressure sores: Nursing management. *J Gerontol Nurs,* 12:17–21.

Brady, SM (1987): Management of pressure sores with occlusive dressings in a select population. *Nurs Manag,* 18:47–50.

Carpendale, MT (1980): Epidemiology of bedsores. Unpublished questionnaire. San Francisco Veterans Administration Medical Center.

Cherry, GW, & Ryan, TJ (1985): Enhanced wound angiogenesis with a new hydrocolloid dressing. *In* Ryan, T.J. (ed): *An Environment for Healing: The Role of Occlusion.* London, Royal Society of Medicine, 61–68.

Chrisp, M (1977): New treatment for pressure sores. *Nurs Times*, 73:1202–1205.

DelaCruz, F, Brown, DH, Leikin, JB, et al. (1987): Iodine absorption after topical administration. *West J Med*, 146:43–45.

Dolezal, R, Cohen, M, & Schultz, RC (1985): The use of Clinitron therapy unit in the immediate postoperative care of pressure ulcers. *Ann Plast Surg*, 14:33–36.

Exton-Smith, AN, Overstall, PW, Wedgwood, J, et al. (1982): Use of the "air wave system" to prevent pressure sores in hospital. *Lancet*, 1:1288–1290.

Exton-Smith, AN, & Sherwin, RW (1961): The prevention of pressure sores: Significance of spontaneous bodily movements. *Lancet*, 2:1124–1126.

Fellin, R (1984): Managing decubitus ulcers—cost savings by substituting hydrocolloid for gauze dressings. *Nurs Manag*, 15:29–30.

Fowler, E (1982): Pressure sores: A deadly nuisance. *J Gerontol Nurs*, 8:680–685.

Gaston, SF (1983): Evaluation of the Norton Scale of risk for the development of pressure ulcers. In Proceedings of Octoberquest: Research: Rising to the challenge. Available from DRW Printing, Los Angeles, CA 90024 (Veterans Administration, District 27).

Gerber, RM, & Van Ort, SR (1981): Topical application of insulin to pressure sores: A questionable therapy. *Am J Nurs*, 81:1159.

Goldstone, LA, & Goldstone, J (1982): The Norton Scale: An early warning of pressure sores? *J Adv Nurs*, 7:419–426.

Gorse, GJ, & Messner, RL (1987): Improved pressure sore healing with hydrocolloid dressing. *Arch Dermatol*, 123:766–771.

Gosnell, DJ (1973): An assessment tool to identify pressure sores. *Nurs Res*, 22:55–59.

Gould, D (1986): Pressure sore prevention and treatment: An example of nurses' failure to implement research findings. *J Adv Nurs*, 11:389–394.

Hutchinson, M (1980): Pressure areas. *Australasian Nurses Journal*, 9:3–4.

Kaada, B (1983): Promoted healing of chronic ulceration by transcutaneous nerve stimulation (TNS). *VASA*, 12:262–269.

Khun, J, & Wygonoski, C (1984): A multidisciplinary team approach to decubitus care. *Nursing Homes*, 33:29–33.

Knutson, RA, Merbitz, LA, Creekmore, MA, et al. (1981): Use of sugar and povidone-iodine to enhance wound healing. *South Med J*, 74:1329–1335.

Kucan, JD, Robson, MC, Heggers, JP, et al. (1981): Comparison of silver sulfadiazine, povidone-iodine and physiologic saline in the treatment of chronic pressure ulcers. *J Am Geriatr Soc*, 29:232–235.

Kurzuk-Howard, G, Simpson, L, & Palmieri, A (1985): Decubitus ulcer care: A comparative study. *West J Nurs Res*, 7:58–79.

Lee, LK, & Ambus, JL (1975): Collagenase therapy for decubitus ulcers. *Geriatrics*, 30:91–98.

Lingner, C, Rolstad, BS, Wetherill, K, et al. (1984): Clinical trial of a moisture vapor-permeable dressing on superficial pressure sores. *J Enterost Ther*, 11:147–149.

Maklebust, J, Mondoux, L, & Sieggreen, M (1986): Pressure relief characteristics of various support surfaces used in prevention and treatment of pressure ulcers. *J Enterost Ther*, 13:85–89.

Mediscus Low Air Loss System, Mediscus Products, Ltd., Derbyshire, England.

Meissner, JE (1980): Which patients on your unit might get a pressure sore? *Nursing '80: 10*:64–65.

Mertz, PM, Marshall, DA, & Eaglstein, WH (1985): Occlusive wound dressing to prevent bacterial invasion and wound infection. *J Am Acad Dermatol*, 12:662–668.

Mulder, G, Albert, SF, & Grimwood, RE (1985): Clinical evaluation of a new occlusive hydrocolloid dressing. *Cutis*, 35:396–400.

Norton, D, McLaren, R, & Exton-Smith, AN (1975): *An Investigation of Geriatric Nursing Problems in Hospital.* Edinburgh, Churchill Livingstone.

Oleske, DM, Smith, XP, White, P, et al. (1986): A randomized clinical trial of two dressing methods for the treatment of low-grade pressure ulcers. *J Enterost Ther*, 13:90–98.

Parish, LC, & Collins, E (1979): Decubitus ulcers: A comparative study. *Cutis*, 23:106–110.

Parish, LC, & Witkowski, JA (1981): Use of dextranomer in decubitus ulcers. *Int J Dermatol*, 20:62–64.

Porreca, RC, & Chagares, RM (1983): Op-Site: A treatment for pressure sores in the orthopaedic patient population. *Orthop Nurs*, 2:30–36.

Rao, DB, Sane, PG, & Georgiev, EL (1975): Collagenase in the treatment of dermal and decubitus ulcers. *J Am Geriatr Soc*, 23:22–30.

Resch, CS, Kerner, E, Robson, MC, et al. (1988): Pressure sore volume measurement. *J Am Geriatr Soc*, 36:444–446.

Roesler, LD (1983): A comparison of two treatments of decubitus ulcers: Op-Site and Bard products. Unpublished report. Palo Alto, CA, Stanford University Hospital.

Ryan, RM (1976): Treatment using Stomahesive. *Nurs Times*, 72:299–301.

Sater, B, Takano-Stone, J, Umeh, L, et al. (1987): Shattering the research mystique. *Geriatr Nurs*, 8:334–337.

Sebern, MD (1986): Pressure ulcer management in home health care: Efficacy and cost effectiveness of moisture vapor permeable dressing. *Arch Phys Med Rehabil*, 67:726–729.

Seiler, WO, Allen, S, & Stahelin, HB (1983): Decubitus ulcer prevention: A new investigative method using transcutaneous oxygen tension measurement. *J Am Geriatr Soc*, 31:786–789.

Shimamoto, Y, Shimamoto, H, Fujihata, H, et al. (1986): Topical application of sugar and povidone-iodine in the management of decubitus ulcers in aged patients. *Hiroshima J Med Sci*, 35:167–169.

Stoneberg, C, Pitcock, N, & Myton, C (1986): Pressure sores in the homebound: One solution. *Am J Nurs*, 86:426–428.

Takano-Stone, J, & Sater, B (1982): Descriptive study of critical factors in pressure sore development. Unpublished report. San Francisco, Veterans Administration Medical Center.

Taylor, BB (1985): Duoderm wafers. *NZ Nurs J*, 78:10–11.

Taylor, V (1980): Decubitus prevention through early assessment. *J Gerontol Nurs*, 6:389–391.

Tooman, T, & Patterson, J (1984): Decubitus ulcer warfare: Product vs process. *Geriatr Nurs, 5:*166–167.

Tudhope, M (1984): Management of pressure ulcers with a hydrocolloid occlusive dressing: Results in twenty-three patients. *J Enterost Ther, 11:*102–105.

Wills, EE, Anderson, TW, Beattie, BL, et al. (1983): A randomized placebo-controlled trial of ultraviolet light in the treatment of superficial pressure sores. *J Am Geriatr Soc, 31:*131–133.

Yarkony, G, Kramer, E, King, R, et al. (1984): Pressure sore management: Efficacy of a moisture reactive occlusive dressing. *Arch Phys Med Rehabil, 65:*597–600.

Yucel, VE, & Basmajian, JV (1974): Controlled study of healing effect of enzymatic spray. *Arch Phys Med Rehabil, 55:*517–519.

CHAPTER
14

The Problem of Falls

JOYCE TAKANO STONE, R.N.C., M.S.
W. CAROLE CHENITZ, R.N., Ed.D.

INTRODUCTION

Falls are a major concern in geriatric care. They occur frequently in the older population and can have severe consequences. Falls create a complex clinical picture; the interacting effects of age-related changes, illness and disease processes, and environmental conditions are the major factors associated with falls. This chapter discusses the problem of falls in the elderly—the scope of the problem, the types and causes of falls, and their consequences.

SCOPE OF THE PROBLEM

Associated with advancing age is a steady rise in the incidence of falls and an increase in the severity of injuries and complications resulting from falls (DeVito, Lambert, Saffin, et al., 1988; Hogue, 1982; Overstall, 1985a; Rubenstein, 1983.) Three-fourths of all falls occur in people over 65 years of age, and falls are the leading cause of fatal and nonfatal injuries in this age group (Rodstein, 1983a; US Department of Commerce, 1985). In the United States, falls cause 9500 deaths annually. For every death resulting from a fall, there are 20 older persons, or 172,000 persons annually, who suffer a fractured hip (Baker & Harvey, 1985).

Falls are a common problem among the elderly at home and in institutions, posing a serious threat to their health and well-being. In the community, about one-third of elderly citizens reported a fall during the previous 12 months (Overstall, 1985a; Prudham & Evans, 1981; Sheldon, 1960). The incidence of falls and injuries also is high in the protected environment of hospitals and residential care facilities. Falls represent the largest cause of accidents, accounting for 40% to 80% of all hospital incidents (Elnicki & Schmitt, 1980; Johnson, 1985; Lee, 1979). Gryfe, Amies, and Ashley (1977) reported in their study that 45% of the ambulatory residents in a residential home reported a fall. Baker and Harvey (1985) found the incidence in their nursing home study to be approximately two falls per resident per year. The high rate in institutions is attributed to the advanced age and frailty of the patients (Baker & Harvey, 1985; Overstall, 1980). (See Table 14–1 for a summary of published studies on falls in hospitals and long-term care institutions.)

The full magnitude of the problem of falls is unknown, since many falls are not reported by the older person or are dismissed as not being significant by health professionals (Nickens, 1985; Overstall, 1985b). Falls are not often listed as a cause of death when, in fact, a fall may have been a major contributor to a series of events that led to death (Baker & Harvey, 1985).

Securing accurate data on falls in the elderly is difficult for a number of reasons. Data on the frequency, causes, and outcome of falls vary from setting to setting with differing study populations and dissimilar methods of data collection (Perry, 1982). Whereas the vast majority of older persons live at home, the number of community-based studies on falls are few (Nickens, 1985). Falls in the home are often unwitnessed, and the older person's recall of the incident is not reliable. Falls are often forgotten by the elderly (Cummings, Nevitt, & Kidd, 1988). Studies on falls in hospitals and nursing homes have been primarily retrospective and often are based on incident reports (Morse, Tylko, & Dixon, 1987). Less than one-fourth of these falls are witnessed (Gibbs, 1982; Morris & Isaacs, 1980; Swartzbeck, 1983).

Carefully designed research studies on falls in the elderly have been limited (Perry, 1982). The lack of a control or non-faller group makes it difficult to determine factors that differentiate those who fall from those who do not. The complex nature of falls, with the multitude of probable causes and contributing factors, adds to the difficulty of studying the problem.

CONSEQUENCES OF FALLS

The majority of people who fall are not injured or they suffer only minor injury and do not seek medical care (Ashley, Gryfe, & Amies, 1977; Brown, 1983; Overstall, 1985b; Swartzbeck, 1983). However, it has been estimated that between 5% and 15% of those who fall sustain fractures or other significant injuries (Cape, 1986). The most common injuries are soft tissue injuries and fractures of the hip, femur, humerus, wrist, and ribs. Subdural hematoma occurs less frequently but should be considered when neurologic changes occur after a fall (Kane, Ouslander, & Abrass, 1984). In the over-65 population falls account for about 172,000 hip fractures annually and are the leading source of injury-related hospital admissions (Baker & Harvey, 1985). Elderly patients who fracture the hip are estimated to require 21 days of hospital care, which is twice the average length of stay for all other causes (Baker & Harvey, 1985). Of special concern are the potential complications of hospitalization and surgery, resulting in a prolonged recovery period, temporary or permanent disability, and institutionalization. Falls can cause a major disruption in life and can markedly reduce its quality. A fall can cost an older person his life, the gravest of all consequences. Fractures result in death in 12% to 20% of cases and in nursing home care for half of those who survive (Riggs & Melton, 1986).

Another consequence of falls is the postfall syndrome. After one or more falls, the older person fears falling again. This fear prevents the older person from remaining fully mobile, active, and functional, adversely affecting their mobility and independence. The postfall syndrome may produce a cycle of increased dependency, social isolation, and depression (Isaacs, 1982). Caregivers also experience the postfall syndrome and often pose unnecessary restrictions on the person who fell.

Older persons who have never experienced a fall may feel it can never happen to them and may not take precautions to prevent a fall. The high morbidity and mortality of falls in the elderly can be greatly reduced by eliminating environmental hazards and adequately evaluating and treating underlying medical problems (Rubenstein, 1983). Fall safety is an issue that should be included in community health education programs, clinics, and the

Text continued on page 297

Table 14–1. SUMMARY OF PUBLISHED STUDIES ON FALLS IN HOSPITALS
AND LONG-TERM CARE INSTITUTIONS*

Author, Location, and Study Design	Population	Data Source	Findings
Ashley, et al. 1977 Toronto, Canada	Elderly residents of home for the aged	Incident report	Examined extrinsic causes: no specific time of day, day of week, or time of year. Most falls occur in "residence" area. The majority of falls caused no injury. The most common activity was going to/returning from toilet.
Baker & Harvey 1985 Baltimore, MD	Nursing home; average census = 270; median age = 82; N = 1078 falls in 2 years	Screening tool developed to identify personal and environmental factors related to falls and injury	Rate of falls approximately 2000 per 1000 patient years, or 2 per patient per year. Of the falls, 2.4% resulted in hip and other fractures. Female patients more likely to fracture hips; 7 times greater than male patients.
Barbieri 1983 San Diego, CA (Descriptive)	Inpatients, VA medical center; N = 25 interviews; N = 420 incident reports	Incident report Patient interview Medical record Patient care plan	Of those interviewed, 96% knew why they fell. Falls were not accidents.
Berry, et al. 1981 Toronto, Canada (Descriptive)	Geriatric/chronic disease VA hospital inpatients; N = 1803 for 3 years	Incident reports	No injury resulted in 61% of falls. Of patients who fell, 42% were "well oriented." Majority used wheelchairs. Average falls were 2.4 per patient; 51% fell more than once and 13 patients had 10 or more falls. Falls on assessment/rehabilitation units were significantly greater than on other units. Patients' room/toilet most common location.
Bright, et al. 1983 South Africa (Descriptive)	Hospital inpatients; N = 54	Statement forms written by nursing staff	Majority of falls resulted in no injury. Medical diagnoses were not contributory. More falls at night.
Brown 1983 (Descriptive)	Inpatients, VA medical center; N = 130	Incident reports	Of 130 falls, two were serious.
Catchen 1983 New York, NY (Descriptive)	Inpatients 65 years or older, large municipal acute-care hospital; N = 392	Accident reports	Of the falls, 36% were associated with beds and 28% with wheelchairs. Night falls were more often associated with beds; 29% of falls occurred during first week; 16% occurred between 12 and 36 weeks; 23% of patients had 2 or more falls; 6 patients had 5 or more; 1 patient had 11. All were restrained after the first accident. Organic mental syndrome or stroke was diagnosis in 40% of repeaters; 10% were recovering from broken bones.
Elnicki and Schmitt 1980 Gainesville, FL (Tested a simple prediction model)	Inpatients, large hospital	Incident reports	Model included 23 patients and hospital environment characteristics. Developed 30 estimated equations. None gave results from which logical policy could be made.

Table continued on following page

Table 14–1. SUMMARY OF PUBLISHED STUDIES ON FALLS IN HOSPITALS
AND LONG-TERM CARE INSTITUTIONS* *Continued*

Author, Location, and Study Design	Population	Data Source	Findings
Gibbs 1982 Melbourne, Australia (Descriptive, prospective)	Inpatients, British university teaching hospital; N = 1 interview, 32 falls from accident forms	Patient interviews Staff interviews Accident reports	Patients were discharged before accident forms available and interviews were not done. Of the falls, 25% were witnessed. No significant correlations between any variables.
Gordon, et al. 1982 Toronto, Canada (Prospective)	Geriatric residential setting; N = 59	Holter monitoring Physical examination	In 16 of 59 residents who were Holter monitored, arrhythmias were a contributing factor in either falls, dizziness, or syncope. Cardiac arrhythmias were present in 12 of 37 patients who fell and 4 of 22 non-fallers.
Granek, et al. 1987 Baltimore, MD (Descriptive, retrospective)	Residents in a 283-bed long-care facility; 184 cases who fell and 184 controls; median age for cases = 83; median age for controls = 81	Incident reports and medical records	Fallers were more often ambulatory; 66% were taking three or more medications, as were 49% of the controls. Odds of being a faller were significant for those taking antidepressants, sedatives/hypnotics, or vasodilators. Odds were higher for patients with osteoarthritis or depression. No significant difference was seen in regard to sex or number of diagnoses. Risk of falling appeared to be more strongly related to drugs.
Gryfe, et al. 1977 Toronto, Canada (Descriptive, longitudinal [5 years])	Geriatric residential ambulatory population; N = 651	Incident reports	Total of 45% of residents fell. Rate of falling was 668 per 1,000 per year. Majority of fallers had more than 1 fall.
Guimarues and Isaacs 1980 Toronto, Canada (Descriptive)	Elderly inpatients; N = 3 elderly fallers, 22 nonfallers, 23 active old people (7 had fallen), and 24 normal young subjects	Observation and examination	Gait of old people who fall is "strikingly abnormal." Resembles *marches a petit pas* seen in Parkinson's disease
Innes and Turman 1983 San Francisco, CA (Descriptive)	Acute hospital; N = 270	Incident reports	Restraints and medications are the most common ways to prevent falls.
Kalchthaler, et al. 1978 Yonkers, NY (Descriptive)	Residents of a nursing home; N = 72	Incident reports	Persons over 85 years had higher incidence. Residents in wheelchairs had the greatest number of falls. Alert residents, those with 3–6 chronic diseases, and those with more than 3 medications were involved in greater number of falls. Area of highest risk was bedside.
Kulikowski 1979 Columbia, SC (Descriptive)	Patients, VA medical center; N = 94 accidents, 79 falls	Incident reports	Falls from a bed (N = 27), falls while transferring from a chair (N = 18), ambulatory (N = 16), and from syncope/seizure (N = 18). Only 6 of 94 accidents were observed by nursing staff.

Table 14–1. SUMMARY OF PUBLISHED STUDIES ON FALLS IN HOSPITALS
AND LONG-TERM CARE INSTITUTIONS* *Continued*

Author, Location, and Study Design	Population	Data Source	Findings
Lee 1979 Great Britain	Emergency department, district geriatric hospital, infirmary, large mental illness hospital, and a specialty hospital; N = 1823 falls	Incident reports	Falls occur when patients leave the bed to go to the toilet. Most falls were not witnessed. Bed rails do not stop patients who want to leave the bed.
MacDonald & MacDonald 1977 Nottingham, Great Britain (Descriptive)	Inpatients with femoral fractures in a geriatric orthopedic unit in a hospital; N = 390	Case notes	Of the 103 patients taking barbiturates, 46 (45%) had a history of frequent falls (over 4 falls/week). Only 64 (22%) of 287 patients not on barbiturates had had frequent falls. Over 90% of patients with nocturnal fractures were taking barbiturate hypnotics compared with 67% of those with morning fractures and none of the afternoon fractures.
Morris and Isaacs 1980 Birmingham, Great Britain	140-bed geriatric hospital	Accident reports for 1 year (1978)	Incidence of 422 falls per 1,000 patients/year or 1 in 5 patients; 1 in 10 fell more than once; 1 in 80 suffered a fracture; and 1 in 100 fractured the hip. Twice as many falls in women (not significant). Falls occurred all hours of the day. Patients who fell were accustomed to being active and independent, whose balance was impaired by recent illness. Hemiplegia patients tended to fall more than once.
Morse, Tylko, & Dixon 1987 Edmonton, Alberta	1200-bed urban hospital (acute and long-term care); N = 100 fallers; N = control group	Interviews Observations Medical records	Patients who fell had more than one diagnosis, were older, confused, had fallen previously during same admission, had nocturia with urgency, had weak or impaired gait, and were on intravenous therapy. Most falls occurred in patient's room or bathroom.
Overstall, et al. 1977 London, England	Elderly people living at home and younger hospital workers; N = 306, 243 elderly and 63 younger	Interviews—fall history and injury; sway measured, drug history obtained, blood pressure measured	Sway increased with age for both sexes. Those who had 5 or more falls swayed more than those who had none to 4 falls. Tripping (47%) was the most common cause of falls.
Sehested and Severin-Nielsen 1977 Naestved, Denmark (Descriptive)	Inpatients in a 97-bed geriatric department who fell in a hospital; N = 134	Brief written report made by nurse on duty	Of the patients who fell, 40% fell more than once. Most falls occurred during the first week of hospitalization. The largest number of falls occurred at the bed (N = 75), ward chair (N = 62), in the corridor (N = 43), in the bathroom (N = 32), and on the floor (N = 15). Many of the patients who fell were weakened by illness.

Table continued on following page

Table 14–1. SUMMARY OF PUBLISHED STUDIES ON FALLS IN HOSPITALS
AND LONG-TERM CARE INSTITUTIONS* *Continued*

Author, Location, and Study Design	Population	Data Source	Findings
Spellbring, et al. 1988 Baltimore, MD (Descriptive, retrospective)	Inpatients in an acute-care hospital	Incident reports and patient records	Established a profile of fallers: history of previous falls, mental status changes, debilitation or weakness, mobility deficits, communication deficits, sensory deficits, multiple medications, urinary alterations, emotional upsets, or loss of a significant other.
Swartzbeck & Milligan 1982 Columbia, SC	Inpatients in a 428-bed general medical/surgical VA hospital Two studies were reviewed: in 1977, N = 94/3 months; in 1978, N = 492/1 year	Incident reports	Majority were alert and oriented. Significantly greater proportion of incidents in those over 65 years. Of the falls, 41% (1977) and 34% (1978) occurred during first week in hospital. Falls increased after the third week of stay. Falls occurred more frequently on medical units, especially the oncology units. No injury occurred in 62% (1977) and 60% (1978) of the falls; 1% had fractures. Time of day, day of week, and month were not significant. Most prevalent falls were from wheelchairs, beds, and while ambulating (respectively).
Swartzbeck 1983 Columbia, SC (Descriptive)	428-bed VA hospital, 120-bed nursing home care unit; N = 443 in acute care hospital, N = 111 in nursing home care unit; combined this data with 1982 study	Incident reports	Significant increase during first week and after third week. More falls on medical service. Of patients who fell, 30% could not recall the incident. Majority had no injury; 1.3% had fracture.
Tinetti, Williams, & Mayewski 1986 Rochester, NY (Descriptive, prospective)	Screened patients admitted for the first time to intermediate care facilities; N = 19; recurrent fallers = 25; fell once or not at all = 54	Questionnaires Examination of patient including balance and gait evaluations Medical records	Common problems associated with one-time faller group: poor mental status, decreased vision, and poor mobility or activities of daily living score. Of the 7 falls, 3 occurred during an acute illness; 3 of the recurrent fallers suffered a fracture; most had no injury or only soft tissue injuries. In comparison to those who fell once or not at all, fallers were significantly less active (56% versus 18%), deteriorated in their activities of daily living score from admission (56% versus 32%), and more likely to become incontinent (50% versus 16%). The risk for falling increased as the number of disabilities increased.

Table 14–1. SUMMARY OF PUBLISHED STUDIES ON FALLS IN HOSPITALS
AND LONG-TERM CARE INSTITUTIONS* *Continued*

Author, Location, and Study Design	Population	Data Source	Findings
Walshe and Rosen 1979 (Descriptive)	Patients in a 300-bed community hospital; N = 106	Incident reports	Equal distribution between normal mental status and disoriented status in patients who fell. One-third fell within 4 days of admission. Profile of patient who fell from bed: over 65, diagnosed with heart problems, side rails up, had not been neglected, questionable mental and ambulatory status.
Watkins and Robson 1981 England (Descriptive)	Rehabilitation unit; N = 386	Incident reports	Of falls in all groups, 87% over 70 years; 74% had no injury; 1% had fractures.
Wong, et al. 1981 Nova Scotia, Canada (Descriptive)	Psychiatric hospital; N = 24	Questionnaires completed by staff after a fall	Falls occurred as follows: 25% getting out of bed; 16.7% standing; 16.7% walking.

*Compiled by Heather Kussman and W. Carole Chenitz.

independent clinician's practice with the elderly.

DEFINITION

A fall is defined as an unintentional change in position (Tinetti, Williams, & Mayewski, 1986). All falls result from a displacement or alteration of the body's center of gravity, causing a loss of balance that is not corrected (Das & Kataria, 1985; Isaacs, 1985).

CONTRIBUTING FACTORS

Falls in the elderly occur under a variety of circumstances and have many causes and contributing factors. Fall-related factors are commonly divided into two categories: intrinsic factors, such as age-related physical changes and a number of pathologic conditions, and extrinsic or environmental factors (Nickens, 1985; Rubenstein, 1983). Nickens (1985) points out that these categories are not mutually exclusive; the "liability to fall" is always bound up with "the opportunity to fall." Table 14–2 lists some of the major contributing factors for falls.

Intrinsic Factors

Intrinsic factors play an important role in falls among the older and more frail elderly. Falls are usually considered a symptom of poor health and a general state of decline (Nickens, 1985; Overstall, 1985b). Several studies have shown a strong relationship between the number of disabilities and illnesses the older person has and the risk of falling (Kalchthaler, Bascom, & Quintos, 1978; Morse, Tylko, & Dixon, 1987; Tinetti, Williams, & Mayewski, 1986). Age-related changes and diseases involving vision, posture, gait, and psychological state are primary contributors to falls (Hogue, 1984; Nickens, 1985; Perry, 1982).

Vision. Poor vision has been associated with those who fall (Overstall, 1985b). Several age-related changes in vision occur that contribute to instability and falls in the elderly. These changes include decreases in visual acuity, depth perception, lateral fields of vision, tolerance for glare, and night vision (Kline &

Table 14–2. CONTRIBUTING FACTORS
FOR FALLS

Intrinsic Factors

Age-related changes in vision, posture, and gait
Poor judgment
Emotional/mental state: agitated, depressed, pressured,
  rushed, distracted, confused, fearful, and anxious
Weakness/deconditioning
Fear of incontinence
Denial of illness, weakness, and dependence
Pain
Podiatric conditions such as ingrown toenails, corns,
  bunions
Adjusting to new environment: recent move, recent
  admission, transfer
Multiple diagnoses: conditions affecting stability,
  mobility, and cognitive function
Drugs: prescribed/over-the-counter/self-prescribed;
  alcohol, sedatives/hypnotics, tricyclic antidepressants,
  antihypertensive agents, analgesics, and diuretics

Extrinsic Factors

Lighting: dark, too dim, glare, shadows
Walking surfaces: uneven, wet and slippery, patterned
  floor
Stairs: inadequate handrails, edges not clearly defined,
  poor step design
Furniture: too low, too soft, tips easily, on wheels
Bathroom: slippery tub or shower, lack of grab rails for
  toilet or tub
Shoes/slippers: too loose, badly worn heels, soles too
  slick
Clothing: too long, loose, and flowing
Equipment: worn out or broken, improper use of
  equipment, use of restraints and siderails

Schieber, 1985). As many as 90% of individuals over 65 years of age wear corrective lenses (Murphey & Myers, 1982). With the decrease in visual acuity and depth perception, the older person may trip and fall because of failure to see a curb or step. With the reduction of visual field size, the older person may not be aware of approaching people or objects.

More light is required for optimal vision because pupillary constriction reduces the amount of light entering the aging eye to only one-third the light received by those under 20 years of age (Kline & Schieber, 1985). Night vision becomes impaired and walking is dangerous in poorly illuminated areas, such as hallways and stairs. With the decreased tolerance for glare, the reflected light from highly polished floors or from large windows may prevent the older person from seeing hazard-

ous objects in the path. The aging eye responds slowly to changes in light intensity, requiring more time to accommodate when entering a dark room from a brighter one.

Among the elderly, there is an increased incidence of conditions that cause a progressive loss of vision, such as cataracts, glaucoma, diabetic retinopathy, and macular degeneration. Visual field deficits resulting from a stroke may also be a contributing factor for falls.

Posture. Upright, vertical posture and balance are maintained by peripheral mechanisms with central integration at the higher centers (Isaacs, 1985; Ochs, Newberry, Lenhardt, et al., 1985; Wolfson, Whipple, Amerman, et al., 1985). Postural sway, the movement while standing in an upright position, increases with age and has been associated with falls due to loss of balance (Overstall, Exton-Smith, Imms, et al., 1977; Lichtenstein, Shields, Shiavi, et al., 1988).

The peripheral mechanisms involved in postural stability include the vestibular, visual, and somatosensory systems (Isaacs, 1985; Ochs, et al., 1985). Degenerative changes have been noted in these systems; the extent due to the aging process or disease is unknown (Ochs, et al., 1985). Sensory input from the three systems is redundant, and postural stability will be maintained if only one or two of the systems are impaired (Nutt, 1984; Ochs, et al., 1985).

Information on the body's position in relation to the line of gravity is provided by the otoliths in the vestibular system (Leibowitz & Shupert, 1985). They play an essential role when the walking surface is uneven or when the stance is unstable (Overstall, 1985a). Closing the eyes or moving the visual environment increases body sway (Ochs, et al., 1985). The oculomotor reflexes maintain gaze stability—the immobilization of the visual image on the retina during head or body movement. Without gaze stability, the image is blurred and distorted and spatial disorientation results (Leibowitz & Shupert, 1985).

Postural reflexes of the somatosensory system maintain postural stability during standing and walking (Leibowitz & Shupert, 1985).

The information on age-related somesthetic changes is limited. Many of the losses in somesthetic sensitivity are not generally found throughout the aged population. Neuropathies due to disease, injury, or circulatory insufficiency may be accountable for these losses. Clinical descriptions indicate that the effect of age on somesthetic acuity is one of general decline in sensitivity (Kenshalo, 1977). The decrease in tactile sensitivity in the elderly varies in relation to the amount of changes in skin thickness and afferent nerve fibers (Kenshalo, 1986; Marsh, 1980). Neuropathies contributed to the loss of sensitivity, especially in the lower extremities (Marsh, 1980).

A significant loss in vibratory sensibility after age 50 years has been reported. The greatest decline is seen in the lower extremities (Ochs, et al., 1985; Wolfson, et al., 1985). Possible causes underlying the decline include changes in circulation, loss of uniform myelination on the nerves, thiamine deficiency, or other disorders such as diabetes (Marsh, 1980). Deficits in kinesthesis—the ability to discern passive movements or position of joints—was shown to exist in the lower limbs. However, this deficit was found in only a small percentage of the older population and is probably not an age-related change (Marsh, 1980).

In the musculoskeletal system, there is a decrease in muscle mass, strength, and coordination. The total number of muscle fibers decreases, reducing the size of the motor unit (Wolfson, et al., 1985). Isometric strength in the proximal and distal muscle decreases 20% to 40% in persons 60 to 70 years of age. In those individuals who fall, a greater decrease in lower extremity muscle function is noted. Of special importance are diminished strength and speed of the ankle muscles, making it difficult for the older person to regain balance by rapidly adjusting the center of gravity (Wolfson, et al., 1985). Tinetti and associates (1986) also found decreased knee strength.

The central integration of sensory input and motor response involves the cerebral hemispheres, basal ganglia, cerebellum, and vestibular nuclei (Nutt, 1984). In the elderly, there is a slowing of those central processes that perceive and integrate input (Ochs, et al.,

1985; Overstall, 1980). For example, an older person is slower to make postural correction to even a small disturbance in balance, such as a minor loss of footing. This slowing is due to the lack of coordination of the early somatosensory reflexes in responding to disruptions and the decreased ability to use visual input to regain postural stability (Leibowitz & Shupert, 1985).

Gait. One of the earliest gait changes that older people notice and frequently complain of is the inability to lift their feet as high as they used to. This change results in tripping when walking on uneven surfaces and stepping up on curbs. With normal age-related changes, there is a reduction in limb coordination and in the movement of the pelvis toward the weight-bearing leg when walking. This allows the other leg to swing forward, but in older persons the swing may be too low to avoid an obstacle, causing them to trip (Overstall, 1980). Elderly women develop a narrow-based, waddling gait, and elderly men have a wide-based, short-stepped gait (Kane, et al., 1984). Fifteen percent of elderly persons have gait disturbances (Koller, Glatt, & Fox, 1985).

Any disease involving the balance systems, that is, proprioception, the vestibular system, or the cerebellar system, affects gait and increases the older person's susceptibility to falls. Conditions associated with gait disturbances include degenerative disorders, such as Alzheimer's or Parkinson's disease; neoplasms; toxic metabolic disorders, such as tardive dyskinesias and metabolic neuropathies of alcoholism or diabetes; diseases with altered immune response, such as myasthenia gravis and polymyositis; episodic events, such as seizures, transient ischemic attacks, postural hypotension, and cardiac arrhythmias; infectious diseases such as general paralysis and Jakob-Creutzfeldt disease; and normal-pressure hydrocephalus, a disorder of spinal fluid flow (Sabin, 1982). The musculoskeletal disorders affecting gait include deconditioning, myopathy, arthritis, and podiatric problems, such as corns, bunions, and ingrown toenails.

Specific gait changes have been identified in fallers. The gait changes seen in hospitalized fallers included extremely short step length, slowness, and variability in the frequency and length of steps (Overstall, 1985a). Impaired gait in the demented elderly population is characterized by shorter step lengths, slower gait, lower stepping frequency, greater step-to-step variability, greater ratio of time when both feet are on the ground in relation to the total time of the stride cycle, and a greater sway path (Overall, 1985a).

It has been noted that older people with established gait disorders generally ambulate safely. Their gait tends to have a consistent pattern. It is the older person with a newly acquired gait disorder resulting from a recent stroke, joint replacement, or amputation who falls as a result of some unexpected event or so-called trivial movement, such as getting out of a chair (Isaacs, 1982).

Psychological Factors. Psychological factors have also been found to play a role in falls in the elderly. Depression, apathy, confusion, and denial of limitation affect alertness, judgment, degree of psychomotor retardation, and motivation (Benton & Strouthides, 1985; Mossey, 1985; Rodstein, 1983b).

Extrinsic Factors

Elderly persons living at home have falls that most frequently occur during the day (Overstall, 1985a; DeVito, et al., 1988), indoors, and usually in the living room or on the stairs (Overstall, 1985a). In his study on falls among the elderly, Sheldon (1960) found that one-third, 63 of 171 falls, occurred on the stairs. Stairs that do not have a clear definition of each step are especially hazardous. Floral prints or confusing patterns, shadows, glare, and similar colors on the stair and tread create hazardous environmental conditions leading to missteps and falls (Archea, 1985; Pastalan, 1982). In another study of community-dwelling elders where elevators, not stairs, were used, over 75% of the falls occurred in the bedroom and bathroom (DeVito, et al., 1988). Hazards in the home environment include loose rugs, stray electrical cords, highly polished floors, poor lighting, and spills on the

floor. Outdoors, predisposing environmental elements are bad weather, uneven terrain, poor condition of sidewalks, and weak illumination from street lights.

In institutional settings, falls frequently occurred when the patient was attempting transfer from bed to chair and while en route to the bathroom (Overstall, 1985a). Inaccessible call lights, TV controls, mobility aids (canes, walkers, and wheelchairs), and toileting equipment, such as urinals and commodes, at the bedside increased the risk for falls. Inadequate lighting may lead to falls, as may restraints and siderails. Beds, tables, and stands with wheels and corridors with moving equipment and people are hazardous for elderly patients. In addition, glare from windows, highly polished floors, objects on the floor, equipment and furniture in need of repair, and absent hand-rails and grab bars create potential safety problems.

Several studies have found that most falls occurred during periods of high activity when the staff was busy. Variations in fall rates by time of day, day, and month have been reported, but these variations were neither explained nor consistent between studies (Morse, et al., 1987).

Factors Associated with Trauma

Several intrinsic and extrinsic factors are associated with increased trauma with falls. These include the speed and force with which the fall occurred (Das & Kataria, 1985), height of the fall, the hardness of the landing surface, frequency of falling, and decreased protective mechanisms, namely slowed reflexes, diminished muscular response, and decreased soft tissue padding. Most falls in the elderly occur at standing height or lower (Melton & Riggs, 1985).

Of special concern is osteoporosis, since falls in the presence of osteoporosis increase the risk of fractures, a serious consequence in the elderly. Osteoporosis, characterized by decreased total bone mass, can lead to fractures after minimal trauma (Riggs & Melton, 1986). Both men and women lose bone mass with advancing age, the onset of trabecular bone loss occurring at age 30 years, a decade earlier than the onset of cortical bone loss (Bellantoni & Blackman, 1988; Riggs & Melton, 1986). The programmed sequence of bone formation and bone resorption is altered by accelerated bone loss, primarily trabecular loss, in postmenopausal women (type I osteoporosis) and by age-dependent impairment in trabecular and cortical bone formation (type II osteoporosis) (Riggs & Melton, 1986). Trabecular bone comprises 20% of the skeleton, including the substance of the vertebrae, the pelvis, much of the neck of the femur, and other flat bones. Cortical or compact bone is found primarily in the peripheral skeleton in the shafts of long bones (Riggs & Melton, 1986; Silverberg & Lindsay, 1987). Aging women lose about 35% of their cortical bone and 50% of their trabecular bone; aging men lose about two-thirds of these amounts (Riggs & Melton, 1986).

Research on the role of estrogen in maintaining normal bone mass and decreasing the severity of osteoporosis has resulted in some new information. Recent studies indicate that estrogen may act directly on the osteoblasts, the bone-forming cells. This new information provides support for estrogen therapy after menopause in the treatment of osteoporosis (Barnes, 1987).

Fractures in older persons with osteoporosis may be viewed as a problem with falls or with loss of bone mass (Riggs & Melton, 1986; Smith, 1987). Fractures usually do not occur until bone mass declines below the critical fracture threshold (Smith, 1987). The propensity of the elderly to fall and the lowered threshold for injury are factors that place the elderly at greater risk for fractures (Riggs & Melton, 1986). While it is believed that occasionally some falls are precipitated by a "pathologic fracture" of the hip, there is no data available on its actual incidence (Baker & Harvey, 1985; Melton & Riggs, 1985).

TYPES OF FALLS AND THEIR CAUSES

Classifying falls and their causes is difficult because of the complexity and overlapping of the many factors associated with falls. Placing the older person at greater risk for falls are age-related physical changes, multiple health problems, and hazards in the environment (Rubenstein & Robbins, 1984). In this chapter, falls have been divided into two major types of categories based on the underlying causes: those due to accidents and those due to illness and disease. Accidental falls occur as a result of intrinsic, age-related changes interacting with extrinsic or environmental factors. Other falls are due primarily to intrinsic factors, the symptoms of underlying pathology.

Accidents account for nearly one-half of all falls in the elderly. Major pathologic causes include syncope, drop attacks, dizziness or vertigo, orthostatic hypotension, central nervous system disorders, and drugs (Rubenstein & Robbins, 1984). The extent to which each of these pathologic entities contributes to the total number of falls is not known. A wide variation is seen in the percentages given for some of these causes—syncope (up to 50%) and drop attacks (12% to 25%) (Overstall, 1985b). Rubenstein and Robbins (1984) summarized the results of several studies on the causes of falls and found the following representative percentages: drop attacks (14%), vertigo/dizziness (11%), central nervous system disorders (7%), postural hypotension (4%), and miscellaneous causes (15%).

Accidental Falls: Slips and Trips

Slips, the sliding on or down a slippery surface, occur when environmental hazards go undetected and the older person fails to regain balance once equilibrium has been disturbed.

The condition of walking surfaces and shoes or slippers is the major extrinsic factor involved in slips. Wet, slippery, or highly polished surfaces are slip hazards. Objects such as pebbles, sand, food on the floor, and scatter rugs make walking areas unsafe. Some shoes, such as those with leather or plastic soles, are slippery on polished surfaces, as are stockings and socks. Table 14–3 summarizes the intrinsic and extrinsic causes of slips.

Table 14–3. CAUSES OF SLIPS

Intrinsic Causes
1. Inability to correct loss of balance secondary to:
   A. Increased reaction time and changes in posture and gait with a forward shift of center of gravity
   B. Pathologic conditions:
      (1) Neurologic dysfunction secondary to alcoholism, diabetes, Parkinson's disease
      (2) Musculoskeletal disorders: deconditioning, myopathy
2. Inability to see hazardous conditions due to changes in vision:
   A. Normal: loss of visual acuity, decrease in peripheral vision and depth perception, increased need for illumination, decreased tolerance for glare
   B. Pathologic: cataracts, glaucoma, diabetic retinopathy, macular degeneration, visual field defects from stroke

Extrinsic Causes
1. Walking with socks on slippery surfaces, such as linoleum, tile, and waxed floors
2. Leather- or plastic-soled shoes/slippers
3. Walking surfaces: wet, slippery, highly polished, and objects on surface, such as sand, pebbles, food, nails, scatter rugs; inadequate cues to differentiate surface of stairs from edge; shadows, glare, poor illumination on surface

Trips, that is, missteps or stumbles, are the result of environmental factors and changes in an older person's gait and vision. Those who trip are usually more posturally stable, less debilitated, and more active than those who fall for other reasons (Overstall, 1985b).

A number of extrinsic factors play a role in trips. Among these are uneven walking surfaces, eyeglasses with two and three corrections, clothing that is too loose and long, and shoes with high heels, no support, or loose fit. A frequent site for trips in the elderly is on stairs. Missteps occur when colors, edges, lines, patterns, and texture do not clearly define the parameters and condition of each step (Archea, 1985). Table 14–4 summarizes the factors associated with trips.

Pathologic Causes

Syncope. Falls in the elderly are frequently associated with syncope (Perry, 1982). Syncope is the "transient loss of consciousness, characterized by unresponsiveness and loss of

postural tone, with spontaneous recovery, not requiring specific resuscitation interventions" (Lipsitz, 1983a). It is caused by a momentary impairment of cerebral perfusion (Kapoor, Snustad, Peterson, et al., 1986). Syncope is a symptom of one or more age- and disease-related processes that impair cerebral perfusion. In 40% to 60% of older patients evaluated for syncope, no diagnosis is determined (Lipsitz, 1983a).

A number of age-related changes affect the compensatory mechanisms that maintain blood pressure and cerebral blood flow. There is a decrease in the sensitivity of the carotid sinus baroreceptors that maintain cerebral perfusion pressure by increasing heart rate and vascular tone in response to hypotension. The elderly are not able to compensate for a sudden drop in blood pressure caused by acute hemorrhage, volume shifts, or abrupt change from a recumbent to an upright position. The heart rate does not increase in response to hypoxia, hypercarbia, exercise, and upright posture (Lipsitz, 1983a). With age, there is a progressive decline in cerebral vasodilatation in response to hypoxia. In the presence of disease or drugs, syncope may be precipitated

Table 14–4. CAUSES OF TRIPS

Intrinsic Causes
1. Not lifting feet high enough secondary to:
   A. Alteration in posture and gait resulting from changes in bone, ligament, and joints
   B. Pathologic conditions, such as Parkinson's disease, stroke, and arthritis
2. Changes in visual acuity and depth perception due to:
   A. Normal changes in the lens, atrophy of the ciliary muscle, pupillary constriction
   B. Pathologic changes, such as cataracts, visual field defects from stroke, macular degeneration
3. Inattention or distraction while ambulating

Extrinsic Causes
1. Walking surfaces: uneven or cracked surfaces, curbs, objects on ground, unexpected changes in level or holes in ground, pets, electrical cords, rugs, patterns on floors, floor-mounted doorstop, shadows, glare, and/or poor illumination
2. Glasses with two or three corrections
3. Clothing too long or too loose
4. Shoes too loose, high heels, backless shoes, shoes with no support, rubber soles sticking to rugs/carpets

when the threshold for ischemic symptoms is reached (Lipsitz, 1985).

Age-related changes in the homeostatic mechanisms that control extracellular volume place the elderly at the risk for rapid volume depletion, drop in blood pressure, and falls. These changes include impairment in the sodium-conserving function of the kidney with the 30% to 50% reduction of plasma renin and aldosterone concentrations (Lipsitz, 1983a; 1985).

Types of Syncope. Approximately one-third of the cases of syncope occurring in the elderly have a cardiovascular cause (Kapoor, et al., 1986). Syncope occurs with cardiac conditions that abruptly or momentarily diminish cardiac output, such as aortic stenosis, mitral valve disease, myocardial infarction, cardiomyopathy, arrhythmias, heart block, and sick sinus syndrome (Kapoor, et al., 1986; Rubenstein, 1983).

A sudden drop in systemic blood pressure may occur with decreased cardiac output caused by the anatomical, myocardial, and electrical abnormalities listed above. Other causes of sudden hypotension include acute volume depletion as seen in hemorrhage, diuresis, third space loss, and dehydration. In these situations, volume depletion reaches a critical point at which the homeostatic mechanisms are not able to compensate to maintain blood pressure.

Carotid sinus hypersensitivity is an abnormality in reflex blood pressure regulation that may lead to syncope. It is defined as a sinus slowing of greater than 50% or systolic blood pressure decline of over 40 mm Hg during carotid sinus massage (Lipsitz, 1983a). Carotid sinus syncope can result from neck turning, a tight collar, and drugs such as digitalis, propranolol, and alpha-methyldopa (Lipsitz, 1983a).

Cough, swallow, micturition, and defecation syncopes are other forms resulting from reflex-mediated blood pressure instability in the older adult. Cough and defecation syncopes occur as a result of the Valsalva maneuver, where cardiac output is diminished by impeded venous return, peripheral vasodilatation is produced by raised intrathoracic pressure that stimulates the baroreceptors, and reduced cerebral perfusion is caused by increases in cerebral spinal fluid and intracranial pressures (Wollner & Spalding, 1985; Lipsitz, 1983a). Hypotension and the decrease in cerebral perfusion cause syncope.

Micturition syncope occurs typically at night with the rapid emptying of a full bladder causing reflex vasodilatation in combination with the sudden assumption of an upright position and peripheral vasodilatation from the warmth of the bed (Lipsitz, 1983a).

Unexplained syncope in the elderly is commonly thought to be vasovagal syncope. It is associated with painful or unpleasant experiences, such as surgery, trauma, hunger, fatigue, and crowding. The person exhibits weakness, pallor, nausea, sweating, sighing, and other signs of intense autonomic nervous system stimulation. Relief from these symptoms occurs when the person lies down. Physiologically, there is a fight or flee type of response, with a sudden increase in heart rate, blood pressure, total systemic resistance, and cardiac output. This phase is quickly followed by peripheral vasodilatation, increase in muscle blood flow, and decrease in venous return to the heart. In the elderly, age-related impairment in cardioacceleration, vasoconstriction, and renin release leads to a fall in blood pressure and decrease in cerebral perfusion (Lipsitz, 1983a).

Consciousness also depends on normal blood composition providing adequate levels of glucose and oxygen to maintain cerebral metabolism. Syncope may occur with anemia and hypoglycemia as well as with respiratory disorders that affect oxygenation, such as acute respiratory failure (Kane, et al., 1984; Lipsitz, 1983a).

In the presence of arteriosclerotic narrowing of the carotid and vertebral arteries, movements of the head may be sufficient to compress the arteries and cause a transient disruption of blood flow to the brain. Falls can occur when lateral head movements compress the carotid arteries or extension of the head compresses the vertebral arteries (Rodstein, 1983).

The onset of a seizure may present as syncope, or syncope may be associated with other seizure-causing disorders. The temporary cessation of cerebral blood flow is caused by tonic-clonic seizure activity (Lipsitz, 1983a).

In a clinical study on syncope, Lipsitz (1985) noted that a disproportionate number of syncopal episodes and falls occurred after a meal. In a followup study, postprandial hypotension, with an average systolic blood pressure fall of 25 mm Hg within 35 minutes after the meal, was noted in one-third of the elderly subjects. The exact mechanism for this reduction in blood pressure is not known, but it is thought to be caused by the hypotensive effect of splanchnic pooling during digestion with inadequate baroreflex compensation (Lipsitz, 1985).

Drop Attacks. Drop attack is a condition described frequently in the British literature and less frequently in the United States. It is unclear whether the drop attack is a separate entity or a symptom of a spectrum of diseases (Lipsitz, 1983b; Cape, 1986). In drop attacks, an older person experiences a sudden buckling of the legs while standing or walking, often after a sudden turn of the head or neck. Loss of consciousness does not occur (Farquharson, 1985). The older person experiences difficulty getting up after a drop attack because of the loss of strength and muscle tone in the legs and trunk. The completely flaccid state of the antigravity muscles may last for several hours. This condition is reported to be totally reversed by putting pressure on the soles of the feet (Lipsitz, 1983b; Pathy, 1985).

As described in the British literature, drop attack is a common, potentially dangerous symptom in the elderly population. Drop attacks increase with age and account for nearly one-quarter of all falls of persons over 85 years of age (Lipsitz, 1983b; Sheldon, 1960). They tend to recur and are unpredictable (Farquharson, 1985). No single explanation exists for drop attacks. A possible underlying cause is believed to be brainstem ischemia resulting from a temporary reduction in vertebrobasilar blood flow or brainstem oxygenation (Lipsitz, 1983b; Pathy, 1985). Conditions that affect blood flow and oxygenation include vertebrobasilar artery insufficiency, structural lesions, and carotid sinus hypersensitivity (Lipsitz,

1983b; Rodstein, 1983b). Contributing factors that are treatable and potentially reversible include anemia, hypoxemia, postural hypotension, arrhythmias, carotid sinus hypersensitivity, and cervical spondylosis (Lipsitz, 1983b). Overstall (1985b) postulates that drop attacks are due to a variety of postural defects rather than a single cause. Possible causes include false interpretation of visual stimulation not corrected by postural feedback, as well as transient and minor physical illness, drug side effects, and psychological upsets (Farquharson, 1985; Overstall, 1985b).

Dizziness or Vertigo. A common complaint of the elderly is dizziness, an abnormal sensation or feeling of imbalance (Ross & Robinson, 1984). It is produced by disturbances in the sensory modalities that provide information on body position and movement. Sensory modalities involved are vision, hearing, vestibular sensation, point-position sense, and touch-pressure sensation (Ross & Robinson, 1984).

Types of Dizziness. Ross and Robinson (1984) identified four common types of dizziness that are due to pathologic conditions. The disequilibrium type of dizziness is caused by neurologic deficits found in patients with Alzheimer's or Parkinson's disease. There is unsteadiness, imbalance, and instability causing problems with walking. In the second type, characterized by an impending faint or a brief loss of consciousness (syncope), the underlying cause is usually a cardiovascular or neurologic condition (discussed earlier in this chapter). The third type is lightheadedness caused by multisensory deficits, anxiety with hyperventilation, and chronic systemic disease. Vertigo, the sensation of rotating in space or spinning, is the fourth type of dizziness. Labyrinthine disturbance due to disease or drug toxicity, rare tumors at the cerebellopontine angle, transient ischemic attacks, and cerebrovascular disease with vascular insufficiency affecting the vestibular nuclei in the brainstem are conditions that may produce vertigo (Kane, et al., 1984; Ross & Robinson, 1984).

Benign positional vertigo is the most common form of vertigo. It is a disorder of the peripheral vestibular system causing hypersensitivity to changes in head position. The duration of the illness is self-limited, lasting for 6 to 8 weeks. The main symptoms are vertigo and nystagmus, the involuntary rhythmic, oscillating movements of the eye. The symptoms usually are paroxysmal, last less than 1 minute, and occur when the head position is turned to the side with the affected ear down (Paulson, 1983; Ross & Robinson, 1984).

Postural or Orthostatic Hypotension. Postural or orthostatic hypotension is found in 30% of the community-dwelling elderly. Its prevalence increases with advanced age and higher basal blood pressure (Lipsitz, 1985). In orthostatic hypotension, there is a drop of 20 mm Hg or more in systolic blood pressure 2 minutes after assuming a standing, upright position (Farquharson, 1985). This transient drop in blood pressure results in underperfusion of the brain, and it is believed to be the cause of many falls by the elderly. Age-related changes in the mechanisms responsible for maintaining adequate blood pressure for cerebral perfusion include a decline in baroreflex sensitivity, progressive decline in cerebral blood flow, and abnormality in excellular volume regulation (Lipsitz, 1985). Orthostatic hypotension is also seen with prolonged inactivity; drugs such as antihypertensives, vasodilators, phenothiazines, and tricyclic antidepressants; central nervous system disorders such as Parkinson's disease, myelopathy, brainstem lesions, and multiple cerebral infarcts; and peripheral and autonomic neuropathies seen in diabetes and alcoholism. In the absence of another cause, orthostatic hypotension may be primary or idiopathic (Kane, et al., 1984; Lipsitz, 1983a).

Central Nervous System Disorders. Falls are caused by gait disturbances, dizziness, and syncope associated with a number of central nervous system diseases. Cerebrovascular diseases (transient ischemic attack, stroke), Parkinson's disease, normal-pressure hydrocephalus, and seizure disorders are neurologic conditions commonly related to falls in the elderly. Cerebellar disorders, lesions, and trauma may also cause instability and falls

(Kane et al., 1984; Rubenstein & Robbins, 1984). Cognitive slowing is an important risk factor in falls. In one study, three times as many individuals diagnosed with severe dementia of Alzheimer's type fell as those who were cognitively healthy (Morris, Rubin, Morris, & Mandel, 1987).

Senile gait disorder is diagnosed when no specific pathogenesis can be found to explain a gait problem. Patients complain that they are weak, unsteady, or afraid of falling (Sabin, 1982). In senile gait disorder, the gait abnormalities are varied and may include dysrhythmic gait with shortened steps, diminished arm swing, difficulty initiating steps, unsteady turns, and disturbances in equilibrium with a tendency toward falling (Koller, et al., 1985; Nutt, 1984). Cerebellar disease, normal-pressure hydrocephalus, or extrapyramidal dysfunction are just some of the many possible underlying causes (Koller, et al., 1985).

Drugs. Polypharmacy is common among the elderly, and drug interactions and adverse reactions are likely to occur. The odds of falling increases when three or more drugs are taken (Granek, Baker, Abbey, et al., 1987; Kalchthaler, Bascom, & Quintos, 1978; McDonald, 1985; Tinetti, et al., 1986). Sedatives, hypnotics, tricyclic antidepressants, nonsteroidal antiinflammatory drugs, analgesics, and diuretics have been associated with increased falls in the elderly (Granek, et al., 1987; Kane, et al., 1984; Louis, 1983; MacDonald, 1985; Sobel & McCart, 1983). The adverse effects of these drugs include sedation, dizziness, blurred vision, confusion, vertigo, ataxia, arrhythmias, orthostatic hypotension, and syncope. While drugs are thought to increase the probability of falls, they do not appear to be the singular cause for falls (Nickens, 1985; Tinetti, et al., 1986).

Alcohol abuse is an underreported problem and should be considered as a possible cause of instability and falls in old people (Rubenstein & Robbins, 1984). Increased sway was found to occur with alcohol consumption in the young population, and it is believed likewise to cause increased sway in the older population. The factor of sway in the presence of physical illness and age-related changes in vision and proprioception increases the risk of falls (MacDonald, 1985).

SUMMARY

Falls are a major concern among the elderly and those caring for them. Falls have potentially serious consequences, such as fractures, hospitalization, surgery, decreased mobility, prolonged recovery, disability, and long-term care at home or in a nursing home. They can decrease the quality and length of life. Age-associated changes, pathologic conditions, and environmental factors affecting stability, mobility, and cognitive function cause older people to fall. All falls have a cause and many are preventable; careful investigation into the cause is critical to prevent future occurrences.

References

Archea, JC (1985): Environmental factors associated with stair accidents by the elderly. *Clin Geriatr Med*, 1:555–569.

Ashley, MJ, Gryfe, CI, & Amies, A (1977): A longitudinal study of falls in an elderly population. II: Some circumstances of falling. *Age Ageing*, 6:211–220.

Baker, SP, & Harvey, AH (1985): Fall injuries in the elderly. *Clin Geriatr Med*, 1:501–512.

Barbieri, E (1983): Patient falls are not patient accidents. *J Gerontol Nurs*, 9:167–173.

Barnes, DM (1987): New leads in osteoporosis. *Science*, 236:915.

Bellantoni, MF, & Blackman, MR (1988): Osteoporosis: Diagnostic screening and its place in current care. *Geriatrics*, 43:63–70.

Benton, KGF, & Strouthides, TM (1985): After the fall. *In* Kataria, MS (ed): *Fits, Faints and Falls in Old Age*. Hingham, MA, Kluwer Academic Publishers, 109–131.

Berry, G, Fisher, RH, & Lang, S (1981): Detrimental incidences, including falls, in an elderly institutional population. *J Am Geriatr Soc*, 29:322–324.

Bright, MI, Minny, LM, Ratsey, GM, et al. (1983): Patients who fall in hospitals: Contributing factors. *Curationis*, 6:52–54.

Brown, B (1983): Study of patient falls in a small busy medical center. *Crit Care Update*, 18:163–166.

Cape, RDT (1986): Falls. *In* Rossman, I (ed): *Clinical Geriatrics*. Philadelphia, JB Lippincott, 683–692.

Catchen, H (1983): Repeaters: Inpatient accidents among the hospitalized elderly. *Gerontologist*, 23:273–276.

Cummings, SR, Nevitt, MC, & Kidd, S (1988): Forgetting falls. The limited accuracy of recall of falls in the elderly. *J Am Geriatr Soc*, 36:613–616.

Das, SK, & Kataria, MS (1985): Stability, movement and posture. *In* Kataria, MS (ed): *Fits, Faints and Falls in Old Age*. Hingham, MA, Kluwer Academic Publishers, 11–13.

DeVito, CA, Lambert, DA, Saffin, RW, et al. (1988): Fall injuries among the elderly: Community-based surveillance. *J Am Geriatr Soc*, 36:1029–1035.

Elnicki, P, & Schmitt, JP (1980): Contributions of patient and hospital characteristics to adverse patient incidents. *Health Serv Res*, 15:397–414.

Farquharson, AJD (1985): Falls in old age: Clinical aspects. *In* Kataria, MS (ed): *Fits, Faints and Falls in Old Age*. Hingham, MA, Kluwer Academic Publishers, 27–43.

Gibbs, J (1982): Bed area falls: A recent report. *Austral Nurs J*, 11:34–37.

Gordon, M, Huang, M, & Gryfe, C (1982): An evaluation of falls, syncope and dizziness by prolonged cardiac monitoring in a geriatric institutional setting. *J Am Geriatr Soc*, 30:6–12.

Granek, E, Baker, SP, Abbey, H, et al. (1987): Medications and diagnoses in relation to falls in a long-term care facility. *J Am Geriatr Soc*, 35:503–511.

Gryfe, CI, Amies, A, & Ashley, MJ (1977): A longitudinal study of falls in an elderly population: Incidence and morbidity. *Age Ageing*, 6:201–210.

Guimarues, RM, & Isaacs, B (1980): Characteristics of gait in old people who fall. *Int Rehabil Med*, 2:177–180.

Hogue, CC (1984): Falls and mobility in late life: An ecological model. *J Am Geriatr Soc*, 32:858–861.

Innes, E, & Turman, W (1983): Evaluation of patient's falls. *Quality Rev Bull*, 9:30–35.

Isaacs, B (1982): *The Clinical Aspects of Falling*. Nutley, NJ, Roche Laboratories.

Isaacs, B (1985): Gait and balance. *In* Pathy, MSJ (ed): *Principles and Practice of Geriatric Medicine*. New York, John Wiley & Sons, 695–699.

Johnson, ET (1985): Accidental falls among geriatric patients: Can more be prevented? *J Natl Med Assoc*, 77:633–639.

Kalchthaler, T, Bascom, RA, & Quintos, V (1978): Falls in the institutionalized elderly. *J Am Geriatr Soc*, 26:424–428.

Kane, RL, Ouslander, JG, & Abrass, IB (1984): *Essentials of Clinical Geriatrics*. New York, McGraw-Hill, 137–151.

Kapoor, W, Snustad, D, Peterson, J, et al. (1986): Syncope in the elderly. *Am J Med*, 80:419–428.

Kenshalo, DR (1977): Age changes in touch, vibration, temperature, kinesthesis, and pain sensitivity. *In* Birren, JE, & Schaie, KW (eds): *Handbook of the Psychology of Aging*. New York, Van Nostrand Reinhold, 562–579.

Kenshalo, DR (1986): Somesthetic sensitivity in young and elderly humans. *J Gerontol*, 41:732–742.

Kline, DW, & Schieber, F (1985): Vision and aging. *In* Birren, JE, Schaie, KW (eds): *Handbook of the Psychology of Aging* (ed 2). New York, Van Nostrand Reinhold, 296–331.

Koller, WC, Glatt, SL, & Fox, JH (1985): Senile gait: A distinct entity. *Clin Geriatr Med*, 1:661–669.

Kulikowski, ES (1979): A study of accidents in a hospital. *Supervisory Nurse*, 10:44–58.

Lee, RG (1979): Health and safety in hospitals. *Med Sci Law*, 29:89–103.

Leibowitz, HW, & Shupert, CL (1985): Spatial orientation mechanisms and their implications for falls. *Clin Geriatr Med*, 1:571–580.

Lichenstein, MJ, Shields, SL, Shiavi, RG, et al. (1988): Clinical determinants of biomechanics platform measures of balance in aged women. *J Am Geriatr Soc*, 36:996–1002.

Lipsitz, LA (1983a): Syncope in the elderly. *Ann Intern Med*, 99:92–105.

Lipsitz, LA (1983b): The drop attack: A common geriatric symptom. *J Am Geriatr Soc*, 31:617–620.

Lipsitz, LA (1985): Abnormalities in blood pressure homeostasis that contribute to falls in the elderly. *Clin Geriatr Med*, 1:637–648.

Louis, M (1983): Falls and their causes. *J Gerontol Nurs*, 9:142–149.

MacDonald, JB (1985): The role of drugs in falls in the elderly. *Clin Geriatr Med*, 1:621–636.

MacDonald, JB, & MacDonald, ET (1977): Nocturnal femoral fracture and continuing widespread use of barbiturate hypnotics. *Br Med J*, 2:483–484.

Marsh, GR (1980): Perceptual changes with aging. *In* Busse, EW, Blazer, DG (eds): *Handbook of Geriatric Psychiatry*. New York, Van Nostrand Reinhold, 147–168.

Melton, LJ, & Riggs, BL (1985): Risk factors for injury after a fall. *Clin Geriatr Med*, 1:525–539.

Morris, EV, & Isaacs, B (1980): The prevention of falls in a geriatric hospital. *Age Ageing*, 9:181–185.

Morris, JC, Rubin, EH, Morris, EJ, et al. (1987): Senile dementia of the Alzheimer's type: An important risk factor for serious falls. *J Gerontol*, 42:412–417.

Morse, JM, Tylko, SJ, & Dixon, HA (1987): Characteristics of the fall-prone patient. *Gerontologist*, 27:516–522.

Mossey, J (1985): Social and psychologic factors related to falls among the elderly. *Clin Geriatr Med*, 1:541–553.

Murphey, M, & Myers, JE (1982): Visual and multiple impairments in older persons. *In* Hull, RH (ed): *Rehabilitation Audiology*. New York, Grune & Stratton, 271–281.

Nickens, H (1985): Intrinsic factors in falling among the elderly. *Arch Intern Med*, 145:1089–1093.

Nutt, JG (1984): Abnormalities of posture and movement. *In* Cassel, CK, & Walsh, JR (eds): *Geriatric Medicine*. Vol. I. New York, Springer-Verlag, 50–60.

Ochs, AL, Newberry, J, Lenhardt, ML, et al. (1985): Neural and vestibular aging associated with falls. *In* Birren, JE, & Schaie, KW (eds): *Handbook of the Psychology of Aging* (ed 2). New York, Van Nostrand Reinhold, 378–399.

Overstall, PW (1980): Prevention of falls in the elderly. *J Am Geriatr Soc*, 28:481–484.

Overstall, PW (1985a): Epidemiology and pathophysiology of falls. *In* Kataria, MS (ed): *Fits, Faints and Falls in Old Age*. Hingham, MA, Kluwer Academic Publishers, 15–26.

Overstall, PW (1985b): Falls. *In* Pathy, MSJ (ed): *Principles and Practice of Geriatric Medicine*. New York, John Wiley & Sons, 701–709.

Overstall, PW, Exton-Smith, AN, Imms, FJ, et al. (1977):

Falls in the elderly related to postural imbalance. *Br Med J*, 1:261–264.

Pastalan, LA (1982): Environmental design and adaptation to the visual environment of the elderly. *In* Sekular, R, Kline, D, & Dismukes, K (eds): *Aging and Human Visual Function*. New York, Alan R Liss, 323–333.

Pathy, MSJ (1985): Clinical presentation and management of neurological disorders in old age. *In* Brocklehurst, JC (ed): *Textbook of Geriatric Medicine and Gerontology* (ed 3). London, Churchill Livingstone, 391–426.

Paulson, GW (1983): Disorders of the central nervous system in the aged. *Med Clin North Am*, 67:345–359.

Perry, BC (1982): Falls among the elderly: A review of the methods and conclusions of epidemiologic studies. *J Am Geriatr Soc*, 30:367–371.

Prudham, D, & Evans, JG (1981): Factors associated with falls in the elderly: A community study. *Age Ageing*, 10:141–146.

Riggs, BL, & Melton, LJ (1986): Involutional osteoporosis. *N Engl J Med*, 314:1676–1686.

Rodstein, M (1983a): Accidents among the aged. *In* Reichel, W (ed): *Clinical Aspects of Aging* (ed 2). Baltimore, Williams & Wilkins, 600–614.

Rodstein, M (1983b): Falls by the aged. *In* Cape, RDT, Coe, RM, & Rossman, I (eds): *Fundamentals of Geriatric Medicine*. New York, Raven Press, 105–116.

Ross, V, & Robinson, B (1984): Dizziness: Causes, prevention and management. *Geriatr Nurs*, 5:289–304.

Rubenstein, LZ (1983): Falls in the elderly: A clinical approach. *West J Med*, 138:273–275.

Rubenstein, LZ, & Robbins, AS (1984): Falls in the elderly: A clinical perspective. *Geriatrics*, 39:67–71, 75–76, 78.

Sabin, TD (1982): Biologic aspects of falls and mobility limitations in the elderly. *J Am Geriatr Soc*, 30:51–58.

Sehested, P, & Severin-Nielson, T (1977): Falls by hospitalized elderly patients: Causes and prevention. *Geriatrics*, 32:101–108.

Sheldon, JH (1960): On the natural history of falls in old age. *Br Med J*, 2:1685–1690.

Silverberg, SJ, & Lindsay, R (1987): Postmenopausal osteoporosis. *Med Clin North Am*, 71:41–57.

Smith, R (1987): Osteoporosis: Cause and management. *Br Med J*, 294:329–332.

Sobel, K, & McCart, G (1983): Drug use and accidental falls in an intermediate care facility. *Drug Intell Clin Pharm*, 17:539–542.

Spellbring, AM, Gannon, ME, Klecker, T, et al.: Improving safety for hospitalized elderly. *J Gerontol Nurs*, 14:31–37.

Swartzbeck, E (1983): The problem of falls in the elderly. *Nurs Management*, 13:34–38.

Swartzbeck, E, & Milligan, WL (1982): A comparative study of hospital incidents. *Nurs Management*, 12:39–43.

Tinetti, ME, Williams, TF, & Mayewski, R (1986): Fall risk index for elderly patients based on number of chronic disabilities. *Am J Med*, 80:429–434.

US Department of Commerce, Bureau of the Census (1985): *Statistical Abstract of the United States 1985* (ed 105). Washington, DC, US Government Printing Office, 74–75.

Walshe, A, & Rosen, H (1979): A study of patient falls from bed. *J Nurs Admin*, 9:31–43.

Watkins, JS, & Robson, P (1981): The hazards of rehabilitation. *Ann R Coll Surg Engl, 63:*386–389.

Wolfson, LI, Whipple, R, Amerman, P, et al (1985): Gait and balance in the elderly: Two functional capacities that link sensory and motor ability to falls. *Clin Geriatr Med, 1:*649–659.

Wollner, L, & Spalding, JMK (1985): The autonomic nervous system. *In* Brocklehurst, JC (ed): *Textbook of Geriatric Medicine and Gerontology* (ed 3). London, Churchill Livingstone, 449–473.

Wong, S, Glennis, K, Muise, M, et al. (1981): An exploration of environmental variables and patient falls. *Dimens Health Serv, 58:*9–11.

CHAPTER
15

Preventing Falls

W. CAROLE CHENITZ, R.N., Ed.D.
HEATHER L. KUSSMAN, R.N.C., M.P.A.
JOYCE TAKANO STONE, R.N.C., M.S.

In this chapter, attention shifts from the causes and the nature of falls (Chapter 14) to preventing them.

EDUCATION AS PREVENTION

The basis of all prevention is to provide the older person and the caregivers, including nursing staff, with information on ways to prevent a fall (Gray-Vickrey, 1984). Prevention techniques for falls are the same, regardless of the type of fall. The educational approach to fall prevention advocated here will require modification from setting to setting. In community settings, nurses may consider instituting fall prevention classes or may conduct informal fall education sessions in the home during routine visits. In hospitals and long-term care settings, one-to-one teaching follows assessment, and assessment requires staff education and awareness. Prevention techniques are presented here for elders at home and in hospitals and other health care institutions. Table 15–1 provides a list that can be given to the client and used as a teaching guide.

Exercise

Tinetti, Speechley, and Ginter (1988) conducted a 1-year prospective study of 336 el-

INTRODUCTION

Falls are the result of intrinsic and extrinsic factors and the interplay between them. Falls are multicausal and require a multifocal approach to prevention (Tinetti & Speechley, 1989). A multifocal approach includes identification and modification of intrinsic and extrinsic factors, along with patient and caregiver education.

Table 15–1. FALL-PREVENTION GUIDELINES FOR THE HOME

Lights and Lighting

1. Eyes tire quickly in improper lighting. Illuminate reading material or the object worked on. Illuminate steps, entranceways, and rooms before entering. Use 70- or 100-watt bulbs, not 60-watt bulbs.
2. Avoid glaring light caused by highly polished floors or large expanses of uncovered glass. Use sunglasses to avoid the glare of highway driving, but use light tints or photoray lenses.
3. Allow more time to adjust to changes in light levels. When going from a dark to a light room or vice versa, allow a minute or two for the eyes to accommodate to the change in light before proceeding.
4. Dirty glasses or outgrown prescription lenses inhibit vision. Keep glasses clean. Have regular eye examinations to identify changes and to get new glasses when needed. If possible, do not use bifocals when walking because you cannot see the ground clearly.
5. Ability to see up, down, and sideways decreases with age. Observe the "lay of the land"; learn to look ahead at the ground to spot and avoid hazards such as cracks in the sidewalks. Use canes, walking sticks, and walkers that are prescribed.
6. At night, keep a nightlight on in your bedroom and bathroom. When getting out of bed at night, put the light on and wait a minute or two for the eyes to adjust before getting up. Have a telephone in the bedroom so you don't have to get out of bed to answer the phone. Before you go out in the evening or late afternoon, turn a light on for your return.

Activity

1. Get up from a chair slowly.
2. When getting out of bed, sit up, then wait a minute or two. Move to the side of the bed and wait another minute. Rise after you have sat for a few minutes.
3. If you are dizzy, sit down immediately. Sit on a step or a chair, or ease yourself to the sidewalk if you are outdoors.
4. Avoid tipping the head backward (extending the neck). Activities to avoid that extend the neck are washing windows, hanging clothes, and getting things from high shelves.
5. Use shelves at eye level. Avoid rapid turning of the head.
6. If weather is rainy and windy, avoid going out.
7. Use alcohol and tranquilizers with caution.
8. Exercise programs keep bodies limber. Consult your physician and then enroll in a senior exercise program.
9. Shoes and slippers should be flat and rubber-soled. Avoid clothing such as long robes and loose-fitting garments that may catch on furniture or door knobs.

Around the House

1. Avoid scatter rugs and small bathroom mats that can slide. Repair loose, torn, wrinkled, or worn carpet.
2. Avoid slick, high polish on floors.
3. Put things in easy reach, and avoid reaching to high shelves.
4. Use nonskid treads on stairs and nonskid mats in tub.
5. May wish to install a grab rail in the bath, shower, and also by the toilet.
6. Install handrails on both sides of the stairs. Paint stair edge in bright contrasting color.
7. Remove door thresholds.
8. Remove low-lying objects, such as coffee tables and extension cords.
9. Wipe up spills immediately.
10. Watch for pets underfoot and scattered pet food.
11. Check for even, nonglare lighting in every room, with easily accessible light switches.
12. Avoid floor coverings with complex patterns.
13. Avoid clutter in living areas.
14. Select furniture that provides stability and support, such as chairs with arms.
15. Check walking aids routinely, such as rubber tips on canes and screws on walkers.

derly people living in the community. During the study period, 32%, or 108 people, fell at least once. Of those who fell, 26 people, or 24%, sustained a serious injury as the result of the fall. Fifty-two of the 108 people who fell, or 48%, reported that they were afraid of falling again, and 28, or 26%, had reduced their activities because they were afraid of falling. The researchers concluded that the risk of falling increased with the number of risk factors present, that is, a fall may result from multiple disabilities. Therefore, the risk for falling can be reduced by modifying risk factors. The goal to prevent and reduce falls is focused on identifying and modifying fall risk factors, increasing stability, and decreasing environmental risks.

Exercise and good general health practices are measures to increase stability and prevent falls in the elderly, although no data exist to support this (Isaacs, 1985). A plan of activity and exercise will help to maintain general limberness, muscle strength, balance, and co-ordination. If health problems occur, proper diagnosis and treatment are essential to prevent complications and disability.

Exercise classes designed for older persons are recommended to improve overall health and stimulate physical, mental and social well-being. Exercise stimulates cardiopulmonary, musculoskeletal, and nervous system functioning, which results in increased alertness, muscle strength, coordination, flexibility, and range of motion. Exercise also increases endurance, confidence, and a sense of well-being (O'Hara-Deveraux, Andrus, & Scott, 1981).

Walking is one of the safest and most popular forms of exercise. Walking in covered shopping malls, individually or in small groups, is becoming a popular way to exercise and avoid weather problems. Other forms of exercise, such as jogging, hiking, swimming, and bicycling, are also enjoyed by older adults. However, a careful assessment and evaluation should be made before the more rigorous forms of exercise are attempted. The elements of an effective exercise program include correct exercise prescription, stepwise progression, adequate supervision, and continuity (Tinetti, 1986). (See Chapter 11, Immobility.)

Disturbances in Equilibrium Related to Aging Changes

To prevent falls, the older person should be taught to move slowly and to avoid any sudden changes in position (Kostopoulos, 1985). Abrupt movements of the head may precipitate syncope and a fall. This can happen when reaching to wash windows, to reach objects on high shelves, to hang up laundry, or during any activity involving tipping the head backward while reaching and stretching upward.

If lying in bed, the person should sit up, wait, then move to the side of the bed and wait again to prevent orthostatic hypotension. If dizziness occurs, the person should ease to a sitting or lying position.

Footgear, Clothing, and Walking Aids

Properly fitting shoes and slippers are important. They should be rubber-soled and even-heeled. Foot problems that cause discomfort should be treated. Long robes, long slacks or trousers, and loose, poorly fitting clothing that can be tripped over or caught on furniture and doorknobs should not be worn (Sehested & Severin-Nielson, 1977).

Walking aids are frequently self-prescribed or given to the person by friends or family members. Each device needs to be a size and type appropriate to the individual's needs. Older people who have hand-me-down canes or walkers may not have received instructions on their use. In such cases, physical therapy consultation may be very useful (Brummel-Smith, Kottke, & Williams, 1988).

Adjusting to Changes in Vision

A safety precaution that should be mentioned to the older person is allowing the eyes to adjust to changes in light level. The older client should be instructed to put the light on when getting up at night and wait a minute or two for the eyes to adjust before getting out of bed. The same rule applies when turning on the light in any room, and especially when using the stairs. A few minutes should also be allowed for the eyes to adjust before walking across a room or hallway, descending or ascending the stairs, or going between indoor and outdoor areas. This allows the eye to accommodate to changes in light, which enables the person to see objects or obstacles on the floor or ground.

Daytime falls that occur in adequately lit areas may be due to changes in peripheral vision. This ability to see up, down, and out of the corners of the eyes prevents stumbling over cracks in the sidewalk, driveway dips, curbs, and that last step in a flight of stairs. Not seeing the ground in proper focus also can be a problem for people who wear bifocals. It will help to have a second pair of glasses with only one correction, that is, for near-sightedness, for outdoor use. Using a cane or walker can help to maintain balance and provides a warning that the ground is uneven or there is a break in the sidewalk.

Dealing with the Environment

Aside from the normal physiologic changes that occur in all people, there are extrinsic or environmental factors that should be taken into account in any discussion of fall prevention. Weather and other geographic conditions are important considerations. When there is rain, snow, ice, or strong winds, older persons should be advised to stay indoors. Many people have arrangements with local grocers or friends to have groceries brought in during winter months or during bad weather. In addition, many pharmacies will deliver prescription medication.

A safe home environment can be maintained by securing the edges on rugs, removing scatter rugs, and paying special attention to furniture placement. Spills should be wiped up immediately and hallways kept free of obstacles. The use of handrails and nonskid material on the stairs and in the bathroom will help keep the older person from losing balance and falling. Any change in the personal environment should be made only after discussion with the elderly person. What may be considered dangerous clutter to caregivers may be familiar, safe furnishings and keepsakes for the older person (Dawson, 1983).

Nightlights are an inexpensive means to decrease nighttime falling at home. They should be used throughout the home, particularly to light the way between the bedroom and the bathroom, the kitchen, and the phone. Readily available in supermarkets and hardware stores, nightlights are inexpensive to use. Moving the telephone or an extension phone

into the bedroom can prevent falls that frequently occur when a person jumps out of bed or runs through a darkened house to answer a ringing telephone (Brummel-Smith, et al., 1988; Dawson, 1983; Lipsitz, 1988; Tinetti & Speechley, 1989).

The hospital and nursing home environment may be hazardous for an older person. The high level of activity, the constant movement of people, and the background noise and equipment in the halls can be disconcerting and may lead to collisions. Highly polished floors, lighting too dim or too bright, spills and splashes, unlocked wheels on tables and beds, and the clutter of special equipment in a small patient unit pose additional dangers. Constant surveillance and correction of environmental hazards are necessary to provide a safe and secure environment for the older patient (Sehested & Severin-Nielson, 1977; Spellbring, Gannon, Kleckner, et al., 1988).

ASSESSMENT FOR FALL PREVENTION IN THE HOSPITAL AND NURSING HOME

The patient must be assessed for risk in order to prevent falls; that is, fall risk may be part of the initial and ongoing nursing assessment (Rowland & Rowland, 1987). Ongoing assessments depend upon changes in patient condition. In long-term care, Johnson (1985) recommends yearly evaluations; however, this may not be frequent enough to account for changes. Assessment at the time of admission to determine risk level should include an exploration of previous falls. This includes the patient's thoughts on the cause of the fall(s), symptoms associated with the fall(s), and the circumstances surrounding the fall(s), such as location and time.

Other questions include: What happened after the fall(s)? Was there loss of consciousness? Was the person able to get up after the fall(s)? Assessment includes inquiring about current neurologic, cardiovascular, or musculoskeletal problems and medications, especially hypnotics, sedatives, tranquilizers, hypotensive drugs, and alcohol. Gait, posture, and postural sway when standing unsupported, and ability to transfer should be observed. If the person uses any ambulatory aids, how well does he or she manage to use them? When and how was the walking aid obtained? Other areas to check include inquiry into normal toileting schedule: Does the person normally get up several times during the night to go to the bathroom? The information that the nurse can glean about the person's patterns and routines may prove helpful in working with the patient and family in preventing future falls or in minimizing injury from a fall.

Assessment must be done continuously throughout hospitalization and nursing home stay because the patient's condition will change over time (Innes & Turman, 1983). The nursing care plan should indicate the potential fall risk and the nursing measures to be taken. Interventions include orienting the older person to the new, unfamiliar environment. The cooperation of the patient and the family is sought to maintain safety precautions. The patient's cooperation should be sought for staying in bed until help arrives or moving slowly from a recumbent to a sitting or standing position. Older patients should be encouraged to achieve the maximal level of activity that they are able to do within the bounds of safety.

Deconditioning, the loss of strength and coordination, can increase the risk of falls. It may be helpful to make an early referral to physical therapy for exercises to maintain muscle strength and balance, for gait assessment, for proper gait training, and for proper prescription and instruction for the use of ambulation aids, such as canes and walkers. An older person may benefit from instruction on how to get in and out of bed or chair when weakness or paralysis is present. In addition to instruction on how to prevent falls, an older person and his or her family should be taught what to do in case of a fall. Physical therapy has helped many older patients to overcome their fear of falling, develop a sense of confidence, and improve their gait.

In the effort to prevent falls, there is a general tendency to use physical restraints and medications to sedate or tranquilize the pa-

tient. Restraints and siderails are not as effective as previously believed. Yet, most hospitals have clearly written policies supporting these measures. In one study conducted in a hospital, 41% of the falls from bed occurred with both siderails raised, and 67% of the patients who fell had been restrained. In 37% of falls from chairs and 60% of falls from wheelchairs, the patients were restrained (Innes & Turman, 1983). In Denmark and England, where the incidence of falls is low, restaints and medications are used only in extreme cases. To prevent falls, patients are moved to where they can be observed or a bell is tied to the siderails so that movement by the patient signals a warning (Kane & Kane, 1976; Kayser-Jones, 1981).

Various types of fall monitoring devices, such as a movement-stimulated alarm band, are available. One device, called the Ambularm, is attached to the thigh of a patient in bed. An intermittent sound is emitted if the leg changes position to one that would allow leaving the bed. This lightweight, battery-operated device has met with some success in acute-care settings (Alert Care, Inc, 1988; Widder, 1985). Figure 15–1 shows the Ambularm.

Another device, called Bed-Check, consists of an alarm and a "sensormat." The unit can

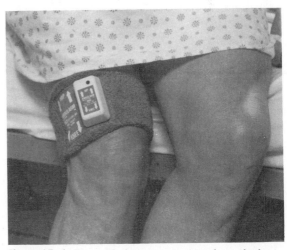

Figure 15–1. The Ambularm is worn just above the knee. The alarm is activated when the patient moves this leg to a vertical position. (Used with permission from AlertCare, Mill Valley, California.)

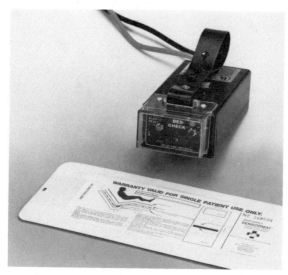

Figure 15–2. Bed-Check system. (Used with permission from Bed-Check Corp., Tulsa, Oklahoma.)

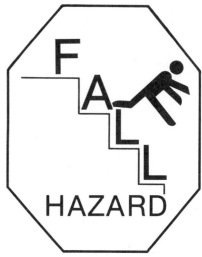

Figure 15–3. Safety alert sticker. The safety alert sticker is designed to signal all staff that this patient is at high risk to fall. It can be placed on the patient's chart or care plan or affixed at the patient's bedside. (Redrawn from Spellbring, AM, et al: Improving safety for hospitalized elderly. J Gerontol Nurs, *14*:36, 1988. With permission.)

be linked to the call light system or can transmit directly to the nurses' station. The sensormat is placed under the patient's hips, and the alarm sounds when the weight is lifted off the sensormat. Again, this device has met with success as a component of a fall-prevention program (Morton, 1989). Figure 15–2 shows the Bed-Check system.

Systematic fall-prevention programs have been initiated by several hospitals. Fall-prevention programs follow a process of development as outlined in Table 15–2.

Fall-prevention programs have resulted in some decrease in the rate of falls within an

Table 15–2. DEVELOPMENT OF A FALL-PREVENTION PROGRAM

Collect and analyze data on falls.
Identify factors related to falls.
Include factors in a fall assessment.
Conduct fall assessments.
Identify the patient at risk.
Correct or minimize factors, when possible.
Alert all staff to risk, e.g., use orange adhesive dot on patient nameband, chart, care plan, door name, and Kardex.
Develop a plan to prevent falls.
Begin interventions, including education to prevent falls. Incorporate family into plan.
Conduct ongoing assessment and revise plan as needed.

institution, as shown in Table 15–3. The differences in rates of falls before and after fall-prevention programs (with the exception of the Fife, Solomon, and Stanton study, 1984) have not been tested for statistical significance. There is no evidence that the rate of falls continues to decrease over time.

In attempts to prevent falls, standard fall-prevention techniques have been developed. These techniques require that nurses continuously assess patients for fall risk factors. Once a patient is determined to be at risk, all staff must be alerted in order to intervene effectively to prevent a fall. The use of an orange adhesive sticker or other eye-catching device on the patient's chart, armband, Kardex, door, or bedside is a popular method to alert staff (Fife, et al., 1984; Spellbring, et al., 1988). Figure 15–3 shows one hospital's fall alert design.

Once risk factors have been identified, efforts are begun to modify the factors. Table 15–4 presents possible interventions to modify intrinsic or patient-related fall risk factors.

Close observation of patients at risk, either by frequent rounds or by moving the patient

Table 15–3. PROGRAMS TO PREVENT FALLS

Author/Date/Location	Population	Program	Findings
Krishna and Van Cleave 1983 Danville, IL	VA medical center	(1) 2 1-hour lectures (2) A video film on falls (3) Informal discussion at patient seminars	32 falls per 10,000 patient days reduced to 20 falls per 10,000
Rainville 1983 Streator, IL	248-bed short-term care facility	Pre-/post-test/group design similar to Innes & Turman, 1983 Developed profile of patient most likely to fall; N = 26 Developed standard care plan from profile High risk assessment Identify high risk patient and place sign on bed	10% decrease in falls. Most of patients who fell during study were not identified as high-risk patients. Need to expand this classification.
Fife, Solomon, and Stanton 1984 Cleveland, OH	410-bed, acute-care hospital	Experimental design care hospital: (1) Developed risk/fall criteria card to identify fall risk patients (2) Implemented standard nursing care plans and procedures for patients at risk (3) Identified patient by orange markers on patient identification band, call box, bed, chart	No statistical difference in falls between control and experimental units. However, on experimental units the number of falls decreased 61% from previous year. (N = 538 patients assessed; 437 [82%] at risk)
Lee and Pash 1983	Hospital	Review 170 incidents on falls Developed assessment form and prevention strategies based on profile of high risk patient *Program Features* (1) Consciousness-raising: nurses use checklist to assess safety precautions (2) Assess and identify high risk patient (3) Teach staff	13% of the patients who fell had fallen more than once.
Hernandez and Miller 1986 Chicago, IL	21-bed geropsychiatric unit	Developed fall assessment tool Developed 3 levels of fall precautions and related interventions based on profiles; N = 60 falls/1 year	Fall rate: 24.98 per 1,000 patient days on study unit, 11.96 per 1,000 patient days in the department. Fall rate on unit decreased 42.3% in first year, 39.4% in second year. Found 20 mm Hg drop in systolic blood pressure from supine to standing position.
Innes and Turman 1983 San Francisco, CA	362-bed acute-care hospital (St. Francis Hospital)	Developed profile of patient most likely to fall from fall data (incident reports) Multidisciplinary workshop on falls Recommendations from workshop implemented and assessment form developed/used on 1 unit Studied 83 falls over 3 months for factors involved in falls Factors involved in at least 33% of falls were: medical admission, abnormal mental status, day 2 or more than 20 days in hospital, over 65 years, central nervous system depressants, need to eliminate, need for protective devices At least 3 factors present in 84% of falls Risk factors added to Kardex Continuing education program on 26 nursing measures for fall prevention Nursing interventions reviewed after each fall Poster campaign included fall risk in change of shift report	31%–41% decrease per month for 3 months compared to previous year. However, falls made up 24.8% of accidents/incidents in 1982, 24.1% in 1983, and 23.1% in 1984.

Table 15–4. INTRINSIC RISK FACTORS FOR FALLING AND POSSIBLE INTERVENTIONS

Risk Factors	Interventions	
	Medical	*Rehabilitative or Environmental*
Reduced visual acuity, dark adaptation, and perception	Refraction; cataract extraction	Home safety assessment
Reduced hearing	Removal of cerumen; audiologic evaluation	Hearing aid if appropriate (with training); reduction in background noise
Vestibular dysfunction	Avoidance of drugs affecting the vestibular system; neurologic or ear, nose, and throat evaluation, if indicated	Habituation exercises
Proprioceptive dysfunction, cervical degenerative disorders, and peripheral neuropathy	Screening for vitamin B_{12} deficiency and cervical spondylosis	Balance exercises; appropriate walking aid; correctly sized footwear with firm soles; home safety assessment
Dementia	Detection of reversible causes; avoidance of sedative or centrally acting drugs	Supervised exercise and ambulation; home safety assessment
Musculoskeletal disorders	Appropriate diagnostic evaluation	Balance-and-gait training; muscle-strengthening exercises; appropriate walking aid; home safety assessment
Foot disorders; (calluses, bunions, deformities)	Shaving of calluses; bunionectomy	Trimming of nails; appropriate footwear
Postural hypotension	Assessment of medications; rehydration; possible alteration in situational factors (e.g., meals, change of position)	Dorsiflexion exercises; pressure-graded stockings; evaluation of head of bed; use of tilt table if condition is severe
Use of medications (sedatives: benzodiazepines, phenothiazines, antidepressants; antihypertensives; others: antiarrhythmics, anticonvulsants, diuretics, alcohol)	Steps to be taken: 1. Attempted reduction in the total number of medications 2. Assessments of risks and benefits of each medication 3. Selection of medication, if needed, that is least centrally acting, least associated with postural hypotension, and has shortest action 4. Prescription of lowest effective dose 5. Frequent reassessment of risks and benefits	

(From Tinetti, ME, and Speechley, M: Prevention of falls among the elderly. N Engl J Med, 320(16):1056, 1989. Reprinted by permission.)

to a room closer to the nurses' station or a place where frequent observation and close supervision are possible, is a standard prevention technique. Additional fall precautions require that nurses use restraints on patients with a fall risk when they are out of bed and siderails and restraints for patients when they are in bed. (This practice is controversial and is not recommended. The reader should read Chapter 16, Physical Restraint of the Elderly.)

Further precautions include the monitoring of environmental factors and correcting these factors as they are found. Standard fall-prevention techniques used in hospitals and nursing homes are presented in Table 15–5.

After an extensive review of the literature on falls, Whedon and Shedd (1989) concluded that, " . . . staff nurses know the basic interventions necessary to prevent patient falls, they just may not incorporate them in their

Table 15–5. FALL-PREVENTION TECHNIQUES USED IN HOSPITALS AND NURSING HOMES*

Patient-Oriented
Restraints/Devices
Posey chest restraints
Soft wrist restraints
Electronic alarm devices, such as Bed-Check, Ambularm
Medications
Note hypnotic/sedative drugs given at night, especially to elderly or postoperative patients.
Note diuretics and laxatives given at night.
Activities of Daily Living
Assist patient to void every 4 hours.
Check for proper slippers/footwear (nonskid footwear).
Keep patient's belongings close to the bed.
Provide rehabilitation training to improve functional ability.

Environment-Oriented
Relocation of patient with high fall risk to room close to nurses' station or in hallway
Nurse call light system in place, e.g., pinned to pillow, within reach
Teach patient and family about the use of call light system, bed controls, bathroom facility, and moveable furniture.
Bed rails up when in bed
Bed in low position
Room light on, light bright and even
Place TV controls within reach.
Clutter-free rooms and hallways

Carpet all hard surfaces.
Nonskid wax
Clean up spills, including urine.
Lock all equipment with wheels.
Keep equipment on one side of hallway.
Maintain equipment in good repair.
Night lights in rooms
Safety (grab) bars in bathroom and hall
Higher-seated lounge chairs and toilets
Use bedside commodes.
Remove wheels from bedside commodes.
Safety posters in room to encourage asking for help

Patient Education
Hand out safety brochure to patient and family on admission.
Teach patient about safety and equipment.
Encourage patient to request help.
Encourage use of bathroom and corridor handrails.
Teach transfer from bed to chair.

Nursing Assessment
Perform assessment at admission and throughout hospital stay.
Assign safety risk.
Frequent rounds/checks/observations

Other
Monitor falls, watch for trends, and conduct in-service when trend emerges.
Have staff move slowly around ambulatory, unsteady patients.

(Data from Sehested & Severin-Nielson, 1977; Swartzbeck, 1983; Innes & Turman, 1983; Kostopoulos, 1985; Johnson, 1985; Hendrich, 1988; Hernandez & Miller, 1986.)
*Inclusion in this list does not imply recommendation by the authors. The use of restraints has *not* been found to reduce falls.

care planning. Instead of focusing on the actions to prevent falls, a study might be designed to measure the effects of raising staff's awareness of the problem since that may be the important factor.'' They suggest that, until there is sufficient empirical evidence, efforts should be focused on raising staff awareness in relation to falls.

Standard assessment forms have been developed to determine a patient's fall risk and to formalize staff awareness and assessment skills. Common factors included in fall-assessment instruments are fall history, mental status, sensory deficits, physical disabilities, postoperative condition, admission or transfer to a hospital or unit in a hospital, drug and alcohol use, gait disturbance, incontinence, attitude, and mood state. Table 15–6 shows

the factors advocated by various authors's assessment instruments.

There are several problems with fall-assessment instruments. The assessments are based on profiles of patients who fell in a hospital. Profiles are most often generated from analysis of incident reports. Incident reports, which form the primary data source for fall profiles, are not the most valid record, since most falls are unwitnessed (Lee, 1979). Further, each institution has developed one profile of the patient at risk from analyses of incident reports, but there may be more than one profile in a given patient population. Items on fall assessments tend to be global rather than specific. In addition, fall-assessment instruments have not been subjected to rigorous testing to determine predictive validity, that

Table 15–6. RISK FACTORS IN FALL ASSESSMENT

Categories of Risk Factors in Fall-Assessment Instrument	Innes & Turman (1983)	Lee & Pash (1983)	Hernandez & Miller (1986)	Tideiksaar (1984)
General Factors				
Fall history	X		X	X
Mental status (confused)	X	X	X	
Sensory deficits	X		X	X
Physical disabilities	X	X		X
Postoperative condition	X	X	X	
Recent change in admission (i.e., admission/ transfer)	X			X
Drugs and/or alcohol	X	X		
Gait disturbance	X		X	
Incontinence			X	X
Attitude/level of cooperation	X		X	
Mood state (agitated, angry, upset)			X	
Diagnoses				
Cerebrovascular accident			X	X
Neurologic problem	X			
Parkinsonism			X	X
Cardiovascular disease			X	
Orthopedic disorders			X	
Diabetes				X
Multiple diagnoses	X			
Medications				
Any medications		X	X	
Sleeping medications				X
Tranquilizers				X
More than five medications				X
Environment				
Footwear	X			
Standard fall precaution implemented		X		

is, whether the instruments can consistently predict a fall in a patient. Without testing, and with nonspecific test criteria, fall-assessment instruments are clearly limited. However, they do formalize the assessment process, and the use of an assessment guide heightens staff awareness and sensitivity, which are key factors in fall prevention.

It is important to note that no assessment for falls is complete without a visual assessment of gait and balance. These fall risk factors are gaining increasing attention in the literature, and there are methods available to determine balance and gait.

The Fall Assessment Scale (FAS; Appendix 15–A) includes a clinical assessment of balance and gait that takes only a few moments to complete. This is called the Get Up and Go test.

The Get Up and Go test, developed by Mathias, Nayak, and Isaacs (1986) in the United Kingdom, is a clinical test designed to measure fall risk by assessing a patient's balance and sway during the performance of a simple set of tasks. A straight-backed, high-seated chair is placed about 10 feet (3 meters) from a wall and facing the wall. The patient is asked to sit comfortably in the chair. The patient is asked to get up, stand still momentarily, walk toward the wall, turn without touching the wall, walk back to the chair, turn around, and sit down. The patient's performance is then rated as 1 = normal; 2 = very slightly abnormal; 3 = mildly abnormal; 4 = moderately abnormal; 5 = severely abnormal.

In order for patients to be rated as normal, they must give no evidence of being at risk for a fall. A severely abnormal rating means that the subject appeared at risk for falling during the test performance. A score in the intermediate range indicates hesitancy, undue slowness, abnormal movements of the trunk or arms, staggering, stumbling, or indicators that the patient is displaying the possibility of falling.

The Get Up and Go test was developed and tested with 40 inpatients, outpatients, and day patients in a hospital in the United Kingdom. The ages of these subjects ranged from 52 to 94 years, with a mean age of 73.8 years. All subjects had some degree of balance disturbance. Subjects were given a trial run to make them familiar with the test. All test runs were videotaped and then reviewed and scored by medical professionals. After completing the Get Up and Go test, subjects stood on a Kistler Force Platform with feet apart and eyes open for 30 seconds while a recording was made of body sway. The mean overall sway path was used as the measure of sway. In addition, automatic recordings were made of the subjects' gait while they walked a short distance on the walkway. Measurements were made of the gait speed, step length, stride width, frequency of stepping, and the ratio of double-support time to stride time. Scores indicate that the Get Up and Go test is a reasonably reliable and consistent test. Sway path was correlated with gait speed, which confirmed the dependence of rapid walking on good balance. Scores on the Get Up and Go test correlated significantly with the total mean sway path, gait speed, and gait parameters. The researchers concluded that the Get Up and Go test is a reliable, simple, practical guide to balance function. A patient with a score of 3 or more on the Get Up and Go test is at risk for a fall.

DEVELOPING A FALL RISK ASSESSMENT GUIDE

The ultimate objective for prevention is to reduce patient falls in hospitals by developing and implementing a program to identify patients' risk for falls and to target interventions on the factors that place patients at risk. The

development of an assessment instrument that can identify hospitalized patients at risk for falling is an important step in a formal fall-prevention program. The literature supports the idea that identification of the high-risk patient is a promising approach to fall prevention.

However, developing a valid and reliable fall-assessment guide can be a complex task. The authors are curently testing a fall-assessment instrument (FAS), and the process of its development is presented to assist others in this work and to demonstrate the complexity of the task (see Appendix 15–A).

The FAS is the result of previous work that attempted to analyze patient falls by developing categories or profiles of patients who fell in one hospital. For this study, 32 alert and oriented hospitalized men were interviewed within 24 hours of their falls in the hospital. Data were also collected on instrinsic and extrinsic factors related to the falls from the patients' medical record, incident report, and nursing time schedule. Five categories of patients who fell were developed and identifying factors in each category were described. The categories of patients who fell are: falls as a way of life, falls as the result of illness and/or treatment, falls in the discharge-ready, falls and denial, and falls as institutionally defined events.

Falls as a way of life characterizes persons with a history of 10 or more falls within the year prior to hospitalization. Falls are not perceived as a problem for them. However, injury from fall is perceived as a problem. They have adapted their home environment and developed personal prevention techniques to avoid injury, if not prevent a fall. This category included 19% or 6 of the 32 patients who fell in this sample.

Falls as part of illness or treatment made up the largest category and included 47% or 15 of the 32 fallers. This category describes patients who are acutely ill and weak, with a recent change in sensory or functional ability, either as a direct consequence of illness or as a side effect of treatment. Typically, there is a change in the physical condition of these patients within the 1 to 2 weeks prior to the fall. They may have fallen recently while at home, and falls may be a reason for the hospital admission. These patients may have periods of disorientation. Cancer and cardiovascular disease were common medical diagnoses.

Discharge-ready patients, or 9% (3 of 32 fallers) of the sample, have been in the hospital for more than 3 weeks and want to prepare themselves for discharge. They are in the active rehabilitation phase of treatment and deliberately take a risk in an attempt to regain or test an ability to walk or perform transfers.

Falls and denial include 19% of patients (6 of 32 fallers). These patients give a vague, nonspecific history of falling. They may not be aware of the reason for hospitalization and are characterized by having medical diagnoses such as alcoholism and cerebrovascular accidents. They use denial to minimize their illness or disability and are not compliant with activity orders.

The final category, falls as institutionally defined events, is used to describe incidents that are not true falls but nevertheless are classified as falls. This category was dropped from further analysis. The specific characteristics in each type of patient category are identified in Table 15–7. The factors identified in each category and the intrinsic factors found in the literature were included to develop a model to describe patient falls. The model for patient falls in a hospital is presented in Figure 15–4.

Morse, Tylko, and Dixon (1987) also found categories of patients who fell. In their study, they compared 100 patients who had fallen in one hospital with 100 randomly selected patients who had not fallen. Data were collected from the patient's medical record, from direct observation, and from patient interviews. Comparison of the two groups revealed several significant differences. The fall group was most likely to be confused, have a secondary diagnosis, be older, be long-term hospital patients, have an abnormal gait, and use furniture or rails for supports rather than a walking aid. Six variables resulted from the discriminant analysis of the group: intravenous therapy, ambulatory aids, presence of secondary

Table 15–7. CHARACTERISTICS OF FALLERS FROM QUALITATIVE ANALYSES

Falls as a Way of Life—18.7%
History of 10 or more falls in 1 year
Adapted to prevent falls/injury

Falls as Part of Illness—46.8%
Recent change in function/sensory ability
May be disoriented
Brief and recent fall history
Cardiac/cancer disease
Weak, debilitated and/or acutely sick

Falls in Discharge-Ready—9%
Oriented
Rehabilitation phase
Take a risk
"Legs gave way"

Falls and Denial—18.7%
Alert
Deny/minimize illness and limitations
No history of falls
Noncompliant with activity restrictions
Alcoholism/cerebrovascular accident

Institutionally Defined—6%
Rolling from bed while asleep
Sitting down on floor to prevent fall

(Data from Chenitz, WC, & Kussman, H: An Analysis of Patient Falls in Hospitals. Paper presented at the 39th annual meeting of the Gerontological Society of America, Chicago, IL, 1986.)

diagnosis, a history of falling, abnormal gait, and mental disorder. In addition, Morse and associates analyzed the data and developed three categories of causes for the "fall-prone patient." These were: psychological, unanticipated, and accidental. The specific variables in these categories are presented in Table 15–8.

The FAS instrument is currently being tested for inter-rater reliability. Once this is completed, testing for predictive validity can begin. This process is time-consuming and expensive. The costs and benefits of this type of undertaking in a clinical setting need to be carefully weighed. It may be determined that staff awareness and sensitivity and a formal assessment are the important components in a fall-prevention program. Further, it may be decided that this can be accomplished using an untested instrument, and the decision may be made to begin a fall-prevention program using the best available instrument.

MODEL OF FALLS IN HOSPITALIZED PATIENTS

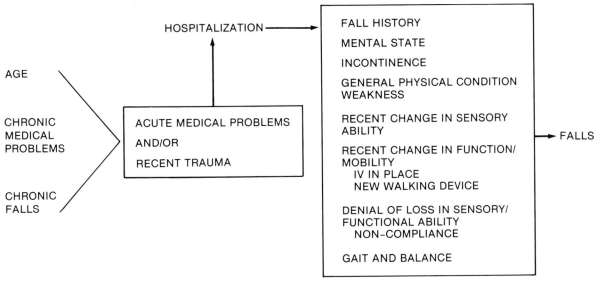

Figure 15—4. Model of falls in hospitalized patients.

IF A FALL OCCURS

In addition to fall-prevention instruction, information should be given on what to do should a fall occur: getting up after a fall, devising a plan of action with the family or

Table 15—8. CHARACTERISTICS OF THE FALL-PRONE PATIENT

Physiologic Anticipated—78%
Impaired gait
Used walking aids
Frequently disoriented
Fallen previously
Had multiple diagnoses
Received IV therapy

Physiologic Unanticipated—8%
Oriented
Fainted
Drug reaction
Seizure
"Knees gave way"

Accidental—14%
Alert
Normal gait

(Data from Morse, JM, Tylko, SJ, & Dixon, HA: Characteristics of the fall-prone patient. *Gerontologist*, 27:516–522.)

neighbors, and learning how to contact the community's emergency system.

Instructions on how to get up after a fall may include any of the following techniques. One method is to have the faller roll onto the right side, bend the right knee, and lever upward to the kneeling position by pressing down on the right forearm. Next, the faller should reach out with the left arm to a nearby chair or bed and, with a twist of the trunk, pull into a sitting position (Isaacs, 1982). A similar method is to roll to a prone position and get up on all fours. Fallers can crawl to a large sturdy chair, couch, or bed, place their hands on it and bring one foot forward, putting the foot flat on the floor. They can then stand up and sit on the chair or bed to recover. This technique is useful for an older person without knee problems (Squires & Bayliss, 1985). If crawling is impossible, the faller can pull to a sitting position, shuffle on the buttocks to a nearby piece of furniture, pull up onto the knees directly in front of a piece of furniture, and then stand (Brummel-Smith, et al., 1988). If these techniques are impossible, the faller may try shuffling to the stairs and gradually moving up and backwards to a height suitable for standing (Squires & Bayliss, 1985). These techniques should be practiced until the person feels confident in managing the problems of falls.

Those who fall frequently might consider keeping flashlights, bells, and even telephone extensions in several locations to call for help. In the event that they cannot get up after a fall, they should be instructed to pull blankets, clothing, or rugs on top of themselves to prevent hypothermia. Frequent fallers may also want to take additional precautions by making arrangements with family and neighbors for a simple reassurance call or by establishing specific signals, such as the window drapes being opened by a predetermined time in the morning, to indicate that all is well. Keys to the house should be left with neighbors or family members for access in the event of emergency. However, some people prefer and can afford an alarm system. There are several types available. Some are radio transmitted devices that can be worn around the neck or placed strategically around the home. A push of the button sends a distress call to a control center and assistance is sent.

Elderly persons should use alcohol and tranquilizers cautiously. While moderation is advisable at all times for all ages, older people may be taking a number of medications for specific chronic conditions. The older person should be cautioned to assess the effects of small doses of alcohol on the general ability to maintain balance and walk with a steady gait.

The first and clearly most important function of a nurse finding a patient who has fallen in an institutional setting is to assess the patient for injury. If injury has occurred, treatment is begun immediately. In most cases this requires notifying physicians, obtaining orders for x-rays and having them performed, and securing ice packs, suture material, and other equipment, depending upon the injury.

During assessment for injury, a description of the fall is obtained from the patient and anyone who witnessed the event (Tideiksaar, 1984). The patient's activity at the time of the fall, state of mind, condition of the floor, hazards in the environment, and factors that might have contributed to the fall are determined (Brummel-Smith, et al., 1988). This information is important not only for the institution's risk management program but also for assessing the cause of the fall. Once the cause is established, intervention is aimed at correction. As Lipsitz (1988) notes, "Falling is a symptom, not a diagnosis, that may result from common, age-related changes that impair homeostatic capacity and may also be a manifestation of any disease process in the elderly." Therefore, after a fall has occurred, it is critical to determine the true cause(s) of the event.

In addition, after assessment and treatment are done, ambulation should be instituted as early as possible and done several times a day. This prevents the hazards of bedrest as well as the fear of falling again, which can severely limit mobility and independence (Brummel-Smith, et al., 1988).

Further, care must be taken to reduce embarrassment and personal ridicule because the older person may feel foolish and responsible for the fall. Reassurance and a matter-of-fact, supportive approach can be helpful. Fall education should be started soon after a fall to prevent falling again. That is, after the analysis of the fall, factors related to the fall should be discussed with staff and corrected when possible, and prevention techniques should be taught to the patient.

Restraints are often used in health care institutions to protect the patient from injury. After a fall, restraints are very commonly used to protect the patient from falling again. Unfortunately, restraints can contribute not only to a fall but to injury sustained during a fall. (See Chapter 16, Physical Restraint of the Elderly, for a full discussion of this complex matter.)

Ideally, each patient needing protection should have one-to-one care. Family members, when available, can be enlisted to provide this service to their kin. However, one-to-one care is not always achievable or realistic. Howe (1985) suggests that the true solution to the problem of restraint is the Four C approach; competent, conscientious, commonsense, and caring staff. Using this approach, staff can balance safety and mobility needs to provide care in the least restrictive environment possible.

SUMMARY

In this chapter, the problem of falls has been presented, with the focus on the importance of nursing assessment in fall prevention. A review of the literature identified numerous factors associated with falls in hospitals, in nursing homes, and in the community. In addition, there were examples of fall-prevention programs and techniques. None of the programs reported offers conclusive evidence that patient falls are being prevented. The use of a validated instrument that can predict fall risk would be beneficial to patients and health care institutions and holds the promise for solutions to this difficult clinical problem. At the present time, falls in the elderly are no longer considered an inevitable consequence of old age (Morse, 1986). Fall prevention through education, assessment, and systematic programs are now considered standard practice.

References

AlertCare, Inc (1988): *News Alert, 1*(2):1–4.

Berryman, E, Gaskin, D, Jones, A, et al. (1989): Point by point: Predicting elders' falls. *Geriatr Nurs, 10*(4):199–201.

Brummel-Smith, K, Kottke, JF, & Williams, GO (1988): When an elderly person falls. *In* Elias, S (ed): *Patient Care, 22*:131–149.

Chenitz, WC, & Kussman, H (1984): An Analysis of Patient Falls in Hospitals. Paper presented at 39th annual meeting of the Gerontological Society of America, Chicago, IL.

Dawson, DE (1983): Take the right steps to prevent slips, trips and falls. *Executive Housekeeping Today, 4*(8):3–4.

Fife, DP, Solomon, P, & Stanton, M (1984): A risk/falls program: Code orange for success. *Nurs Manag, 15*:50–53.

Gray-Vickrey, M (1984): Education to prevent falls. *Geriatr Nurs, 5*(3):179–183.

Hendrich, AL (1988): Unit-based fall prevention. *J Qual Assur, 10*(1):15–17.

Hernandez, M, & Miller, S (1986): How to reduce falls. *Geriatr Nurs, 7*(2):97–102.

Hill, BA, Johnson, R, & Garret, BJ (1988): Reducing the incidence of falls in high risk patients. *J Nurs Admin, 18*(7–8):24–28.

Innes, EM, & Turman, WG (1983): Evaluation of patient falls. *Qual Rev Bull, 9*(2):30–35.

Isaacs, B (1982): *The Clinical Aspects of Falling*. Nutley, NJ, Roche Laboratories.

Isaacs, B (1985): Clinical and laboratory studies of falls in old people: Prospects for prevention. *In* Radebaugh, TS, Hadley, E, & Suzman, R (eds): Symposium of Falls in the Elderly, *Clin Geriatr Med, 1*(3):513–524.

Janken, JK, Reynolds BA, & Sweich, K (1986): Patient falls in the acute care setting: Identifying risk factors. *Nurs Res, 35*(4):215–219.

Johnson, ET (1985): Accidental falls among geriatric patients: Can more be prevented? *J Natl Med Assoc, 77*(8):633–637.

Kane, RA, & Kane, RL (1976): *Long-term care in six countries: Implications for the United States* (DHEW Publication No. NIH 76-1207). Washington, DC, US Government Printing Office.

Kayser-Jones, J (1981): *Old, Alone and Neglected: Care of the Aged in Scotland and the United States*. Berkeley, CA, University of California Press.

Kostopoulos, MR (1985): Reducing patient falls. *Orthop Nurs, 4*(6):14–15.

Krishna, KM, & Van Cleave, RJ (1983): Decrease in the incidence of patient falls in a geriatric hospital after education programs (letter). *J Am Geriatr Soc, 31*:187.

Lee, RG (1979): Health and safety in hospitals. *Med Sci Law, 29*:89–103.

Lee, PS, & Pash, JH (1983): Preventing patient falls. *Nurs '83, 13*:118, 120.

Lipsitz, LA (1988): Falls and syncope. *In* Rowe, JW, & Besdine, RW (eds): *Geriatric Medicine*. Boston, Little, Brown.

Lowe, AS (1985): *Anatomy of a Fall*. Burkeville, Va. Piedmont Geriatric Institute.

Mader, SL, Josephson, KR, & Rubenstein, LZ (1987): Low prevalence of postural hypotension among community dwelling elderly. *JAMA, 258*:1511–1514.

Mathias, S, Nayak, USL, & Isaacs, B (1986): Balance in elderly patients: The "Get Up and Go" test. *Arch Phys Med Rehabil, 67*:387–389.

Morse, JM (1986): Computerized evaluation of a scale to identify the fall-prone patient. *Can J Public Health, 77*:21–25.

Morse, JM, Tylko, SJ, & Dixon, HA (1987): Characteristics of the fall-prone patient. *Gerontologist, 27*:516–522.

Morton, D (1989): Five years of fewer falls. *Am J Nurs, 89*:204–205.

O'Hara-Deveraux, M, Andrus, LH, & Scott, CD (eds) (1981): *Eldercare*. New York, Grune & Stratton.

Overstall, PW (1980): Prevention of falls in the elderly. *J Am Geriatr Soc, 28*:481–484.

Perry, BC (1982): Falls among the elderly: A review of the methods and conclusions of epidemiological studies. *J Am Geriatr Soc, 30*:367–371.

Rainville, NG (1983): Effect of an implemented fall prevention program on the frequency of patient falls. *QRB, 10*:287–291.

Raz, T, & Baretich, BF (1987): Factors affecting the incidence of patient falls in hospitals. *Med Care*, 25(3):185–195.

Rowland, HS, & Rowland, BL (1987): *The Manual of Nursing Quality Assurance*. Rockville, MD, Aspen.

Rubenstein, LZ, Robbins, AS, Schulman, BL, et al. (1988): Falls and instability in the elderly. *J Am Geriatr Soc*, 36:266–278.

Sehested, P, & Severin-Nielson, T (1977): Falls by hospitalized elderly patients: Cause and prevention. *Geriatrics*, 32:101–108.

Spellbring, AM, Gannon, ME, Kleckner, T, et al. (1988): Improving safety for hospitalized elderly. *J Gerontol Nurs*, 14:31–37.

Squires, A, & Bayliss, DE (1985): Rehabilitation of fallers. *In* Kataria, MS (ed): *Fits, Faints and Falls in Old Age*. Hingham, MA, Kluwer Academic Publishers, 15–26.

Swartzbeck, E (1983): The problems of falls in the elderly. *Nurs Manag*, 13:34–43.

Tideiksaar, R (1984): An assessment form for falls. *J Am Geriatr Soc*, 32:538–539.

Tinetti, ME (1986): Performance-oriented assessment of mobility problems in elderly patients. *J Am Geriatr Soc*, 34:119–126.

Tinetti, ME, & Ginter, SF (1988): Identifying mobility dysfunctions in elderly patients: Standard neuromuscular examination or direct assessment? *JAMA*, 259:1190–1193.

Tinetti, ME, & Speechley, M (1989): Prevention of falls among the elderly. *N Engl J Med*, 329(16):1055–1059.

Tinetti, ME, Speechley, M, & Ginter, S (1988): Risk factors for falls among elderly persons living in the community. *N Engl J Med*, 319(26):1701–1707.

Whedon, MD, & Shedd, P (1989): Prediction and prevention of patient falls. *Image*, 21(2):108–114.

Widder, B (1985): A new device to decrease falls. *Geriatr Nurs*, 6(5):287–288.

APPENDIX 15–A

Fall Assessment Scale (FAS) Guide

Purpose: This guide provides instructions and definitions required to assess patient fall risk using the FAS.

Supplies: Pencil
FAS

INSTRUCTIONS

1. Utilize any resources including patient's medical record, Nursing Care Plan, and the patient himself/herself to complete the FAS.

2. Read the following definitions to clarify the meaning of terms in FAS prior to completing the FAS.

DEFINITIONS

1. *Age*—the patient's chronological age in years lived.

2. Check any of the following *diagnoses* that are applicable to this patient at this time:

   Alcoholism—continued excessive or compulsive use of alcohol.

   Cancer—a malignant tumor of potentially unlimited growth that expands locally by invasion and systemically by metastasis.

   CVA (stroke)—sudden loss of consciousness followed by paralysis caused by hemorrhage into the brain, formation of an embolus or thrombus that occludes an artery, or rupture of an extracerebral artery causing subarachnoid hemorrhage.

   Drug Addiction—physical and/or psychological dependence on the use of mind-altering drugs.

   AIDS—the occurrence of immune deficiency in previously healthy individuals in the presence of an indicator disease.

   Unstable cardiac condition—a state of cardiac functioning marked by fluctuation or change from normal.

3. *History of falls prior to hospitalization*—the experience of leaving an erect position suddenly and involuntarily at some point *before* becoming hospitalized.

325

4. *Falls in hospital*—the experience of leaving an erect position suddenly and involuntarily at some point *during* hospitalization.

5. *Physical condition*—the state of fitness of the body:
   Good—appears healthy and sound for age.
   Fair—average condition for age.
   Poor—is sick/weak.

6. *Able to give correct reason for hospitalization*—the patient is able to provide a reasonable and accurate explanation for why he/she is hospitalized currently.

7. *IV in place*—The presence of an infusion device within the vein of a patient. (This might include angiocath, heparin lock, infuse-a-port, or any other venous access device.)

8. *Patient complies with activity order*—patient cooperates with the recommendation for physical movement as prescribed by physician or nursing staff.

9. *Ability to walk:*
   No problem/normal gait—there is no problem with gait.

   Walks with helper/impaired gait—a disturbance with the way in which person walks. May require another person or assistance while walking.

   Cannot walk—person lacks the ability to walk even with assistance.

Note: The following relate to conditions/assessments of the patient within the 24 hours preceding the time of assessment.

10. *Alert and oriented at all times:*

    Alert—quick to perceive and act.

    and

    Oriented—being intellectually and emotionally directed.

11. *Up at night to void*—the need to get up at night to urinate.

12. *Incontinent of urine:*

    Incontinent—the inability to control urination.
    Frequency—the need to urinate at short intervals.
    Urgency—the feeling of needing to urinate immediately.

13. *Incontinent of feces:*
    Diarrhea—frequent passage of unformed, watery bowel movements.
    Incontinent at least once—the inability to control defecation.

14. *Mental status changed from oriented to disoriented*, that is, a shift in the person's thinking and response that reflects an inability to report accurately person, place, and/or time.

15. *Mental status changed from oriented to confused*, that is, a shift in the person's thinking and behavior that reflects inappropriate response to stimuli.

Note: The following relate to any changes in the patient during the last week.

16. *Ability to walk*—any recent change in the patient's balance, gait, and ambulation.

17. *Vision*—any recent change in the patient's ability to see.

Fall Assessment Scale

Complete the following items with all available information you have on this patient. Rate the patient as he/she appears to you now.

(1) STATE AGE IN YEARS. _____

(2) CHECK ANY OF THE FOLLOWING DI-AGNOSES THAT ARE APPLICABLE TO THIS PATIENT.

_____ 1. Alcoholism
_____ 2. Cancer
_____ 3. CVA
_____ 4. Drug addiction
_____ 5. AIDS
_____ 6. Unstable cardiac condition

(3) HISTORY OF FALLS PRIOR TO HOS-PITALIZATION

_____ 1. No
_____ 2. Yes
_____ 3. Don't know

(4) FALLS IN HOSPITAL
_____ 1. No
_____ 2. Yes
_____ 3. Don't know

(5) PHYSICAL CONDITION

_____ 1. Good
_____ 2. Fair
_____ 3. Poor

(6) ABLE TO GIVE CORRECT REASON FOR HOSPITALIZATION

_____ 1. No
_____ 2. Yes
_____ 3. Don't know

(7) IV IN PLACE

_____ 1. No
_____ 2. Yes
_____ 3. Don't know

(8) PATIENT COMPLIES WITH ACTIVITY ORDER

_____ 1. No
_____ 2. Yes
_____ 3. Don't know

(9) ABILITY TO WALK

_____ 1. No problem/normal gait
_____ 2. Walk with cane, walker, crutches, brace or other device/weak gait
_____ 3. Walk with a helper/impaired gait
_____ 4. Cannot walk
_____ 5. Don't know

RATE THE FOLLOWING ITEMS FOR THE PAST 24 HOURS

(10) ALERT AND ORIENTED AT ALL TIMES

_____ 1. No
_____ 2. Yes
_____ 3. Don't know

(11) UP AT NIGHT TO VOID

_____ 1. No
_____ 2. Yes
_____ 3. Don't know

(12) INCONTINENT OF URINE

_____ 1. No
_____ 2. Frequency/urgency
_____ 3. Catheter in place
_____ 4. Incontinent at least once
_____ 5. Don't know

(13) INCONTINENT OF FECES

_____ 1. No
_____ 2. Diarrhea
_____ 3. Incontinent at least once
_____ 4. Don't know

MENTAL STATUS CHANGES

(14) ORIENTED TO DISORIENTED

_____ 1. No
_____ 2. Yes
_____ 3. Don't know

(15) ORIENTED TO CONFUSED

_____ 1. No
_____ 2. Yes
_____ 3. Don't know

Within the last week has there been a change in the patient's

(16) ABILITY TO WALK?

_____ 1. No
_____ 2. Yes
_____ 3. Don't know

(17) VISION?

_____ 1. No
_____ 2. Yes
_____ 3. Don't know

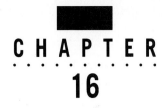

CHAPTER
16

Physical Restraint of the Elderly

NEVILLE E. STRUMPF, R.N, Ph.D., F.A.A.N.
LOIS K. EVANS, R.N., D.N.Sc., F.A.A.N.
DORIS SCHWARTZ, R.N., M.A., F.A.A.N.

INTRODUCTION

The authors' growing interest in the problem of physical restraint of older people is the result, in part, of several encounters with residents of one life-care community, all of whom were interviewed concerning their experiences in the hospital. The first, an 84-year-old woman, provided the following account of a previous hospitalization, several months earlier:

> I was taken by ambulance to the hospital emergency room because of palpitations; there I received lidocaine to which I was "allergic." Apparently it caused me to misbehave badly and I tried to climb out of bed. I don't remember misbehaving, but I may have been deranged from all the pills they gave me. Normally I am spirited, but I am also good and obedient. Nevertheless, the nurse tied me down, like Jesus on the cross, by bandaging both wrists and ankles. As I lay there I wondered if His arms and legs had ached like mine. I said, "My hands and ankles will swell." It felt awful, I hurt, and I worried "What if I get leg cramps, what will I do then if I can't move?" It was miserable, not being able to move, and an awful shock. It was unfair of the hospital to tie me. I felt terrible, aching pain and numbness; I wondered now how I ate; no one fed me that I know of. And I don't think I slept at night. Because I am a cooperative person, I felt so resentful. Callers, including men friends, saw me like that and I lost something; I lost a little personal prestige. I was embarrassed, like a child placed in a corner for being bad. I had been important, and well, and to be tied down in bed took a big toll.

> Even though I apologized for badly misbehaving, the nurse was unsympathetic; in fact, I think she was told to restrain me. It could have been done differently; a nurse or companion should have been assigned to watch me if I was misbehaving, but they said they didn't know if I could afford it. With gentle talk I wouldn't have

done anything and could have been tied for a shorter period. I'm not sure how long the restraints were left on, but it seemed like a very long time. I just couldn't see how tying me down could help my situation—my idea of restraint is the state hospital—I wasn't going to hurt anybody. I asked everyone to remove the restraint. I pleaded with the nurse, promising to stay in bed, and I begged my son, who had just come from Texas. I said to him, "Fix yourself a drink, you must need one." Of course, there wasn't any liquor in my room and the nurse took that as further evidence that my mind wasn't working. I know there were a lot of time lapses, but I was rational when I felt that the restraints should be taken off or not put on in the first place.

People assumed I needed a restraint. When I told the doctor about it on the day of discharge, he said, "You're glad to be alive, aren't you? You have to trust us to take care of you the way we think is best." But many gaps and questions about the experience remain. For weeks I couldn't look at this wrist (*she holds up right arm*) without feeling pain, psychological pain. Sometimes I feel my wrists still hurt. I told the nurse I would write a story about being restrained if I could, but it would scare people. Usually I meet life by trying to forget the bad things, but this was such a vivid experience. I haven't forgotten the pain and the indignity of being tied.

Two other residents of the same life-care community also recalled for the authors their experiences with physical restraints during a recent hospitalization. Although less detailed than the above account, striking similarities concerning responses to the restraint emerged in their narratives. One 80-year-old woman, a retired nurse, referred to the restraint as a "belt with chains and movable buckles." Throughout the experience she recalled feeling "incarcerated," "terrible," and as if she would "go mad." She remembered the device as "uncomfortable" and "too tight," but felt that to "get home in one piece," one had to "be obedient." She expressed the sentiment, "It did something to me," adding that reassurance in the form of a "little pat" from the staff indicating "we're together on this" would have made a big difference. She concluded, "Nurses need more training in personal relations; it is not enough to be concerned with just techniques."

The third resident, a 90-year-old woman, described her experience in a critical care unit following a stroke:

I was not exactly out of contact; I realized what was going on. Both of my feet were restrained, making it impossible to turn over or even to pull myself up. If anyone tried to explain, I don't remember, but I can still hear myself saying, "Please, oh, please undo my feet." Queer things happened to me. They say it was dreams, but I think I had hallucinations.

Each of these vignettes has several themes in common: a vivid recollection of the experience, despite transient confusion during the hospitalization; a lingering sense of physical and psychological distress for months following discharge; a belief that explanations and treatment by the staff were inadequate; and finally, considerable conviction that the restraint was unnecessary. It was apparent to the authors, on the basis of such potent descriptions, that the response of patients to mechanical restraint deserved greater scrutiny. This recognition led, in turn, to a "call for help" letter in *Geriatric Nursing* (Schwartz, 1985a), an exhaustive search of the literature, and the development of a series of research projects on physical restraint of older people. The remainder of this chapter provides a brief review of the literature, describes one study conducted by two of the investigators (Strumpf & Evans, 1988) on restraint experiences of hospitalized patients and their primary nurses, discusses the implications for nursing practice, and concludes with alternatives to this significant clinical and ethical problem.

REVIEW OF THE LITERATURE

Schwartz's "Call for Help" elicited 126 relevant references to published literature on restraints of older people (Schwartz, 1985b). A conventional literature search by the authors followed, which yielded only references to auto safety equipment, restraint use in psychiatry, and devices for immobilizing research animals. Use of reference lists from articles on falls, confusion, and wandering produced additional information on restraints. Considerable material concerning physical restraints was summarized, synthesized, and analyzed, including reasons for use, historical perspectives, opinions, prevalance, effects and consequences, alternatives, guidelines and policies, legal and ethical aspects, nursing responses and decision-making, and environmental considerations (Evans & Strumpf, 1989). The lack of any systematic review, organization of material, or conceptual framework on the problem, as well as a paucity of actual research studies on physical restraint, was apparent. Only nine articles could be classified strictly as research (Applebaum & Roth, 1984; Cape, 1985; Farnsworth, 1973; Frengley & Mion, 1986; Lichtenstein & Stone, 1987; Mitchell-Pederson, Edmund, Fingerote, et al., 1985; Morrison, Crinklaw-Wiancko, King, et al., 1987; Robbins, Boyko, Lane, et al., 1987; Yarmesch & Sheafor, 1984).

The major findings of this literature review are summarized below, with special emphasis on historical background, reasons for restraint, prevalence, effects, and legal implications.

History

Various forms of physical restraint have, for centuries, been used to manage violent behavior, particularly in the mentally ill (Soloff, 1984). In the 1950s and 1960s, however, efforts to increase the protection of individual human rights led to several landmark decisions by United States courts on behalf of the mentally ill, especially with regard to guaranteeing the right to refuse treatment and restricting involuntary use of seclusion, mechanical restraint, and psychotropic medication (Shindul & Snyder, 1981). In psychiatric care, the decade of the 1970s was characterized by growing recognition that present-day restraints were little more than minor modifications of the humiliating, restrictive devices applied in the past (Guirguis & Durost, 1978). Thus, the modern therapeutic community stood in direct philosophical opposition to physical restraints (Soloff, 1978), and a number of studies demon-

strated that the use of restraints with psychiatric patients could be decreased or eliminated (Cohen, 1977; Hay & Cromwell, 1980; Jacoby, Babilian, McLamb, et al., 1958). At best, restraints were designated a treatment of last resort (Rosen & DiGiacomo, 1978; Soloff, 1979).

If, as Soloff (1984) suggests, the use of physical means to manage behavior is bound to the cultural framework of an era, parallel development of restraint use with older people during a time of reduction with psychiatric patients is both curious and disturbing. It is not entirely clear when the use of physical restraints became routine and widespread with this population, but the first textbook devoted entirely to geriatric nursing (Newton, 1950) never mentions the use of restraint, not even in the section on care of "senile patients." Two references to physical restraint had appeared in United States journals, however, by the latter half of the next decade. Patrick (1967) noted that the confused "elderly" patient is "frequently restrained either by physical means or by drugs, both of which can contribute to his confusion by hindering communication." The author went on to say that restraints are usually interpreted as punitive and lead to struggle, which can cause skin damage as well as predispose the patient to problems with elimination, pneumonia, or other complications of immobility. Patrick further described the case of an 82-year-old man whose so-called confusion disappeared when he was relieved of restraints, and she urged that the nurse intervene with the physician as soon as possible to discontinue the order for restraints. In a similar article on confused or delirious hospitalized "elderly patients," Gerdes (1968) warned that restraints "seem to intensify the disorganized behavior of many patients . . . . Restraints, in themselves, contribute to sensory deprivation and a loss of self-image." In Great Britain, Cubbin (1970) declared that, "It is the duty of each individual nurse to make every effort to see that restraint is kept to a minimum and we would then perhaps see fewer reports of ill-treatment and cruelty in the national press." It was also her observation that the "effect of restraining many patients who are mentally well but physically poor can undoubtedly lead to a deterioration in the patient's mental condition." These injunctions notwithstanding, it was Schwab's (1975) contention that pressure from United States agencies to prevent falls or wandering away led to overuse and abuse of restraints, siderails, and medications.

In a poll by mailed questionnaire of restraint use in 500 randomly selected nursing homes in the United States, Farnsworth (1973) received 183 responses, with 181 reporting regular use of some form of restraint, including vests (137), waist ties (135), mitts (34), wrist/ankle ties (21), and wrist/elbow restraints (2). In the 1977 national survey of nursing homes, 25% of residents, more than 300,000 persons, were regularly restrained by geriatric chairs, cuffs, belts, or similar devices (Department of Health, Education and Welfare [DHEW], 1979); a decade later, the Health Care Financing Administration (HCFA, 1988) reported 41% of all skilled nursing home residents and 31% of all intermediate care facility residents restrained at some point during the day, placing the number of those restrained daily at least at 500,000. As the frequency of physical restraints mounted in the United States, their prevalence declined in Great Britain where policies and philosophy apparently discouraged their use (Editorial, 1980).

Throughout the 1970s, the literature demonstrates a modest but growing concern for the problems created by the application of physical restraints. Miller (1975) and Oster (1976) describe the myriad adverse effects of restraints and immobilization in older people, especially declines in central nervous system activity and problems with sensory deprivation. Earlier classic immobilization studies by Zubek and others (1963, 1966, 1969) provide strong theoretical support for the numerous hazards associated with any form of restriction in bodily movement, regardless of age or health status. Nevertheless, Covert, Rodrigues, and Solomon (1977) describe the frequency with which displays of socially deviant behavior meet with physical or chemical restraints in nursing homes. Trockman (1978) explicitly advised siderails for mildly confused

hospitalized older persons who suffer sundown syndrome; mitts and restraints to protect severely agitated patients and their intravenous lines, tubes, dressings, and so on; and nightly vest restraints for the chronically confused who might wander or fall out of bed. Yet in a study of hospitalized older patients with hip fractures, Williams and others (1979) indicated that while restraint use was common, it was a potential risk factor in developing or worsening confusion. Throughout the 1980s, the literature increasingly demonstrated the marked usage of restraints, perhaps prompting Burnside's (1984) editorial, "Are Nurses Taught to Tie People Down?" Regardless of the answer, the prevalence of restraints and the oft-quoted reasons for their application speak to a sense of inevitability and acquiescence regarding their use. The recorded history of restraint usage with older Americans may be short, but the practice seems deeply entrenched.

Prevalence

Precise figures on the prevalence of restraint use among older persons are difficult to obtain, but recent surveys in both hospitals and nursing homes indicate that the practice remains common and widespread. Statistics from studies conducted in several hospitals suggest that from 6% to 50% of older adults are restrained for some period during their hospitalization (Frengley & Mion, 1986; Katz, Weber, & Dodge, 1981; MacLean, Shamian, Butcher, et al., 1982; Mion, Frengley, & Adams, 1986; Morrison, et al., 1987; Robbins, 1986; Robbins, et al., 1987; Stilwell, 1983; Warshaw, 1983). In those instances where hospitalized elders are deemed confused or at risk of falling, the likelihood of physical restraint often exceeds 50% (Appelbaum & Roth, 1984; Gillick, Serrell, & Gillick, 1982; Inness & Turman, 1983). Other than the reports cited earlier (Farnsworth, 1973; DHEW, 1979; HCFA, 1988), only one study was found indicating prevalence of restraint use in a nursing home (Zimmer, Watson, & Treat, 1984). In a random sample of skilled nursing facility residents in upstate New York, the authors found that 47% of those with serious behavioral problems had been restrained during the past 30 days. Of those persons noted to have moderate behavioral problems, 46% had orders on record for a physical restraint. One report compared prevalence of restraint use in continuing-care hospitals in London, Ontario, and London, England. In Ontario, 84.6% of the residents had a restraint in use, the most common device being a "seatbelt," and all had bedrails. In England, however, only 11.6% of residents had a bedrail in use and 8.1% had another type of restraint. The literature does not suggest any discernible difference in characteristics between institutionalized elders in the United Kingdom and those in the United States or Canada.

Reasons

A common rationale for the widespread use of restraints with older people is repeatedly reported: to protect from injury, to prevent interference with treatment, or to control disruptive behavior. Frengley and Mion (1986) identified protection of the patient, equipment, or others from harm, including prevention of falls from bed or chair and wandering, as the common reasons given for restraint. Similarly, Appelbaum and Roth (1984) found that restraint was employed against a patient's will when harm seemed likely (falls from bed, other self-injury, interferences with treatment) or when disturbances to others took place (wandering, shouting). Precipitating incidents involved patients' attempts to get out of bed or resist treatment while confused or disoriented. Similar observations have been made regarding application of restraints to reduce risk of injury (Warshaw, 1983), to control patients exhibiting confusion (Gillick, et al., 1982; Wolanin & Phillips, 1980); to prevent injuires and maintain integrity of treatment plans with the confused and agitated (Cohen-Mansfield & Billig, 1986; MacLean, et al., 1982); and to prevent injury, provide physical security, and limit movement to the extent necessary for treatment, examination, or protection (Katz, et al., 1981). In skilled nursing homes, restraints are often employed in instances of aggressive behavior, physical resistance to care, uncontrolled wandering, self-abuse (including removal of catheters), physical disruption (throwing food), and taking others' belongings (Zimmer, et al., 1984). Wandering is clearly perceived as a major reason for restraint (Burnside, 1980; Fisk, 1984). Misik (1981) suggests that symptoms like vagueness, listlessness, anxiety, agitation, and hostility may warrant a restraint.

Lichtenstein and Stone (1987) found that nurses in one Veterans Administration medical center tried to avoid physical restraints, but ultimately resorted to them for problematic behaviors (confusion, agitation, restlessness, combativeness); concerns about mobility (history or risk of falling, ataxia); and attempts to remove intravenous lines and catheters. To understand nurses' decisions to restrain, Yarmesch and Sheafor (1984) asked 23 nurses in a hospital and a long-term care setting to complete a questionnaire containing four patient vignettes. The nurses made 81 decisions to use restraint and only 10 decisions to withhold it in favor of an alternate nursing action. Their reasons to restrain were most often to protect the patient or others and to control behavior.

Effects

Supportive evidence for the effectiveness of physical restraint in preventing falls, promoting treatment, or controlling behavior is sparse. Paradoxically, "protective devices" like siderails or physical restraints may actually exacerbate many of the problems for which the devices are customarily applied. In a study at one acute-care facility, Kustaborder and Rigney (1983) identified the number and circumstances of accidents among older patients and concluded that restraint measures might, but do not always, prevent the risk of injury. The effectiveness of restraints in the prevention of falls and injuries is increasingly questioned (Barbieri, 1983; Coyle, 1979; Feist, 1978; Innes & Turman, 1983; Janken, Reynolds, &

Swiech, 1986; Lund & Sheafor, 1985; Lynn, 1980; Sehested & Severin-Nielson, 1977; Walshe & Rosen, 1979). Catchen (1983) notes that once a patient falls, even without undue physical harm, the negative consequences often include some form of restraint or confinement. Although most accidents result in only minor injuries, nursing personnel are much more likely to restrain older than younger patients, as confirmed by Kulikowski (1979), in the mistaken belief that the elderly will always injure themselves seriously. Nevertheless, Morgan and others (1985) caution that "restrictions in activity present greater hazards than the risk of falls, even among the elderly for whom falls have the most serious consequences."

No support could be found in the literature to document the efficacy of physical restraints in facilitating treatment or controlling behavior in older people. Greater use of physical restraints has been noted, however, during periods of short staffing (Cubbin, 1970; Rose, 1987), presumably when no one is available to monitor patient activity. Furthermore, Cubbin states that the constant use of restraints on a given care unit becomes habitual and makes it increasingly difficult to reduce their prevalence. Rather than preventing undesirable behavior, application of a restraint may intensify disorganized behavior (Lipowski, 1983) and may contribute to sensory deprivation, loss of a positive self-image, and growing dependency (Gerdes, 1968). Restraints may also increase confusion by limiting communication (Patrick, 1967), heightening degree of disorientation (Castleberry & Seither, 1982; Cohen-Mansfield, 1986), and precipitating regressive behavior and withdrawal (Rose, 1987). Edelson and Lyons (1985) observed that many patients are incapable of understanding or accepting the restraint and become increasingly agitated. In addition, the restrained person tends to be viewed by others as disturbed, dangerous, or mentally incompetent (Mitchell-Pederson, et al., 1985).

Other potential consequences of restraints include incontinence (Gillick, et al., 1982), diminished functional capacity leading to poor potential for rehabilitation (Warshaw, 1983),

and grave physical complications like deep vein thrombosis and embolus (Gillick, et al., 1982) or contractures, edema, skin abrasion, pressure sores, reduced muscle mass, bone loss, and cardiac and respiratory impairment (Gutheil & Tardiff, 1984; Lofgren, Mac-Pherson, Granieri, et al., 1989; Miller, 1975; Rader, Doan, & Schwab, 1985; Straker, 1984). Additional psychological sequelae include sensory deprivation (Roslaniec & Fitzpatrick, 1979), as well as fear, panic, and combativeness (LaPorte, 1982). For combative patients, physical restraints are, in fact, clearly contraindicated (Dietsche & Pollmann, 1982). Prolonged length of stay in the health facility and increased death rate have been observed for restrained patients (Frengley & Mion, 1986; Robbins, et al., 1987). That physical restraints may clearly do more harm than good is evidenced by reports of accidental strangulation by these devices (Cape, 1985; Dube & Mitchell, 1986; Katz, et al., 1981; MacLean, et al., 1982).

LEGAL IMPLICATIONS

Physical restraints are known to have potential ill-effects and are rarely used in the United Kingdom (Editorial, 1980). In the United States, federal and state regulations ensure nursing home residents freedom from unnecessary restraint (Selye, 1985). Thus, clues to explain rising use in the United States must be sought in the literature. Fear of litigation and pressure from administrators and regulatory agencies to prevent falls or wandering have no doubt become significant factors in the growing abuse of physical restraints, siderails, and medications (Editorial, 1984; Rubenstein, Miller, Postel, et al., 1983; Schwab, 1975). Legal guidelines appearing in professional journals make it clear that (1) considerable burden rests with staff to apply as much restraint as necessary to protect patients from hurting themselves or others (Cushing, 1985; Regan, 1982, 1983); (2) incident reports serve as regular alerts to administrators of potential legal action (Sklar, 1985); and (3) courts are finding that hospitals have a duty to any patient capable of self-injury to prevent such injuries (Creighton, 1982; Halpert & Connors, 1986; Northrop, 1987). Ethical considerations concerning patient rights, self-determination, and personal autonomy notwithstanding, the most compelling reasons to restrain appear to be fear of litigation, administrative pressure, and unavailable alternatives.

Virtual silence in the literature on the subjective impact of the restraint experience on patients and their nurses may also have contributed markedly to a practice that in most cases appears to be neither benign nor humane. The magnitude of the problem (as noted earlier) and this gap in the literature led us to study the restraint experiences of hospitalized older people and their nurses (Strumpf & Evans, 1988).

RESTRAINT EXPERIENCES OF HOSPITALIZED OLDER PATIENTS AND THEIR NURSES

This descriptive exploratory study of patients' subjective experiences, nurses' beliefs and decision-making, and patterns of restraint use in one tertiary-care institution was conducted to answer the following questions:

1. What reasons are offered by patients and their nurses for physical restraint?

2. Are there differences between patients' and primary nurses' perceptions of responses, effects, coping strategies, and alternatives to physical restraint?

3. What characterizes the decision-making process in the application of a physical restraint?

Method

Setting, Sample and Instruments. The sample consisted of 20 patients ranging in age from 60 to 81 years (x = 73.3 years) on three general medical units at a 694-bed metropolitan teaching hospital. The patients were judged sufficiently oriented to speak to the interviewer, and all either were or had been physically restrained at some point during the current admission. Patient consents and interviews were tape recorded. Restraints were defined as mechanical devices such as vests, belts, or ties applied to the patient's body and restricting movement in some way. Each patient's primary nurse was also interviewed, and medical records were reviewed to obtain diagnosis, mental status, restraint documentation, length of hospitalization, medications, and pertinent physical and laboratory data.

The investigators developed three instruments for the study: (1) a 19-item semistructured interview guide, the Subjective Experience of Being Restrained (SEBR), used to elicit patients' perceptions and understanding of the restraint experience, including reasons, coping behaviors, effects, and alternatives; (2) a nine-item, self-administered Perceptions of Restraint Use Questionnaire (PRUQ) to ascertain the relative importance the patients' nurses ascribed to commonly asserted reasons for using physical restraints with the elderly (Cronbach's alpha of 0.80); and (3) an 11-item investigator-developed semistructured guide, Primary Nurse Questionnaire (PNQ), to elicit data regarding the perceptions of the patients' nurses as to reasons for and outcomes of restraint use, including decision-making processes, personal feelings, and knowledge of alternatives.

Results

Profile of Restrained Patients. For the 20 patients in the study, the period of restraint ranged from 1 to 121 days with a mean of 23.3 days, median of 11 days, and mode of 4 days. Omitting the patient with 121 days in restraint, the average length of time in restraint was 17.8 days. A high correlation existed between length of stay (x = 30.8 days, omitting the two patients with lengths of stay exceeding 100 days) and the number of days in restraint (r = 0.7933, p = 0.0005). The vest was the most frequently used device, applied at least once, according to the chart, to 19 of 20 patients. Records also indicated that 13 of the patients at some point were restrained with wrist or ankle ties, and 2 patients were restrained with leather restraints. Some patients were restrained with multiple devices.

Thirteen different terms for the restraint device were reported by patients, including a "harness," "chains," or a "clamp." In labelling the restraints used for their patients, 13 nurses chose words like "soft," "vest," or "jacket" to describe the devices that they had applied. These words were also frequently encountered in the progress notes; only leather restraints were characterized as "hard."

Reasons for Restraint. Reasons for physical restraint offered by patients and their primary nurses did not always coincide. Regardless of the reasons for restraint verbalized by patients and nurses, prevention of falls or compensation for changes in mental status was consistently recorded by the nurses as rationale in the progress notes.

Patients were less likely than nurses to report a perceived need for physical restraint. A few indicated the need for its use to prevent falls (20%); to enhance safety due to wandering, elopement, or potential self-injury (25%); because of impaired mental status (15%); or other reasons (15%). "Other" reasons included "being real sick," "to keep me out of mischief," "to keep me quiet," or involvement in an "incident requiring restraint." None of the patients saw facilitation of treatment as a reason for restraint.

The patients' nurses most often gave the following reasons for restraint: impaired mental status (65%), such as confusion, agitation, restlessness, disorientation, poor judgment, and inappropriateness; prevention of falls (60%), especially when there was a history of falls or general concern that they were likely to occur; and facilitation of treatment (40%). In progress notes, the reasons for restraint application were given as prevention of falls (90%), mental status changes (90%), facilitation of treatment (60%),and other safety (25%).

Comparison of Patient and Nurse Perceptions. Analysis of the SEBR suggested nine categories of response by the patients to physical restraint: anger, fear, resistance, humiliation, demoralization, discomfort, resignation, denial, and agreement. These categories were determined primarily from replies to three questions: (1) What do/did you feel when having the (device) applied?; (2) How did/do you deal with being restrained? and (3) Have you had any immediate effects from this (device)? The data demonstrate a range of responses by the patients to the physical, emotional, and behavioral effects of restraints. In addition, other selected comments from patients indicate that some awareness of the relationship between mental state and application of a restraint exists:

"They told me I was confused when I was perfectly sane; when people are confused they do not need a restraint—that drives them over the wall."

"I may not have remembered what the nurse told me (*not to get out of bed*), but I was fully aware of being tied. I didn't feel confused, but the nurse kept asking me if I was confused and the longer I took to answer I guess the more confused she thought I was."

"It's hard to be in bed (*restrained*)—you can't move. It's terrible—you don't know what's going to happen. You look around and you hardly know where you are. It makes your mind go a little bit."

The PNQ revealed that the patients' primary nurses also experienced personal responses to the experience of physical restraint. Considerable discomfort and ambivalence about the practice were demonstrated by selected responses addressing both the conflicts and the coping strategies for those faced with the decision to restrain:

"I'd rather use a restraint than have her fall."

"Safety is my ultimate responsibility."

"I tell myself it's for their safety. I can't allow myself to feel sorry for the patient."

"Everyone hated to restrain him; he was such a nice man. But he seemed to accept it and he became used to it, which helped the staff."

"Sometimes it bothers me when the patient can't understand the need for restraint. I wonder if it's really for his own good."

"There may not be any other choice."

"It drives me crazy to restrain so many patients. I feel like a jailer rather than a nurse."

"I feel guilty at times because you take away the patient's freedom and that bothers me."

Effects of Physical Restraint. Both patients and nurses indicated some awareness of behavioral, emotional, physical, and other effects of physical restraint on patients. Behavioral effects, noted by 11 of the nurses and none of the patients, included attempts to remove the restraint (one patient repeatedly asked to be released and, in fact, tried to cut off the vest restraint with his table knife), and signs of increased anger, combativeness, agitation, resistance, or even hallucination. Two patients and five nurses reported emotional effects of unhappiness and anger. Six patients were described by their nurses as either cooperating, not resisting, or being aware of restraint. For two patients restraints were reported to be effective in "slowing them down" or "decreasing agitation and pulling out tubes."

Coping with Physical Restraint. When asked "What do/did you do when the (device) is/was applied?" and "How did/do you deal with being restrained?" patients reported up to three coping strategies, including doing nothing or giving up (30%); thinking, praying, or trying to forget (20%); attempting removal (15%); and making verbal requests to discontinue the restraint (10%). Seven (35%) tried "good" behavior or other responses; no one reported the use of physical means like hitting or striking out to deal with the situation. Recognizing that employment of coping strategies might be influenced by patient expectations regarding duration of the restraint experience, patients were asked how long they (had) expected to wear the restraint. The majority (55%) reported having expected to be restrained only "hours"; 10% felt it might be days; 10% were unable to predict the length of time, and one patient felt it would be "forever."

When asked how they dealt with the experience, nurses reported that it helped them cope if the patient did not object to, or agreed with the need for, restraint, as did being able to talk with the patient, other nurses, and friends about the experience, especially since the duration of restraint ranged from several days to weeks at a time.

Alternatives to Physical Restraint. Eleven alternatives to restraints were proposed by seven of the patients, including greater availability of nursing staff, more explanations, easier access to the bathroom and toileting, a device that would be "softer and easier," increase in diversionary activity, and discharge from the hospital altogether. Nurses, on the other hand, gave none at all or only a limited number of alternatives to restraint use, most of which focused on frequent monitoring or greater availability of staff for direct supervision; medication; increased activity; attempts at stimulation or reasoning; and environmental considerations (e.g., room location, mattress on floor). Nurses seldom suggested that restraints could or should be eliminated.

Decision to Apply a Restraint. To gain further understanding regarding the nurses' willingness to use a physical restraint in patient care management, data from the PRUQ were analyzed. Nurses believed the most important reasons for restraining an older person were to (1) provide for safety; (2) protect from falling out of bed or chair; and (3) prevent from getting into dangerous places or supplies. Rated as the least important reason for restraint of an older person was to prevent taking things from others.

In general, documentation of the initial need for restraint, nurse or physician orders, patient response, progress, and reassessment was consistently made by the nurse; such documentation, however, was scarce or nonexistent from the physician. Despite a hospital policy requiring written orders by either nurse or physician and appropriate documentation, seven patients (35%) had no written orders for restraint. Whether or not an order was present, data from the PNQ indicated that in 19 of 20 cases the nurse made the actual decision to apply a restraint. In only six cases was the patients' response to the restraint described in the progress note; the only documentation that occurred 100% of the time was a daily note by the nurse that a physical restraint was in use.

Seven criteria by which nurses made judgments to discontinue restraints were given: improved mental status, capacity to adhere to a contract regarding expected behavior, improved ambulation with little further risk of falling, reduced wandering or inappropriate climbing out of bed, availability of direct supervision, discontinuation of various tubes or lines, and elimination of restrictions in activity. Improvement in mental status was given most frequently as a reason for discontinuation of restraints. Exceptions to restraint usage were few, but they included physician orders against it, adamant refusal by the patient, and presence of fever or any of the above-mentioned criteria for discontinuation. One nurse noted that restraints should never be used simply for staff convenience. None of the nurses gave a wholly accurate description of the hospital's restraint policy.

Discussion

This descriptive study revealed the heretofore largely unreported complexity and impact of the restraint experience on both older medical patients and their nurses. Although the reasons, responses, awareness of effects, coping strategies, and alternatives described by patients and their primary nurses frequently lacked congruence, they were nevertheless revealing, poignant, and insightful. For the patients, cognitive impairment was no barrier to awareness of the discomfort associated with restraining devices. Physical and psychological impact was apparent in patients' assessments of length of time the restraint would remain in place and in the coping strategies employed to deal with a sometimes unbearable situation. Patients were remarkable in their suggestions for alternatives and were often more creative than their caregivers, who saw few options unless constant supervision was available. Patients found many words or phrases to describe their restraints and struggled to understand the reasons for their application. Clearly, this was a memorable, often troubling experience resulting in a wide spectrum of emotions, ranging in temporality and intensity. Among the most articulate was the following account by one 74-year-old man who became "confused" after a single dose of Ativan:

It's all one long dream, but as I recall, I was somewhat depressed that my hospitalization had been very tenuous; one day I was told by the doctors "maybe we'll do this or that," "maybe we'll operate," but nothing definite seemed to happen. I told the doctor I was depressed and he said we can take care of that. Soon after a nurse came and offered me a little white pill which I was told was ordered by the doctor to "keep me in better spirits." I agreed to take it around 3:00 p.m., I think. My next recollection is of the passing (*death*) of my room partner and of being questioned in an inquisitorial way by a tall statuesque character, questions which I tried to answer humorously. The next thing I remember is of being bound left and right and of working very hard to get out of bed—I have a very clear recollection of trying to loosen my hands. As I became aware of the restraints I experienced a great deal of resentment—and I resisted—I could see no reason for doing that to me. I assume I behaved as any human being would—I resented the use of such methods against my person. Once freed I walked to the nurses' station and began to argue—"I shouldn't have been bound," and I pleaded with them never to do it again. I was told I'd had an "incident" requiring restraint but I was unsure what the incident was—I thought it was a conspiracy. I couldn't see myself as confused; I view myself as a rational person. I have no nightmares because of it, I assure you. But I have an ongoing curiosity to know the real events as they occurred and in what sequence of time. I would have liked someone to clue me in on the events that took place and to restore to me the nature of that experience . . . . I think that that's something the hospital owes to the individual.

This patient's story shows the degree of conflict and uncertainty engendered by the application of a restraint, as well as the range of emotional responses, including anger, discomfort, and resistance. The desire for resolution remains extremely potent and patients' need for staff to constantly explain, reassure, and "debrief" becomes obvious.

In analyzing the nurses' beliefs and decision-making process, it became evident that staff felt a need to respond to concerns about patient safety, especially reflecting administrative pressures to minimize any risks that might precipitate legal action. At the same time, staff also continually struggled to reconcile restraint decisions with concerns about patient autonomy and beliefs about professional integrity, as evidenced in the following vignette:

> Mr. M.G., a married 72-year-old black male, was admitted from home to the hospital with a change in mental status secondary to dehydration. The problem list included "chronic progressive dementia," hypertension, urinary incontinence, nutritional cachexia, and need for nursing home placement. Mental status at the time of admission was recorded as "alert and oriented times two, speech difficult to understand but coherent." Over the next several days, the patient was described as more restless, especially at night, with frequent attempts to get out of bed to the bathroom. It was known to the nursing staff that Mr. G. had fallen during a previous hospitalization, injuring his hip. A decision was made by a nurse on the night shift to apply a vest and soft wrist restraint for "increased agitation and for safety," and these were used intermittently on all three shifts for the next 23 days. Progress notes by the nursing staff indicated that the patient often resisted the restraints verbally and physically, at times managing to free himself and wander from his room into the hall and onto the elevator. After being returned to his bed and restrained following one such incident, Mr. G. said to his nurse, "I just want to die." When Mr. G. was allowed out of bed, he was placed in a "geri-chair," although his usual response was to beg not to be placed in "that chair" and not to be "tied down" because it made him "feel like dirt." When Mr. G. was judged no longer confused by the nursing staff, restraints were discontinued. No falls occurred during this admission and Mr. G. was sent to a nursing home, alert and oriented and with some improvement in his overall status.

Although beyond the scope of this chapter, many questions remain unanswered, including whether the above circumstances warranted restraint, who is responsible (patient, nurse, agency) in the event of a fall, how much autonomy can be given to patients judged to be frail and at risk of injury, and whose rights are the most important. Selected responses from the primary nurse questionnaire clearly reflect competing loyalties and conflicts among institutional policies, patient rights, and morally justifiable professional behavior. Although nurses offered some alternatives to restraints, these did not take precedence over deeply rooted fears about potential liability. As one nurse put it, "A patient fall is an *incident* requiring a written report; psychologic repercussions from application of a restraint are not." The message is a clear one: "Don't let anyone fall."

Dimensions of the decision-making process involved in applying and maintaining a physical restraint were clarified, and several observations about the way in which the nurses made decisions and interpreted the institution's restraint policy were noteworthy. In every case the progress note reflected a judgment by the nurse that a patient's behavior warranted restraint and a note was written, without fail, on every shift for as long as the restraint was in place. In this study, notes appeared on the interdisciplinary progress notes; the patients' physicians, however, seldom mentioned the presence of a restraint, although general references were often made about a patient's mental status. A psychiatric consultation was unusual.

Reading the entire record revealed two parallel sets of observations: the nurses always noted that a restraint was in place, and physicians rarely mentioned restraints or the associated behaviors or consequences. For whatever reasons, physical restraints appeared to be the nurses' problem. The complexity of potential causes of behavior precipitating the initial need for restraint, as well as the seriousness of possible sequelae, strongly suggests the need for interdisciplinary collaboration, especially in situations where restraints are in place continuously for days, weeks, or, in the case of one patient, months. Furthermore, it is reasonable to propose that a restrained patient deserves especially attentive monitoring.

IMPLICATIONS FOR NURSING PRACTICE

The existing evidence on the potential harmfulness of restraints (described in the preceding review of the literature) and the subjective experiences ascertained by the study reported above, add persuasively to an argument for alternatives to restraint. Alternatives need to be more consistent with ethical practice and should guarantee a higher quality of care for the frail, institutionalized older person. What seems particularly urgent is the careful testing of alternative interventions and the reformulation of restraint policies. Except for the most serious circumstances, it is our opinion that the use of restraint devices should be avoided.

The literature provides recommended guidelines for use of restraints with older people; these are similar to those for psychiatric patients (Guirguis, 1978; Roper, Coutts, Sather, et al., 1978; Straker, 1984). A review of these articles reveals common standards for practice (Katz, et al., 1981; MacLean, et al., 1982; Morrison, et al., 1987; Robbins, 1986; Tadsen & Brandt, 1973). In general, the authors agree that restraints should be used only when absolutely necessary and never as a substitute for surveillance; that the rare decision to restrain should be a collaborative one between nurse and physician; that any problematic behavior should trigger investigation, treatment, and elimination of the underlying cause, as opposed to immediate application of a physical restraint; that patients and families should be informed and involved in all care decisions; that restraints should be used only as a last resort on a short-term basis; and that staff be trained in alternative measures.

Research on alternatives to restraint is, unfortunately, somewhat limited (Schwartz, 1985b), especially for management of allegedly unsafe behavior. Lichtenstein and Stone (1987) found nurses' efforts to avoid physical restraints included explanations (86%), family cooperation (22%), and medication (16%). Williams and associates (1979), in a hospital study of risk factors for confusion in older hip fracture patients, reported several effective nursing interventions to prevent or treat confusional episodes. Their interventions were aimed at an approach that is appropriate to the individual, including incorporation of orienting information as part of the conversation; keeping patients informed about and giving rationale for treatment and procedures; correcting sensory deficits; overseeing continuity of care; providing time pieces; maintaining

adequate pain control; minimizing the number of hospital personnel interacting with the patient; encouraging family visits; and assisting the patient to have a sense of control.

General guidelines for any problematic behavior known to precipitate restraint use should include the following steps:

- Complete baseline and ongoing assessment of any physical or psychologic impairment.
- Identify and document any problematic behaviors that present potential problems.
- Investigate causes as completely as possible.
- Collaborate with other members of the health care team, and include family or significant others whenever possible.
- Use restraint only as a temporary and emergency means for managing behavior.

In the rare event that a physical restraint is applied:

- Select the least restrictive device of the proper type and size.
- Observe frequently.
- Assess physical and emotional response every hour; determine continuing need for restraint.
- Release a minimum of every 2 hours for 10 to 20 minutes and perform range of motion exercises.
- Maintain proper body alignment and patient comfort.
- Avoid isolation; continue interacting frequently with the patient.
- Anticipate and meet needs for fluids and nourishment, toileting, and access to essential items like a call bell, tissues, and the telephone.
- Remove restraints as soon as possible.
- Help patient verbalize recollection of the restraint experience and associated anxiety; clarify and validate the experience for the patient.

Although further research is certainly needed, the literature, nevertheless, provides a countless supply of alternatives to physical restraint. These include:

1. *Specific nursing care* (Code, 1984):
   a. General comfort measures
   b. Positioning with pillows, recliners, etc.
   c. Changes in form of treatment, e.g., substituting oral feedings for intravenous or nasogastric tubes and removal of catheters or external urinary drains
2. *Psychosocial intervention* (Covert, et al., 1977; LaPorte, 1982; Massachusetts Nurses' Association, 1983; Misik, 1981; Prehn, 1982; Rader, et al., 1985; Rose, 1987):
   a. Reality orientation
   b. Remotivation therapy
   c. Behavior modification
   d. Therapeutic touch
   e. Active listening
   f. Allowance for and attention to expression of feelings and concerns
   g. Companionship and supervision (staff, family, friends, volunteers), especially at night
3. *Activities* (Code, 1984; Covert, et al., 1977; Schwab, et al., 1985):
   a. Distraction by television, radio, record, or tape player
   b. Social-recreational-physical activity
   c. Training in activities of daily living
4. *Environmental manipulation* (Cohen, 1977; Davidson, Hemingway, & Wysorki, 1984; Editorial, 1980; Hay & Cromwell, 1980; Hernandez & Miller, 1986; Jacoby, et al., 1958; Lichtenstein & Stone, 1987; Lipowski, 1983; Mitchell-Pederson, et al., 1985; Olsen, 1985):
   a. Removal of restraint devices from the unit/facility
   b. Circular or semicircular room arrangement around nursing station for maximal visiblity
   c. Redesign of furniture, e.g., lower beds and removal of wheels from furniture
   d. Increased light
   e. Color-orienting cues
   f. Available quiet room
   g. Accessible call light or other means of communication
   h. Bedrails in down position
   i. Commode at bedside
   j. Mattress on floor
   k. Transfer to home or familiar surroundings
5. *Staff, administrative, and policy interventions* (Editorial, 1980; Huey, 1985; Robbins, 1986; Rovner, Kafonek, Filipp, et al., 1986):
   a. Training and emotional support for staff who work with persons having behavioral disturbances
   b. Education of staff to accept a broader range of potentially bothersome behaviors
   c. Change in policy and staff expectations
   d. Implementation of an interdisciplinary restraint-monitoring team
   e. Administrative support to decrease staff fear of malpractice suit or other repercussions

Wandering is the only problematic behavior for which a developing literature is available concerning environmental, cognitive, social, and nursing interventions (Cornbleth, 1977; Dawson & Reid, 1987; Dietsche & Pollmann, 1982; Fennelly, 1985; Gaffney, 1986; Hiatt, 1980, 1985, 1986; Huey, 1985; Mitchell-Pederson, et al., 1985; Rader, et al., 1985; Snyder, Rupprecht, Pyrek, et al., 1978), including the following measures: locked or closed unit, door alarm systems, sheltered courts and gardens with irregular space for exploring, camouflage for doors, reduction in messages over public address system, broad-based rockers, easily identified garments (shirts, sweaters) or other special means of identification, cognitive improvement activities, recreational and social activity and exercise, appropriate outlets for industrious or anxious behavior, routines for those who awaken and wander (e.g., night-time activities), deliberate attempts to meet the patient's specific agenda, treatment of incontinence, and occasional glass of beer or wine.

It is obvious from the above-named interventions that an approach to care emphasizing observation and engagement between individual patients and staff is most likely to prevent application of a physical restraint. Our observations in facilities throughout Scotland confirm that a combination of the above strategies, appropriately employed, do indeed reduce dramatically the use of restraining devices.

What remains astounding, however, is that despite regular reporting of possible alternatives, the impact on restraint use in the United States has been slight. This may be due to "abuse of litigation" (Editorial, 1984), of which the legal community in the United States is also aware. As Rubenstein and associates (1983) report, the fear of litigation for negligence has led to nearly routine use of bedrails.

At the same time that every hospital and nursing home in the United States is expected to adhere to some version of the Patient's Bill of Rights, they are also required to have a policy regarding use of restraints. Although an assumption is made throughout these documents that alternatives are preferred, many obstacles, not the least of which is habit, stand in the way of a significant reduction in restraint use. Only in those instances where written policy makes it explicitly difficult to use a physical restraint (e.g., requiring a written medical order within 15 minutes and checks every 15 minutes by a registered nurse) has there been much evidence of decreased use (Cohen, 1977; Mitchell-Pederson, et al., 1985). The authors have identified several long-term care facilities with protocols requiring that every effort to limit the use of restraints be undertaken. These facilities, regularly reported in a publication prepared by the Kendal Corporation (1989), have apparently succeeded because of a uniformly shared philosophy of care and an understanding that in the event of falls or injuries, staff decisions will be supported by administration. Without such support, genuine concern on the part of nurses about potential liability will, unfortunately, continue to take precedence over attempts to employ alternatives to restraint. For the nurse, the dilemma is great: Concerns about patient safety, especially in the face of actual or perceived administrative pressures to minimize any risks that might precipitate legal action, competes with concerns for patient autonomy, ethical practice, and professional integrity. We are convinced that the best protection for patient, caregiver, and agency is care delivered with dignity and humanity, using knowledge currently available.

SUMMARY

Review of the literature and recent research indicates that application of a physical restraint is far from a benign procedure, especially in its physical and psychological impact on older people. In addition, it poses a critical ethical dilemma for all providers of health care. The foregoing discussion demonstrates the need for alternatives that are consistent with standards of professional practice and that guarantee individualized, dignified care for frail, institutionalized older people. It is our recommendation that, inasmuch as possible, use of restraining devices be severely limited or entirely eliminated. Alternatives exist and are known to succeed in other countries and at restraint-free facilities in the United States. This task must be accomplished if we are to be true to our responsibilities for patient autonomy, personal safety, and quality of life. Without question, this is one of the great challenges for those who nurse, and care deeply about, older people in our society.

References

Applebaum, PS, & Roth, LH (1984): Involuntary treatment in medicine and psychiatry. *Am J Psychiatry,* 141(2):202–205.

Barbieri, EB (1983): Patient falls are not patient accidents. *J Gerontol Nurs,* 9(3):165–173.

Burnside, IM (1980): Wandering behavior. *In* Burnside, IM (ed): *Psychosocial Nursing Care of the Aged.* New York, McGraw-Hill.

Burnside, IM (1984): Are nurses taught to tie people down? *J Gerontol Nurs,* 10(5):6.

Cape, RDT (1985): Avoiding restraints. XIII International Congress of Gerontology, Book of Abstracts, 401.

Castleberry, K, & Seither, F (1982): Disorientation. *In* Norris, CM (ed): *Concept Clarification in Nursing.* Rockville, MD, Aspen.

Catchen, H (1983): Repeaters: Inpatient accidents among the hospitalized elderly. *Gerontologist,* 23(3):273–276.

Cohen, SI (1977): The first year at the New Esrath Nashim Hospital, Jerusalem 1968–69: Abolition of physical restraints. *Br J Psychiatry,* 130:544–547.

Cohen-Mansfield, J (1986): Agitated behaviors in the elderly II: Preliminary results in the cognitively deteriorated. *J Am Geriatr Soc,* 34(10):722–727.

Cohen-Mansfield, J, & Billig, N (1986): Agitated behaviors in the elderly I: A conceptual review. *J Am Geriatr Soc,* 34(10):711–721.

Cornbleth, T (1977): Effects of a protective hospital ward

area on wandering and non-wandering geriatric patients. *J Gerontol, 32*(5):573–577.

Covert, AB, Rodrigues, T, & Solomon, K (1977): The use of mechanical and chemical restraints in nursing homes. *J Am Geriatr Soc, 25*(2):85–89.

Coyle, N (1979): A problem-focused approach to nursing audit: Patient falls. *Cancer Nurs, 2*(10):389–391.

Creighton, H (1982): Are siderails necessary? *Nurs Manag, 13*(6):45–48.

Cubbin, JK (1970): Mechanical restraints: To use or not to use? *Nurs Times, 66*(24):752.

Cushing, M (1985): First, anticipate the harm. *Am J Nurs, 85*(2):137–138.

Davidson, NA, Hemingway, MA, Wysorki, T (1984): Reducing the use of restrictive procedures in a residential facility. *Hosp Community Psychiatry, 35*(2):164–167.

Dawson, P, & Reid, DW (1987): Behavioral dimensions of patients at risk of wandering. *Gerontologist, 27*(1):104–107.

Department of Health, Education and Welfare (DHEW) (1979): National Nursing Home Survey: 1977. PHS 79:1794. Hyattsville, MD, National Center for Health Statistics.

Dietsche, LM, & Pollmann, JN (1982): Alzheimer's disease: Advances in clinical nursing. *J Gerontol Nurs, 8*(2):97–100.

Dube, AH, & Mitchell, EK (1986): Accidental strangulation from vest restraints. *JAMA, 256*(19):2725–2726.

Edelson, JS, & Lyons, WH (1985): *Institutional Care of the Mentally Impaired Elderly.* New York, Van Nostrand Reinhold.

Editorial (1980): Restrained in Canada—Free in Britain. *Health Care, 22*(7):22.

Editorial (1984): Cotsides—Protecting whom against what? *Lancet, 35*(18 August):383–384.

Evans, LK, & Strumpf, NE (1989): Tying down the elderly: A review of the literature on physical restraint. *J Am Geriatr Soc, 37*(1):65–74.

Farnsworth, EL (1973): Nursing homes use caution when they use restraints. *Mod Nurs Home, 30*(3):4, 9–10.

Feist, R (1978): A survey of accidental falls in a small home for the aged. *J Gerontol Nurs, 4*(6):15–17.

Fennelly, AL (1985): Making it safe for the patient to wander. *Am Health Care Assoc J 11*(7):29–30.

Fisk, VR (1984): When nurses' aides care. *J Gerontol Nurs, 10*(3):119–127.

Frengley, JD, & Mion, LC (1986): Incidence of physical restraints on acute general medical wards. *J Am Geriatr Soc, 34*(8):565–568.

Gaffney, J (1986): Toward a less restrictive environment. *Geriatric Nursing, 7*(2):94–96.

Gerdes, L (1968): The confused or delirious patient. *Am J Nurs, 68*(6):1228–1233.

Gillick, MR, Serrell, NA, & Gillick, LS (1982): Adverse consequences of hospitalization in the elderly. *Soc Sci Med, 16*:1033–1038.

Guirguis, EF (1978): Management of disturbed patients: An alternative to the use of mechanical restraints. *J Clin Psychiatry, 39*(4):295–303.

Guirguis, EF, & Durost, HB (1978): The role of mechanical restraints in the management of disturbed patients. *Can Psychiatr Assoc J, 23*(4):209–218.

Gutheil, TG, & Tardiff, K (1984): Indication and contraindication for seclusion and restraint. *In* Tardiff, K (ed): *The Psychiatric Uses of Seclusion and Restraint.* Washington, DC, APA Press.

Halpert, A, & Connors, JP (1986): Prevention of patient falls through perceived control and other techniques. *Law Med Health Care, 14*(1):20–24.

Hay, D, & Cromwell, R (1980): Reducing the use of full-leather restraints in an acute adult inpatient ward. *Hosp Community Psychiatry, 31*(3):198–200.

Health Care Financing Administration (HCFA) (1988): *Medicare/Medicaid Nursing Home Information: 1987–1988.* Washington, DC, US Government Printing Office.

Hernandez, M, & Miller, J (1986): How to reduce falls. *Geriatr Nurs, 7*(2):97–102.

Hiatt, LG (1980): The happy wanderer. *Nurs Home, 29*(2):27–31.

Hiatt, LG (1985): Understanding the physical environment. *Pride Institute J, 4*(2):12–22.

Hiatt, LG (1986): Effective trends in interior design. *Provider, 12*(4):28–30.

Huey, FL (1985): What teaching nursing homes are teaching us. *Am J Nurs, 85*(6):678–683.

Innes, EM, & Turman, WG (1983): Evolution of patient falls. *Qual Rev Bull, 9*(2):30–35.

Jacoby, MG, Babilian, H, McLamb, E, et al. (1958): A study in non-restraint. *Am J Psychiatry, 115*(8):114–120.

Janken, JK, Reynolds, BA, & Swiech, K (1986): Patient falls in the acute care setting: Identifying risk factors. *Nursing Res, 35*(4):215–219.

Katz, L, Weber, F, & Dodge, P (1981): Patient restraint and safety vests: Minimizing the hazards. *Dimens Health Serv, 58*(5):10–11.

Kendal Corporation (1989): *Unite the Elderly, 1*(1). (Available from Kendal Corporation, P.O. Box # 100, Kennett Square, PA 19348).

Kulikowski, ES (1979): A study of accidents in a hospital. *Supervisor Nurse, 10*(7):44–58.

Kustaborder, MJ, & Rigney, M (1983): Intervention for safety. *J Gerontol Nurs, 9*(3):159–162, 173.

LaPorte, HJ (1982): Reversible causes of dementia: A nursing challenge. *J Gerontol Nurs, 8*(2):74–80.

Lichtenstein, H, & Stone, JT (1987): *Restraints in the Elderly.* Paper presented at American Society on Aging, Salt Lake City, UT, March.

Lipowski, Z (1983): Transient cognitive disorders (delirium, acute confusional states) in the elderly. *Am J Psychiatry, 140*(11):1426–1436.

Lofgren, RP, MacPherson, DS, Granieri, R, et al. (1989): Mechanical restraints on the medical wards: Are protective devices safe? *Am J Public Health, 79*:735–738.

Lund, C, & Sheafor, ML (1985): Is your patient about to fall? *J Gerontol Nurs, 11*(4):37–41.

Lynn, FH (1980): Incidents—Need they be accidents? *Am J Nurs, 80*(6):1098–1101.

MacLean, J, Shamian, J, Butcher, P, et al. (1982): Restraining the elderly agitated patient. *Canadian Nurse, 78*(6):44–46.

Massachusetts Nurses' Association (1983): Nursing guidelines for the use of restraints in non-psychiatric settings. *J Gerontol Nurs, 9*(3):180–181.

Miller, M (1975): Iatrogenic and nursigenic effects of

prolonged immobilization of the ill aged. *J Am Geriatr Soc*, 23:360–369.

Mion, L, Frengley, JD, & Adams, M (1986): Nursing patients 75 years and older. *Nurs Manag*, 17(9):24–28.

Misik, I (1981): About using restraints with restraint. *Nursing 81*, 11(8):50–55.

Mitchell-Pederson, L, Edmund, L, Fingerote, E, et al. (1985): Let's unite the elderly. *OAHA Quarterly*, 21(10):10–14.

Morgan, VR, Mathison, JH, Rice, JC, & Clemmer, DI (1985): Hospital falls: A persistent problem. *Am J Public Health*, 75(7):775–777.

Morrison, J, Crinklaw-Wiancko, D, King, D, et al. (1987): Formulating a restraint use policy for adults based on the research process. *J Nurs Admin*, 17(3):39–42.

Newton, K (1950): *Geriatric Nursing*. St. Louis, CV Mosby.

Northrop, CE (1987): A question of restraints. *Nursing '87*, 17(2):41.

Olsen, LP (1985): A nurse-administered long term care unit. *J Gerontol Nurs*, 6(10):616–621.

Oster, C (1976): Sensory deprivation in geriatric patients. *J Am Geriatr Soc*, 24(10):461–463.

Patrick, ML (1967): Care of the confused elderly. *Am J Nurs*, 67(12):2536–2539.

Prehn, RA (1982): Applied behavioral analysis for disturbed elderly patients. *J Gerontol Nurs*, 8(5):286–288.

Rader, J, Doan, J, & Schwab, Sr M (1985): How to decrease wandering: A form of agenda behavior. *Geriatr Nurs*, 6(4):196–199.

Regan, WA (1982): Restrain as needed: Nursing judgment required. *Regan Report on Nursing Law*, 23(3):4.

Regan, WA (1983): Restraints and bedfalls: Most frequent accidents. *Regan Report on Nursing Law*, 23(10):4.

Robbins, LJ (1986): Restraining the elderly patient. *Clin Geriatr Med*, 2(3):591–599.

Robbins, LJ, Boyko, E, Lane, J, et al. (1987): Binding the elderly: A prospective study of the use of mechanical restraints in an acute care hospital. *J Am Geriatr Soc*, 35(4):290–296.

Roper, JM, Coutts, A, Sather, J, et al. (1978): Restraint and seclusion: A standard and standard care plan. *J Psychsoc Nurs*, 23(6):18–23.

Rose, J (1987): When the care plan says restrain. *Geriatr Nurs*, 8(1):20–21.

Rosen, H, & DiGiacomo, JN (1978): The role of physical restraints in the treatment of psychiatric illness. *J Clin Psychiatry*, 39(3):228–232.

Roslaniec, A, & Fitzpatrick, JJ (1979): Changes in mental status in older adults with four days of hospitalization. *Res Nurs Health*, 2:177–187.

Rovner, BW, Kafonek, S, Fillipp, L, et al. (1986): Prevalence of mental illness in a community nursing home. *Am J Psychiatry*, 143(11):1446–1449.

Rubenstein, HS, Miller, FH, Postel, S, et al. (1983): Standards of medical care based on consensus rather than evidence: The case of routine bedrail use for the elderly. *Law Med Health Care*, 11(6):271–276.

Schwab, Sr M (1975): Nursing care in nursing homes. *Am J Nurs*, 75(10):1812–1815.

Schwartz, D (1985a): Call for help. *Geriatr Nurs*, 6(1):9.

Schwartz, D (1985b): Replies to a "Call for help." *Geriatr Nurs*, 6(6):250–251.

Sehested, P, & Severin-Nielsen, T (1977): Falls by hospitalized elderly patients: Causes, prevention. *Geriatrics*, 32(4):101–108.

Selye, JH (1985): Privacy rights and rights related to physical security. *Am Health Care Assoc J*, 11(3):20–22.

Shindul, JA, & Snyder, ME (1981): Legal restraints on restraint. *Am J Nurs*, 81(2):393–394.

Sklar, C (1985): Liability for a fall. *Canadian Nurs*, 81(5):15–16.

Snyder, LH, Rupprecht, P, Pyrek, J, et al (1978): Wandering. *Gerontologist*, 18(3):272–280.

Soloff, PH (1978): Behavioral precipitants of restraint in the modern milieu. *Compr Psychiatry*, 19(2):179–184.

Soloff, PH (1979): Physical restraint and the non-psychotic patient: Clinical and legal perspectives. *J Clin Psychiatry*, 40(7):302–305.

Soloff, PH (1984): Historical notes on seclusion and restraint. *In* Tardiff, K (ed): *The Psychiatric Uses of Seclusion and Restraint*. Washington, DC, APA Press.

Stilwell, E (1983): Nurses' use of physical restraint on hospitalized aged. Paper presented at Potomac '83, Washington, DC, November 17.

Straker, M (1984): Guidelines for the elderly. *In* Tardiff, K (ed): *The Psychiatric Uses of Seclusion and Restraint*. Washington, DC, APA Press.

Strumpf, N, & Evans, L (1988): Physical restraint of the hospitalized elderly: Perceptions of patients and nurses. *Nurs Res*, 37(3):132–137.

Tadsen, J, & Brandt, RW (1973): Rules for restraints: Hygiene and humanity. *Mod Nurs Home*, 30(3):57–58.

Trockman, G (1978): Caring for the confused or delirious patient. *Am J Nurs*, 78(9):1495–1499.

Walshe, A, & Rosen, H (1979): A study of patient falls from bed. *J Nurs Admin*, 9(5):31–35.

Warshaw, GA (1983): Hospital care for the elderly patients. *Center Reports on Advances in Research*, 7(3).

Williams, MA, Holloway, JR, Winn, MC, et al. (1979): Nursing action and acute confusional states. *Nurs Res*, 28(1):25–35.

Wolanin, MO, & Phillips, LF (1980): Who's confused here? *Geriatr Nurs*, 1(2):122–125.

Yarmesch, M, & Sheafor, M (1984): The decision to restrain. *Geriatr Nurs*, 5(4):242–244.

Zimmer, JG, Watson, N, & Treat, A (1984): Behavioral problems among patients in skilled nursing facilities. *Am J Public Health*, 74(10):1118–1121.

Zubek, JP, Boyer, L, Milstein, S, et al. (1969): Behavioral and physiological changes during prolonged immobilization plus perceptual deprivation. *J Abnorm Psychol*, 74(2):230–236.

Zubek, JP, & Wilgosh, L (1963): Prolonged immobilization of the body: Changes in performance and in the EEG. *Science*, 140:306–308.

Zubek, JP, & MacNeill, M (1966): The effects of immobilization: Behavioral and EEG changes. *Can J Psychol*, 20(3):316–336.

The Sundown Syndrome: A Nursing Management Problem

LOIS K. EVANS, R.N., D.N.Sc., F.A.A.N.

INTRODUCTION

Among health care professionals who work with the elderly, the term "sundown syndrome" is used to describe the occurrence or exacerbation of symptoms of confusion during the late afternoon and early evening hours. This is the time of day when even mildly impaired older people may become dis-oriented, agitated, or restless and may begin to wander about or scream. Whether these behaviors actually increase in the evening or are merely more noticeable at that time of day is not known from research; regardless, the behaviors pose tremendous management problems for caregivers, both in the home and in health care institutions.

Despite acknowledgment of its common clinical occurrence in acute-care hospitals, psychiatric hospitals, nursing homes, and the community, little research on the sundown syndrome has been reported in the literature, with two exceptions: the syndrome can apparently be precipitated by placing an elderly demented subject in a darkened room during the daytime (Cameron, 1941), and administering caffeine has no apparent effect on quality or quantity of sleep among sundown syndrome sufferers (Ginsburg & Weintraub, 1976). Thus, little is known about sundown syndrome itself, factors related to its occurrence, or how it may be prevented, alleviated, or managed.

An exploratory study was undertaken to describe the phenomenon of sundown syndrome, to examine its prevalence in a nursing home population, and to identify physiologic, psychosocial, and environmental factors associated with the phenomenon. Specifically, the aims were to (1) determine the prevalence of sundown syndrome among a typical intermediate and skilled nursing facility population; (2) identify and quantify behavioral components and patterns of the syndrome; (3) identify associated medical diagnoses; and (4) determine the relationship of other variables to sundown syndrome, including age, sex, body temperature, blood pressure, morale, mental status, presence of organic mental impairment, sensory function, medication use, time of day, mealtime, length of stay, patient-staff ratio, and environmental variables.

This chapter discusses literature relevant to understanding sundown syndrome, summarizes the methods and findings of the exploratory study, and suggests implications for further study and for nursing practice with elders at risk for the phenomenon.

BACKGROUND

In dementia, there is a progressive decline in cognitive function, especially marked by short-term memory loss. Ability to function may be retained for some time unless additional stressors, such as illness, hospitalization, or other crises, are superimposed. With the lowered cerebral reserve in dementia, such stress may precipitate an acute confusional state or delirium (Lipowski, 1983; Prinz & Raskind, 1978; Warshaw, Moore, Friedman, et al., 1982).

Sundown syndrome resembles delirium in that patients with either condition may present with disordered cognition, attention, sleep-wake pattern, and psychomotor behavior, and the symptoms tend to be more pronounced at night. However, delirium ordinarily resolves in less than 1 month or ends in death; sundown syndrome does not appear to follow this pattern. As Lipowski (1980) states, "It is not known if nocturnal confusion in a patient with senile dementia really represents delirium or a similar syndrome, possibly with different pathophysiology."

The work of Cameron (1941) on sundown syndrome appears to have been accepted by clinicians as definitive. To test the onset of darkness as a precipitating factor, he placed known sundown patients in a darkened room during the earlier part of the day. In each instance, symptoms of delirium appeared within 1 hour of imposed darkness and subsided within 1 hour of light. Cameron believed that this finding supported the importance of darkness as opposed to fatigue as a causative factor. In subsequent tests he found that subjects with severe loss of recent memory had extremely impaired orienting capacity when blindfolded. He postulated that sundown syndrome, or "nocturnal delirium," in persons with severe recent memory impairment resulted from loss of orienting capacity imposed by darkness.

Sundown syndrome continues to be recognized as a clinical problem (Barnes, Raskind, Scott, et al., 1981; Jahnigen, Hannon, Laxson, et al., 1982; Mace & Rabins, 1981; Prinz & Raskind, 1978; Sherman & Libow, 1981; Snyder, Rupprecht, Pyrek, et al., 1978). Yet, except for the previously mentioned caffeine study (Ginsburg & Weintraub, 1976), no further research has been reported. Therefore, selected findings from related areas, such as acute confusional states or delirium, biological rhythms, and depression, along with hypotheses from clinical practice, are summarized here in three categories: psychosocial, physiologic, and environmental factors.

Psychosocial Factors

Depression, which is prevalent among demented patients (Miller, 1980), frequently masquerades as confusion and is referred to as pseudodementia (Warshaw, et al., 1982) or dementia of depression (Reynolds, Kupfer, Hoch, et al., 1986). Stress (Kral, 1962), fear, loneliness, and social isolation (Burnside, 1981; Ernst, Beran, Safford, et al., 1978; Fowler & Fordyce, 1972; Regestein, 1980; Wolanin & Phillips, 1981) have all been postulated as causes of confusion and sundown syndrome. Conversely, Williams, Holloway, Winn, and associates (1979) found that elderly hospitalized patients in single rooms had better memory 1 and 3 days following surgical repair of hip fractures than those in multiple occupancy rooms.

Physiologic Factors

Generalized confusion is known to result from hypoxia from any origin (toxic conditions, nutritional disorders, infections, endocrine disorders, cerebral disease [Schneck, Reisberg, & Ferris, 1982]); disturbances in the sleep-wake cycle, which are so common among the demented (Feinberg, Koresko, & Shaffner, 1965; Dement, Miles, & Carskadon, 1982; Reynolds, Spiker, Hanin, et al., 1983); immobility (Miller, 1975; Williams, et al., 1979; Zubek, Boyer, Milstein, et al., 1969); dehydration (Snyder, et al., 1978); and pain (Wolanin & Phillips, 1981). Sensory deprivation, sensory overload, and exposure to unfamiliar situations in combination with altered sensory acuity and memory loss are viewed as possible factors in precipitating acute confusional states and sundown syndrome (Butler & Lewis, 1977; Castleberry & Seither, 1982; Oster, 1979; Trockman, 1978; verWoerdt, 1981). Patients with impaired hearing or vision have a great need for extrasensory stimulation (Drummond, Kirchhoff, & Scarbrough, 1978), yet responsiveness to touch decreases as mental status declines (Langland & Panicucci, 1982). Finally, given the periodicity of sundown syndrome itself, disturbances in circadian rhythms are possible factors; in normal elderly men, for instance, the modal peak for physiologic variables is 5:00 p.m. (Cahn, Folk, & Huston, 1968). Thus, if desynchronization occurs, evening confusion might logically be a result.

Environmental Factors

Dwindling environmental light as evening approaches (Bartol, 1983; Burnside, 1981; Butler & Lewis, 1977; Cameron, 1941); noisiness in the environment or too much silence (Wolanin & Phillips, 1981); lack of orienting cues (Williams, et al., 1979); use of physical restraints (Burnside & Moehrlin, 1980; verWoerdt, 1981); and reduced patient-to-staff ratios and lowered unit activity levels common in institutions in the evening (Fowler & Fordyce, 1972; Lawton, 1981) may also contribute

to periodic disorientation. In addition, clinicians and caregivers observe that sundown syndrome seems to increase with extreme changes in atmospheric pressure and during a full moon (Snyder, et al., 1978).

Despite its common occurrence and the wealth of data supporting possible causative factors, little is actually known about the specific causes, prevalence, prevention, and management of sundown syndrome.

SUMMARY OF AN EXPLORATORY STUDY OF SUNDOWN SYNDROME

Methods

The sample consisted of 89 randomly selected residents of the Health Care Institute, a 180-bed teaching nursing home affiliated with Georgetown University, Washington, DC. (See Evans, 1987, for a more detailed description of the study.) Fifty-nine residents were judged from medical or nursing documentation to be demented, and 30 others served as a nonimpaired comparison group. The 89 subjects had an average age of 80 years; were 89% black, predominantly female, and currently single; had lived in the facility an average of 14 months; and were most likely to have a nonskilled labor or homemaker occupational history and a ninth grade education. Seventy percent had been admitted from an acute-care facility. Subjects had an average of five medical diagnoses and seven prescribed medications. The mean score on Pfeiffer's Short Portable Mental Status Questionnaire was 5.4 (moderately impaired), and over 65% failed the Face-Hand Test, indicating an organic basis for cognitive impairment. One-third were totally dependent for mobility.

Presence of sundown syndrome was determined through use of a structured observation tool, the Confusion Inventory (Tables 17–1 and 17–2). The observer indicated the presence or absence of each of 48 psychomotor and psychosocial behaviors indicative of confusion during 10-minute observation sessions in the morning and evening on 2 consecutive days. Those subjects who displayed more behaviors

Table 17–1. SUNDOWN SYNDROME CONFUSION INVENTORY*

Date: Day I _____ Day II _____ Observation Period: AM _____ PM _____

Time: Day I _____ Day II _____ Subject # _____ Observer _____

Instructions: Locate the subject on the unit. (NOTE: If off the unit, await his/her return if expected during the allowable observation time period.) Situate self in as comfortable and unobtrusive a manner as possible so as to facilitate observation of the subject for a 10-minute period. During this period, *circle as many items per category as observed*. Try to refrain from engaging in conversation with the subject or other patients, staff, or visitors during this period. Record the Day I observations in column I and the Day II observations in column II, as appropriate.

1. **Psychomotor Activity** (circle all that apply)		Day I	Day II
a. Gross motor activity:	rocking	1	1
	wheeling	1	1
b. Restless activity:	tapping with feet/fingers	1	1
	picking at clothing/bedclothes	1	1
	scratching self	1	1
	touching/pursing lips	1	1
	moving extremities randomly/aimlessly	1	1
	banging self/furniture	1	1
	chewing/grinding teeth	1	1
	rubbing self/object	1	1
	other restless behavior	1	1
c. Security-seeking/other behavior:	hoarding	1	1
	striking out/hitting	1	1
	kicking	1	1
	spitting	1	1
	carrying security object	1	1
	rummaging in drawers/closet	1	1
	undressing inappropriately	1	1
d. Escape behavior:	attempting to get out of bed/chair	1	1
	attempting to remove restraints	1	1
2. **Psychosocial Activity** (circle all that apply)		Day I	Day II
a. Behavioral appearance:	searching	1	1
	intense/driven/sense of urgency	1	1
b. Expression of feelings:	crying	1	1
	laughing	1	1
	smiling	1	1
	complaining	1	1
	cursing	1	1
	demanding	1	1
	temper outburst	1	1
c. Other verbalizations:	sucking	1	1
	muttering/mumbling	1	1
	moaning	1	1
	humming	1	1
d. Interactive behavior:	social/personal	1	1
	calling for help	1	1
	asking questions	1	1
	perseveration	1	1

Table 17–1. SUNDOWN SYNDROME CONFUSION INVENTORY* *Continued*

3. At the end of the 10-minute observation period, rate the subject in the following areas (circle one rank for each area).

Agitation Rating Scale	Day I Observation				Day II Observation			
	Not at All	Just a Little	Pretty Much	Very Much	Not at All	Just a Little	Pretty Much	Very Much
agitation/restlessness	0	1	2	3	0	1	2	3
destructiveness/combativeness	0	1	2	3	0	1	2	3
loudness/noiseness	0	1	2	3	0	1	2	3
isolation/deprivation	0	1	2	3	0	1	2	3
fear/worry	0	1	2	3	0	1	2	3
intensity/urgency	0	1	2	3	0	1	2	3

4. From your observation of the subject, do you consider this patient to be:†

	Day I	Day II
rational	1	1
moderately confused	2	2
severely confused	3	3

*The Sundown Syndrome Confusion Inventory contains 37 of the original 48 behavioral items that were tested in the Evans (1987) study. Only the factors that positively discriminated sundown syndrome patients from nonsundown patients were retained in the present tool. Sources of behaviors include Norris (1975); Pfeiffer (1978); Dement, Miles, & Carskadon (1982); and Greene, Smith, Gardiner, et al. (1982).

†Matron's Overall Assessment of Confusion, from Slater & Lipman (1977).

in the evening than in the morning were labeled sundown syndrome patients. These 11 subjects represented 12.4% or 1 in 8 of the population age 60 years and older in this nursing home. Mental status was measured by Pfeiffer's (1975) 10-item Short Portable Mental Status Questionnaire (SPMSQ); the Face-Hand Test (Fink, Green, & Bender, 1952) was used to screen for organicity; and morale was measured by the 17-item Philadelphia Geriatric Center Morale Scale (Lawton, 1972). Data regarding medical diagnoses, medications, and nighttime sleep habits were obtained from health care records and a nursing staff questionnaire. Each subject was screened for vision, hearing, and light touch. Environmental light intensity, blood pressure, oral temperature, and observation for odor of urine (a gross proxy measure of level of hydration [Acee, 1984; Taylor & Henderson, 1986]) were obtained immediately following each observation period.

Findings

Several factors were related to the appearance of sundown syndrome in this population (Table 17–3).

Mental Status. All but two of the sundown syndrome patients came from the demented group; thus, while the syndrome was seen to be more than twice as likely to occur among demented patients, only 15% of the demented subjects displayed the phenomenon. However, sundown syndrome patients had significantly greater impairment in mental function (SPMSQ) and all failed the Face-Hand Test of organicity, as compared with 61% who did not display the syndrome. Although mental impairment would appear to be an important risk factor, the fact that so many impaired elders did not display sundown syndrome indicated that there are other factors at work.

Psychosocial Factors. Sundown syndrome patients had been in the facility a shorter length of time and were more likely to have been relocated within the facility during the past month. Further, these patients were observed to be relatively isolated from others, had few visitors, and were engaged in few activities in the afternoon.

Physiologic Factors. All but one patient with sundown syndrome had a cardiovascular or cerebrovascular disorder; in addition, nine of the 11 were diagnosed with dementia and the other two had cerebrovascular disorders. The

Table 17–2. GUIDE TO USE OF CONFUSION INVENTORY

Purpose: This guide specifies supplies, instructions and definitions required to accomplish reliable observation of confused behavior.

Supplies: Assemble the following:
2 pencils
Confusion Inventory/subject
Clipboard
Timing device

Instructions:
1. Plan to observe each subject over a minimum of 2 consecutive days during a 10-minute period in the morning and late afternoon or evening.
2. Use one Sundown Syndrome Confusion Inventory form for the two morning observation periods and a separate form for the two afternoon periods in order to reduce observer bias. Record in pencil.
3. If possible, position yourself so that your observation of the resident is unobtrusive. Try to refrain from engaging in verbal interaction with subject or other residents during this time. If necessary, you may acknowledge the subject with a nod and smile. If necessary to observe resident in the room, ask permission to enter, indicating that you would like to sit with the resident for a few minutes. If asked, you may state that you are interested in observing how the resident is getting along.
4. Set the timing device for 10 minutes. Observe the resident, taking a "mental photograph" of his or her location and behavior.
5. Record any behavior in appropriate sections 1 and 2. Resume observation of the resident. Record any additional or new behavior observed. You may observe and record several times during the 10-minute period. When the timer sounds, stop; review each observation category one more time, adding any additional observations. Move to sections 3 and 4 and complete rating scales. Unless otherwise indicated on form, circle *every* behavior observed in each category during the observation period.
6. Subjects are *not* to be observed in toilet or bathing areas or behind closed doors or curtains.
7. If a subject is off the unit (e.g., having dinner) and is not likely to return during the allowable observation period, you may locate the resident off the unit (e.g., in the dining room) and make your observations there. So indicate in margin.

Definitions:
1. Psychomotor Activity
   a. Gross motor activity
      Rocking: Self-propelled back and forth movement in chair or while standing
      Wheeling: Propelling oneself in a wheelchair
   b. Restless activity
      As per items on tool. Refers to behavior directed toward self, e.g., scratching, banging, rubbing.
      Other: may include clapping hands, pill-rolling, grasping, shifting position, wriggling body part, wringing hands, etc.
   c. Security-seeking
      Hoarding: placing or keeping food or other objects on or about the person (inside pocket, bra, or clothing), in purse or bag to carry, or in bed or furniture, e.g., wheelchair
      Striking out/hitting: flailing limbs with or without apparent purpose (i.e., intention to harm another)
      Kicking: striking another with foot with apparent intention
      Spitting: expectorating toward another, into container, or on furniture or floor
      Carrying security object: keeping special object on person, e.g., blanket, doll, purse, bag
      Rummaging in drawers or closet: may or may not be emptying contents
      Undressing inappropriately: i.e., publicly and/or not in preparation for bed, hygiene, etc.; implies *action* on part of subject
   d. Escape behavior (Attempts to . . .)
      Get out of bed/chair: e.g., shaking bedrails, placing limbs over sides of bedrails or chair arms, pushing as to rise out of chair; refers only to situation in which subject is in some way restrained or immobilized
      Remove restraints: picking or pulling at restraints, shaking mitts
2. Psychosocial activity
   a. Behavioral appearance
      Searching: looking as if hunting for someone/something
      Intense/driven/urgent: compelled, unable to stop, frantic, compulsive, "life and death," earnest

Table 17–2. GUIDE TO USE OF CONFUSION INVENTORY *Continued*

   b. Expression of feelings
      Crying: uttering weeping, wailing, or sobbing sounds, usually accompanied by tears
      Laughing: uttering chortling/chuckling sounds
      Smiling: mouth turned up, no sound
      Complaining: verbal statement of complaint
      Cursing: using profanity
      Demanding: calling for something in authoritative voice
      Temper outburst: sudden show of anger, accompanied by verbal and/or physical behavior
   c. Other verbalization
      Sucking: licking or smacking noises ordinarily accompanying the act of drawing liquid into mouth
      Muttering/mumbling: mouth is moving as though speaking, but voice is so low words are indistinct
      Moan/groan: a deep or low murmur of pain or distress
      Humming: singing with closed lips
   d. Interactive behavior
      Social/personal: ritual social comments initiated in greeting/farewell or by a focus on an event with relevance
         to the individual; "good morning"; "you are pretty"; "it is cold"
      Calling for help: verbally requesting assistance of another, whether present or not, e.g., "please turn on the
         light"; "nurse! nurse! nurse!"; "I want a drink"
      Asking questions: inquiring of another other than social amenities
      Perseveration: continuing repetition of meaningless word or phrase or of questions that have already been
         answered
3. Agitation rating scale
   Agitated/restless: degree of excited, disturbed, fidgety, nervous behavior
   Destructiveness/combativeness: degree of destroying or ruining objects, striking out at others, especially in response to
   an approach by the other
   Loudness/noisiness: decibel of sound, turbulence, or disturbing sound
   Isolation/deprivation: degree to which subject is insulated from interpersonal and sensory stimulation
   Fear/worry: degree of expressed alarm or uneasiness
   Intensity/urgency: degree of frantic compulsiveness in behavior
4. Base rating on the 10 minutes of observed behavior.
Scoring:
1. Every behavior 1a through 2d is scored 1 if present, zero if not present, *with the exception of laughing and smiling*,
   which are scored in the reverse (expecting them to be absent in confusional states). The morning score is subtracted
   from the evening score for each of the 37 items to obtain a change score. Subjects who exhibit a given behavior in the
   morning but not in the evening will have a negative change score; subjects who exhibit the behavior only in the
   evening will have a positive change score; and subjects who either never or always display the behavior score zero.
   Each pair of change scores for all 37 behaviors is summed and a mean is calculated for the two days of observation.
   To determine patients with sundown syndrome, the frequency distribution should be examined. In the Evans (1987)
   study, subjects who scored 2.5 and over were classified as having sundown syndrome.
2. Similarly calculate a mean change score for each component of the Agitation Rating Scale over the 2-day period. In
   the Evans (1987) study, sundown syndrome patients had significantly higher evening agitation. With further
   refinement, this short scale may be useful as a measure of observed confusion variability over a 24-hour period.
3. Calculate a mean change score for the Matron's Confusion Scale over the 2-day period. In the Evans (1987) study,
   sundown syndrome patients were significantly more likely to be rated with greater confusion in the evening.

sundown syndrome patients had a much lower average number of diagnoses than non-sundowners (3.9 vs. 5.1). Very few residents in the facility were taking drugs commonly associated with confusion: hypnotics/sedatives, tranquilizers, antidepressants, and analgesics. No particular medication type was statistically associated with sundowning. Patients with sundown syndrome were more likely to have an odor of urine (suggesting possible dehydration) in the afternoon and were awakened frequently during the night for routine nursing care and monitoring. Although not statistically significant, sundown syndrome patients tended to have normal hearing but impaired vision, and, in several, blood pressure dropped in the afternoon.

Environmental Factors. Although not significantly related to sundown syndrome, a majority of these patients were observed to be in dim light in the late afternoon, especially those found in their own bedrooms. Lights

Table 17–3. FACTORS THAT DIFFERENTIATED SUNDOWNERS FROM NON-SUNDOWNERS*

Factor	Sundown Syndrome Trait
Psychosocial	
Mental status	Greater impairment
Organicity	All organically impaired
Degree of confusion	Increased in afternoon
Length of stay	Shorter
Room transfer	Recent
Physiologic	
Medical diagnoses	Fewer total diagnoses
Urine odor	Increased in afternoon
Sleep disturbance	Awakened every 2 hours during night
Environmental	
None	
Demographic	
None	

*Only factors that achieved statistical significance are included.

were frequently not turned on until the dinner hour, which occurred after sunset during the weeks of this study. Eight of the 11 sundown syndrome patients were physically restrained; in fact, they were more than three times as likely to be restrained as the others. However, an expected increase in restraint use in the evening was not found to be associated with sundown syndrome.

Discussion

These findings and the review of literature revealed several possible explanations for certain patients developing sundown syndrome. Presence of an organic dementia, together with severe cognitive impairment, appears to be an important risk factor, but it is not sufficient to predict who will develop or display the syndrome.

Psychosocial Stressors. We all depend to some degree on social cues, such as regular mealtime, ringing of noontime church bells, the evening news program, bathing and bedtime patterns, for regulation of our biologic rhythms (Czeisler, Richardson, Zimmerman, et al., 1981). When these are disrupted, such as during travel or on admission to an institution, rhythm desynchrony and confusion

may result (Armstrong-Esther, 1978). In this patient population, sundowning may have been a response to problems in adapting to a new environment with different or absent social cues. Sundown syndrome patients had lived a shorter time in the facility and were more likely to have been recently relocated to a new room or unit within the facility. Five of the patients were identified by nursing staff as having had a stressful environmental change in the past month, including a change in roommate or a transfer to the hospital. That no sundown syndrome patients had been in the facility for less than 5 months, however, suggests that some cognitively impaired elders may need more time than others to adjust to a new environment. Further, their orientation to time and place may have been hampered by the observed lack of activities and social contacts in the afternoon (Lawton, 1981). Visual impairment, low environmental light, and short-term memory deficits (Cameron, 1941) may also have combined to contribute to disorientation at this time of day. While morale, as an indicator of depression (Morris, Wolf, & Klerman, 1975), did not significantly differentiate sundown syndrome patients from others, depression is a possible component for some patients and should be considered.

Delirium. There is some support from these findings for considering sundown syndrome as a form of delirium. Risk of delirium increases with advanced age, and all sundown syndrome patients were over age 74 years (average age 83 years). Among disorders that are known to pose particular risk for delirium, cardiovascular, cerebrovascular, or organic brain disorders were likewise present in all sundown syndrome patients. Disturbed sleep cycles and dehydration, found in this group, are also known to precipitate delirium. It is likely that the low incidence of sundown syndrome in this sample may be related to the lack of polypharmacy and low level use of drugs commonly associated with delirium. Institutionalized elderly are estimated to take between 5 and 12 prescription drugs, the most prevalent of which are tranquilizers (Lamy, 1980). In this sample, the low level of drug use in part results from the collaborative efforts of gerontological nurse clinicians and physicians in this teaching nursing home to evaluate and discontinue potentially harmful drugs when possible.

Circadian Rhythm Desynchrony. The periodicity of sundown syndrome itself raises the question of a disturbance in circadian rhythms as a possible factor. Higher oral temperature but lower blood pressure in the afternoon among the sundown syndrome patients may indicate a change in rhythms, since normally a peak is expected in both parameters in the late afternoon. An increased dissociation of circadian rhythm peaks with advancing age has already been noted (Cahn, et al., 1968); sundown patients' average age was 83 years. Others have also documented an earlier peaking of blood pressure in nondemented hypertensive elderly (Drayer, Weber, DeYoung, et al., 1982) and some instability in temperature regulation in demented patients (Prinz, Christie, Smallwood, et al., 1984). terHaar (1977) has suggested that hypotension may be implicated in day-evening confusional displays. Without 24-hour data it was not possible to explicate these patterns of the sundown syndrome patients.

Potential Underdiagnosis. One interesting finding is that sundown syndrome patients had fewer diagnosed medical conditions than others. Hoffman (1982) found that 63% of elderly people with suspected dementia actually had treatable conditions, in addition to or instead of dementia. Thus, one should wonder whether these sundown syndrome patients, labeled as demented, were suffering additional but undiagnosed medical conditions that may have contributed to their impaired mental status and delirium-like symptoms. Regardless, dementia itself interferes with patients' ability to report signs and symptoms and to seek help appropriately, placing the onus on nursing staff to closely observe and verify changes in health status.

Sensory Deprivation or Overload. In experiments with normal adults, both sensory deprivation and overload have been shown to produce disorientation and confusion. By 5:00 p.m. most nonnursing personnel had gone home, and there were commonly fewer nursing staff per patient on the evening shift. Thus, decreased social activities and interaction were typical. Further, sundown syndrome patients had normal hearing but impaired vision and touch senses, which may both limit and distort sensory intake. In the normal circadian cycle, steroid levels decline and sensory acuity increases to a peak between 5:00 and 7:00 p.m. (Luce, 1970). For some residents, the increased sensitivity to auditory stimuli at that time of day, together with visual deficits that interfered with correct interpretation of the source of auditory stimuli, may have contributed to an increase in agitation and confusion. Regardless, visual impairment among sundown syndrome patients may have been a predisposing factor (Cameron, 1941).

Rest-Activity Cycle. The rest-activity cycle is believed to be a strong regulator of biologic rhythms in humans. The prevalence of sleep-wake cycle disturbance in dementia and its relation to delirium is well established (Feinberg, et al., 1965; Prinz & Raskind, 1978; Reynolds, et al., 1983). In this study it is not known whether subjects also suffered from sleep apnea, which together with cardiovascular disorders, would increase vulnerability to hypoxia and resultant confusional states (Reynolds, Kupfer, Hoch, et al., 1985). The finding that routine "good" nursing care, that is, the frequent monitoring of patients throughout the night to prevent skin breakdown from incontinence, might contribute to sundown syndrome is extremely interesting in this regard and certainly warrants further study. Would a monitoring schedule that more closely approximates the normal 90-minute sleep cycle be less disruptive?

Dehydration. Dehydration is common among the elderly, especially those with impaired mobility or memory, those with chronic diseases, and those taking diuretics. Hospital admissions for nursing home patients with hypernatremic dehydration occur with relative frequency (Himmelstein, Jones, & Woolhandler, 1983). Recently it was found that the sense of thirst may decline in normal older adults, thereby interfering with maintaining an optimal level of hydration (Phillips, Phil, Rolls, et al., 1984). Dehydration precipitates delirium as a result of electrolyte imbalance and is highly correlated with mental confusion (Seymour, Henscheke, Cape, et al., 1980). Level of hydration was not measured directly in the present study. However, clinicians commonly agree that concentrated urine has a particularly strong odor (Acee, 1984; Taylor & Henderson, 1986). Thus, the appearance of a strong urine odor in the late afternoon among sundown syndrome patients is suggestive of dehydration. Further, the tendency for increased body temperature and decreased diastolic blood pressure in the evening lends support to the possible influence of dehydration in the sundown syndrome patients in this sample. Whether the observation of urine odor in the afternoon indicates higher incidence of incontinence associated with sundowner syndrome patient's progressive dementia or staff inattention to the toileting and hygiene needs of these residents in the late afternoon, rather than more concentrated urine, is not known. However, any of these factors might predispose to greater confusion (Lawton, 1981; Lipowski, 1980).

Light-Dark Cycle. The light-dark cycle is also responsible for regulating biologic rhythms in humans. Cameron's early description of nocturnal delirium implicates the approaching darkness of evening as a precipitating factor. Although a decrease in room light was not a significant factor in this study, the fact that room lights were not turned on until after sunset may have affected these patients, especially those who were placed in their bedrooms in the afternoon. Room light intensity in the afternoon, rather than a change in light over the course of a day, may be a more important factor to examine.

Restraint Use. Physical restraints are known to precipitate agitation and confusion, especially in delirious or demented patients (LaPorte, 1982; MacLean, Shamian, Butcher, et al., 1982). Many authors caution against their use in these populations (Burnside, 1979). While sundown syndrome patients were three times more likely to be restrained at some point during the day, their sundowning behavior did not appear to precipitate an increase in restraint use during the late afternoon hours. The possible association of restraint use and sundowning warrants further examination, especially since immobilization is known to produce confusion and agitation in the elderly (Miller, 1975).

Implications for Further Study

To better document the occurrence of sundown syndrome, including the late night (2:00 a.m.) exacerbation in confusion frequently described by clinicians, systematic round-the-clock observation of sleep-wake behavior (including electroencephalographic monitoring), confusion, and agitation should be undertaken over a longer period of time, for example, 1 month. It is important to document whether sundowning behavior, once it occurs, continues on a daily basis or waxes and wanes. If sundown syndrome is really delirium, then it should resolve in a few days or weeks, although the patient may be vulnerable to its recurrence. In additional studies, more precise measures of depression, hydration, and biologic rhythms should be used. Also, other population groups (i.e., Caucasian and Asian elders, those at home and in acute-care settings) should be studied to determine patterns and precipitating and predisposing factors. Finally, studies to test the effects of nursing measures on the incidence and management of sundown syndrome should be undertaken.

Implications for Practice

These study results are not conclusive about the nature of sundown syndrome; many questions were raised and remain unanswered. However, we have moved a few steps beyond folklore. Based on study findings and the existing literature, several nursing strategies can be recommended for prevention and management of sundown syndrome. The range of individual differences displayed by the 11 patients with sundown syndrome supports the notion that there is no one cause for the phenomenon. Nor will a particular intervention necessarily be effective for a given patient.

Therefore, the following strategies are suggested for use on a trial-and-error basis, depending on individual patient assessment.

Assessment. On admission to the facility and periodically thereafter, it is advisable to assess each individual for risk factors for the development of sundown syndrome. Sources of data include the transfer record, medical records, patient and family interviews, and nursing observation and evaluation. The nurse should attempt to answer the following questions:

1. Has the patient ever had the experience of becoming more confused or restless in the evening? This could have occurred during a prior hospitalization or at home. Response to previous relocation experiences is important.

2. If so, how would the behavior best be described? Did/does the patient wander and try to leave the house or facility "to go home?" Was/is there verbal calling out or repetitive asking of questions? Was/is there agitation, pacing, crying, etc.?

3. Does the patient have any of the following risk factors for delirium: Older age (e.g., over 74 years)? Cardiovascular disease, cerebrovascular disease, dementia? Polypharmacy (especially with sedatives/hypnotics, tranquilizers, antidepressants, analgesics, diuretics)? Electrolyte imbalance, dehydration? Limited mobility?

4. Does the patient have impaired vision, hearing, or touch sensation?

5. Does the patient experience hypotension in the afternoon or evening?

6. Is the patient's mental status greatly impaired? Is there organicity?

7. Has the patient experienced any psychosocial losses or crises in the recent past?

8. What is the patient's normal sleep pattern?

Prevention and Management. For patients with a past history of sundown syndrome or those with risk factors, the following measures will help them become and remain oriented to the new environment, will help staff prevent or treat delirium, and will support the older person's remaining strengths.

Psychosocial Interventions
1. Orient the resident several times over a period of days to the room, toilet, common areas, unit, and facility.

2. Assist the resident to participate in arrangement of room furnishings and storage of personal belongings.

3. Encourage the family to bring in photos and other mementos of home to keep at the bedside or in the resident's room.

4. Do not relocate this resident within the facility without good reason; if a room change is *absolutely* necessary, involve the resident in the decision, orient the resident to the new room prior to the move, and provide additional environmental orienting cues (Pablo, 1977).

5. Consider room placement near the nurses' station, if possible, to facilitate monitoring as well as to increase the likelihood of social interaction.

6. Involve the resident in organized activities in the afternoon.

7. Use soft music, singing, and other social sensory stimulation in the late afternoon. If possible, arrange activity staff or volunteer schedules to cover the late afternoon and early evening period.

Physiologic Interventions
1. Offer fluids frequently, especially to demented and less mobile patients.

2. Offer high carbohydrate snacks in the afternoon.

3. Provide extra touch stimulation to patients with lowered touch sensation.

4. Evaluate the need for monitoring continency every 2 hours during the night, especially for elderly with sleep-wake disturbance; coordinate such assessments with the 90-minute sleep cycle.

5. Continue to monitor and decrease unnecessary drugs that may cause delirium.

6. Consider demented patients with cardiovascular and cerebrovascular disease particularly at risk for sundown syndrome.

7. If there is evidence that the patient may be experiencing hallucinations or other psychotic symptoms, a low dose of a neuroleptic drug may be tried on a short-term basis. Haloperidol, from 0.125 to 0.5 mg once or twice a day, is often recommended because it is a low-dose, high-potency drug with low sedating

and anticholinergic side effects. The drug need not be continued indefinitely, since the patient's condition may change. Therefore a drug-free period should be tried intermittently.

Environmental Interventions

1. Make sure that environmental orienting cues are in place: large clock and large-print calendar in every room at eye level, distinguishing characteristics on each corridor, labels (with graphics) on important doors such as toilet, dining room, patients' rooms.

2. Turn on the lights before dark; if possible install a sensor to maintain an even level of light intensity. Have night lights in resident rooms.

3. Consider placement in a single rather than double room (Williams, et al., 1979).

4. Use alternatives to physical restraint, such as one-to-one supervision (involve family or volunteers), supervised activity, Adirondack or beanbag chairs. (See Chapter 16 for additional alternatives.)

To clearly assess and document that a resident is experiencing sundown syndrome, a modified version of the Confusion Inventory may be used. This checklist includes the psychomotor and psychosocial behaviors that are most predictive of sundown syndrome (Evans, 1987). Using the Confusion Inventory before and after instituting a preventive or management strategy or program aimed at decreasing the extent of sundowning in a patient or unit would assist in evaluating effectiveness. The modified Confusion Inventory and instructions for its use are found in Tables 17–1 and 17–2.

These suggested interventions, although described for a long-term care setting, can be modified for use in the home or an acute-care facility. Sudden appearance or exacerbation of evening confusion should be presumed to be delirium and should trigger a search for a cause in any setting.

SUMMARY

Sundown syndrome can be a frightening experience for patients and families and a serious management problem for nursing staff in acute-care and long-term care facilities. Recognition of potential risk factors and institution of environmental and programmatic changes that may prevent or assist in management of the syndrome are well within the purview of nursing. As Jahnigen and associates (1982) have stated, symptoms of sundown syndrome may "emerge under stress and fear, change in routine, sleep deprivation, or immobilization. If so, it may be possible to identify susceptible patients on admission and to take measures to reduce the frequency of such events." Thus, the challenge exists to develop, test, and refine interventions that will preserve function and contribute to the quality of life of these elders.

References

Acee, S (1984): Helping patients breathe more easily. *Geriatr Nurs,* 5(6):230–233.

Armstrong-Esther, C (1978): Day for night. *Nurs Times,* 78(30):1263–1265.

Barnes, R, Raskind, M, Scott, M, et al. (1981): Problems of families caring for Alzheimer's patients: Use of a support group. *J Am Geriatr Soc,* 29(2):80–85.

Bartol, M (1983): Alzheimer's disease: Reaching the patient. *Geriatr Nurs,* 4(4):234–236.

Burnside, I (1979): Alzheimer's disease: An overview. *J Gerontol Nurs,* 5(4):14–20.

Burnside, I (1981): *Nursing and the Aged.* New York, McGraw-Hill.

Burnside, I, & Moehrlin, B (1980): Health care of the confused elderly at home. *Nurs Clin North Am,* 15(2):389–402.

Butler, R, & Lewis, M (1977): *Aging and Mental Health.* St. Louis, CV Mosby.

Cahn, A, Folk, G, & Huston, P (1968): Age comparison of human day-night physiological differences. *Aerospace Med,* 39(6):608–610.

Cameron, O (1941): Studies in senile nocturnal delirium. *Psychiatr Q,* 15:47–53.

Castleberry, K, & Seither, F (1982): Disorientation. *In* Norris, CM (ed): *Concept Clarification in Nursing.* Rockville, MD, Aspen, 309–323.

Czeisler, C, Richardson, G, Zimmerman, J, et al. (1981): Entrainment of human circadian rhythms by light-dark cycles: A reassessment. *Photochem Photobiol,* 34(1):239–247.

Dement, W, Miles, L, & Carskadon, M (1982): "White paper" on sleep and aging. *J Am Geriatr Soc,* 30(1):25–50.

Drayer, J, Weber, M, DeYoung, J, et al. (1982): Circadian blood pressure patterns in ambulatory hypertensive patients. *Am J Med,* 73(4):493–499.

Drummond, L, Kirchhoff, L, & Scarbrough, D (1978): A practical guide to reality orientation: A treatment approach for confusion and disorientation. *Gerontologist,* 18(6):568–573.

Ernst, P, Beran, B, Safford, F, et al. (1978): Isolation and the symptoms of chronic brain syndrome. *Gerontologist,* 18(5):468–474.

Evans, L (1987): Sundown syndrome in institutionalized elderly. *J Am Geriatr Soc,* 35(2):101–108.

Feinberg, I, Koresko, R, & Shaffner, I (1965): Sleep electroencephalographic and eye movement patterns in patients with chronic brain syndrome. *J Psychiatr Res,* 3:11–26.

Fink, M, Green, M, & Bender, MB (1952): The face-hand test as a diagnostic sign of organic mental syndrome. *Neurology,* 2:46–58.

Fowler, R, & Fordyce, W (1972): Adapting care for the brain-damaged patient. *Am J Nurs,* 72(11):2056–2059.

Ginsburg, R, & Weintraub, M (1976): Caffeine in the "sundown syndrome": Report of negative results. *J Gerontol,* 31(4):419–420.

Greene, J, Smith, R, Gardiner, M, et al. (1982): Measuring behavioral disturbance of elderly demented patients in the community and its effect on relatives: A factor analysis. *Age Ageing,* 11:121–126.

Himmelstein, D, Jones, A, & Woolhandler, S (1983): Hypernatremic dehydration in nursing home patients: An indicator of neglect. *J Am Geriatr Soc,* 31(8):466–471.

Hoffman, R (1982): Diagnostic errors in the evaluation of behavioral disorders. *JAMA,* 248(8):964–967.

Jahnigen, D, Hannon, D, Laxson, L, et al. (1982): Iatrogenic diseases in hospitalized elderly veterans. *J Am Geriatr Soc,* 30(6):387–390.

Kral, V (1962): Stress and mental disorder. *Med Serv J Can,* 18(2):363–369.

Lamy, P (1980): *Prescribing for the Elderly.* Boston, John Wright.

Langland, R, & Panicucci, C (1982): Effects of touch on communicating with elderly confused clients. *J Gerontol Nurs,* 8(3):152–155.

LaPorte, H (1982): Reversible causes of dementia: A nursing challenge. *J Gerontol Nurs,* 8(2):74–80.

Lawton, M (1981): Sensory deprivation and the effect of the environment on management of the patient with senile dementia. *In* Miller, N, & Cohen, G (eds): *Clinical Aspects of Alzheimer's Disease and Senile Dementia.* New York, Raven Press, 227–249.

Lawton, M (1972): The dimensions of morale. *In* Kent, D, Kastenbaum, R, & Sherwood, S (eds): *Research Planning and Action.* New York, Behavioral Publications.

Lipowski, Z (1983): Transient cognitive disorders (delirium, acute confusional states) in the elderly. *Am J Psychiatry,* 140(11):1426–1436.

Lipowski, Z (1980): *Delirium.* Springfield, IL, Charles C Thomas, 542.

Luce, G (1970): Biological rhythms in psychiatry and medicine (ADAMHA Publication). Washington, DC, US Government Printing Office.

Mace, N, & Rabins, P (1981): *The 36-Hour Day.* Baltimore, Johns Hopkins University Press.

MacLean, J, Shamian, J, Butcher, P, et al. (1982): Restraining the elderly agitated patient. *Canadian Nurse,* 78(6):44–46.

Miller, M (1975): Iatrogenic and nursigenic effects of prolonged immobilization of the ill aged. *J Am Geriatr Soc,* 23:360–369.

Miller, N (1980): The measurement of mood in senile brain disease: Examiner ratings and self-reports. *In* Cole, J, & Barrett, J (eds): *Psychopathology in the Aged.* New York, Raven Press, 97–118.

Morris, J, Wolf, R, & Klerman, L (1975): Common themes among morale and depression scales. *J Gerontol,* 30:209–215.

Norris, C (1975): Restlessness: A nursing phenomenon in search of meaning. *Nurs Outlook,* 23(2):103–107.

Oster, C (1979): Sensory deprivation and homeostasis. *J Am Geriatr Soc,* 27(8):364–367.

Pablo, R (1977): Intra-institutional relocation: Its impact on long-term care patients. *Gerontologist,* 17(5):426–435.

Pfeiffer, E (1978): Clinical manifestations of senile dementia. *In* Kalidas, N (ed): *Senile Dementia: A Biomedical Approach.* New York, Elsevier/North-Holland Biomedical Press, 171–184.

Pfeiffer, E (1975): A short portable mental status questionnaire for the assessment of organic brain deficit in elderly patients. J Am Geriatr Soc, 23(10):433–441.

Phillips, P, Phil, D, Rolls, B et al. (1984): Reduced thirst after water deprivation in healthy elderly men. *N Engl J Med,* 311:753–759.

Prinz, P, & Raskind, M (1978): Aging and sleep disorders. *In* Williams, R, & Karacan, I (eds): *Sleep Disorders: Diagnosis and Treatment.* New York, John Wiley & Sons, 303–321.

Prinz, R, Christie, C, Smallwood, R, et al. (1984): Circadian temperature variation in health, aged and in Alzheimer's disease. *J Gerontol,* 39(1):30–35.

Regestein, Q (1980): Insomnia and sleep disturbances in the aged. *J Geriatr Psychiatry,* 13(2):153–171.

Reynolds, C, Kupfer, D, Hoch, C, et al. (1986): Two-year follow-up of elderly patients with mixed depression and dementia. *J Am Geriatr Soc,* 34(11):793–799.

Reynolds, C, Kupfer, D, Hoch, C, et al. (1985): Sleeping pills for the elderly: Are they ever justified? *Psychiatry,* 46(2, Sec. 2):9–12.

Reynolds, C, Spiker, D, Hanin, I, et al. (1983): Electroencephalographic sleep, aging and psychopathology: New data and state of the art. *Biol Psychiatry,* 18(2):139–155.

Schneck, M, Reisberg, B, & Ferris, S (1982): An overview of current concepts of Alzheimer's disease. *Am J Psychiatry,* 139(2):165–173.

Seymour, D, Henscheke, P, Cape, R, et al. (1980): Acute confusional states and dementia in the elderly: The role of dehydration/volume depletion, physical illness, and old age. *Age Ageing,* 9(3):137–146.

Sherman, F, & Libow, L (1981): Pharmacology and medication. *In* Libow, L, & Sherman, F (eds): *The Core of Geriatric Medicine.* St. Louis, CV Mosby.

Slater, R, & Lipman, A (1977): Staff assessments of confusion and the situation of confused residents in homes for old people. *Gerontologist,* 17(6):523–530.

Snyder, L, Rupprecht, P, Pyrek, J, et al. (1978): Wandering. *Gerontologist,* 18(3):272–280.

Taylor, K, & Henderson, J (1986): Effects of biofeedback

on urinary stress incontinence in older women. *J Gerontol Nurs, 12*(9):25–30.

terHaar, H (1977): The relief of restlessness in the elderly. *Age Ageing, 6*(Suppl):73–77.

Trockman, G (1978): Caring for the confused or delirous patient. *Am J Nurs, 78*(9):1495–1499.

verWoerdt, A (1981): *Clinical Geropsychiatry.* Baltimore, Williams & Wilkins.

Warshaw, G, Moore, J, Friedman, W, et al. (1982): Functional disability in the hospitalized elderly. *JAMA, 248*(7):847–850.

Williams, M, Holloway, J, Winn, M, et al. (1979): Nursing action and acute confusional states. *Nurs Res, 28*(1):25–35.

Wolanin, M, & Phillips, L, (1981): *Confusion: Prevention and Care.* St. Louis, CV Mosby.

Zubek, J, Boyer, L, Milstein, S, et al. (1969): Behavioral and physiological changes during prolonged immobilization plus perceptual deprivation. *J Abnorm Psychol, 74*(2):230–236.

CHAPTER
18

Preventing Physical Iatrogenic Problems

JOYCE TAKANO STONE, R.N.C., M.S.

INTRODUCTION

A frequently encountered problem in the health care of the elderly is iatrogenic illnesses, disorders resulting from medical diagnosis or therapy (Jahnigen, Hannon, Laxson, et al. 1982; Patterson, 1986). The older person often experiences multiple chronic conditions requiring a complex regimen of care, frequent visits to the physician, and hospitalization. This increased exposure to the health care system increases the risk for iatrogenic illness. Age has been implicated as a major risk factor for iatrogenic conditions (Jahnigen, et al., 1982). Studies report that 30% to 40% of hospitalized elderly experience iatrogenic complications (Jahnigen, et al., 1982; Reichel, 1965; Steel, Gertman, Crescenzi, et al., 1981). There is a diminished physiologic capacity to compensate and adapt to changes and a diminished physiologic reserve. The individual variations between elderly persons increase the difficulty in prescribing care and predicting

359

outcomes; the role of aging in iatrogenic illnesses requires further exploration and study. This chapter will focus on common iatrogenic events involving physiologic processes. The iatrogenic conditions to be discussed are infection, malnutrition, incontinence, adverse incidents, disturbances of the sleep/wake cycle, immobility, and drug-related problems.

IATROGENIC INFECTIONS

The elderly have an increased incidence and severity of many infectious diseases. They are more susceptible to infections, and although the exact mechanism underlying this increased susceptibility is not known, it appears that multiple factors are involved.

Predisposing Factors

Age. There are alterations in the structure and function of many tissues and organs, diminishing the older person's ability to respond to stresses such as infections. For example, in the respiratory system the increased rigidity of the chest wall and decreased strength of the expiratory muscles result in a less effective cough. With impairment of the cilia lining the respiratory tract, secretions are not cleared readily, and inhaled air is not cleansed as well (Goldman, 1979). Susceptibility to infections is increased as a result of age-related changes in the skin, an important barrier to microorganisms. Increased vulnerability to trauma and a slower rate of healing result from the thinning of the epidermis, a slowing of cell replacement in the stratum corneum, loss of subcutaneous fat, and diminished blood flow (Tonnesen & Weston, 1982; Yoshikawa, 1983). The susceptibility of older persons to bacterial infections may be the result of altered mucosal defense barriers, making them more susceptible to the attachment of and colonization by bacterial pathogens (Schneider, 1983). This tendency for colonization with common pathogens, such as gram-negative bacilli, was noted in the elderly in

both hospital and skilled nursing facilities (Powers, Nagel, Hoh, et al., 1987; Yoshikawa, 1983).

There are age-related changes in the immune system, resulting in a decreased capacity to resist bacterial, fungal, and viral infections, an increased risk of reactivating latent infection, and an altered immune response to immunization or infection (Finkelstein, 1985). It is not unusual to find that the classic signs and symptoms of inflammation are absent in the elderly. Often there is no fever or only a low grade fever and little pain, and the presenting signs and symptoms are not specific enough to localize the site of infection (Finkelstein, 1985).

A change in the immune system found universally among aging individuals is thymic involution, with progressive decline in serum thymic hormone activity (Fox, 1985). The thymus gland plays a crucial role in the generation of mature peripheral lymphoid cells. As a result of the gradual involution of the thymus gland, there is an increase in immature T lymphocytes in the thymus and in peripheral blood. The total number of lymphocytes in the peripheral blood does not change with age, but there are changes in surface receptor function and defects in proliferative capacity (Hausman & Weksler, 1985). Normal immune response requires a proliferation of lymphocytes. Macrophages and B cell function remain relatively intact.

With age, specific antibody responses to foreign antigens are significantly impaired. For example, the response to vaccines is less in the older population. Despite this decline in response, there may be only slight alterations in the total amount of antibody formed following antigenic stimulation. It is postulated that other immunoglobulins, such as autoantibodies, are produced by the aged to make up for the decrease in specific antibody production. Studies of healthy older persons show that host defenses appear to remain the same or slightly diminished. Alterations in the host defenses are seen in the presence of chronic illness or malnutrition (Besedine & Rose, 1982).

Disease States. Some disease states frequently seen in the elderly are associated with a high incidence of infections (Fox, 1985). Urinary tract infection, candidiasis, and skin and soft tissue infections are seen in persons with diabetes mellitus, a common disorder among the elderly. Infections are common in patients with a malignancy because of associated malnutrition and impaired immunity (Fox, 1985). The enlarged prostate predisposes the older male patient to urinary retention and genitourinary instrumentation (Yoshikawa, 1981). Poor functional status has been associated with a higher incidence of infections (Alvarez, Shell, Woolley, et al., 1988).

Certain vitamin deficiencies, notably cyanocobalamin, folate, and pyridoxine, and zinc deficiency have produced a decline in immunologic response (Schneider, 1983). Other nutrient deficiencies may also contribute, and further research is needed to understand the role nutrition plays in immunologic response.

Types of Infections

The most devastating infections are frequently acquired by the hospitalized elderly. The risk of nosocomial infections in the elderly is three times greater than in the general population. This increase in nosocomial infection rates with age reflects the more frequent hospitalizations and longer hospital stays of the elderly, as compared to younger patients (Steel, 1984; Yoshikawa, 1983). In extended care facilities, 5% to 10% of the residents acquire an infection during a given month (Smith, 1988). The incidence of pneumonia, urinary tract infection, surgical wound infection, and bacteremia increases with age (Haley, Hooten, & Culver, 1981).

The information available on nosocomial infections in nursing homes is limited. Surveys have indicated that the greatest prevalence of infections in nursing homes is in infections of the urinary tract, respiratory tract, and skin (Alvarez, et al., 1988; Jackson & Fierer, 1985; Schneider, 1983; Smith, 1988). Factors contributing to the problem of nosocomial infections include high turnover rate of staff, the high number of nonprofessional staff, understaffing, the lack of a trained infection control practitioner, minimal education of personnel in infection control, substandard practices, and inadequate facilities for isolation or handwashing. There is clearly a need for more research on nursing home-acquired infections (LeClair, Schicker, Duthie, et al., 1988; Setia, Serventi, & Lorenz, 1985; Smith, 1985).

Urinary Tract Infection. The urinary tract is the most common site of infection in the elderly, both in the community and in the hospital (Besedine & Rose, 1982; Schneider, 1983). The prevalence of asymptomatic bacteriuria rises from 3% in middle age to over 20% after 70 years and nearly 30% in the institutionalized elderly. Asymptomatic bacteriuria is defined as greater than 10^5 of the same organism per milliliter of urine on two consecutive, aseptically collected urine cultures in an individual without fever or symptoms referable to the urinary tract (Besedine & Rose, 1982; Mostow, 1982). Predisposing factors include poor hygiene, decreased immune competence, and residual urine with stasis and bacterial growth. This condition rarely leads to serious acute illness or loss of renal function, and antibiotic treatment is not indicated. However, in hospitalized patients, nosocomial gram-negative bacteremia often originates in the urinary tract. Due to its high mortality rate, treatment is indicated. In the hospitalized elderly or the elderly at home, bacteriuria and infection in the presence of an indwelling catheter requires attention to both proper care of the catheter and treatment of the infection (Besedine & Rose, 1982).

Pneumonia. Pneumonia in the older population often goes undiagnosed. Instead of the expected fever, cough, increased sputum production, pleuritic chest pain, and elevated white blood cell count, pneumonia in the elderly presents as cognitive changes, usually confusion, lethargy, anorexia, tachypnea, and deterioration of preexisting conditions, such as congestive heart failure and chronic obstructive pulmonary disease. Breath sounds are diminished and rales may be difficult to hear on auscultation (Hill & Stamm, 1982; Mostow, 1982; Raju & Khan, 1988).

The most common cause of pneumonia is the aspiration of bacteria-laden secretions from the oropharynx into the lungs (Besedine & Rose, 1982). The organism of nosocomial pneumonia, the enteric gram-negative aerobic bacteria (EGNAB), tends to colonize in the chronically and seriously ill elderly. Colonization results from contamination of the patient's own gastrointestinal flora, presumably by the fecal-oral route. Persons who are incontinent, immobile, debilitated from malignant, cardiac, and respiratory diseases, and those in deteriorating or preterminal states are at greatest risk for EGNAB pneumonia. Immobility and respiratory disease are the major contributors to colonization (Besedine & Rose, 1982).

Aspiration pneumonia occurs when drugs or anesthesia interferes with normal swallowing and protective mechanisms. Improper positioning during mealtimes or nasogastric feeding can also cause aspiration pneumonia.

Other contributing factors to pneumonia include poor technique during procedures such as tracheal intubation, inadequate provision of fluids to keep bronchial secretions thin and loose, keeping the older person on prolonged bedrest, and neglect of deep breathing exercises.

In addition to antibiotic therapy based on culture and sensitivity tests, careful respiratory care is indicated. Included in the program of care is adequate fluid intake, chest physical therapy, adequate humidification of inspired air, cough and deep breathing exercises, gentle mechanical suctioning when auscultation indicates accumulation of secretions, and careful administration of oxygen for hypoxemic elderly patients, with special attention to the risk of ablating the hypoxic drive to respiration (Besedine & Rose, 1982).

Preventive Measures

Prevention of infections is critical. Pneumococcal and influenza immunizations are recommended to prevent serious respiratory disease in the older population (Mostow, 1982; Raju & Kahn, 1988). Knowledge of infection control principles, especially handwashing and aseptic technique, plays an important role in the prevention and control of iatrogenic infections. Identifying sources of infection, such as indwelling urinary catheters and prolonged immobility, and eliminating these practices will do much to reduce the incidence rate. Understanding the atypical presentation of infectious conditions in the elderly, such as vague, nonspecific symptoms and changes in mental status, as opposed to fever, chills, and leukocytosis, allows for early recognition and prompt treatment. While the suggested interventions are considered basic and fundamental, they are all important in the prevention of infections.

IATROGENIC MALNUTRITION

Factors Leading to Iatrogenic Malnutrition

Nutritional health is commonly affected by illness, hospitalization, and entry into a nursing home. Often, disruptions occur in the usual diet, mealtime, and social aspects of eating. Older persons are especially at risk for nutrition-related problems if they have a prior history of inadequate nutrition resulting from a decrease in income, poor health, loneliness, and isolation (Guigoz & Munro, 1985). The high incidence of polypharmacy in the elderly contributes to poor nutrition. Drugs may interfere or interact with nutrients, may cause anorexia, or may result in dryness of the mouth.

The food served in hospitals and nursing homes may not meet the cultural or personal preferences of the older person. Set mealtimes of the institution may be different from those at home. Other factors, such as food wrapped in difficult-to-open containers; absence of family members to share the mealtime; environmental factors such as unpleasant sights, sounds, and smells; use of uncomfortable restraints; the lack of opportunity for oral hygiene and hand washing; inaccessibility of dentures, glasses, and hearing aids; the inaccessibility of food and fluids between meals all contribute to potentially poor nutritional intake. Activities such as physical therapy, tests and procedures, bathing and routine

Table 18–1. FACTORS LEADING TO
IATROGENIC MALNUTRITION

Illness
Polypharmacy
Pain
Decreased mobility and activity
Anorexia
Special diets, dietary restrictions
Poorly fitting dentures
Hospital/Nursing Home
Unmet cultural or personal preferences in diet
Change in usual mealtimes
Absence of family members
Packaging of food and utensils
Unpleasant environment
Lack of opportunity for oral care, handwashing
Without dentures, glasses, hearing aid
Use of restraints
Multiple activities resulting in fatigue
Prolonged use of glucose and saline intravenous fluids
NPO for diagnostic tests and procedures
Failure to recognize increased metabolic needs with
   illness/injury

care, dressing change of wounds with foul drainage, or painful treatments have to be scheduled so as not to interfere with mealtimes or make the older patient too tired to eat.

Several practices in hospitals can lead to inadequate intake of nutrients and fluids. Such practices include the prolonged use of glucose and saline intravenous fluids, withholding meals for diagnostic tests and procedures, keeping patients on nothing by mouth (NPO) status for prolonged periods, failure to recognize the increased metabolic needs resulting from injury or illness, and failure to provide nutritional support until depletion is corrected (Table 18–1) (Grant, 1979; Patterson, 1986).

Preventive Measures

Nurses play an important role in coordinating nutrition with the dietitian and others on the health team. Careful assessment, recording of height and weight, observation of intake, and continued surveillance of nutritional status during hospitalization or nursing home care are necessary to maintain nutritional health.

IATROGENIC INCONTINENCE

Causes

Incontinence may result from multiple practices carried out in the hospital or other health care facilities (Table 18–2). An older person is in an unfamiliar environment, not knowing or remembering where the bathroom is. Transportation from one test or appointment to another may not include a bathroom stop. Restraints and tubing of all types are major barriers to getting to the bathroom. A restrained patient may desperately try to escape the restraints but fail to do so in time. Delayed response to a call light of a person requiring assistance to the bathroom and failure to provide a urinal within reach or a commode for the older person on bedrest or limited activity status may result in incontinence. In the home, hospital, or other settings, prescribed medications, such as diuretics or laxatives, may precipitate incontinence. If these medications are administered without consideration of the time of peak action, problems might occur during the night. Hypnotics or sedatives may make the older person too drowsy to be aware of toileting needs. Prolonged bedrest or inactivity and weakness from illness may prevent an older person from getting to the bathroom in time (see Table 18–2).

Preventive Measures

Recognition of the possible iatrogenic factors of incontinence and taking measures to avoid poor practices will do much to eliminate this preventable type of incontinence.

Table 18–2. CAUSES OF IATROGENIC
INCONTINENCE

Unable to locate bathroom
Inaccessible urinal or commode
Delayed response to call light
No bathroom stop between tests, procedures, etc.
Restraints
Medications
Prolonged bedrest and inactivity

IATROGENIC ADVERSE INCIDENTS

Factors Leading to Adverse Incidents

The hospital or nursing home environment creates special problems for safety of an older person, especially at a time when that person is vulnerable to the effects of illness and treatment, including sedation, restricted mobility, and pain. Special attention to the environment can prevent or reduce iatrogenic accidents and possible injuries. Potential hazards for a hospitalized older person are listed in Table 18–3.

Initially, an unfamiliar environment poses special problems. The first week of hospitalization has been identified as a time of high accident frequency for elderly hospitalized patients (Catchen, 1983). An elderly person will not find things in their usual places, and maneuvering around a strange hospital environment may prove awkward, difficult, and

Table 18–3. POTENTIAL HAZARDS

Floor
Slippery due to wax or spills
Light
Inadequate lighting
Glare
Corridors
Cluttered corridors
Human traffic
Equipment
Wheels not locked on wheelchair, commode, bedside
    stand and table, and bed
Bed not in low position
Objects and obstacles
    Siderails
    Trapeze bar
    Tubing
    Cords
    Special equipment, e.g., IV poles
Defective or broken equipment
Patient
Clothing
    Poorly fitting clothes
    Poorly fitting shoes or slippers
    Shoes or slippers not placed under bed, bedside
        stand, or in closet
Medications
    Sedatives/hypnotics
    Diuretics
    Antihypertensive agents
    Laxatives

hazardous. The older person may be surprised to find the bedside table and stand are on wheels and do not provide the support of the furniture at home. The bed may not sit as low as the one at home, making it more difficult to get in and out. Unexpected objects and obstacles, such as siderails, trapeze bars, nasogastric tubes, oxygen tubing, catheters, and intravenous lines, interfere with movement and ambulation. Other sources of potential accidents and injuries include spilled liquids, highly polished floors, ill-fitting hospital garments, human traffic moving at rapid speed, unrepaired or defective equipment, sharp instruments inadvertently left at the bedside, and cluttered corridors.

Elderly patients with musculoskeletal or cognitive impairments are particularly at risk for accidents. Medications such as sedatives, hypnotics, analgesics, and antihypertensive agents may cause sedation, orthostatic hypotension, decreased coordination, and instability in the elderly.

Preventive Measures

Careful, systematic assessment of the older person with consideration of causative factors, such as a history of falls, incontinence, and weakness, will identify the patient at risk for adverse incidents. Providing a clean, safe environment requires the awareness and cooperation of all personnel to identify potentially dangerous situations and to intervene before an incident occurs. The patient will need orientation to the new surroundings, explanations about equipment, and education about special precautions necessary due to illness or treatment.

IATROGENIC DISTURBANCES OF THE SLEEP/WAKE CYCLE

There are two distinct components in the normal sleep/wake cycle. There is rapid eye movement (REM) sleep and nonREM (NREM) sleep, a continuum from light sleep (stage 1) to deep sleep (stage 4). During the night, most people go through four or five cycles of the four stages of NREM and REM sleep, each lasting 85 to 110 minutes. This rhythm plays an important role in learning, memory, and adaptation, and stage 4 sleep gives a restorative boost (Hoch & Reynolds, 1986; Pacini & Fitzpatrick, 1982). Duration of REM sleep remains constant throughout adulthood. A decline is seen around the eighth decade or in extreme old age. It is also noted in the presence of organic brain syndrome and changes in cerebral blood flow. Elderly people experience an increased total duration of stage 1 sleep and an increase in the number of shifts into stage 1 sleep. A decrease or no change in sleep stages 2 and decreases in stages 3 and 4 are seen in the elderly (Dement, Miles, & Carskadon, 1982; Pressman & Fry, 1988; Woodruff, 1985).

The elderly spend more time in bed, take longer to fall asleep, have increased nocturnal wakefulness, and experience more sleepiness during the day than do younger adults. Elevated levels of norepinephrine and age-related respiratory dysfunction may be responsible for sleep fragmentation (Dement, Richardson, Prinz, et al., 1985; Woodruff, 1985). About one-third of the elderly population experience increased incidence of sleep apnea, and this problem is exacerbated by the use of sleep medications (Pressman & Fry, 1988; Woodruff, 1985). It has been suggested that the quality of sleep in the elderly might be improved by spending less time in bed during the day and avoiding pharmacologic intervention. Daytime sleepiness is associated with frequent nighttime awakenings, and it is reported that the elderly take naps to compensate for inadequate nighttime sleep. Napping may be contraindicated, since studies have shown the sleep loss actually improved the quality of sleep the next night (Woodruff, 1985). However, Hayter (1985) and Regestein and Morris (1987) found no evidence that naps decreased nighttime sleep.

Disruption of Sleep Patterns

Adjustment to any change in the normal sleep/wake pattern takes longer in older persons (Dement, et al., 1982; Pacini & Fitzpatrick, 1982). Disruption of the normal sleep pattern frequently results when an older person becomes ill, requires hospitalization, or enters a nursing home. Table 18–4 lists some of the causes of disturbances in sleep pattern. The state of health has a significant impact on sleep patterns (Pacini & Fitzpatrick, 1982). Illnesses can be aggravated by sleep, such as the respiratory disturbance that is experienced by an older person with severe chronic bronchitis. Sleep disturbances can occur as a result of illness, for example, pain and discomfort from arthritis or the nocturnal dyspnea accompanying congestive heart failure (Dement, et al., 1982).

In a study comparing sleep patterns of hospitalized and nonhospitalized elders, hospitalization was found to affect two quantitative measures of sleep, nocturnal sleep time and other sleep time (Pacini & Fitzpatrick, 1982). There are many reasons why hospitalization can create problems with sleep. There is often a lack of light and dark cues and a lack of activity and exercise due to bedrest or limitations posed by the illness (Dement, et al., 1982). Other disturbances of sleep during hospitalization include a higher level of light, noise, and activity during the normal hours of sleep and frequent awakening for a variety of nursing and other activities, such as determining daily weights, taking vital signs, administering medications, drawing blood, and early

Table 18–4. CAUSES OF DISTURBANCES IN SLEEP PATTERNS

Disruption of normal sleep pattern
Illness
Pain
Respiratory disturbances
Fatigue
Medications
Sedatives/hypnotics
Diuretics
Laxatives
Hunger
Anxiety, worry, tension
Boredom, inactivity, monotony
Environment
Lack of light/dark cues
Excessive light, noise
Room temperature too hot or too cold

breakfast service. A new environment with a strange bed, different sounds and lights, as well as a different schedule of activities may interfere with sleep. Medications, especially sedatives, hypnotics, and diuretics, also interfere with the sleep/wake cycle. Inadequate attention to pain, cold, and hunger may cause the older person to experience poor sleep. Boredom, inactivity, and monotony during the day lead to frequent naps and possible wakefulness at night.

While the hospital environment causes some sleep problem, the major factors for the differences in the quality of sleep between hospitalized and nonhospitalized elderly people include state of health, state of mind, and state of fatigue. A hospitalized older person experiences a poorer state of health and more worry, anxiety, tension, and fatigue than a nonhospitalized older adult (Pacini & Fitzpatrick, 1982).

Preventive Measures

There is wide variation in sleep patterns of older persons. Careful history-taking with an assessment of usual sleep patterns helps to direct the nursing care of older persons. Every effort should be made to maintain the normal sleep pattern. The changing sleep cycle of older adults has to be taken into consideration in the plan of care. There is the danger of administering hypnotics in the attempt to make the older adult's sleep pattern more like that of younger adults.

Measures to ensure sleep include placing an extra blanket on the bed, putting socks on the feet, decreasing the amount of fluids taken after the evening meal, providing a late evening snack, encouraging toileting before bedtime, administering pain medication prior to the hour of sleep, carefully timing medications such as laxatives and diuretics, and encouraging relaxing, restful activities prior to bedtime. In addition, careful explanation about tests, procedures, and the illness may allay some worry and concern, improve the state of mind, and, thereby, improve the quality of sleep.

IATROGENIC IMMOBILITY

Factors Leading to Immobility

The hospital experience may result in the older person being more debilitated and disabled than is warranted by the primary illness. Functional disabilities increase with age, and there is a high percentage of functional disability in the hospitalized older population (Warshaw, Moore, Friedman, et al., 1982). This situation is further aggravated by many hospital practices, such as keeping older patients in bed or in one position for an extended period of time. Improper positioning contributes to muscle atrophy and contracture, tight Achilles tendon, and pressure sores (Wolcott, 1981). Hospital and nursing home design may interfere with mobility and independence. There may be limited areas to ambulate, and hurried, busy hallways may prove dangerous. Sometimes inadequate numbers of personnel to provide assistance and inadequate or inappropriate assistive devices and environmental support keep the older person less active.

Restraints are often applied to prevent patient falls and injury, to protect staff when a patient is combative, and to prevent the interruption of treatment measures, such as intravenous lines, oxygen apparatus, and indwelling catheters. The use of restraints results in limitation of general body movement or movement of a body part. Care must be taken to properly apply the restraints. Improper use of restraints has resulted in injury and deaths (Katz, Weber, & Dodge, 1981). Ongoing assessment is done to determine the continued need for restraints; their use should be discontinued as soon as possible. Continuous observation of the restrained patient is necessary to ensure that restraints have not twisted or tightened, to remove the restraint and exercise the extremity, and to check the circulation and skin.

Neuroleptic drugs are frequently administered for management of agitation and assaultiveness in older patients. The dose, administration, and effects of neuroleptics must be carefully calculated and monitored because of the high incidence of side effects associated with this group of drugs. Neurologic side effects, such as sedation, orthostatic hypotension, and extrapyramidal symptoms, are particularly hazardous to the elderly, hampering their safe mobility (Salzman, 1982). Nonpharmacologic therapy should be tried first (Risse & Barnes, 1986). If drugs are used, the dosage should be low enough to prevent oversedation and other side effects.

Restorative activities are often overlooked or delayed, with resultant complications, as discussed in Chapter 11 on immobility. In a survey of 312 hospitalized patients 70 years of age or older, 65% were not able to ambulate independently. The majority were found in bed during the survey. Physical therapy was ordered for only 30% of these patients. The others had no program planned on the ward to promote and improve ambulation (Warshaw, et al., 1982). Confinement to bed or to sitting in a chair for even a short period over a few days results in decreased physical strength and loss of steadiness and balance (Coni, Davison, & Webster, 1977).

Delayed referral for physical rehabilitation results in increased disability and dependence. Parry (1983) reported that well-planned physical rehabilitation is effective in the very old patient. In his study on 97 patients over 85 years of age, 79% showed improvement and were able to return to the same setting as before hospitalization or were able to move in with family members, 18% remained the same, and 3% worsened. Acute illness and hospitalization often upset the delicate balance between independent functioning and dependence (Parry, 1983). The older person may benefit from 2 to 3 weeks of rehabilitation to recuperate, mobilize emotional and physical resources, and regain functional status.

Preventive Measures

Increased awareness of the effects on mobility of common practices, such as use of restraints and administration of neuroleptics, will help to prevent some of their negative consequences. Early referral for physical rehabilitation and development of a clearly de-

fined plan of care are critical elements. Good communication must be established between the rehabilitation medicine service and the staff on the ward. The goals and treatment program have to be understood by all who are involved in the care of the patient, or else the program developed in physical therapy may not be carried out when the patient returns to the ward or home. The physical therapy program must be integrated into the activities on the ward in order to prevent unnecessary restriction of activity and to allow gradual resumption of the desired level of function. Older persons and their families need explanations and clear instructions about limitations of movement or activity required by their illness. Unless such information is given, unnecessary restriction may be imposed on the patient.

IATROGENIC PROBLEMS RELATED TO DRUGS

Iatrogenic illness resulting from adverse drug reactions is common among the elderly. Adverse reactions are defined as undesirable or unwanted consequences that occur when drugs are used to diagnose or treat disease states (Friesen, 1983). A number of factors make persons over 65 years of age particularly vulnerable to drug-induced iatrogenesis. Factors influencing safe and effective drug therapy in the elderly include incorrect diagnosis, multiple conditions and polypharmacy, age-related changes affecting pharmacokinetics and pharmacodynamics, changes in nutritional status, and poor communication between older adults and health care providers (Friesen, 1983; Hazzard, 1985; Michocki & Lamy, 1988; Ouslander, 1981).

Factors Influencing Drug Therapy

Incorrect Diagnosis. The elderly often present with multiple vague and nonspecific symptoms, making it difficult to arrive at an accurate diagnosis and prescribe appropriate drug therapy. These symptoms represent a variety of medical and psychiatric disorders, such as dementia, depression, or infections. The "giants of geriatrics," confusion, falls, immobility, and urinary incontinence, are often the presenting manifestations of many illnesses (Fox, 1985).

There is a high prevalence of symptoms and disease in the elderly. Difficulties occur in utilizing symptoms to establish a diagnosis because some symptoms are so commonly found in the older age group that they lose diagnostic significance. For example, Hale, Perkins, May, and associates (1986) found that nocturia was a symptom reported by 80.4% of the women and 79.8% of the men in their sample of 1927 women and 1140 men over 65 years of age. Misdiagnosis may occur due to medication side effects that mimic symptoms of a variety of conditions. There is generally a low level of suspicion among clinicians that symptoms are due to drugs. The tendency is to ascribe new symptoms to a new disease state, exacerbation of an existing condition, or to aging, with a result that more drugs are prescribed, adding to the problem (Friesen, 1983). On the other hand, physicians misdiagnose also by mistakenly attributing complaints in the elderly to the side effects of medications. Studies have shown that many older persons complaining of symptoms were taking no medications (Foxall, 1982; Hale, et al., 1986). Unrecognized conditions or incorrect diagnoses may result in nontreatment or inappropriate drug therapy.

Multiple Conditions and Polypharmacy. The elderly are heavy users of drugs, receiving a disproportionately high percentage of drugs compared to other segments of the population. While comprising 12% of the population, the elderly account for 20% to 25% of all prescription and nonprescription medications, spending about $3 billion per year (Vestal, 1985). The elderly are likely to have one or more chronic illnesses, and drugs are viewed as a major component of chronic disease management (Lamy, 1984).

Surveys of elderly people in the community indicate that up to 90% take at least one medication and most take two or more. The most commonly used drugs in this segment of the population are cardiovascular agents and antihypertensives, analgesics and antiarthritic preparations, sedatives and tranquilizers, and gastrointestinal preparations, such as laxatives and antacids (Roberts & Tumer, 1988; Vestal, 1985).

In long-term care facilities, two-thirds of the residents received three or more drugs (Vestal, 1985). Another survey showed one-third of the residents received 8 to 16 drugs daily (Lamy, 1984). Psychotropics were prescribed to nearly 75% of the residents (Vestal, 1985), followed in frequency by cardiovascular agents, laxatives, analgesics, and vitamins (Lamy, 1984; Vestal, 1985).

The incidence of medication errors and adverse reactions or interactions increases as the number of prescribed drugs rises (Patterson, 1986). The incidence of adverse reactions in the elderly rises from 15% among the 60-plus group to 24% among those over age 80 years (Vestal, 1982). An estimated 1.5 million persons are hospitalized each year as a result of adverse drug reactions (Lamy, 1984).

Age-Related Changes in Pharmacokinetics and Pharmacodynamics. Age-related changes in two basic mechanisms, pharmacokinetics and pharmacodynamics, help to explain the differences seen in drug disposition and response in the elderly.

Pharmacokinetics. Pharmacokinetics is the study of the time course of drug action in the body and includes the quantitative study of drug absorption, distribution, metabolism, and excretion (Robertson, 1985; Vestal, 1985). Age-related physiological changes affect pharmacokinetics of drugs, and these are summarized in Table 18–5. Some of the changes will be discussed using the drugs commonly taken by the elderly as examples.

Absorption. Most drugs are prescribed for oral administration. The increase of gastric pH may affect the ionization and solubility of drugs. Slower gastric emptying rates may affect the onset of action. Elderly people lose approximately 20% of absorption surface with aging, which may lower drug bioavailability, the amount of drug administered that enters the systemic circulation. However, many studies show that these changes minimally affect

Table 18–5. AGE-RELATED PHYSIOLOGIC
CHANGES AND PHARMACOKINETICS

Age-related Physiologic Changes	Pharmacokinetic Parameter
Increased gastric pH Decreased absorptive surface Decreased splanchnic blood flow Altered gastrointestinal motility	Absorption
Decreased cardiac output Decreased total body water Decreased lean body mass Increased body fat Decreased serum albumin Altered protein binding	Distribution
Decreased hepatic mass Decreased hepatic blood flow Decreased enzyme activity Decreased enzyme inducibility	Metabolism
Decreased renal blood flow Decreased glomerular filtration rate Decreased tubular secretory function	Excretion

Data from Kane, Ouslander, & Abrass, 1984; Lamy, 1982; Vestal, 1985.)

drug absorption in the elderly (Greenblatt, Divoll, Abernethy, et al., 1982; Vestal & Dawson, 1985).

Distribution. Changes in body composition may alter cellular distribution of drugs. There is a decrease in total body water and in muscles and lean body mass. Fat content approximately doubles, from 18% to 36%, in older men and increases 1.5 times, from 33% to 45%, in older women (Greenblatt, et al., 1982; Vestal & Dawson, 1985). Drugs that are distributed in body water or lean body mass, such as ethanol, digoxin, and acetaminophen, will result in higher blood levels of the drug in the elderly. With the increase in body fat with age, highly lipid soluble drugs, such as diazepam, chlorpromazine, and phenobarbital, may be stored in fatty tissue, thus prolonging and possibly increasing their effects (Goldberg & Roberts, 1983).

Free drug concentration is an important factor in drug distribution and elimination. Alterations in the binding of drugs to plasma protein, red blood cells, and other body tissues may be a source of altered pharmacokinetics in old age. Serum albumin is reduced by 10% to 20%, meaning less albumin is available for drug binding and more free drug is available for pharmacologic action (Ouslander, 1981; Vestal & Dawson, 1985). Drugs that are protein bound include phenytoin, warfarin, phenylbutazone, and tolbutamide. Binding of drugs to red cells has not been studied extensively. Meperidine was found to bind to red cells more in older persons (Goldberg & Roberts, 1983).

Metabolism. The liver is the site of metabolism for most drugs. Enzymatic action is responsible for biotransformation, the conversion of drugs into metabolites enhancing drug elimination (Oppeneer & Vervoren, 1983). There is evidence of a decline in hepatic drug metabolism with increasing age (Schmuker, 1979). Drugs eliminated primarily by hepatic metabolism have longer half-lives (amount of time required for elimination of one-half the amount of drug distributed in the body) and reduced clearances (Michocki & Lamy, 1988; Vestal, 1985). The enzymatic action in the liver can be affected by some drugs, causing drug toxicities or reduced activity and requiring adjustments in dosage.

Excretion. Drugs are usually eliminated via the kidney into the urine or via the liver into the feces (Oppeneer & Vervoren, 1983). Diminished renal function is common among the elderly. In people between 20 and 90 years of age, glomerular filtration rate may fall as much as 50%, with an average of 35%; renal plasma flow declines 1.9% per year (Vestal & Dawson, 1985). The rate of elimination is reduced for drugs such as digoxin, cimetidine, lithium, procainamide, chlorpropamide, and most common antimicrobials (Greenblatt, et al., 1982; Patterson, 1986). Age differences in pharmacokinetics are unlikely when renal function is determined to be normal (>80 ml/min/1.73 m^2) (Vestal & Dawson, 1985). Creatinine clearance, rather than serum creatinine concentration, should be used to estimate renal function. In the elderly, renal function may decline without a change in serum creatinine. This is due to the fact that endogenous creatinine production decreases in the elderly as a result of a generalized reduction in muscle mass with age (Greenblatt, et al., 1982; Lamy & Vestal, 1976).

Pharmacodynamics. Pharmacodynamics refers to the biologic and therapeutic effect of drugs or the physiological or psychological response to drugs (Robertson, 1985; Vestal, 1985). Information on pharmacodynamics in the elderly is limited, and studies on response to specific drugs have produced conflicting results (Vestal, 1985).

It is known that the elderly are not necessarily more sensitive to the effect of drugs than are younger persons. For example, while older persons are more sensitive to the effects of potent analgesics and sedatives than are younger persons, they are more resistant to isoproterenol and propranolol (Vestal, 1985). Age differences in responsiveness are thought to be due, in part, to alterations in receptor numbers or affinity (Pagliaro & Pagliaro, 1983; Roberts & Tumer, 1988).

Nutritional Status. Drug-nutrient interactions are common in older persons, leading to adverse consequences such as nutritional deficiency or drug toxicity.

Dietary Effects on Drugs. Drug metabolism and efficacy may be affected by changes in the older person's diet. For example, an increase in protein intake can affect the bioavailability of certain drugs and increase the rate of drug metabolism (Roe, 1986). Tea and coffee have been found to weaken the effects of antipsychotics by precipitating the active constituents of the drugs (Lamy, 1982). Caffeine-containing beverages may potentiate the effects of theophylline, commonly used for chronic obstructive pulmonary disease (Smith & Bidlack, 1982). The absorption of many antibiotics is delayed if they are taken with foods and beverages other than water (Smith & Bidlack, 1982). The timing of drug intake in relation to food intake, the manner in which food is cooked, and the consumption of alcohol, vegetables, high-fiber or low-fiber diet, and other dietary factors may alter drug response (Roe, 1985). The practice of suggesting that older persons take their medications with meals, as a memory cue, can add to the problem of drug-nutrient interactions.

Drug Effects on Nutrition. The frail elderly in poor health and on marginal diets are especially at risk for drug-induced nutritional deficiencies. Roe (1986) identified four basic ways in which drugs may interfere with the nutritional status of the older adult. These four basic ways are (1) suppression or stimulation of appetite, (2) alteration in the digestion and absorption of nutrients, (3) alteration in nutrient metabolism or utilization, and (4) alteration in excretion of the nutrient. For example, antipsychotic medications, such as lithium or the phenothiazines, can stimulate the appetite. Digoxin or chemotherapy drugs can cause anorexia or food aversion, thus reducing food intake. Aluminum antacids can impair absorption of phosphate, calcium, and vitamin D (Roe, 1985). Alcohol can affect both digestion and absorption (Roe, 1986).

Poor Communication. Poor communication between the older adult and health care professionals is responsible for inadequate drug histories of older patients, lack of information about alternatives to drug therapy, insufficient information about drugs, and the lack of reporting of adverse effects by elders (American Association of Retired Persons [AARP], 1984). Confusing labeling language, difficult-to-read print on labels and drug information leaflets, and confusing pill shapes and colors contribute to the problems associated with medications (Hazzard, 1985).

Information should be given about safe, proper self-administration of prescribed medications and over-the-counter preparations used by older persons. Helping older persons to understand their drug regimen is critical in compliance and in reducing adverse effects. Noncompliance on the part of older patients is usually intentional. They do not obtain prescription refills when they do not believe that the drugs are beneficial, or if they experience side effects, or if symptoms have improved (AARP, 1984). An older person may supplement prescription medications with over-the-counter drugs or borrowed medications. The potential hazards of these practices need to be explained.

Problem Drugs

While a large number of drugs pose particular risk for the elderly, a few of the most frequently used drugs have been selected for discussion. Several excellent review articles written on problem drugs are cited in the references for this chapter.

The Cardiovascular Drugs

Digitalis. Digitalis must be used carefully in the elderly due to its narrow therapeutic index and potentially life-threatening toxicity (Roffman, 1984). Older persons require lower-than-normal doses of digitalis because the drug is distributed primarily in lean body mass and decreased renal function will elevate serum concentration of digoxin (Gerber, 1982; Roberts & Tumer, 1988). Other factors predispose the elderly to digitalis toxicity, such as the presence of hypokalemia, hypercalcemia, hypomagnesemia, metabolic acidosis or alkalosis, or hypoxia. The addition of quinidine may increase serum digoxin concentration by as much as 100%, and concurrent administration of antibiotics such as erythromycin or tetracycline can raise serum digoxin concentration as much as twofold (Roffman, 1984). Evaluating renal function and measuring serum digoxin concentration are important to determine correct dosage (therapeutic range for digoxin is 0.5 to 2.0 ng/ml) (Roffman, 1984).

The clinical manifestations of digitalis toxicity are different in the elderly. Gastrointestinal disturbances, such as anorexia, nausea, and vomiting, are seen in about 75% to 100% of older persons with digitalis toxicity. However, these symptoms may not be attributed to the medication and instead may be believed to be due to other causes. The central nervous system manifestations of disorientation, agitation, restlessness, hallucinations, color vision disturbances, and changes in behavior are more frequently seen in older patients than in younger patients (Roberts & Tumer, 1988). The cardiac arrhythmias that may result are the most serious; any new change in rhythm in a patient on digitalis should be considered digitalis toxicity until proved otherwise (Roffman, 1984).

Diuretics. Diuretics, especially the rapid-acting loop diuretics, can lead to volume contraction, dehydration, postural hypotension, and hypokalemia (Robertson, 1985). Potassium supplements or potassium-sparing diuretics create problems of hyperkalemia in elderly persons with impaired renal function. Potassium levels, renal function, and blood pressure measurements, taken while the patient is both recumbent and standing, should be monitored (Nattel, 1981; Roberts & Tumer, 1988).

Antihypertensives. Antihypertensive agents can cause severe orthostasis and syncope in older adults unless the dosage is carefully titrated. Because the elderly are very sensitive to the central nervous depressant effects of antihypertensive agents such as methyldopa, clonidine, and reserpine, these drugs should be avoided (Goldberg & Roberts, 1983; Nattel, 1981). Beta-blockers are the preferred drugs, although there are increased risks of adverse reactions to drugs like propranolol for older adults (Robertson, 1985).

Psychotropic Drugs. Adverse side effects frequently develop in the elderly because of age-related changes in the distribution and elimination of these drugs and the increased sensitivity to them. Psychotropic drugs should be used with caution in the elderly. Dosages are usually only 30% to 50% as high as those for younger people (Salzman, 1982; Thompson, Moran, & Nies, 1983a).

Antianxiety Agents—Minor Tranquilizers. The most frequently prescribed anxiolytic agents are the benzodiazepines, which include oxazepam, diazepam, and lorazepam. These drugs produce greater effects on the central nervous system in the elderly, partly due to increased target organ sensitivity and partly due to impaired drug disposition and elimination (Thompson, et al., 1983a). For example, diazepam has a longer half-life in the elderly, from 20 hours in the 20-year-old person to 90 hours in the 80-year-old person. The reason for the prolonged half-life is delayed elimination and increased volume of distribution. Repeated doses of benzodiazepines may result in accumulation of the drug; this can produce excessive sedation, diminished sexual desire, and lowered energy level (Thompson et al., 1983a).

Sedative-Hypnotics. Frequent complaints about sleep from elderly persons often result in sedative-hypnotics being prescribed. The elderly receive almost 40% of all sedative-hypnotic prescriptions, with the benzodiazepines being the drug class most frequently prescribed. Unless dosages are adjusted for age, however, side effects may occur, such as excess daytime sedation and decrease in stages 3 and 4 sleep and REM sleep. Excessive dosage results in central nervous system dysfunction, which may predispose the elderly to prolonged sedation, impaired motor coordination, perceptual disturbances, and delirium (Salzman, 1982; Thompson, et al., 1983a).

The use of barbiturates in the elderly should be avoided because they tend to produce paradoxical excitement and suppress REM sleep, as well as because of their habituating qualities, low therapeutic ratio, and risks associated with overdose (Hicks, Dysken, Davis, et al., 1981).

Antidepressants. Depression is seen in at least 10% of the elderly. The tricyclic antidepressants (amitriptyline, doxepin, imipramine, nortriptyline, desipramine) are often prescribed and have potentially serious side effects, such as arrhythmias, orthostatic hypotension, and anticholinergic effects (Vestal & Dawson, 1985). Anticholinergic effects frequently cause changes in mentation, impaired visual accommodation, delayed gastric emptying, urinary retention, and decreased sweating and hyperthermic response (Levinson, 1981; Thompson, et al., 1983b). Sexual dysfunction is another distressing side effect (Van Arsdalen & Wein, 1984).

Antipsychotics—Major Tranquilizers. Antipsychotics are used for chronic schizophrenia, psychotic paranoid states, manic-depressive disorders, and agitated states of depression, delirium, and dementia (Thompson, et al., 1983b). Antipsychotic agents are equal in therapeutic efficacy if prescribed according to dose equivalent potency. The drugs differ in number of side effects, the more potent agents, such as haloperidol and fluphenazine, causing the highest incidence of extrapyramidal symptoms. Extrapyramidal side effects, which include drug-induced parkinsonism, akathisias, and dystonia, are common in the elderly (Vestal & Dawson, 1985). The least potent antipsychotics, chlorpromazine and thioridazine, are sedating and have the most marked anticholinergic effects, such as urinary retention, constipation, confusion, disorientation, and hallucinations (Robertson, 1985; Thompson, et al., 1983a). Autonomic side effects also occur with the less potent neuroleptics, causing hypotensive episodes and predisposing the elderly to falls, myocardial infarction, and cerebrovascular accidents. In the elderly, there is an increased incidence of tardive dyskinesia, a serious, debilitating side effect that occurs with long-term use of anticholinergic medications (Thompson, et al., 1983b). Tapering the dose or discontinuing the drugs may eliminate or reduce the adverse reactions, except for tardive dyskinesia (Robertson, 1985). To prevent as many of the problems associated with antipsychotics as possible, it is important to prescribe antipsychotic medications in the lowest effective dose (Patterson, 1986).

Lithium Carbonate-Antimanic Agent. Lithium is used to treat the manic episodes associated with manic-depressive illness. It is often used in conjunction with antipsychotic medications for short-term management (Thompson, et al., 1983b). Lithium clearance decreases with age because the drug is excreted by the kidney. The half-life increases from 18 to 30 hours in the younger age group to 36 hours in the elderly. Toxicity commonly manifests in the elderly as tremors, indigestion, nausea, abdominal pain, and frequent stools. Serious problems that may occur with lithium include nephrotoxicity, central nervous system toxicity, and cardiac toxicity. Serum lithium levels should be checked monthly and even more frequently if toxic symptoms appear (Thompson, et al., 1983b).

Preventive Measures

Many adverse drug reactions arise from excessive doses, excessive duration, and the use of unnecessary drugs (Lamy, 1980). Measures can be taken to prevent iatrogenic problems related to drugs (Table 18–6). Adverse reac-

Table 18–6. PREVENTIVE MEASURES FOR IATROGENIC DRUG-RELATED PROBLEMS

Accurate diagnosis
Using nonpharmaceutical approach to treatment
Taking a careful drug history
Ensuring drug therapy is appropriate to the individual patient
Being aware of drug-induced illnesses
Simplifying medication regimen
Periodically reviewing drug therapy
Ongoing assessment and evaluation of drug regimen

tions can be greatly reduced by ensuring accurate diagnosis, using a nonpharmaceutical approach to treatment whenever possible, tailoring drug therapy to the patient, and being aware of the frequency in which drug-induced illness occurs (Friesen, 1983).

Prevention of iatrogenic drug-related problems requires the coordinated effort of all involved in the care of the older person. Drug histories are important. Fewer problems occur when medication regimens are minimal and simplified. A periodic review of drug therapy to identify potential drug interactions and therapeutic redundancy will reduce the incidence of drug-induced iatrogenesis (Vestal, 1985). There is also a need for ongoing assessment of drug effectiveness, monitoring of adverse reactions, and evaluation for the continued need of each medication.

While there has been steady, increasing interest and study of drugs and the elderly, few generalizations can be made about age-related effects of drug disposition and response (Plein & Plein, 1981; Vestal, 1985). The extent to which age alone may predispose to drug interactions is not known. The extent to which disease, diet, and environmental factors such as smoking affect drug distribution, drug elimination, and drug action is also unknown (Vestal, 1985). Many drugs are not tested on aged populations; when they are tested, they are rarely tested on persons with multiple illnesses and multiple prescriptions (Hazzard, 1985). Insufficient information on appropriate drugs and doses for older adults is a major source of problems related to drugs. Another complicating factor is the marked individual variation in the aging process, requiring care-

ful design of each person's drug treatment program (Vestal, 1985).

Research continues on pharmacokinetics, pharmacodynamics, and aging. New drugs will be introduced. While it is difficult to keep abreast of new information, it is important that our knowledge and practice remain current in order to prevent or significantly reduce iatrogenic problems related to drugs.

SUMMARY

Iatrogenic complications bring distress to all involved. There are costs in terms of economic and human expenses. For the older person, iatrogenic complications may mean increased suffering from disability, discomfort, pain, another illness or injury to be added to the existing long list of conditions, prolonged recovery period, hospitalization or institutionalization, or even death. For health care professionals, questions arise about errors, misjudgment, or lack of knowledge and skill.

Prevention of iatrogenesis is foremost. It is critical that susceptible patients be identified and measures taken to reduce practices and events that are known to cause iatrogenic conditions. Health care professionals must develop the ability to accurately weigh the risk-benefit ratio of a proposed approach to care. This ratio improves with increased knowledge, understanding, and predictability of the elderly person's response to illness, treatment, and environment for care. Health care providers need to continue to critically review and analyze their practice to prevent the occurrence of iatrogenic complications.

References

Alvarez, S, Shell, CG, Woolley, TW, et al. (1988): Nosocomial infections in long-term facilities. *J Gerontol*, 43:M9–M17.

American Association of Retired Persons (AARP) (1984): *Prescription Drugs: A Survey of Consumer Use, Attitudes, and Behavior*. Washington, DC, American Association of Retired Persons.

Besedine, R, & Rose, RM (1982): Aspects of infection in the elderly. *In* Eisdorfer, C (ed): *Annual Review of Gerontology and Geriatrics*. New York, Springer, 181–227.

Catchen, H (1983): Repeaters: Inpatient accidents among hospitalized elderly. *Gerontologist*, 23:273–276.

Coni, N, Davison, W, & Webster, S (1977): *Lecture Notes on Geriatrics*. Oxford, Blackwell Scientific Publications.

Dement, WC, Miles, LE, & Carskadon, MA (1982): "White paper" on sleep and aging. *J Am Geriatr Soc*, 30:25–50.

Dement, W, Richardson, G, Prinz, P, et al. (1985): Changes in sleep and wakefulness with age. *In* Finch, CE, & Schneider, EL (eds): *Handbook of the Biology of Aging* (ed 2). New York, Van Nostrand Reinhold, 692–717.

Finkelstein, MS (1985): Aging immunocytes and immunity. Characteristics and significance. *Clin Geriatr Med*, 4:899–911.

Fox, RA (1985): Immunology of aging. *In* Brocklehurst JC (ed): *Textbook of Geriatric Medicine and Gerontology* (ed 3). Edinburgh, Churchill Livingstone, 82–104.

Foxall, MJH (1982): Elderly patients at risk of potential drug interactions in long-term care facilities. *West J Nurs Res*, 4:133–152.

Friesen, AJD (1983): Adverse drug reactions in the geriatric client. *In* Pagliaro, LA, & Pagliaro, AM (eds): *Pharmacologic Aspects of Aging*. St. Louis, CV Mosby, 257–293.

Gerber, JG (1982): Drug usage in the elderly. *In* Schrier, RW (ed): *Clinical Internal Medicine in the Aged*. Philadelphia, WB Saunders, 51–65.

Goldberg, PB, & Roberts, J (1983): Pharmacologic basis for developing rational drug regimens for elderly patients. *Med Clin North Am*, 67:315–328.

Goldman, R (1976): Decline in organ function with aging. *In* Rossman, I (ed): *Clinical Geriatrics* (ed 2). Philadelphia, JB Lippincott, 23–59.

Grant, A (1979): *Nutritional Assessment Guidelines* (ed 2). Seattle, Author. Available through Anne Grant, Box 25057, Northgate Station, Seattle, WA 98125.

Greenblatt, DJ, Divoll, M, Abernethy, DR, et al. (1982): Physiologic changes in old age: Relation to altered drug disposition. *J Am Geriatr Soc*, 30(Suppl):S6–S10.

Guigoz, Y, & Munro, HN (1985): Nutrition and aging. *In* Finch, CE, & Schneider, EL (eds): *Handbook on the Biology of Aging*. (ed 2). New York, Van Nostrand Reinhold, 878–893.

Hale, WE, Perkins, LL, May, FE, et al. (1986): Symptom prevalence in the elderly. An evaluation of age, sex, disease, and medication use. *J Am Geriatr Soc*, 34:333–340.

Haley, RW, Hooten, TM, & Culver, DH (1981): Nosocomial infections in U. S. hospitals, 1975–1976. Estimated frequency by selected characteristics of patients. *Am J Med*, 70:947–959.

Hausman, PB, & Weksler, ME (1985): Changes in the immune response with age. *In* Finch, CE, & Schneider, EL (eds): *Handbook of the Biology of Aging* (ed 2). New York, Van Nostrand Reinhold, 414–432.

Hayter, J (1985): To nap or not to nap? *Geriatr Nurs*, 6:104–106.

Hazzard, WR (1985): *A State of the Art Review of Preventive Strategies and Health Promotion for the Elderly*. A report submitted by Geriatrics and Gerontology Advisory Committee. Washington, DC, Veterans Administration.

Hicks, R, Dysken, MW, Davis, JM, et al. (1981): The pharmacokinetics of psychotropic medication in the elderly: A review. *J Clin Psychiatry*, 42:374–385.

Hill, CD, & Stamm, WE (1982): Pneumonia in the elderly: The fatal complication. *Geriatrics*, 37:40–50.

Hoch, C, & Reynolds, III, C (1986): Sleep disturbances and what to do about them. *Geriatr Nurs*, 7:24–27.

Jackson, MM, & Fierer, J (1985): Infections and infection risk in residents of long-term care facilities: A review of the literature, 1970–1984. *Am J Infect Control*, 13(2):63–77.

Jahnigen, D, Hannon, C, Laxson, L, et al. (1982): Iatrogenic disease in hospitalized elderly veterans. *J Am Geriatr Soc*, 30:387–390.

Kane, RL, Ouslander, JG, & Abrass, IB (1984): *Essentials of Clinical Geriatrics*. New York, McGraw-Hill.

Katz, L, Weber, F, & Dodge, P (1981): Patient restraint and safety vests: Minimizing the hazards. *Dimens Health Serv*, 58(5):10–11.

Lamy, PP (1980): Misuse and abuse of drugs by the elderly: Another view. *Am Pharmacist*, 20(5):14–17.

Lamy, PP (1982): Effects of diet and nutrition on drug therapy. *J Am Geriatr Soc*, 30(Suppl.):S99–S112.

Lamy, PP (1984): Hazards of drug use in the elderly. *Postgrad Med*, 76:50–53, 56–57, 60–61.

Lamy, PP, & Vestal, RE (1976): Drug prescribing for the elderly. *Hosp Pract*, 11:111–118.

LeClair, SM, Schicker, JM, Duthie, EH, et al. (1988): Survey of nursing personnel attitudes towards infections and their control in the elderly. *Am J Infect Control*, 16:159–166.

Levinson, AJ (1981): Psychotropic drug use in the elderly: An overview. *Am Fam Physician*, 24:194–199.

Michocki, RJ, & Lamy, PP (1988): A "risk" approach to adverse drug reactions. *J Am Geriatr Soc*, 36:79–81.

Mostow, SR (1982): Infectious diseases in the aged. *In* Schrier, RW (ed): *Clinical Internal Medicine in the Aged*. Philadelphia, WB Saunders, 256–273.

Nattel, S (1981): Playing it safe with drugs for the elderly. *Consultant*, 21:87–89, 92.

Oppeneer, JE, & Vervoren, TM (1983): *Gerontological Pharmacology*. St. Louis, CV Mosby.

Ouslander, JG (1981): Drug therapy in the elderly. *Ann Intern Med*, 95:711–722.

Pacini, CM, & Fitzpatrick, JJ (1982): Sleep patterns of hospitalized and nonhospitalized aged individuals. *J Gerontol Nurs*, 8:327–332.

Pagliaro, LA, & Pagliaro, AM (1983): *Pharmacologic Aspects of Aging*. St. Louis, CV Mosby.

Parry, F, (1983): Physical rehabilitation of the old, old patient. *J Am Geriatr Soc*, 31:182–184.

Patterson, C (1986): Iatrogenic disease in late life. *Clin Geriatr Med*, 2:121–137.

Plein, JB, & Plein, EM (1981): Aging and drug therapy. *In* Eisdorfer, C (ed): *Annual Review of Gerontology and Geriatrics*, Vol. 2. New York, Springer, 211–254.

Powers, DC, Nagel, JE, Hoh, J, et al. (1987): Immune function in the elderly. *Postgrad Med*, 81:355–359.

Pressman, MR, & Fry, JM (1988): What is normal sleep in the elderly? *Clin Geriatr Med*, 4:71–81.

Raju, L, & Khan, F (1988): Pneumonia in the elderly: A review. *Geriatrics*, 43(10):51–52, 55–57, 59–62.

Regestein, QR, & Morris, J (1987): Daily sleep patterns

observed among institutionalized elderly residents. *J Am Geriatr Soc*, 35:767–772.

Reichel, W (1965): Complications in the care of five hundred elderly hospitalized patients. *J Am Geriatr Soc*, 13:973–981.

Risse, SC, & Barnes, R (1986): Pharmacologic treatment of agitation associated with dementia. *J Am Geriatr Soc*, 34:368–376.

Roberts, J, & Tumer, N (1988): Pharmacodynamic basis for altered drug action in the elderly. *Clin Geriatr Med*, 4:127–149.

Robertson, D (1985): Pharmacology and aging—pharmacokinetics and pharmacodynamics. *In* Brocklehurst, JC (ed): *Textbook of Geriatric Medicine and Gerontology* (ed 3). Edinburgh, Churchill Livingstone, 145–156.

Roe, DA (1985): Therapeutic effects of drug-nutrient interactions in the elderly. *Continuing Education*, 85:174–181.

Roe, DA (1986): Drug-nutrient interactions in the elderly. *Geriatrics*, 41:57–59, 63–64, 74.

Roffman, DS (1984): Special concerns of digitalis use in elderly patients. *Geriatrics*, 39:97–105.

Salzman, C (1982): A primer on geriatric psychopharmacology. *Am J Psychiatry*, 139:67–74.

Schmucker, DL (1979): Age related changes in drug disposition. *Pharmacol Rev*, 30:445–456.

Schneider, EL (1983): Infectious diseases in the elderly. *Ann Intern Med*, 98:395–400.

Setia, U, Serventi, I, & Lorenz, P (1985): Nosocomial infections among patients in a long-term care facility: Spectrum, prevalence, and risk factors. *Am J Infect Control*, 13(2):57–62.

Smith, CH, & Bidlack, WR (1982): Nutrition and the elderly: Food and drug interactions. *Nutrition and the M.D.*, 8:1–3.

Smith, PW (1985): Infections in long-term care facilities. *Infect Control*, 6:435–436.

Smith, PW (1988): Infections in extended care facilities: Prevalence, problems, and prevention. *Asepsis*, 10:2–5.

Steel, K (1984): Iatrogenic disease on a medical service. *J Am Geriatr Soc*, 32:445–449.

Steel, K, Gertman, PM, Crescenzi, C, et al. (1981): Iatrogenic illness on a general medical service at a university hospital. *N Engl J Med*, 304:638–642.

Thompson, TL, Moran, MG, & Nies, AS (1983a): Psychotropic drug use in the elderly—Part I. *N Engl J Med*, 308:134–138.

Thompson, TL, Moran, MG, & Nies, AS (1983b): Psychotropic drug use in the elderly—Part II. *N Engl J Med*, 308:194–199.

Tonnesen, MG, & Weston, WL (1982): Aging of skin. *In* Schrier, RW (ed): *Clinical Internal Medicine in the Aged*. Philadelphia, WB Saunders, 296–304.

Van Arsdalen, KN, & Wein, AJ (1984): Drug-induced sexual dysfunction in older men. *Geriatrics*, 39:63–67, 70.

Vestal, RE (1982): Pharmacology and aging. *J Am Geriatr Soc*, 30:191–200.

Vestal, RE (1985): Clinical pharmacology. *In* Andes, R, Bierman, EL, & Hazzard, WR (eds): *Principles of Geriatric Medicine*. New York, McGraw-Hill, 424–443.

Vestal, RE, & Dawson, GW (1985): Pharmacology and aging. *In* Finch, CE, & Schneider, EL (eds): *Handbook of the Biology of Aging* (ed 2). New York, Van Nostrand Reinhold, 744–819.

Warshaw, GA, Moore, JT, Friedman, W, et al. (1982): Functional disability in the hospitalized elderly. *JAMA*, 248:847–850.

Wolcott, LE (1981): Rehabilitation and the aged. *In* Reichel, W (ed): *Topics in Aging and Long Term Care*. Baltimore, Williams & Wilkins, 87–110.

Woodruff, DS (1985): Arousal, sleep, and aging. *In* Birren, JE, & Schaie, KW (eds): *Handbook of the Psychology of Aging* (ed 2). New York, Van Nostrand Reinhold, 261–295.

Yoshikawa, TT (1981): Important infections in elderly persons. *West J Med*, 135:441–445.

Yoshikawa, TT (1983): Geriatric infectious diseases: An emerging problem. *J Am Geriatr Soc*, 31:34–39.

CHAPTER
19

Monitoring the Effects of Anticholinergic Drugs

GINETTE A. PEPPER, R.N. G.N.P., Ph.D.

INTRODUCTION

Observation for adverse drug effects is a fundamental nursing responsibility. In the time of Florence Nightingale so few drugs actually were beneficial in disease treatment that drug therapy required little more of nurses than accuracy in administration and recognition of adverse drug effects. However, the current nursing role in drug therapy has expanded to include many complex functions, such as evaluation for therapeutic response, patient education, dosage titration, diverse drug administration techniques, and even prescriptive authority in some states. These new functions have tended to overshadow the importance of detecting and ameliorating adverse drug effects (Schiff, 1984).

ADVERSE DRUG EFFECTS

Adverse drug effects are any effects attributable to a drug other than the specific therapeutic effects for which the drug was prescribed. Although elderly people may not report adverse effects unless specifically questioned, they are two to seven times more likely to experience adverse drug effects than are younger adults (Hollister, 1977; Hurwitz, 1969; Siedl, Thornton, & Smith, 1966; Williamson & Chopin, 1980). In part this is attributable to prolonged half-lives and elevated serum levels secondary to pharmacokinetic changes associated with aging (Bressler, 1982; Jennings, Tourville, & Pepper, 1985).

Because homeostatic mechanisms respond

slowly and are less competent in the elderly, adverse effects that are innocuous to a young adult might be catastrophic for a person in the eighth or ninth decade of life. Elderly people are more likely than younger people to be hospitalized for a drug-induced illness (Caranasos, Stewart, & Cluff, 1974). Even "minor" effects can affect quality of life for the elderly. Examples of common adverse effects considered minor inconveniences by most prescribers are dizziness and dry mouth. Yet many elderly persons severely curtail activity when they are dizzy because they fear falling (MacDonald, 1985; Mossey, 1985). Dry mouth contributes to denture intolerance, impaired taste and swallowing, oral infections, and difficult speech; some elders with dry mouth avoid social contact because conversation is so uncomfortable (Baum, 1981; Epstein, 1982; Lyons, 1972; Navazesh & Ship, 1983; Todd, 1982).

Barriers to Management

The morbidity and mortality associated with adverse drug effects are not fully appreciated by many health care providers (Mellville, 1984). These effects may be difficult to distinguish from disease symptoms, particularly among the elderly in whom identification of adverse drug effects is complicated by the existence of multiple concurrent diseases and age-related physiologic changes. Adverse effects are easily dismissed as signs of aging or symptoms of disease processes.

Basen (1977) identified additional impediments to the management of adverse effects in the elderly. First, little is known regarding specific adverse effects during chronic drug therapy, since most toxicity studies are based on a single dose or on short-term dosing. Although many pharmacology references purport that most adverse effects abate with prolonged therapy, there is little systematic research to support this contention. Accumulated clinical experience suggests that many adverse effects persist throughout the duration of therapy and that the elderly often learn to cope with the effects of modifying their activities

and adopting compensating behavior. A second impediment to identification and amelioration of adverse drug effects in the elderly is lack of studies about the characteristics of those at highest risk for these effects. Finally, the relationship of multiple drug therapy to the incidence and severity of adverse drug effects is not understood. For example, if an elderly patient takes several drugs with overlapping adverse effects, will the adverse reaction be intensified, additive, or even multiplicative?

Significant Adverse Effects

Table 19–1 outlines selected adverse effects to which the elderly are particularly susceptible. As reflected in this table, management of adverse drug effects involves interventions to detect, prevent, or ameliorate the effect. One group of adverse drug reactions, the anticholinergic (atropine-like) effects, are probably the most thoroughly studied, although much further study is indicated. As a result, more is known about the risk factors, response to chronic therapy, and effects of multidrug therapy with this group than with others. This chapter focuses on anticholinergic adverse drug effects, which are particularly problematic for older patients. The mechanism, detection, and prevention of anticholinergic effects are described, followed by a brief discussion of approaches for ameliorating these adverse effects.

MECHANISM OF ANTICHOLINERGIC EFFECTS

Neurotransmitters are chemicals released from a neuron to convey a message across the synaptic cleft to a target cell, which may be a muscle fiber, a gland, or another neuron (Figure 19–1). The neurotransmitter interacts with a chemical configuration known as a receptor on the target cell. Acetylcholine is a major neurotransmitter, and the receptors for acetylcholine are called *cholinergic receptors*. Anticholinergic effects are caused by blockade of cho-

Table 19–1. ADVERSE DRUG EFFECTS COMMON AMONG THE ELDERLY

Effect	Major Drugs	Management
Memory and/or psychomotor deficit	anticholinergics benzodiazepines barbiturates beta blockers digoxin	Standard mental status questionnaire 1. Baseline 2. Routine reevaluation Modulate sensory input Exercise (with safety precautions)
Depression	*Antihypertensives* reserpine clonidine (Catapres) methyldopa (Aldomet) guanethidine (Ismelin) *Steroids* corticosteroids estrogens ACTH *Beta blockers* propranolol (Inderal) metoprolol (Lopressor) *Antiparkinsonians* amantadine (Symmetrel) levodopa *Other* digoxin procainamide (Pronestyl) appetite suppressants antineoplastics analgesics	Assess somatic and psychosocial signs 1. Baseline 2. Routine reevaluation Change drug if signs of depression Suicide precautions Exercise Family involvement Pet therapy
Delirium/confusion	See Memory and/or psychomotor deficit, above benzodiazepines digoxin oral hypoglycemics antiarrhythmics levodopa depressants (narcotics, benzodiazepines, anticonvulsants, hypnotics) beta blockers cimetidine (Tagamet) diuretics See Fluid retention, below	See Memory and/or psychomotor deficit, above Change drug or reduce dose Assess temporal aspects (sundowning, relation to dosing, etc.) Rule out depression ("pseudodementia") Reality orientation Resocialization
Postural hypotension	antihypertensives antipsychotic agents diuretics	Postural blood pressures 1. Baseline 2. Routine reevaluation Assess risk factors: dehydration, anemia, heart failure Avoid standing for long periods Move slowly to upright position Increases risk for deep vein thrombosis, embolism

Table continued on following page

linergic receptors by drugs, which prevents acetylcholine from interacting with the receptors.

Drugs with anticholinergic properties can be divided into those employed clinically for their anticholinergic properties and those used for other pharmacologic effects. For example, anticholinergic antiulcer agents exert their therapeutic effects by decreasing gastrointestinal motility and secretions through blockade of cholinergic synapses, while the antipsychotic activity of phenothiazine drugs like

Table 19–1. ADVERSE DRUG EFFECTS COMMON AMONG THE ELDERLY *Continued*

Effect	Major Drugs	Management

Fluid retention	*Antihypertensives*
	    reserpine
	    prazosin (Minipress)
	    terazosin (Hytrin)
	    diazoxide (Hyperstat)
	    hydralazine (Apresoline)
	Steroids
	    estrogens
	    androgens
	    progestins
	    corticosteroids
	Antiarthritis agents
	    aspirin
	    ibuprofen (Motrin, Advil)
	    indomethacin (Indocin)
	    sulindac (Clinoril)
	    naproxen (Anaprox, Naprosyn)
	    fenoprofen (Nalfon)
	    piroxicam (Feldene)
		Weight, hematocrit
		    1. Baseline
		    2. Routine reevaluation
		    3. Ascertain dry weight if edematous
		Low salt intake
		Positioning to promote drainage of extremities and prevent restricted circulation

Tardive dyskinesia	antipsychotic drugs	Assess tongue movements for fasciculations
		    1. Baseline
		    2. Reevaluate every 3 months
		Lowest effective dose
		Drug holidays
		Avoid routine use of anticholinergic antiparkinsonian drugs
		Risk factors: female, older, anticholinergic use, other neurologic deficit

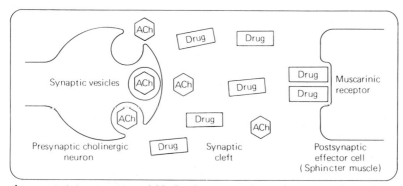

Figure 19–1. This schematic representation shows the mechanism of muscarinic blockade in a cholinergic synapse. The neurotransmitter acetylcholine (ACh) is normally released on stimulation of the presynaptic neuron and crosses the synapse to interact with the muscarinic receptor on the postsynaptic effector cell (in this case a sphincter muscle cell in the iris of the eye). This interaction causes contraction of the muscle, which is manifested as pupil constriction. When a chemical with anticholinergic properties is present (Drug), it interacts with the muscarinic receptor and blocks the action of acetylcholine, resulting in pupil dilation. (Modified from Boyd, EH, Karch, AH: Parasympathetic blocking drugs. *In* Wiener, MB, Pepper, GA (eds). Clinical Pharmacology and Therapeutics in Nursing (ed 2). New York, McGraw-Hill, 1985, p 179. Reprinted with permission.)

chlorpromazine (Thorazine) is thought to be through blockade of dopamine receptors; it is exclusive of the capacity of phenothiazines to block cholinergic receptors as well. Both types of drugs, however, cause undesirable anticholinergic adverse effects.

Types of Receptors

There are two major types of cholinergic receptors, nicotinic and muscarinic. The excitatory effects of acetylcholine on striated muscle and in ganglia can be simulated by nicotine, so these receptors are called *nicotine receptors*. These receptors are not significantly related to the anticholinergic effects described in this chapter. Muscarine reproduces the effects of acetylcholine at parasympathetic cholinergic receptors on smooth muscle, glands, and cardiac muscle, so these receptors are called *muscarinic receptors*. In the central nervous system most cholinergic receptors are muscarinic. Atropine blocks muscarinic receptors. Whether the primary therapeutic mechanism of a drug is muscarinic blockade or some other mechanism, such as the dopamine-receptor blockade of the antipsychotic drugs, the undesirable effects caused by muscarinic receptor blockade are referred to as *anticholinergic, antimuscarinic, parasympatholytic,* or *atropine-like* adverse drug effects.

Anticholinergic Effects

Drugs that block muscarinic receptors affect almost every organ system. Blockade of muscarinic receptors in the brain and spinal cord, such as those in the hippocampus associated with memory and those in the striatum associated with movement, results in central anticholinergic adverse effects. Central anticholinergic syndrome is an acute delirium manifested as memory loss, disorientation, confusion, and even coma. Peripheral anticholinergic adverse drug effects reflect antagonism of parasympathetic nervous system effects on target cells in the iris, ciliary muscle, lacrimal glands, salivary glands, heart, bronchi, gastrointes-

tinal tract, urinary bladder, corpora cavernosa, and sweat glands.

Anticholinergic adverse effects, which are outlined in Table 19–2, constitute a particular risk for the elderly because the effects often overlap with age-related physiologic and neuropsychiatric changes and because muscarinic blockade can exacerbate or mimic diseases common in the elderly (Busse & Simpson, 1983; Kendrick, 1982; Nelson, Jatlow, Bock, et al., 1982; Robinson, 1983; Salzman, 1982; Weiner, 1982). The potential hazards of drugs with anticholinergic activity to the elderly are highlighted by evidence from biochemical and pharmacologic studies indicating that anticholinergic drugs impair memory and that central cholinergic activity is decreased in aging and the senile dementias (Bartus, 1981; Carlsson, 1981; Davies & Maloney, 1976; Drachman & Leavitt, 1974; Ghoneim & Mewaldt, 1977; Smith & Swash, 1978). Hence, anticholinergic drugs might compound the biochemical mechanisms of memory loss and dementia. On the other hand, there are some anticholinergic effects that are less applicable to the elderly, such as paralysis of visual accommodation; since accommodation is normally absent after about age 65 years, use of anticholinergic drugs cannot increase this effect in the elderly.

Research indicates that anticholinergic drugs are associated with decreased self-care capacity in the elderly (Rovner, David, Lucas-Blaustein, et al., 1988). Risk of hip fracture is greater in those taking psychotropic drugs with anticholinergic effects (Ray, Griffin, Schaffer, et al., 1987).

Receptor Sensitivity

Muscarinic receptors in different organs are not equally sensitive to anticholinergic agents; for example, muscarinic receptors in the gastrointestinal system are more sensitive than those in the urinary bladder. Atropine dosages of 0.5 mg elicit slowed pulse, dry mouth, thirst, and decreased sweating. Dosages of 1.0 mg cause acceleration of the heart and pupillary changes. At 5.0 mg, speech and swallowing disturbances occur, accompanied by difficult

Table 19–2. MECHANISM AND CONSEQUENCES OF ANTICHOLINERGIC EFFECTS

Adverse Effect	Receptor Location	Potential Consequences
Central		
Sedation	Unknown (? brainstem)	Accidents, falls, social withdrawal, physical deterioration
Cognitive impairment, disorientation, memory loss	Hippocampus	Reversible dementia, developing into irreversible dementia if not corrected
Ataxia, imbalance	Brain, spinal cord, basal ganglia	Falls, resulting in fracture; fear of falling, resulting in self-imposed activity restriction
Other central symptoms: hallucinations, agitation, tremors, increased susceptibility to tardive dyskinesia	Brain (striatum, hippocampus)	Dementia, psychosis, tardive dyskinesia, stereotypy
Peripheral		
Dry mouth	Salivary glands	Dental caries, denture intolerance, reduced sense of taste, difficult speech, mucosal infection and lesions, dysphagia, dysphasia, anorexia, malnutrition, parasthesias of tongue
Impaired sweating	Sweat glands	Dry skin, fever, heatstroke, increased susceptibility to hyperthermia
Eye effects: dilated, nonreactive pupils; paralysis of accommodation	Iris, ciliary muscle, lacrimal glands	Blurred vision, glare intolerance, precipitate acute angle-closure glaucoma attack, falls, accidents, keratoconjunctivitis sicca, lesions of cornea, contact lens intolerance, blindness
Tachycardia	Sinoatrial node	Increased cardiac workload leading to angina or congestive heart failure
Decreased bowel motility	Smooth muscle of bowel	Constipation, fecal impaction, paralytic ileus
Decreased tone of bladder and increased tone of sphincters	Detrusor muscle and sphincters	Urinary hesitancy: urinary retention leading to renal damage, overflow or stress incontinence
Failure of penile erection	Corpora cavernosa	Impotence, sexual dysfunction
Decreased bronchial secretions	Bronchial glands	Mucous plugs, pneumonia
Drug interactions	Small intestine, stomach	Delayed stomach emptying, slowed absorption of many drugs

micturition, headache, decreased peristalsis, and fatigue. Increasing the atropine dosage to 10 mg or more results in severe peripheral symptoms and the appearance of central symptoms of ataxia and confusion. The usual adult preoperative dose of atropine for the person weighing 40 kg or more is 0.4 to 0.6 mg. Thus, most of these effects are found at doses in excess of the usual therapeutic dose, although when a patient is taking several anticholinergic agents the effective dose may greatly exceed this amount.

The following list shows anticholinergic effects in the usual order of appearance with increasing atropine dosage. As dosage increases, additional effects occur and the effects already present become more marked (Weiner, 1980).

Bradycardia
Dry mouth
Decreased sweating
Tachycardia
Dilated pupils
Blurred near vision
Decreased intestinal peristalsis
Dysphasia
Dysphagia
Urinary retention
Hyperthermia, flushing
Ataxia
Hallucinations
Delirium
Coma

This sequence can be a useful guide for clinical observation. For example, the fact that the confusion typical of central anticholinergic syndrome is accompanied by peripheral anticholinergic effects such as dilated, poorly reactive pupil; flushing, dry mucous membranes; urinary retention; and ataxia permits the clinician to differentiate this syndrome from other causes of confusion. Further, the nurse can use this sequence to gauge if drug accumulation is occurring, since patients will display gradually increasing symptoms. However, this sequence was established by studies on young subjects, and it is possible that it may be somewhat different in the elderly due to changes in receptor sensitivity or responsiveness that occur with aging.

Drugs with Anticholinergic Properties

Examples of drug classes and specific agents with anticholinergic properties are listed in Table 19–3. Belladonna alkaloids, gastrointestinal antispasmodics, genitourinary antispasmodics, many psychotropic agents (antidepressants, antipsychotics), antiparkinsonian drugs, antihistamines, some opththalmologic agents, two muscle relaxants, and one antiarrhythmic drug have anticholinergic activity.

Anticholinergic Potency. Anticholinergic drugs share a common chemical structure that permits them to bind to muscarinic receptors. How potent a particular drug is depends upon how well its specific structure binds to the receptor, which is called its receptor *affinity*. Drugs with high receptor affinity tend to be more potent, that is, less drug is required to elicit a particular effect. Conversely, drugs with low receptor affinity are generally less potent and a higher dosage is required to achieve the particular effect. Drugs with very low affinity may not elicit the full desired response no matter how much drug is used.

Within a particular drug class, agents vary in their anticholinergic potency. For example, among the antidepressants, amitriptyline (Elavil, Endep) has high anticholinergic potency; nortriptyline (Aventyl, Pamelor) has moderate anticholinergic potency; amoxapine (Asendin) has low anticholinergic potency. Among the antihistamines, diphenhydramine (Benadryl) has high anticholinergic potency; chlorpheniramine (Chlor-Trimeton) has mod-

Table 19–3. EXAMPLES OF DRUGS WITH ANTICHOLINERGIC ACTIVITY

Drug Class	Selected Examples*
Belladonna alkaloids	atropine, diphenoxylate with atropine (Lomotil), scopolamine, belladonna (Bellergal)
Antipsychotic agents	chlorpromazine (Thorazine), thioridazine (Mellaril), haloperidol (Haldol)
Antiparkinsonian agents	trihexphenidyl (Artane), benztropine (Cogentin)
Antidepressants	amitriptyline (Elavil), imipramine (Tofranil), amoxapine (Asendin)
Antispasmodics (gastrointestinal)	dicyclomine (Bentyl), propantheline (Pro-Banthine), clidinium (Quarzan), glycopyrrolate (Robinul)
Antispasmodics (genitourinary)	oxybutynin (Ditropan), L-hyoscyamine (Levsin, Cystospaz)
Antihistamines	diphenhydramine (Benadryl), cyclizine (Marezine), chlorpheniramine (Chlor-Trimeton), hydroxyzine (Vistaril)
Ophthalmologic cycloplegics and mydriatics	homatropine, cyclopentolate (Cyclogel)
Antiarrhythmic	disopyramide (Norpace)
Skeletal muscle relaxants	orphenadrine (Norflex), cyclobenzaprine (Flexeril)
Analgesics	Methotrimeprazine (Levoprome), droperidol (Inapsine, Innovar)

*Some agents include an anticholinergic drug as one component of a multidrug preparation.

erate anticholinergic potency; terfenadine (Seldane) has low anticholinergic potency. Relative ranking of drugs by potency of anticholinergic effects is frequently found in drug references or pharmacology textbooks. These rankings permit prescribers to choose the agent with the least anticholinergic effect in the class if the patient seems to be at particular risk for an anticholinergic effect or previously has shown susceptibility to these effects. However, these rankings do not allow comparison of drugs across classes; thus, a high-potency antidepressant may not be comparable to a high-potency antihistamine in terms of the severity of anticholinergic effects elicited.

Technologic developments have produced radioreceptor assay procedures to permit scientists to measure the receptor affinity of anticholinergic drugs in the laboratory (Shein & Smith, 1978; Snyder, Greenburg, & Yamamura, 1974; Snyder & Yamamura, 1977). Atropine is used as the standard against which these drugs are compared. Using this method, the antiparkinsonian agents such as benztropine (Cogentin) and trihexphenidyl (Artane) are about half as potent as atropine. Amitriptyline (Elavil), the most potent anticholinergic of the antidepressants, is only 1/25th as active as atropine; that is, 25 mg of amitriptyline would have the same anticholinergic effects as 1 mg of atropine. The most potent anticholinergic of the antipsychotics, thioridazine (Mellaril), is less than 1/10th as potent as amitriptyline (or 1/300th as potent as atropine). When comparing the potency of various agents, it is important to consider usual dosage. For example, although amitriptyline is less than 5% as potent as atropine, it can be expected to cause considerable anticholinergic effect because its usual dosage is 100 or more times larger than that for atropine.

Although radioreceptor binding studies have been performed for relatively few drugs, it is possible to extrapolate the available data from clinical and laboratory studies to a classification of drugs with anticholinergic activity (Table 19–4) and to assign a numerical value to each class, representing relative anticholinergic potency compared to atropine (Pepper, 1985).

CLINICAL ASSESSMENT OF ANTICHOLINERGIC RISK

Drugs with anticholinergic properties are among those most frequently prescribed for the elderly and are components of many over-the-counter products. Studies show that 30% to 60% of elderly daily receive drugs with anticholinergic activity; between 9% and 32% simultaneously take two or more of these anticholinergic agents (Blazer, Felderspeil, Ray, et al., 1983; Pepper, 1985; Seifert, Jamieson, & Gardner, 1983). Because anticholinergic

adverse effects can cause reactions ranging from discomfort to death, the clinician must be able to judge the threat a particular drug regimen poses for a specific patient. The magnitude of the threat depends upon the total anticholinergic dosage of all drugs in the regimen with anticholinergic activity and the unique risk factors characteristic of the patient. If the threat is great and the consequences of one or more anticholinergic adverse drug effects are serious or significantly disruptive (see Table 19–2), preventive action is required. If the risk factors cannot be modified, the drug therapy should be adjusted by reducing the dosage, substituting an agent from another drug class, or using an agent within the same class that has very low anticholinergic potency.

Temporal Aspects

Most adverse effects occur relatively early in drug therapy. Patients unable to tolerate a particular effect will usually report the effect when it first occurs; likewise, clinicians are more likely to specifically question the patient about anticholinergic effects during the first visit after the drug is initiated. However, anticholinergic adverse effects, such as constipation, dry mouth, and postural instability, do persist with chronic therapy (Pepper, 1985). Further, prolonged half-lives of most drugs in the elderly mean that it takes much longer for blood levels to reach steady state in the elderly, so that adverse effects often commence much later than in younger adults (Jennings, Tourville, & Pepper, 1985). A change in the physical condition of an elderly person, such as exacerbation of congestive heart failure (which decreases drug metabolism), may cause a previously latent adverse effect to become manifest. Anticholinergic effects may appear suddenly when a new prescription or over-the-counter drug with anticholinergic properties is added to the drug regimen, because of the additive effects of the old and new agents. In summary, while most anticholinergic adverse effects appear soon after a drug is initiated, the nurse must remain vigi-

Table 19–4. ESTIMATION OF ANTICHOLINERGIC EXPOSURE

Approximate Atropine Equivalent Factors (AEF)*
Very High Potency Drugs (AEF = 1 to 5)

atropine† (1)	cyclopentolate† (1)	L-hyoscyamine (1)
belladonna alkaloid (1)	glycopyrrolate‡ (3)	oxybutynin (5)
benztropine (4)	homatropine† (1)	tropicamide† (1)
		trihexphenidyl (3)

High Potency Drugs (AEF = 10)

amitriptyline	diphenhydramine	propantheline‡
anisotropine‡	doxepin	protriptyline
biperidin	hexocyclium‡	
carbinoxamine	isopropamide‡	
clemastine	mepenzolate‡	
clidinium‡	methscopolamine‡	
dimenhydrinate	oxyphenonium‡	
	procyclidine	

Medium Potency Drugs (AEF = 100)

chlorphenoxamine	mesoridazine	promethazine
desipramine	methantheline‡	triflupromazine
ethopropazine	methdilazine	trimeprazine
imipramine	nortriptyline	trimipramine
maprotiline	orphenadrine	thioridazine
	promazine	

Low Potency Drugs (AEF = 1000)

amoxapine	cyproheptadine	phenindamine
azatadine	dexchlorpheniramine	promazine
brompheniramine	diphenylpyraline	pyrilamine
buclizine	disopyramide	trazodone
chlorpheniramine	hydroxyzine	tripelennamine
chlorpromazine	methotrimeprazine	triprolidine
chlorprothixene	meclizine	
cyclizine		

Very Low Potency Drugs (AEF = 10,000)

acetophenazine	loxapine	terfenadine
dicyclomine	molindone	thiothixene
droperidol	oxyphencyclimine	trifluoperazine
fluphenazine	perphenazine	
haloperidol	prochlorperazine	

Anticholinergic Exposure Estimate

Computed total anticholinergic dose in atropine equivalents mg/kg/day	Average daily dose comparable to (mg) atropine	Level of anticholinergic exposure
>0.030	>2	Very high
0.009 to 0.030	>0.6 to 2	High
0.003 to 0.009	>0.2 to 0.6	Moderate
<0.003	<0.2	Low

*Number in parentheses indicates the AEF for drugs in this group.
†When given topically in an ophthalmologic solution, about 20% of the dose may be absorbed.
‡Quaternary amine drug that does not cross the blood-brain barrier, so it causes negligible central anticholinergic effects.

lant for anticholinergic adverse effects throughout the duration of therapy.

Estimating Anticholinergic Exposure

Information in Table 19–4 can be used to estimate the total anticholinergic activity in atropine equivalents of all of the drugs in a patient's regimen and to rank this total dosage from low to very high. Because the patient's weight is an important determinant of a given dosage, it is also considered in this calculation. The steps for estimating a patient's anticholinergic exposure are as follows:

1. Find the *generic* name of the first anticholinergic drug in Table 19–4 that the patient is taking. Divide the patient's total (or average) daily dosage by the Atropine Equivalent Factor (AEF) listed for the group or specific agent. If the medication is a multidrug combination, use a reference or the package insert to ascertain the amount of the anticholinergic agent in the preparation.

2. Repeat no. 1, above, for each anticholinergic drug the patient is taking. Add the results of all of these calculations.

3. Divide the sum by the patient's weight in kilograms.

4. Compare the result to the ranges given on the bottom of Table 19–4 to classify the patient as having low, moderate, high, or very high anticholinergic exposure.

Thus, if a female patient who weighs 40 kg (88 lb) has a regimen of Ditropan 5 mg BID and Mellaril 25 mg TID, she would have a daily dosage comparable to 2.75 mg of atropine or 0.069 mg/kg/day, which would place her in the very high anticholinergic exposure group, indicating that she is likely to demonstrate a number of anticholinergic effects. This is computed as follows:

Step 1. Since the AEF of oxybutynin (Ditropan) is 5 (from the Very High Group) and the daily dosage is 10 mg (2×5 mg), the atropine equivalence for this drug is 2.0.

Step 2. The AEF for thioridazine (Mellaril) is 100 (from the Medium Group) and the total daily dosage is 75 mg (3×25 mg), so the atropine equivalence for this drug is 0.75. The patient's comparable atropine dosage is 2.75 ($2.0 + 0.75$). (If the Mellaril has been ordered TID PRN and the patient did not take the drug three times every day, an average dosage could be calculated by adding the dosage over several days and dividing by the number of days surveyed.)

Step 3. When the total atropine equivalent dosage is divided by the patient's weight, the computed total anticholinergic dose is 0.069 mg/kg/day.

Step 4. From the chart at the bottom of Table 19–4, the patient's drug regimen ranks in the Very High Exposure Group.

Determining Risk Factors

Knowledge of a patient's anticholinergic exposure is a major factor in predicting the incidence and severity of adverse effects, but individual characteristics can significantly increase the risk associated with a particular exposure level. Many physical characteristics and pathologic conditions increase the risk for development of adverse effects. For example, since the average elderly person weighs less than the average young adult and yet usually is prescribed similar dosages, the weight-adjusted dose for the elderly person is often greater. Benign prostatic hypertrophy, which is common among elderly males, increases the risk of urinary retention when drugs with anticholinergic properties are taken. The incidence of angle-closure glaucoma rises sharply after the age of 40 years, so acute angle closure can be anticipated to occur more frequently among those in this age group who take anticholinergic drugs.

Recently, researchers and clinicians began to recognize that psychosocial characteristics are also predictive of both positive and negative responses to therapy (Gyrell & Katahan, 1978; Pepper, 1985; Rowe & Kahn, 1987; Schwartz, Wang, Zeitz, et al., 1962). Studies

Table 19–5. RISK FACTORS AND MANAGEMENT FOR COMMON ANTICHOLINERGIC ADVERSE DRUG EFFECTS

Adverse Effect	Risk Factors for Developing the Effect	Risk Factors for Serious Sequelae	Interventions to Ameliorate Adverse Effect
Sedation	Other central nervous system depressant drugs Dementia	Coma, impaired neurologic function Prone to pneumonia Hazardous environment or tasks	Minimize dosage and give two-thirds at bedtime and one-third during day Exercise and social stimulation Ensure safe environment Avoid driving and hazardous activities
Confusion, memory impairment	Organic brain syndrome Sensory deprivation Low educational level	Undetected for long period Dementia	Minimize dosage Exercise and social stimulation Environmental reminders (clocks and calendars; color-coded rooms) In crisis give physostigmine 1–2 mg parenterally
Ataxia, imbalance	Postural hypotension Poor muscle strength Proprioceptive deficit Visual deficit	Prior history of falls Osteoporosis Fear of falling	Exercises for strength and balance Ensure safe environment and good lighting Encourage activity in spite of fear, giving maximal reassurance
Visual effects: dilated pupils, precipitate acute angle closure, dry eyes	Visual deficits (cataracts, presbyopia) Steroids and other drugs that increase ocular pressure	Narrow-angle glaucoma Contact lens use	Regular glaucoma evaluation after age 40 Indirect lighting without glare Allow time to accommodate when going from dark to bright areas Careful handwashing when using contact lenses or other eye care; environmental humidification and lubricating eye drops (compatible with contact lenses if used)
Dry mouth	Women Nonsmoker or heavy smoker Poor hydration Clonidine therapy	Oral infection Chemotherapy or immunosuppressants	Good oral hygiene including regular dental visits Good hydration including frequent sips of water or electrolyte drink Suck hard sugarless candy Use artificial saliva
Tachycardia	Women Angina	Coronary artery disease Heart failure Arrhythmias	Monitor pulse at time of peak drug effects Organize activities to minimize exertion
Skin changes: decreased sweating, dry skin	Dehydration Diuretic therapy	Excessive environmental heat Scratching, leading to lesions and infection	Minimize washing, especially with soaps; use lotions and oils Air conditioning during heat waves Environmental humidification in winter
Decreased bowel motility	Polypharmacy Dehydration Poor diet Inactivity	Toxic megacolon Paralytic ileus	Adequate dietary fluid, fat, and roughage Exercise and regular routine Keep bowel record in order to prevent unrecognized impaction
Decreased bladder motility	Prostatic enlargement Multiparity	Prostatic enlargement Renal impairment	Void before taking dose Use commode or stand to void Kegel exercises Good hydration

show that the risk factors for adverse drug effects in general are age over 75 years, white, female, living alone, and having multiple diagnoses and therapies (Lamy, 1980). Risk factors for anticholinergic adverse effects as a group are advanced age, female gender, poor cognitive function, multiple drug orders (both anticholinergic and other drugs), lower expectations for benefit from drug therapy, and negative reference group influences (Pepper, 1985). The person's reference group (social support systems), both formal (doctors, nurses, other professional caregivers) and informal (family, friends, significant others), seems to influence the person's expectations for positive or negative outcomes of therapy, which in turn is related to the prevalence of adverse effects. Risk factors for specific anticholinergic adverse effects are shown in Table 19–5.

AMELIORATING ANTICHOLINERGIC EFFECTS

At times, anticholinergic adverse effects are unavoidable, since some therapeutic effects cannot be separated from the adverse effects. In these cases the usual preventative strategies (decreasing the dose or changing to another drug class or a lower-potency anticholinergic) result in loss of desired effects. The responsibility of the nurse is then to assist the patient to ameliorate the adverse effects, reducing their severity or the degree of discomfort and danger posed. Interventions should be efficient and associated with minimal risk of additional adverse effects, and should conserve the elderly patient's resources. For example, dry mouth may be managed by having the patient suck on hard candies, but the sugar in the candy actually further dries the mucous membranes and increases the incidence of dental caries by supplying a substrate for bacterial growth. Artificial salivas are products that are very effective in treating dry mouth, but these products are expensive and can pose a financial burden to the elderly patient. Frequent sips of water or electrolyte solution (e.g., Gatorade), environmental humidifica-

tion, and good oral hygiene may be the most feasible management of dry mouth. Table 19–5 outlines strategies for ameliorating anticholinergic adverse effects.

SUMMARY

Adverse drug effects are more common in the elderly and can cause significant morbidity and mortality. By being aware of the most common types of adverse effects, nurses can participate in prevention, detection, and management of these problems. Anticholinergic adverse effects are particularly important for the elderly, since this group of effects can exacerbate or mimic several age-related or disease-related problems, such as memory loss, confusion, imbalance, dry mouth, abnormal cardiac rate or rhythm, dry skin, keratoconjunctivitis sicca ("dry eye"), hyperthermia, urinary retention, constipation, and sexual dysfunction. Drug groups containing agents with anticholinergic properties include antipsychotics, antidepressants, antiparkinsonian agents, antispasmodics, ophthalmologic mydriatics and cycloplegics, and antihistamines. Although agents vary widely in potency and patients often take several different agents with anticholinergic activity, the total dosage can be estimated in atropine equivalents, based upon laboratory studies of the receptor affinity of various drugs. The likelihood that a specific patient will develop anticholinergic adverse effects can be predicted from this estimated atropine equivalent dosage and awareness of physical and psychosocial risk factors. For patients at high risk of anticholinergic adverse effects, interventions to prevent, detect, or ameliorate the effects should be initiated.

References

Bartus, RT (1981): Age-related memory loss and cholinergic dysfunction: Possible directions based on animal models. *In* Crooks, T, & Gershon, S (eds): *Strategies for the Development of Effective Treatment for Senile Dementia.* New Canaan, CT, Mark Powley, 71–92.
Basen, MM (1977): The elderly and drugs: Problem over-

view and program strategy. *Public Health Rep, 92*(1):43–48.

Baum, BJ (1981): Research on aging and oral health: An assessment of current status and future needs. *Spec Care Dentistry*, 1:156–165.

Blazer, DG, Felderspeil, CF, Ray, WA, et al. (1983): The risk of anticholinergic toxicity in the elderly: A study of the prescribing practices of two populations. *J Gerontol*, 38:31–35.

Boyd, EH, & Karch, AH: Parasympathetic blocking drugs. *In* Weiner, MB, & Pepper, GA (eds): *Clinical Pharmacology and Therapeutics in Nursing* (ed 2). New York, McGraw-Hill, 1985.

Bressler, R (1982): Adverse drug reactions. *In* Conrad, KA, & Bressler, R (eds): *Drug Therapy for the Elderly*. St Louis, CV Mosby, 64–85.

Busse, E, & Simpson, D (1983): Depression and antidepressants in the elderly. *J Clin Psychiatry*, 44(Sec. 2):35–39.

Caranasos, GJ, Stewart, RB, & Cluff, LE (1974): Drug-induced illness leading to hospitalization. *JAMA*, 228:713–717.

Carlsson, A (1981): Aging and brain neurotransmitters. *In* Crook, T, & Gershon, S (eds): *Strategies for the Development of Effective Treatment for Senile Dementia*. New Canaan, CT, Mark Powley, 93–106.

Davies, RK, & Maloney, AJF (1976): Selective loss of central cholinergic neurons in Alzheimer's disease. *Lancet*, 2:1403.

Drachman, DA, & Leavitt, J (1974): Human memory and the cholinergic nervous system: A relationship to aging? *Arch Neurol*, 30:113–121.

Epstein, JB (1982): Clinical trials of a sialogogue in humans: A preliminary report. *Spec Care Dentistry*, 2:17–19.

Ghoneim, M, & Mewaldt, S (1977): Studies on human memory: The interactions of diazepam, scopolamine, and physostigmine. *Psychopharmacology*, 52:1–6.

Gyrell, SH, & Katahan, M (1978): Situational factors contributory to the placebo effect. *Psychopharmacology*, 57:253–262.

Hollister, LE (1977): Prescribing drugs for the elderly. *Geriatrics*, 32 (2, 11):71–73.

Hurwitz, N (1969): Predisposing factors in adverse reactions to drugs. *Br Med J*, 1:536.

Jennings, B, Tourville, JF, & Pepper, GA (1985): Pharmacokinetics through the life span. *In* Wiener, MB, & Pepper, GA (eds): *Clinical Pharmacology and Therapeutics in Nursing* (ed 2). New York, McGraw-Hill, 107–133.

Kendrick, DC (1982): Why assess the aged? A clinical psychologist's view. *Br J Clin Psychol*, 21:47–54.

Lamy, PP (1980): *Prescribing for the Elderly*. Littleton, MA, PSG.

Lyons, DC (1972): The dry mouth adverse reaction syndrome in the geriatric patient. *J Oral Med*, 27(4):110–111.

MacDonald, JB (1985): The role of drugs in falls in the elderly. *Clin Geriatr Med*, 1:621–631.

Mellville, A (1984): Set and serendipity in the detection of drug hazards. *Soc Sci Med*, 14(4):391–396.

Mossey, JM (1985): Social and psychologic factors related to falls in the elderly. *Clin Geriatr Med*, 1:541–553.

Navazesh, M, & Ship, I (1983): Xerostomia: Diagnosis and treatment. *Am J Otolaryngol*, 4:283–292.

Nelson, JC, Jatlow, PI, Bock, J, et al. (1982): Major adverse reactions during desipramine treatment. *Arch Gen Psychiatry*, 39:1055–1061.

Pepper, GA (1985): *Central and Peripheral Anticholinergic Adverse Drug Effects in the Institutionalized Elderly*. Unpublished doctoral dissertation, University of Colorado Health Sciences Center, Denver.

Ray, WA, Griffin, MR, Schaffner, W, et al. (1987): Psychotropic drug use and the risk of hip fracture. *N Engl J Med*, 316:363–369.

Robinson, DS (1983): Aging and neuropharmacology. *In* Yetiv, JZ, & Bianchine, JR (eds): *Recent Advances in Clinical Therapeutics*. New York, Grune & Stratton, 127–139.

Rovner, BW, David, A, Lucas-Blaustein, J, et al. (1988): Self-care capacity and anticholinergic drug levels in nursing home patients. *Am J Psychiatry*, 145:107–109.

Rowe, JW, & Kahn, RL (1987): Human aging: Usual and successful. *Science*, 237:143–149.

Salzman, C (1982): Basic principles of psychotropic drug prescription for the elderly. *Hosp Community Psychiatry*, 33:133–136.

Schiff, G (1984): Adverse drug reactions: Recognition of the problem. *Drug Newsletter*, 3:49–50.

Schwartz, D, Wang, M, Zeitz, L, et al. (1962): Medication errors made by elderly chronically ill patients. *Am J Public Health*, 12:2018–2028.

Seifert, R, Jamieson, J, & Gardner, R Jr (1983): Use of anticholinergics in the nursing home: An empirical study and review. *Drug Intell Clin Pharm*, 17:471–473.

Shein, K, & Smith, SE (1978): Structure-activity relationships for the anticholinoceptor action of tricyclic antidepressants. *Br J Pharmacol*, 62:567–571.

Siedl, LG, Thornton, GF, & Smith, JW (1966): Studies on the epidemiology of adverse drug reactions: III. Reactions in patients on general medical service. *Bull Johns Hopkins Hosp*, 119:299–315.

Smith, CM, & Swash, M (1978): Possible biochemical basis of memory disorder in Alzheimer's disease. *Ann Neurol*, 3:471–473.

Snyder, SH, Greenburg, D, & Yamamura, HH (1974): Antischizophrenic drugs and brain cholinergic receptors. *Arch Gen Psychiatry*, 31:58–61.

Snyder, SH, & Yamamura, HH (1977): Antidepressants and the muscarinic acetylcholine receptor. *Arch Gen Psychiatry*, 31:58–61.

Todd, B (1982): Dry mouth—Causes and cures. *Geriatr Nurs*, 5:122–123.

Weiner, N (1982): Update on antiparkinsonian agents. *Geriatrics*, 37:81–84, 89–91.

Weiner, N (1980): Atropine, scopolamine, and related antimuscarinic drugs. *In* Gilman, AG, Goodman, LS, & Gilman, A (eds): *Goodman and Gilman's the Pharmacological Basis of Therapeutics* (ed 6). New York, Macmillan, 120–137.

Williamson, J, & Chopin, JM (1980): Adverse reactions to prescribed drugs in the elderly: A multicenter investigation. *Age Ageing*, 9:73.

CHAPTER
20

Preventing Excess Disability

SALLY A. SALISBURY, R.N.C.S., M.S.

"You know how it is, when people learn that you are 83 years old they automatically expect you to be enfeebled, weak, and incapable. I forget things but I'm not a cripple. My family is crippling me with their caring."

An Alzheimer's patient

"My doctor just says, 'Well you have to expect those things at your age. Get a cane.' But I don't feel old. It is always a shock to me when I see myself in the mirror, because I don't feel like I look."

An 81-year-old woman being treated for tendinitis

Chapter 19 discussed the physical causes of iatrogenic illness. Illness involves more than a series of pathophysiologic changes. The meaning and impact of illness for a person are the result of pathophysiology and the social and interactional processes that accompany it. The style and content of interactions accompanying treatment and caregiving may themselves have a negative effect on health and well-being. The social and interactional context of an illness may result in excess disability. In this chapter, the related concepts of locus of control, sick role, and learned helplessness are used to examine excess disability as it may occur in acute- or long-term care environments. This chapter addresses indirect self-destructive behaviors of patients and labeling behavior of staff as contributors to excess disability. Interventions to prevent or ameliorate excess disability in acute-care and long-term care settings are defined.

EXCESS DISABILITY

Definition

Excess disability is the failure of patients to perform cognitive and self-care tasks when they have the physical and mental ability to do so (Kahn, 1965). Some patients do not do as much for themselves as they are capable of doing. Excess disability is a reversible deficit that may be more disabling than the primary

391

disability (Dawson, Kline, Crinklaw, et al., 1986). It represents the gap between actual function and potential function (Brody, Kleban, Lawton, et al., 1974). Brody, Kleban, Powell, and associates (1971), working with a population of mentally impaired elderly persons, identified seven categories in which excess disability appears. They are mobility, self-care, social relationships, family relationships, organized activities, individualized activities, and emotional discomfort, anxiety, or depression (Brody, et al., 1971). The construct of excess disability received scholarly attention by social and behavioral scientists in the late 1960s and early 1970s. More recently, with the medical emphasis on chronic and long-term care, the concept of excess disability has received less attention. However, for nurses who work with this population and who must be concerned more with function than with cure, the prevention of excess disability is an integral part of nursing practice.

Causes

Excess disability may be mitigated or exacerbated by a person's locus of control belief, by the constraints and expectations of the sick role, and by learned helplessness. These factors, combined with real helplessness resulting from physical impairment, may create disability. The degree of disability is also affected by a person's support system, learned survival skills, and the ability to adapt to a new and demanding situation.

Locus of Control. Locus of control is a concept that relates to an individual's beliefs about the amount of personal control that he or she exercises over important events in life and the personal environment. Persons whose perception is that they have the ability to regulate or direct situations or events are said to have an internal locus of control. Those who perceive that the course of events that influence their lives and the situations in which they find themselves are caused by external authorities or fate are said to have an external locus of control (Lefcourt, 1976). People with an internal locus of control have a

highly developed sense of their own self-efficacy and are characterized by being active and assertive. Self-efficacy refers to an individual's belief that his or her actions are effective in achieving personal goals. It implies a sense of mastery over body, environment, and fortune and a high degree of independence. Those with an external locus of control are thought to have decreased self-efficacy and are characterized by being withdrawn and passive (Woodward & Wallston, 1987; Lefcourt, 1976). Internal locus of control defines if a person feels personal responsibility for what happens to him or her in life.

The questions of how locus of control and self-efficacy mediate adaptation to both illness and aging has been addressed by researchers. An individual with an external locus of control is more likely to blame an illness on germs or bad luck and to come to a health care professional with a request that the illness be fixed (Bieliauskas, 1983). Since these people attribute the cause of illness to something apart from their own behavior, it is difficult to convince them of the usefulness of avoiding or curing illness by certain self-help behaviors, such as stopping smoking. People with an internal locus of control may avoid the physician when ill, since "he can't do anything" or "if I wait long enough I will get better myself." However, such a person may be more likely to take preventive self-help health actions (Bieliauskas, 1983) and, when ill, may have fewer days in bed and briefer illnesses. These suppositions were supported in a longitudinal study of 931 subjects who were drawn from a random probability, urban community sample. Locus of control and health history and behavior were assessed separately over a 1-year timespan. The sample contained persons of both sexes and all ages. Those with an internal locus of control were found to practice more preventive health measures; they tried to quit smoking, were more sanguine about early treatment for cancer, rated their self-perceived health level higher, stayed in bed less once illness was diagnosed, and were less dependent on physicians than on other subjects (Seeman & Seeman, 1983).

Barusch (1988) reports that a personal style

that includes doing things on one's own (having an internal locus of control), while effective in youth, may actually interfere with adjustment in aging. Her study found that the elderly caregivers of Alzheimer's patients were inhibited from seeking help, even when such help was needed, because of the high degree of satisfaction they derived from handling the situation independently. Consequences were a higher level of stress for the caregivers and a higher incidence of behavior problems in their patients. However, in a study relating to patients rather than caregivers, Smith, Wallston, Forsberg, and associates (1984) found that individuals over 60 years of age had a lower desire to have control over their health than did younger adults. In another study, those individuals most vulnerable to illness and most likely to enter the health care system were most likely to see themselves as less competent regarding health, and more likely to give up in terms of health care and health care decision-making (Woodward & Wallston, 1987). In this sense, a low level of perceived self-efficacy may be detrimental to effective coping (Bandura, 1982), since the individual may not seek needed help or may participate only passively in treatment.

Moch (1988) has broadened the concepts of external locus of control and low self-efficacy, which she calls "uncontrol." She defines uncontrol as "the acceptance that one does not have power over all, or even many events, people or conditions that affect one's life" (Moch, 1988). This may include belief in a higher power than the self, a power that may be perceived in religious or philosophical terms. Her contention is that effective nursing involves assisting the patient to achieve a balance between control and uncontrol.

The Sick Role. Role theory offers a plausible explanation for the presence of a greater incapacity than is warranted by the severity of the disease. Role theory postulates that we are who we are and we do what we do as a result of the roles we have taken throughout our lives. As we age and become infirm, we lose former roles and take on new ones. The process of role-taking is complex. People take into account what others are doing and interpret the behavior and communication of others. They then form their own behaviors and concepts of self on the basis of this interpretation. This process is ongoing, not static, and our ideas of ourselves and the roles we take on are continually evolving as long as we are living in social groups (Blumer, 1969). In our culture the role of the elderly is defined negatively in terms of loss of economic and social utility and changed identity (Rosow, 1973). As a result, many elderly occupy a deviant role wherein they are exempted from responsibility. The elderly may even ascribe this role to themselves as a group, while not accepting the role prescription as individuals. To themselves they are not what society expects them to be (Thomas, 1981). The elderly sick are often socialized to the sick role by the role casting of physicians, nurses, and family. Role casting refers to expectations of behavior such as inactivity, nonproductivity, and dependence for reasons of health or age (Nuttbrock, 1986). The quotations at the beginning of this chapter attest to elderly women's view of themselves as different from others' views of them, and they describe the experience of being cast into the sick role. Disability and learned helplessness are intrinsic to the sick role, which is defined as the extent to which a person perceives himself to resemble sick persons with regard to worthiness, power, activity, and independence (Brown & Rawlinson, 1979).

There are times when the sick role is appropriate. When a person has an acute illness, such as congestive heart failure, that person requires the technical professional help of specially trained medical and nursing personnel. The patient's survival depends on his or her acceptance of the sick role, with its attendant behaviors of submitting to treatment and following the dictates of others regarding activity, medical regimen, and place of treatment, i.e., cardiac care unit or step-down unit. Accepting the sick role enables the person to utilize the skills of others to achieve recovery. Thus, the sick role has its compensations. It becomes disabling only when a person is cast into the role without relevant supporting clinical observations.

People believing themselves dependent and powerless will function as though they are, actual physical condition notwithstanding. This is one compensation of the sick role. Less is expected of sick people; they are permitted a certain level of dependence and irresponsibility, and others offer aid and assistance. Nuttbrock (1986) found that those elderly experiencing social strain were more likely to be cast into the sick role than those who were not, regardless of the degree of infirmity. He postulates that elderly people who perceive their present social roles as overly demanding in effect convince others to define them as sick. When patients accept the sick role, they accept that they are at the mercy of the medical skills and expertise of the health care professional. The sick role reinforces stereotypes of the elderly and gives the patient permission to give up responsibility. The health care professional is then in a position to manipulate rewards for appropriate sick role behavior. Since all power is held by the professional, the professional's response and rewards may be totally independent of the patient's needs and responses (Solomon, 1982). As health care professionals increase distance between themselves and the patient, they increase their own power and the patient's sense of helplessness. The following professional behaviors all increase distance between professional and patient. In each of the interchanges, the staff response appears to be unrelated to the prior patient behavior.

1. Answering a question with an unrelated statement: *Patient:* "Have you seen my doctor today?" *Nurse:* "Your breakfast is here."

2. Interrupting the patient: one study noted that physicians, in 52 of 74 videotaped interviews, interrupted their patients within 18 seconds of the time the patients began stating their complaints (Pfeiffer, 1986).

3. Doing physical care without speaking: e.g., coming into a room, hanging an IV, and leaving.

4. Minimizing the patient's concerns: *Patient:* "What if my leg ulcer doesn't heal?" *Nurse:* "Of course it will heal, what a worrywart you are."

5. Talking about the patient as if he weren't there: *Nurse to physician, speaking across patient in bed:* "His skin turgor is poor and his weight is down, do you think he should be getting supplemental feedings?" *Physician:* "That's a good idea, I'll order some."

6. Making decisions for the patient: *Nurse to visitor in front of patient:* "He has been up long enough, we are going to put him in bed now and you can come back later."

Learned Helplessness. As patients repeatedly see themselves as powerless, they learn helplessness. Seligman (1975) maintained that learned helplessness develops when a person experiences noncontingent responses. When patients' behaviors are either not responded to or are responded to in a haphazard or inappropriate manner, they come to believe that the responses of those in their environment are totally beyond their control. They expect that nothing they do will influence the outcome of their actions. Rather than engage in actions they believe to be futile to change outcome, they simply give up. The construct of learned helplessness has been associated with increased depression in the elderly. In a study that examined the relationships between rehabilitation outcome and psychological functioning on a medical rehabilitation unit, high levels of perceived helplessness were associated with poor rehabilitative outcomes (Mermelstein & Lopez, 1985).

Learned helplessness can also be acquired from observation. If a person observes others in a situation where they have no power to influence outcome, that person may infer that he or she too is helpless (DeVellis, DeVellis, & McCauley, 1978). Helplessness and a belief in one's incompetence may be inferred from the situational context of the activities in which one is engaged (Langer & Benevento, 1978). If people no longer perform tasks they formerly did, are assigned a label that connotes inferiority, or allow others to do something for them, and if these matters are important and uncomfortable to them, these people may see themselves as helpless.

All of the above circumstances are present in long-term care institutions. It is well recognized that geriatric nurses who do too much for their patients rather than encourage patients to retain or regain self-care skills may actually push patients into unnecessary dependence. Dependency is a strong predictor of mortality, whether patients live in the community or in institutions, regardless of their age (Campbell, 1986). Using an operant conditioning theoretical framework, Baltes and Skinner (1983) found that dependent behaviors of nursing home residents were followed by dependence-supporting behavior by staff. In contrast, independent behavior on the part of residents was either not responded to or was responded to by staff behavior that was incongruent with the preceding behavior of the resident (a series of behaviors called noncontingent reinforcement). Relatives likewise were observed to positively reinforce dependent behavior. The author recently observed the following example of dependency-enforcing behavior. The patient was sitting in his wheelchair next to his bed. The nurse had just finished shaving the patient. She lifted the patient's comb from his bedside stand, and the patient reached out his hand to take the comb. The nurse did not respond to the patient's gesture and proceeded to comb his hair. In this way, staff actively participate in teaching patients to be "good," when good is defined as passively accepting care ministrations and relinquishing troublesome independent actions in the nursing tasks of bathing, feeding, or grooming. Miller (1985) compared patient outcomes over time on wards that used a traditional task assignment method of delivering care with those that employed individually focused care and encouraged self-care. Her study patients had similar dependency levels on admission. Long-term care patients on traditional wards were more physically dependent, had more communication difficulty, and had information orientation scores lower than their cohorts on self-care wards after 1 year.

Other more subtle ways of increasing or reinforcing dependency involve interacting with patients or residents in a manner that communicates indirectly that they are in a one-down position. One resident in a long-term care setting complained bitterly that two aides talked to each other, "over me, as if I were a sack of potatoes," during her bed bath. She continued angrily, "And as if that isn't bad enough, I have to listen to the details of the porno films they are going to rent for their boyfriends!" The aides, who gave meticulous physical care to this very difficult and demanding patient, were amazed that she even listened, much less remembered what they discussed. They meant no harm, yet by their conversation they communicated to the resident that she was less than a person, reminded her of her own lack of relationships, and offended her sensibilities. Other staff behaviors that place patients in a one-down position of relative helplessness are (1) ascribing to selected patients the role of pet or mascot; (2) criticizing a resident's behavior in front of other residents; (3) encouraging tale-bearing by residents; and (4) arbitrating disputes between residents so that one wins and one loses (Peplau, 1978).

It is one of the economic ironies of our time that units that care for a large number of patients who must be fed, bathed, and wheeled about are often allocated more staff. If nurses are successful in increasing independence in self-care of their institutionalized patients, they may find they lose staff allocation. Patient dependency is not a desired outcome criterion, but it is made legitimate as a criterion for resource allocation. If one accepts that self-care skills must be used to be maintained and that increased dependency is correlated with longer length of stay, higher mortality, and lower discharge rate, it is ethically imperative to alter the method of nursing care delivery to encourage and reward independent rather than dependent functioning.

INDIRECT SELF-DESTRUCTIVE BEHAVIOR

Definition, Examples, and Purpose

Indirect self-destructive behaviors are those that have as their result further illness or injury and the ultimate shortening of life. Nelson and Faberow (1980) studied the indirect self-destructive behavior of nursing home residents. They identified the following behaviors as frequent, problematic to staff, and indirectly self-destructive to the resident: failing to take medications; signing out against medical advice; refusing to get out of bed although able to; abusing alcohol; refusing to eat; and engaging in conflict with staff or other residents. At first glance, these behaviors appear irrational and futile, yet all behaviors have meaning.

Indirect self-destructive behavior may serve the dual purposes of expressing anger and frustration and establishing some control over one's own life. Often the benefits or comfort patients derive from apparently destructive behavior outweigh, in their opinion, the negative effects. Patients may perceive a treatment, intervention, or intended therapeutic interaction as a threat to their well-being and autonomy. If so, they will act to protect themselves by thwarting the perceived threat.

Patients who engage in indirect self-destructive behavior are the bane of every health care service. They frustrate the best efforts to cure disease and promote health. Examples are the patient with chronic obstructive pulmonary disease (COPD) who continues to smoke two packs of cigarettes a day, the diabetic patient who refuses to adhere to a diet and often is brought to the emergency room in diabetic coma, and the patient with bipolar affective disorder who stops taking prescribed lithium, is evicted from housing, and is jailed. No amount of health education seems to break the pattern, and each episode of noncompliance and exacerbation of illness leaves the patient more weakened and debilitated. The following case study illustrates indirect self-destructive behavior.

THE CASE OF IRENE: "CIGARETTES ARE MY ONLY FRIENDS"

Irene, a patient with a long history of chronic schizophrenia in remission and severe COPD, was admitted to a psychiatric service from her residential care home. She was subsequently transferred twice to medical units, when her pO_2 was 42 mm Hg. While she was not psychotic, her intrusiveness, overly demanding behavior, and agitation were worsened by her poor cerebral oxygenation and the anxiety that accompanies respiratory insufficiency. Irene continued to chain-smoke while on the psychiatric ward, and no staff intervention directed at reducing her smoking accomplished more than increasing her agitation.

Irene has led a life characterized by long hospitalizations interspersed with periods of community living in various placements. She stated, "Cigarettes have been my only friends for 40 years. I'm not trying to kill myself, but if I die sooner, so be it." She was also angry at what she perceived to be control and abandonment by others. Her only outside contacts were her elderly sister and conservator and her 96-year-old mother. As Irene's family aged, they became less tolerant of her obstreperous personality.

It takes time and skill to determine the causes for indirect self-destructive behavior and its meaning to the patient. Such patients are antagonistic and difficult. They evoke strong feelings of frustration, guilt, and even disgust in staff who attempt to care for them. The specific problem behaviors become lost in sweeping generalities, such as "he is just an old crock" or "nothing will ever work with her." Staff need to be treated also if the cycle of antagonistic behavior and response is to be broken. They need permission to vent their anger, and they need recognition that they have performed well under adverse circumstances. When staff reach the point of no longer reacting to a patient's behavior and have achieved some detachment, they can be taught to interpret the behavior and plan strategies for intervention.

Successful interventions with Irene were those that did not focus on her smoking directly but, rather, those that addressed the feelings and needs she was communicating with her incessant smoking. She expressed considerable anger at being, as she put it, "shoved, pushed, blood drawn, and hollered at." She felt out of control and threatened by what she perceived as overwhelming demands to cooperate and behave. In addition, Irene was feeling real and anticipatory grief over the loss of her placement and her family. She literally clung to cigarettes as a source of primitive nurture and solace, much as a child clings to a transitional object like a blanket or teddy bear. Irene was allowed to have input into the scheduling of her tests, an intervention that greatly reduced her anxiety. Her nurse case manager from the community was encouraged to maintain a relationship with Irene during her hospitalization, since the nurse represented the only really enduring relationship Irene had. Pending placement, Irene was even allowed to choose her hospital unit, a previously unheard-of accommodation. Interestingly, Irene elected to remain on the medical unit, where "it is harder for me to get smokes and I don't have to go to all those groups where they yell at me for interrupting." At the time of transfer to a new board-and-care home, Irene was smoking less than a half a pack of cigarettes a day and had no further episodes of acute respiratory decompensation.

LABELING

Definition and Impact of Labeling

Labeling is the process of ascribing characteristics and expectations for certain behaviors to a person without regard for objective assessment. The term "label," as it is used here, has a negative connotation. Labels may be added to a certain diagnosis or may take the form of a patient reputation. A diagnosis made with inadequate information may be in itself a label. In one study nurses were presented with case study vignettes in which the only variable was age, either 28 years or 68 years. The nurses were much more likely to diagnose the elderly patient as having organic brain syndrome rather than functional psychosis and to choose nursing home placement over psychotherapy. They also tended to give the elderly patient a much poorer prognosis than the younger cohort, even though symptom presentations were identical (Ciliberto, Levin, & Arluke, 1981). Labels represent real barriers to care and may result in exacerbation of or failure to treat illness. Every patient care service has patient labels that connote a sense of staff frustration and serve as barriers to accurate perceptions of the patient. "Gomers," get out of my emergency room, is used to refer to emergency room repeaters who present with nonemergency, ill-defined complaints. "Druggies," "lungers," "dements," and "vegetables" are some of the more demeaning terms used to label, stereotype, and cast patient roles. The roles that are assigned to these patients are not the sick roles but ones suggesting the patient is hopelessly and possibly deservedly sick. Terms borrowed from the language of psychiatry, "manipulative" or "resistant," have been overused and may also be labels. The following clinical example demonstrates the negative impact of a label on treatment planning.

THE CASE OF SAM

Sam, a 68-year-old inpatient on an acute psychiatric ward, was in the discharge planning phase of treatment. His therapist became frustrated when he repeatedly requested passes to go and look for housing in the city but then failed to keep his appointments with hotel managers. Sam was labeled as "resistant to discharge." The treatment team decided to set a definite discharge date and discharge Sam on that date, regardless of the arrangements he had made for his housing. This was done. Sam was readmitted through the psychiatric emergency service within 48 hours, tired, unkempt, and hungry. The "resistant to discharge" label reemerged and a similar treatment plan was decided on. At this point, Sam's primary nurse did some exploration with Sam, who suffered from severe emphysema as well as paranoid schizophrenia. She learned that because Sam had to stop so often to regain his breath, he was unable to take the bus across town to the hotel, look at a room, and return in the time his passes allowed. On the one occasion he made it all the way to his destination, his respirations were so labored that he was afraid to meet the manager of the residential hotel. "He will think I'm going to kick off at any minute, and he won't rent to me because he'll be afraid of finding a stiff in his room," was how Sam imagined the interview would have gone.

Once the treatment staff could see beyond their label of Sam, they were able to interpret his behavior in a new light. Discharge planning in line with Sam's physical ability was successful. Labels such as "psychiatric patient," "unmotivated," or "demented" may serve as barriers to placement or services. This negative effect can be neutralized if each professional who comes in contact with the patient takes the time to make an objective appraisal of the patient's abilities, needs, and wants, independent of prior judgments.

Certain diagnoses carry with them an intrinsic expectation for poor performance. Schizophrenia, depression, dementia, chronic obstructive pulmonary disease, alcoholism, and peripheral vascular disease are diagnoses to avoid if one wishes to receive impartial care. Clinicians recognize the truth in this statement, but little research has been done to identify stereotypes and lowered expectations linked to specific diagnoses.

INTERVENTIONS TO PREVENT EXCESS DISABILITY

Acute-care Settings

Acute-care settings are highly structured environments with many organizational constraints. The good patient is defined by staff as the one who follows the rules and passively cooperates in all aspects of care. The nurse can help the elderly patient adjust to the hospital setting by determining his or her locus of control and adjusting treatment conditions to take advantage of this belief system (Ciricelli, 1987). The individual with an external locus of control may be better adapted to the hospital environment with its high level of perceived objective constraints than a person with high self-efficacy and a belief in an internal locus of control (Ciricelli, 1987). For the patient with an external locus of control, interventions that foster the formation of an alliance between the patient and a recognized health expert, such as a clinical nurse specialist, will build on the patient's system of belief and may foster cooperation. Those patients whose internal locus of control style interferes with their acceptance of treatment can be helped by interventions that enhance personal uncontrol. Examples of these are teaching me-

diation, supporting the use of prayer, and fostering interpersonal relationships that reveal personal vulnerability (Moch, 1988). Reid's (1984) idea of participatory control achieves a balance between control and uncontrol. When health professionals and patients relate to each other in the framework of participatory control, the patient participates in limited decision-making concerning his or her care and voluntarily delegates authority for some aspects of care and treatment to the professional whose expertise is trusted and acknowledged. Patients who believe that their health care outcomes are governed mainly by chance benefit most from a predictable and consistent environment. In such an environment, patients begin to learn the relationship between behavior and health outcomes. All of these interventions have as their goal increasing and enhancing patient participation in the health care process.

Although most elderly patients are admitted to hospitals because of an acute illness or the exacerbation of a chronic disease, they often also have other chronic illnesses that may or may not be related to the cause of hospitalization but that must be managed. The patient's participation in all aspects of care and treatment is needed to stabilize chronic conditions during acute illness if further disability is to be avoided. Patient participation is defined as knowing what questions to ask and whom to ask, recognizing the relationship between behavior and health outcome, and being willing to learn aspects of care in order to assume responsibility after discharge. Davis (1980) identified structural and organizational features of a rehabilitation ward in an acute-care hospital that she believes facilitate patient participation.

1. Staff-patient interactions that involve the patient and the family in setting realistic short-term goals and reinforcing expectations for patient performance.

2. High visibility among patients and staff, which fosters patients' ongoing learning from both staff and patient role models.

3. An explicitly formulated philosophy of care that emphasizes rehabilitation and deemphasizes focus only on the acute illness.

4. A shift away from the traditional medical model hierarchical structure, so that the physician participates with nurses, occupational therapists, and social workers in decisions about admission, discharge, and treatment.

5. The primary nurse serves as an ideology-bearer, teaching the unit philosophy to all new and temporary staff (Davis, 1980).

Long-term Care Settings

Tobin and Lieberman (1978) studied relatively healthy elderly persons who were on the waiting list for admission to homes for the aged; they studied them again during admission and 1 year after admission. Although many variables were examined, only passivity was not linked to survival; rather, it correlated with increased disability and death. In an expanded longitudinal study of 253 elderly persons entering long-term care facilities, Kahana, Kahana, and Young (1987) concluded that active behavioral coping styles, which included strategies of getting information and doing something definite, were linked to high morale and good cognitive functioning. Affective coping methods, defined as withdrawal, blaming, expressions of anger, and expecting the worst, were linked to low self-esteem, low morale, and poor cognitive functioning (Kahana, Kahana, & Young, 1987).

A perception of control in long-term care settings has been positively linked to improved morale (Ryden, 1984). Individuals with perceived greater choice in the institution and those who spend more time socializing are more satisfied and less lonely (Pohl & Fuller, 1980). Chang (1978) found that the morale for persons in a nursing home with high perceived self-determination regarding their daily activities had better morale than those with low self-determination, regardless of their locus of control belief. The inference can be drawn that control over decisions in long-term care institutions is associated with improved morale and psychological well-being, which is in turn associated with decreased morbidity.

Interventions can be made in health care institutions to increase both the objective ex-

tent of patient control and the subjective perception of control. Chang (1978) devised an assessment instrument, the Situational Control of Daily Activities (SCDA), that nurses can use to measure patients' perception of situational control and to devise a basis for action. Various constraints may prohibit patients from determining how often they bathe and what they eat, but limited choice can be offered. "Do you prefer to eat in bed or in the dining room?" All patient requests can be responded to appropriately if nurses realize that an appropriate response does not have to mean granting the request. For example, one can imagine a patient asking the nurse to be taken to the telephone. Rather than say, "No, I have no one available to take you to the phone now," the nurse can respond, "I know going to the phone is important to you. I can't take you right now, but let's make a point to go at the start of the next shift. Why don't you remind me at 3 p.m." This response acknowledges the need and puts a demand on the patient for active participation in getting needs met. Even within the constraints of the sick role, it endows the patient with potency and responsibility.

Nurses in leadership roles in institutions of long-term and acute care occupy a prime position in teaching the effects of interactions on the behavior and self-concept of residents. To do this effectively, nurses must remain gentle and nonjudgmental. It is one thing to examine one's interactions with patients when occupying the role of expert. It is quite another to be cognizant of overt and unconscious communications while attempting to bathe, medicate, or toilet many residents in a given period of time, which is never quite long enough. Ryden (1985) found that while caregivers preferred more resident control, they wanted to maintain a considerable share of the decision-making concerning daily activities, such as feeding and grooming. Staff attitudes about the extent of control allowed to residents should be explored before staff behavior can be influenced and changed. In order to examine their interactions, staff need to feel safe and have a time to ventilate their own frustrations, fears, and concerns. Nurses in leadership roles need to openly acknowledge that staff irritability and insensitivity may be a result of unrealistic performance expectations, and they must be willing to examine those expectations. It is important to recognize that provocative and demeaning patient behavior plays a role in evoking hostile or avoidant staff response. If the nursing leader can be objective and neutral, the patterns of maladaptive interactions with the cycles of dependency-inducing responses and increased patient helplessness can be identified and changed.

Strategies that facilitate this process are those that increase each person's awareness of how his or her behavior is perceived by others. Some methods are staff role-playing, videotaping or films with discussion, and staff support groups. One of the most effective ways of changing patterns of interactions is to meet with select staff and residents and assume the role of interpreter and facilitator to clarify misperceptions and help people see how their behavior is interpreted by others. As this is done, the nurse in a leadership role can observe actual interactions and identify the patterns as they occur. Nurses in leadership roles can work to make staff goals (that is, pleasant and less stressful patient care) congruent with patient goals (that is, respectful care with maximal personal control).

SUMMARY

Excess disability can be prevented when the elderly individual is encouraged to participate in his or her own care and when interpersonal and organizational factors serve to increase and maintain the elderly person's control over daily activities. People may practice independent self-care through acting on their own motivations or from compliance with external authority figures (Riesch & Hauck, 1988). This chapter has illustrated strategies for enhancing self-worth and perceived control in different settings. The debilitating effects of the sick role and learned helplessness can be mitigated by those interventions that teach and foster self-care and decrease dependence for patients of any age, regardless of diagnosis.

References

Baltes, MM, Hohn, S, Barton, E, et al. (1983): On the social ecology of dependence and independence in elderly nursing home residents, a replication and extension. *J Gerontol, 38*:556–564.

Baltes, MM, & Skinner, EH (1983): Cognitive performance deficits and hospitalization: Learned helplessness, instrumental passivity or what? *J Pers Soc Psychol, 45*:1013–1016.

Bandura, A (1982): Self efficacy in human agency. *Am Psychol, 37*:122–147.

Barusch, A (1988): Problems and coping strategies of elderly spouse caregivers. *Gerontologist, 28*:677–683.

Bieliauskas, L (1983): *The Influence of Individual Differences in Health and Illness.* Boulder, CO, Westview Press.

Blumer, H (1969): *Symbolic Interactionism.* Englewood Cliffs, NJ, Prentice-Hall.

Brody, E, Kleban, M, Lawton, M, et al. (1974): A longitudinal look at excess disabilities in the mentally impaired aged. *J Gerontol, 29*(1):79–84.

Brody, E, Kleban, M, Powell, M, et al. (1971): Excess disabilities of mentally impaired aged: Impact of individualized treatment. *Gerontologist, 2*(1):124–133.

Brown, JS, & Rawlinson, ME (1979): Sick role acceptance measure. *In Psychosocial Instruments,* Vol. 1. New York, American Psychological Association, 212–215.

Campbell, J (1986): Changes in levels of dependency and predictors of mortality in elderly people in institutional care in Dunedin. *N Zeal Med J, 99*:507–509.

Chang, B (1978): Perceived situational control of daily activities: A new tool. *Res Nurs Health, 1*:181–188.

Ciliberto, D, Levin, J, & Arluke, A (1981): Nurses' diagnostic stereotyping of the elderly. *Res Aging, 3*:299–310.

Ciricelli, V (1987): Locus of control and patient role adjustments of the elderly in acute care hospitals. *Psychol Aging, 2*:138–143.

Davis, M (1980): The organizational, interactional and care oriented conditions for patient participation in continuity of care: A framework for staff interventions. *Soc Sci Med, 14A*:39–47.

Dawson, P, Kline, K, Crinklaw, DC, et al. (1986): Preventing excess disability in patients with Alzheimer's disease. *Geriatr Nurs, 7*(6):298–301.

DeVellis, F, DeVellis, BM, & McCauley, M (1978): Vicarious acquisition of learned helplessness. *J Pers Soc Psychol, 36*:894–899.

Kahana, E, Kahana, B, & Young, R (1987): Strategies of coping and postinstitutional outcomes. *Res Aging, 9*:182–197.

Kahn, RS (1965): Comments. *In Proceedings of the York House Institute on the Mentally Impaired Aged.* Philadelphia, Philadelphia Geriatric Center.

Langer, EJ, & Benevento, A (1968): Self induced dependence. *J Pers Soc Psychol, 36*:886–893.

Lefcourt, H (1976): *Locus of Control: Current Trends in Theory and Research.* New York, John Wiley & Sons.

Mermelstein, RJ, & Lopez, MA (November, 1985): Psychological complaints and problems as predictors of outcome on a geriatric physical rehabilitation unit. Paper presented at the 38th Annual Scientific Meeting of the Gerontological Society of America, New Orleans.

Miller, A (1985): Nurse-patient dependency: Is it iatrogenic? *J Adv Nurs*, 10:63–69.

Moch, S (1988): Towards a personal control/uncontrol balance. *J Adv Nurs*, 13:119–123.

Nelson, EF, & Faberow, R (1980): Indirect self destructive behavior in nursing home residents. *J Gerontol*, 35:362–370.

Nuttbrock, L (1986): Socialization to the chronic sick role in later life: An interactionist view. *Res Aging*, 8:368–387.

Peplau, H (1978): Psychiatric nursing: Role of nurses and psychiatric nurses. *Int Nurs Rev*, 25:41–47.

Pfeiffer, J (1986): Listening for emotions. *Science 86*, 7:14–16.

Pohl, J, & Fuller, S (1980): Perceived choice, social interaction and dimensions of morale of residents in a home for the aged. *Res Nurs Health*, 3(3):147–157.

Reid, D (1984): Participatory control and chronic illness adjustment process. *In* Lefcourt, HM (ed): *Research with the Locus of Control Construct: Vol. 3, Extensions and Limitations*. Orlando, FL, Academic Press, 361–389.

Riesch, S, & Hauck, M (1988): The exercise of self care agency: An analysis of construct and discrimination validity. *Res Nurs Health*, 11(4):245–255.

Rosow, I (1973): The social context of the aging self. *Gerontologist*, 13:82–87.

Ryden, M (1984): Morale and perceived control in institutionalized elderly. *Nurs Res*, 33:130–138.

Ryden, M (1985): Environmental support for autonomy in the institutionalized elderly. *Res Nurs Health*, 8(2):363–371.

Seeman, M, & Seeman, T (1983): Health behavior and personal autonomy: A longitudinal study of the sense of control in illness. *J Health Soc Behav*, 24(2):144–159.

Seligman, M (1975): *Helplessness: On Depression, Development and Death*. San Francisco, WH Freeman.

Smith, R, Wallston, B, Forsberg, P, et al. (1984): Measuring desire for control of health care processes. *J Pers Soc Psychol*, 47(2):415–426.

Solomon, K (1982): The social antecedents of learned helplessness in the health care setting. *Gerontologist*, 22:282–287.

Thomas, WC (1981): The expectation gap and the stereotype of the stereotype: Images of old people. *Gerontologist*, 21:402–407.

Tobin, S, & Lieberman, M (1978): *Last Home for the Aged*. San Francisco, Jossey-Bass.

Woodward, N, & Wallston, B (1987): Age and health care beliefs, self efficacy as a mediator of low desire for control. *Psychol Aging*, 2(1):3–8.

CHAPTER
21

Managing Behavioral Problems

SALLY A. SALISBURY, R.N.C.S., M.S.
JOYCE TAKANO STONE, R.N.C., M.S.

DEFINITION OF A BEHAVIORAL PROBLEM

This chapter addresses the nursing management of behavioral problems of the elderly client. A behavioral problem is defined as a recurring behavior that is deviant from that which is commonly regarded as acceptable by societal norms. These behaviors, while not of the same clinical significance as acute illness or medical diagnostic problems, are a source of consternation and distress to family caregivers and professional health care providers. Their management (or nonmanagement) may have serious financial, legal, and medical consequences for the individual performing the behavior.

Specific behavioral problems addressed in this chapter are:

1. Demanding
2. Wandering
3. Repetitious, annoying, persistent behaviors
4. Resistance to physical care
5. Nocturnal restlessness
6. Paranoid and suspicious behavior
7. Assaultive behavior
8. Inappropriate sexual behavior

These behaviors will be defined and their etiology discussed. Specific behavioral management strategies will be presented for each of the behaviors, which may be applied in home or institutional settings.

THE PROCESS OF BEHAVIORAL MANAGEMENT

Behavioral management, as the term is used here, means a systematic series of observations

403

of human behavior, analysis and interpretation of observations, and planning and implementing of interventions that have as their goal a discernible behavioral change. The process of behavioral management may be applied in any situation in which disturbed behavior occurs. When a person exhibits positive change and his or her responses to the behavior become more predictable and consistent, that person perceives an increased sense of self-efficacy and self-worth. The process of behavioral management is summarized in Table 21–1.

Behavioral management is often more effective than medications in producing desired change. It may be used alone or in conjunction with medications. A detailed discussion on the use of psychotropic medications for behavioral management is beyond the scope of this chapter, but a summary table (Table 21–2) is provided to identify specific behavioral problems where medications are of demonstrated value, including the type and dose of medication. Table 21–3 provides a list of terms used in behavioral management and their definitions.

Defining the Problem

An elderly patient with a problem behavior is not usually the one seeking help with behavioral management. Family, friends, or staff

Table 21–1. THE PROCESS OF BEHAVIORAL MANAGEMENT

1. **Definition of the problem**
   A. Who is the person with the problematic behavior?
   B. What is the behavior?
   C. What does the behavior mean?
   D. Where does the behavior occur?
   E. Who are the significant others involved?
   F. What is the time and frequency of the behavior?
   G. What is the pattern and sequence of the behavior and the events that precede it?
   H. What is the usual outcome of the behavior?
2. **What is the desired change?**
   A. Change the meaning of the behavior.
   B. Change the response to the behavior.
   C. Change the specific behavior itself.
3. **Determine the type of intervention strategy that will be appropriate and effective.**

are the ones who bring their concerns to the gerontological nurse. Consequently, the first information one hears about the "problem" is someone else's perception of it. The first step in the process of behavioral management, therefore, is to determine if a problem exists and, if so, whose problem it is. Is the behavior itself problematic? Is it a recurring behavior that is deviant from that which is commonly regarded as acceptable by societal norms?

Mrs. B was brought to the Alzheimer's Center for an evaluation of her cognitive deficits by her distraught daughter, Jane. Three months prior to the evaluation, Jane had insisted Mrs. B give up her own apartment and move in with Jane and Jane's adolescent daughter because, as Jane stated, "Mother just cannot be trusted alone." Although Mrs. B did in fact have mild global cognitive deficits, a functional assessment done with her in her recently vacated apartment determined that she was able to perform all the activities of daily living, as well as instrumental activities of daily living necessary to stay safely alone. When this was explained to Jane, she exclaimed, "How can you say that? Just today she took two baths and she needs me to balance her checkbook!" In an aside to the nurse who did the assessment, Mrs. B said, "Jane always had a perfect mother who could do everything, and she can't forgive me a little forgetfulness." Mrs. B was subsequently returned to her apartment with arrangements for an in-home care worker three times a week, and Jane was referred for counseling, which she accepted.

Mrs. B's "problem" existed not in her behavior, but in the meaning her forgetful behavior had for her daughter. In this case, the proper intervention was to change the way the daughter responded to the behavior, not the behavior itself. The remainder of this section deals with only those situations in which the behavior of the identified patient itself is the focus of the intervention.

Who Is the Person with the Problematic Behavior? To gain an understanding of the problem, once it has been determined that a problem exists, something must be known about the person performing the behavior. Other chapters in this text (see Chapters 3 to 7) provide detailed guidelines for comprehen-

Table 21–2. PHARMACOLOGIC INTERVENTION IN BEHAVIORAL MANAGEMENT

Behavior	Drug	Dose Range	Adverse Effects and Special Precautions
Mild to moderate agitation	Mild tranquilizers— anxiolytics Short-acting benzodiazepines		May cause paradoxic behavioral actions such as increased confusion and agitation
	alprazolam (Xanax)	0.75 to 1.5 mg/day	Accumulates with repeated doses, but less likely with short-acting benzodiazepines
	lorazepam (Ativan)	0.5 to 2 mg/day	Oversedation, ataxia, lightheadedness, confusion, vertigo
	oxazepam (Serax)	10 mg 3 times/day	Avoid alcohol, sedatives, narcotics, hypnotics
			Slowly taper to discontinue. Withdrawal reactions may occur when drugs are suddenly discontinued
			Psychological dependence may develop with long-term use
	buspirone (BuSpar)	5 to 10 mg 1 to 3 times/ day	7- to 10-day lag period before therapeutic effects seen
			Full effect may not be seen for several months
Wandering	Low-dose neuroleptics haloperidol (Haldol)	0.25 to 2 mg/day	Low sedative effect High extrapyramidal effect
	thioridazine (Mellaril)	10 to 25 mg 2 to 3 times/day	High sedative effect Orthostatic hypotension Low extrapyramidal effect Anticholinergic effect
Nocturnal restlessness	chloral hydrate (Noctec)	500 mg to 1.0 gm HS	Gastric irritation, lightheadedness, ataxia Relatively potent displacer of acidic drugs such as warfarin and phenytoin from plasma proteins; may cause sudden increase in concentration of these drugs
	diphenhydramine (Benadryl)	25 to 50 mg HS	Anticholinergic effect
	Short-acting hypnotics		Avoid alcohol, narcotics, tranquilizers, barbiturates, antidepressants, and other medications for sleep
	triazolam (Halcion)	0.125 mg HS	Short half-life; may lead to rebound insomnia
	temazepam (Restoril)	15 mg HS	Half-life of 5 to 15 hours; needs to be administered 1 to 2 hours before bedtime to ensure sedation Causes rebound insomnia if withdrawn abruptly May lose clinical effect after 20 to 30 days of continued use

Table continued on following page

sive assessment. In this context, information is gathered about the following:

1. Name, age, sex, place of residence
2. Significant active medical and psychiatric problems
3. Functional and cognitive ability
4. The person's understanding of the situation that others have defined as a problem

This information is best obtained from the patient, and can be learned in a private, 15-minute informal interview as part of a physical assessment in the home or at the bedside.

What Is the Behavior? Behavior refers to any observable action or sequence of actions. It does not refer to a description or interpretation. Behaviors are always stated as verbs. Whenever possible, the professional should

Table 21–2. PHARMACOLOGIC INTERVENTION IN BEHAVIORAL MANAGEMENT *Continued*

Behavior	Drug	Dose Range	Adverse Effects and Special Precautions
Severe agitation, assaultive			
Due to high anxiety without thought disorder	Anxiolytics Short-acting benzodiazepines		See under Mild to moderate agitation, above
With thought disorder, hallucinations, delusions	Major tranquilizers— neuroleptics, antipsychotics		
	thioridazine (Mellaril)	10 to 25 mg 2 to 3 times/day	Sedating Orthostatic hypotension Anticholinergic effects High incidence of cardiotoxicity
Paranoia	chlorpromazine (Thorazine)	10 to 25 mg 2 to 3 times/day	Highly sedating High degree of anticholinergic properties Hypotension
Inappropriate sexual behavior	loxapine (Loxitane)	5 to 100 mg/day	Moderate sedation, anticholinergic, and extrapyramidal effects
	propranolol (Inderal)	30 to 320 mg/day	Hypotension, bradycardia, depression
	haloperidol (Haldol)	0.25 to 6 mg/day	High incidence of extrapyramidal symptoms Negligible cardiovascular side effects
	fluphenazine (Prolixin)	0.5 to 2 mg/day	Extrapyramidal symptoms
	trazodone	50 mg 1 to 4 times/day	Gastric discomfort; should be taken with food rather than on an empty stomach

Data from Kane, Ouslander, & Abrass, 1984; Friesen, 1983; Jenike, 1988; Risse & Barnes, 1986; Salzman, 1985, 1987, 1988; Thompson, Moran, & Nies, 1983a, 1983b; U'Ren, 1984.

observe the behavior. If this is not feasible, questions to a caregiver should elicit specific behavioral definitions. A nursing assistant's complaint of "she is just a mean, ungrateful person," should be stated specifically, perhaps as "she calls out 'help me, help me' repeatedly every few minutes. This happens when she is tied in her wheelchair in the late afternoon and when she wakes up at night."

What Does the Behavior Mean to the Individual? In the course of one evening shift in an acute-care unit, two elderly male patients may be apprehended attempting to leave the unit. One patient may be deliberately trying to leave the hospital and return to his hotel because he believes that further treatment will only cause him further discomfort and bring him no gains. The other may be confused and think that he has to get home and do his milking, even though he has not lived on a farm for 20 years. Thus, the observed behavior can have different meanings to those performing it. The meaning of the behavior can seldom be accurately inferred without exploration and assessment.

Where Does the Behavior Occur? As an aging person gradually becomes less competent, dependency on the physical and social environment is greater and he or she becomes more vulnerable to demands and limitations of the environment (Lawton, 1970). In the context of managing behavioral problems, any possible relationship between the behavior and the environment must be explored. Is the behavior environmentally determined, that is, does it occur in one place only? If the patient is confined to an institution, does the disordered behavior relate to any specific environmental event? When studying violent behavior, Jones (1985) found that 28% of all incidents occurred during periods of high activity, between 9:00 and 10:00 a.m., when baths, treatments, and medication dispensing were all in progress. Are the behavioral norms and expectations of the setting congruent with the patient's ability and functional level? The problem behavior in a retirement community may not be a problem in a board-and-care home, where more supervision is provided and less is expected of the resident. In some

Table 21–3. DEFINITION OF TERMS USED IN BEHAVIORAL MANAGEMENT

Reinforcement. A reinforcement is the sequential response to a behavior. Positive reinforcement is the application of a pleasant stimulus following a behavior. An example would be rewarding a patient with praise and attention for independently completing a hygiene task.

Noncontingent Reinforcement. A noncontingent reinforcer is one that is a random and unpredictable response to a behavior that is experienced as unrelated to the behavior and beyond the control of the person performing the behavior (Seligman, 1975).

Shaping. Shaping involves selecting intermediate goals that approximate the desired behavior and positively reinforce them. For example, if the goal is to maintain as much independence as possible in areas of activities of daily living, behaviors that approximate self-care are positively reinforced, even if they fall short of optimal performance.

Reward/punishment. Positive reinforcements serve as rewards for desired behavior. The concept of punishment is a difficult one for nurses to accept; punishment seems antithetical to nurses and their work. Punishment, in this context, means the withdrawal of positive reinforcers. This technique has proved to be an effective means of managing behavior that is harmful to misbehaving patients and seriously infringes on the well-being of others. If combined with methods that foster constructive alternatives, this form of behavioral management can produce enduring changes in social behavior (Bandura, 1969). The form of punishment most accepted is "time out." In using time out, the patient is removed to a quiet room and, if it can be done safely, left alone for a specific length of time. This is done each time the patient performs the deleterious behavior. The patient is informed of the plan in advance. If such patients cannot be safely left alone, staff are assigned to sit with them, but not to speak to them or provide any stimulation. Other forms of punishment may be withholding pleasant activities, such as television or snacks.

Extinction. Extinction, as used here, refers to the technique of avoiding reinforcement of a behavior by showing no response at all, that is, by simply ignoring the behavior.

---

cases, changing the environment is a more humane and effective intervention than attempting to bring behavior in line with a setting.

Who Are the Significant Others Involved? Does the behavioral problem occur regardless of who is present and interacting with the patient, or is it manifested only when the patient interacts with some persons and never with others? This is a critical question. The elderly patient may have active racial prejudices or age biases that make it difficult for him or her to accept help from some and not from others. In the interest of expediency, it may be more pragmatic to note and accommodate these factors, rather than to embark on a reeducation process.

Some family members have a history of conflict, or unresolved issues, that interferes with effective caregiving and precipitates disturbed behavior. The chapter, Social Support of the Older Client, elaborates on the relationship between elderly and their caregivers. Just as the clinician can intervene by changing the environment, interventions can be aimed at changing the designated caregiver, rather than dealing with deep-seated interpersonal issues. The decision is guided by factors such as time, resources, urgency, and probability of success.

In some families, long-standing patterns of relating according to mutually accepted family roles interfere with the members' ability to care for the impaired elder. Professional health care staff who work with adult children of cognitively impaired elders are often struck by the way in which children seem immobilized in situations that call for action. If mother insists that she does not want or need help, children often stand by helplessly, while mother, who lives alone, continues to drive at her peril, goes without adequate food, and neglects to pay her bills. In these instances, interventions are directed at the children. They are helped and supported in giving up outdated, inappropriate roles and assuming new ones—those of responsible decision-making adults. The behavioral problem of resistance to care is managed indirectly by changing the response of significant others in the environment.

What Is the Time and Frequency of the Behavior? When and how often the behavior occurs may determine the severity of the problem. A patient who has nocturnal restlessness every night and keeps his spouse awake obviously is more of a problem than someone who occasionally awakens at night. For caregivers, any behavioral problem is more significant if it occurs at night. Behavioral problems that are continuous or frequent are more problematic than those that rarely occur.

What Are the Pattern and Sequence of the Behavior and the Events That Precede It? Can a definite precipitant be established for the behavior? If so, interventions can be anticipatory, with staff or family placed in a proactive position rather than a reactive one. Does the behavior follow a pattern and established sequence? If so, interventions may be chosen to interrupt the pattern or accommodate it. The care plan for wandering is an example of an intervention based on a known pattern or sequence. Not all behavioral problems fall into such clear delineations, however. Observations of the patient over time and history-taking from the patient and caretakers may reveal more obscure behavior patterns that can then be addressed. The following is an example:

Mr. L, who lived in a single room occupancy hotel, became more inappropriate in his dress and slovenly toward the end of every month. He also appeared confused at these times, a situation that was brought to the attention of his county case manager by the hotel operator. By the third week of every month, Mr. L's finances were depleted and he subsisted on gleanings from trash cans and panhandling. His malnourishment was contributing to his confusion and disorganization. The case manager took a more active role in managing the distribution of funds, spreading them over time, and the problem was resolved.

What Is the Usual Outcome of the Behavior? All behavior has meaning and purpose, although these may not be readily apparent. A part of any behavioral analysis is observing the behavior over time and noting the responses that tend to maintain it (Prehn, 1982). The consequences of behavior provide the patient with some gratification of needs or accomplishment of goals, which in turn maintains the behavior.

An analysis of a behavioral problem involves identifying the person with the behavior and knowing where, how often, and with whom the behavior occurs. Over time, the problem is studied to ascertain any consistent triggering events or interactions and the responses that follow. In applying this methodology it is ascertained first whether, in fact, there is a problem, and if so, whose it is, and what is the severity and risk involved.

Determining the Desired Change

Change the Meaning of the Behavior. Behavior does not occur in a vacuum. All behavior has meaning. The meaning of behavior is derived from people's perceptions of it. There are times when it may not be possible to change the behavior itself; then intervention focuses on changing people's perceptions of the behavior, which changes its meaning and significance. An example follows:

An aging spouse caring for a patient with Alzheimer's disease described his wife's behavior in the following way: "I do everything; all the cleaning, cooking, shopping, gardening. Then when the children come over she tells them how tired she is from all the housework and laundry she did all day. She doesn't appreciate anything I do for her; she lies about who does what and makes me look lazy, like I'm mean to her." The caregiver was taught to understand the extent of his wife's cognitive deficits and how these were manifested in behavior. He came to understand that her "lying" was an attempt on her part to deny her illness and save face with others. He became tolerant of her distortions of their household routine and no longer felt badly when she described her workload.

The meaning of this patient's behavior was changed from one of negating him to one of attempting to salvage her self-esteem.

Change the Response to the Behavior. This is related to and follows naturally from changing the meaning of the behavior. When the behavior is understood in a new light by others, their response to it will be different. In the above example, the caretaker no longer angrily disputed his wife's statements in front of their children, but replied instead, "Yes, your mother is a wonderful housekeeper. I don't know what I'd do without her."

Change a Specific Behavior. This intervention identifies and targets a specific behavior and eliminates or modifies it. The method by which this is done may deal only with the behavior or with the behavior and the cognitive processes that accompany it.

INTERVENTION STRATEGIES FOR SPECIFIC BEHAVIORAL PROBLEMS

The selection of the intervention depends on the information obtained in the assessment phases of behavioral management. An intervention must be appropriate to the cognitive and functional ability of the patient and the setting in which he or she lives. Its aim must be realistic in terms of the behavior itself, the place where it occurs, and the people whom it affects. Any intervention should be made with flexibility, with an understanding that failure is possible. This attitude allows for objective evaluation of the results and a willingness to move on and try something else, without experiencing needless self-criticism and feelings of failure on the part of the manager.

Demanding

Sometimes, sadly, those who need the care of others are unable to accept it gracefully. Those who are dependent and yet demanding, overcritical, and controlling in their interactions with caregivers interfere with the process of caregiving and may exacerbate their existing health problems.

Definition. Specific behaviors associated with the patient classified as demanding are:

1. Refusing to accept assistance
2. Being mean, cantankerous, obstreperous
3. Complaining excessively about medical, social, or material needs, along with resistance and failure to cooperate with corrective interventions
4. Lacking appreciation for what is done
5. Exhibiting occasionally hostile behavior, screaming or striking out at those who are attempting to provide care

6. Engaging in spiteful acts such as soiling right after toileting (Verwoerdt, 1981)

Etiology. Older people who all their lives survived and succeeded by trusting only themselves may be unable to surrender control of their lives to others and adapt to dependency. These people carry with them a lifetime of disappointment (real or imagined) in others and a belief that no one really cares for them or is worthy of their trust. At the same time, they are burdened by a reservoir of unmet dependency needs, covered with a veneer of hostility that hardens and thickens with age. Thus, they deny and by their behavior repel the kind of response from others that they most crave and need, and they deny to themselves and to others that these needs exist at all.

Behavior—Complaining. Excessive complaining about any care is given. The patient shows a lack of appreciation for any effort on the part of caretakers.

Possible Causes. These include an inability to accept a dependent role or intense ambivalence about being in a dependent position. Anger, frustration, and resentment may be the dominant emotions governing behavior.

Intervention. Accept that nothing will be good enough; resist attempts to try and do "the right thing the right way." Explore the feelings underlying the behavior. Support staff or family caretakers in being nonreactive, detached, but supportive. A behavioral program may be instituted in which the complaining is not reinforced and more acceptable methods of communicating are shaped.

Behavior—Spiteful Acts. The patient may engage in spiteful acts, soiling just after being put to bed or dumping food trays.

Possible Causes. The patient may be trying to maintain control over the environment and salvage a sense of self; he or she may be feeling overwhelmed and out of control.

Intervention. Provide caregivers with an outlet for their anger away from the patient. In a nonreactive way, simply correct the situation without comment, e.g., change the bed, get a new tray. Set up a program that rewards refraining from spiteful acts, such as an extra dessert tray if the meal tray is not spilled or extra staff time if the bed remains dry for 30 minutes after the patient is put to bed, for example.

Behavior—Resistance to Care. The patient may vociferously refuse all assistance and may threaten or verbally abuse potential helpers.

Possible Causes. These are the same as for spiteful acts, above.

Intervention. Approach the patient quietly, without making a demand. Elicit the patient's perception of the situation. Negotiate a system for care with the active participation of the patient. Adhere to it, and ensure that others do so also.

Wandering

Wandering is a serious problem, often resulting in dangerous consequences for the wanderer. Wandering behavior may be the reason families decide they can no longer care for the older person at home, and it is often the reason for nonacceptance by nursing homes, day health centers, and respite programs. This behavior is generally associated with dementing illness.

Definition. Wandering is defined as the tendency "to move about, either in a seemingly aimless or disoriented fashion, or in pursuit of an indefinable or untouchable goal" (Snyder, Rupprecht, Pyrek, et al., 1978).

Etiology. In studies comparing wanderers to nonwanderers, wanderers scored lower on mental status tests, had deficits in recent and remote memory and orientation, and had less ability to communicate appropriately (Snyder, et al., 1978; Hussian, 1981). Monsour and Robb (1982) found that wanderers tended to show more motor behavior than nonwanderers when experiencing stress and that they had previously been very active with social and leisure activities. Hussian (1981) noted a direct relationship between time spent in restraints and time spent wandering. Wandering decreased when periods of free ambulation were allowed.

Some wandering is thought to be a response to boredom (Burnside, 1980). The wanderer may be in pursuit of some stimulation, and other self-stimulating behaviors such as rattling door knobs, rocking, and touching walls and furniture may be observed in conjunction with the wandering. Wandering away from an unfamiliar place, such as a hospital or adult day health center, may be due to fear of an unfamiliar place and a desire to return home. Wandering away may also be the older person's attempt to get to someplace else, which may be a place that no longer exists except in memory, or a patient may forget where he or she is attempting to go. In the cognitively impaired patient wandering may be an attempt to recapture old situations that are associated with feelings of safety and belonging (Rader, Doan, & Schwab, 1985).

Behavior—Pacing. Pacing, usually in a repetitive predictable pattern, may occur at times of confusion, heightened noise in the environment, or at predictable times of the day. The patient may perform other self-stimulating actions, such as rattling door knobs or rubbing furniture.

Possible Causes. The demented patient may be bored and engaging in self-stimulation or may be using gross motor activity to deal with feelings of restlessness, tension, or anxiety.

Intervention. Map the route of the wandering to be sure that it is hazard-free. Place barriers at exits to contain the behavior. These may be doors with latches in unusual places, such as at the top or bottom of the door, gates with latches on the outside, or stop signs. Place articles to catch interest along the route, tables with objects to handle, snacks, rocking chairs with wide bases. If the wandering results from overstimulation, try to provide a quiet room or outdoor space. Determine if the patient is hungry or needs toileting.

Behavior—Inappropriate Destination. The patient will appear determined but bewildered. He or she may try to leave home or the treatment setting and may become combative if intercepted. The patient may verbalize a goal that is inappropriate to the present situation; for example, a 96-year-old woman may state she must get home to take care of her babies. This behavior may occur at predictable times, such as at early evening or just after a visit from the patient's family.

Possible Causes. The patient may be disoriented and confused. He may be trying to reach a place he associates with comfort and security to ease feelings of loneliness, abandonment, or fear. The place he wants to find may no longer exist or may not be reachable.

Intervention. Try to interpret the feeling behind the behavior. Attempt to have the patient verbalize this feeling. Gently provide reassurance and reality feedback. Offer substitute gratification by providing interpersonal contact, empathy, and environmental niceties, such as soft music or a warm nourishing snack. If possible, anticipate patterns and provide gratification before wandering begins. (For example, one man arranged to leave work early so that he could be home with his demented wife at the time their children used to return home from school.) Alert all staff to the patient's potential for leaving; be sure that doors are fastened. If the patient is in the home, alert neighbors or the local police, and provide them with a description or photograph of the patient and the name and address of the caretaker. If the patient is out in the street and will not willingly return, walk along with him until he can be led back, or stay with him and summon help.

Behavior—Escape Attempts. The patient may make a determined attempt to leave the treatment setting or the home of a relative and may threaten to become violent if physically restrained.

Possible Causes. The patient may not be confused or disoriented but may be simply trying to leave a situation he or she finds unfamiliar and return home or to another more acceptable place. The patient may show impaired judgment in that his or her plans are contrary to health and well-being.

Intervention. As above, be sure that exits are secured. Attempt to dissuade the patient from leaving. Empathize with the patient's plight and try to establish an agreement to stay for a defined period of time, such as until the physician arrives or until morning. Assess whether the patient legally can be held against his or her will. Bargain.

Repetitious, Annoying, Persistent Behaviors

Although the behaviors in this category are relatively benign and threaten little danger for the patient and caregivers, they are extremely problematic because of the irritation and frustration they engender in caregivers.

Definition. Repetitious, annoying, persistent behaviors as defined here are those that (1) appear to serve no functional purpose; (2) disrupt the environment; (3) interfere with normal communication in the family or institution; (4) occur continuously; (5) require a verbal or behavioral response from the caregiver; (6) disturb the order of things, wherein the patient is piling, moving, or rearranging objects in an irrational, untidy way.

Etiology. These behaviors are commonly associated with middle and late stage Alzheimer's disease. Speculations as to the underlying motivation for them are included below. The same behaviors infrequently occur in geriatric patients with long-standing chronic mental illness. In these instances, they may be a manifestation of agitation or motor restlessness. In both cases, the patient is suffering from diminished capacity to interact appropriately with others or to plan and implement goal-directed action. The interventions described, therefore, are appropriately uncomplicated.

Behavior—Questioning. The patient asks the same question over and over.

Possible Causes. The patient may be needing information but may have a recent memory loss that prevents remembering or retrieving the information given.

Intervention. Simply give the information. If the patient is cognitively able to use them, provide memory aids such as notes, signs pasted on doors, clocks, or calendars. (Be sure that if notes are used they are kept current and accurate.) Digital clocks that give the day, date, and time are effective because they do not require problem-solving skills.

Behavior—Repeating Content. The patient repeats a few phrases endlessly.

Possible Causes. The patient may be seeking contact and conversation but may have lost the skills necessary for conversation.

Intervention. Provide conversation or verbal input that places few demands on the patient, such as a running monologue of what you are doing. Offer verbal and nonverbal messages that the patient is included in group conversations.

Behavior—Redoing Tasks. The patient may perform a task correctly but repetitiously, such as ironing the same clothes over and over or watering a plant repeatedly.

Possible Causes. The patient may be bored and restless. The patient may believe that he or she is supposed to be busy doing something but may have forgotten how to do it or what is to be done. The behavior may be an attempt to accomplish a task that was formerly a part of the patient's routine or an attempt by the patient to establish order and control of the situation.

Intervention. Coach the caregiver to permit and tolerate this behavior by defining it as the patient's attempt to remain the same contributing member of the household.

Behavior—Disrupting Objects. The patient may take objects in the house and disrupt them in a bizarre way, such as moving all clothes onto the dining room table, piling books on the floor, or hiding objects in peculiar places.

Possible Causes. These are the same as for redoing tasks, above.

Intervention. Substitute a repetitious, nonannoying activity, such as the sorting of cards and beads or folding and refolding clothes. Try media distractors that are appropriate for the patient's cognitive level for severely impaired persons. Videotapes of "Sesame Street," "Mr. Rogers," or musical movies have been successful. Include the patient in chores without putting demands for task performance on him. Allow the patient to wash dishes or make salad, even if the task must be done over by the caretaker. Put away any important or unnecessary objects, or lock drawers or closets that should not be disturbed. One wife caretaker of a former attorney with late stage Alzheimer's disease provided him with a desk

and typewriter but kept the bills and papers in a separate locked desk.

Behavior—Trailing Caregiver. The patient may constantly follow the caregiver, either at home or in an institution.

Possible Causes. The patient may be insecure and afraid of being lost or abandoned.

Intervention. The above interventions may be successful. In addition, try to structure the environment so that the patient is always in eye contact with the caretaker. Place seats around the nurses' station in institutions. At home, dutch or screen doors at the kitchen or den may allow the caregiver to work and still allow the patient to feel he or she is not alone. A special chair for the patient in the kitchen or den may accomplish the same. If dealing with a family caregiver, plan for respite from constant vigilance by using inhome attendants, sitters, or respite care.

Resistance to Physical Care

Definition. Resistance to physical care, as the term is used here, refers to patient behaviors that impede the accomplishment of self-care tasks necessary for the maintenance of health and prevention of opportunistic secondary disease. By some action, the patient resists bathing, changing, and eating, and by resistance incurs a real physical risk. Caution is needed to accurately assess the degree of risk before labeling this resistance a behavioral problem. One patient who was identified by her children's family, her caretakers, as being resistant to bathing was, in fact, adhering to her lifelong habit of a once-weekly bath and shampoo after her illness forced her move to her daughter's home. Her son-in-law took strong exception to this, saying, "In this house we all shower every night."

Etiology. Patients in the advanced stages of dementing illness may be confused and frightened by the physical objects and activity that accompany bathing. Since they no longer remember what bathing is, they often are frightened of water, of their own reflection in the mirror, or of being asked to disrobe. They may misinterpret the objectives of staff or family, particularly if the person attempting care is of the opposite sex.

Patients who are severely, clinically depressed lack the initiative and energy to engage in a task that to them is futile. In addition, their passive noncompliance with hygiene and nutritional tasks frustrates and worries both staff and families. By stymieing the attempts of their caretakers to keep them alive and well, patients achieve an indirect expression of anger, both at themselves and those around them.

Resistance to physical care is discussed in more depth in Chapter 20, in the section on indirect self-destructive behavior.

Behavior—Passive Refusal. The patient refuses to cooperate with hygiene tasks, passively standing and not helping.

Possible Causes. In the later stages of Alzheimer's disease, patients may resist bathing. They may be afraid of water or of falling and may not understand what is expected of them. They may be overwhelmed by the demands of a complex task for which they no longer remember the purpose.

Intervention. The patient may need step-by-step instructions to break the task down into simple steps. Initiate the tasks, for example, by placing the washcloth in the patient's hand, if you want the patient to begin to wash.

Behavior—Active Refusal. Some patients engage in active refusal, clutching clothes to the body if staff try to undress them, striking out, refusing to get into the shower, and yelling for help.

Possible Causes. These are the same as for passive refusal, above.

Intervention. Evaluate the need for a bath and the amount of effort required to achieve the goal. Consider whether a sink and towel bath might meet hygienic needs as well. Choose a time when the staff and caregiver are not hurried. If possible, select the patient's "good" time of day. Determine which gender of caregiver the patient is most comfortable with and use that person as the helper. If a bath or shower must be accomplished without the patient's cooperation and against active resistance, select a time when sufficient staff are available to provide enough physical control so that injury to the patient and staff is prevented. Have an exact plan of how to proceed and who will perform specific tasks. Designate one staff member only to speak to the patient during the procedure. If possible, remove other patients from the area where you will be transporting and bathing the patient. If other patients or visitors are in the area, explain ahead of time what is going to be done and what they may expect to see and hear. After the procedure is over, have one person stay with the patient and offer verbal or nonverbal reassurance and support in the form of pleasant discourse. Do this only if it does not further anger and agitate the patient. Use special aids such as a tub or shower chair to decrease fear of falling. Install grab bars and grips. A spray attachment to the tub or shower is helpful, but it may need to be introduced slowly and carefully to the patient each time it is used.

Behavior—Conflicting Statements. The patient may agree to comply with expectations but passively not do so. The patient may state in a complaining tone that he or she cannot comply or that it is of no use.

Possible Causes. It may be a symptom of a depressive illness. It may be the patient's way of expressing self-loathing.

Intervention. Use a gentle, firm, matter-of-fact approach. Do not try to elicit cooperation by being jovial or by offering assurance. Acknowledge that the task at hand seems futile but gently insist that it is necessary. Use hands-on assistance if needed to accomplish goals. Use a program of shaping desired behavior and substitute more acceptable expressions of negative feedings. These patients will most likely require pharmacologic intervention.

Behavior—Refusing to Eat. The patient may refuse meals or toy with food. He or she may show a marked rapid weight loss. The patient may claim to be full or unable to swallow in the absence of dysphagia.

Possible Causes. It may be a symptom of depression.

Intervention. Assess for clinical depression, and refer for active psychopharmacologic treatment. Avoid power struggles over food.

Offer small, frequent feedings and dietary supplements. These patients may need parenteral nutrition or nasogastric feedings.

Behavior—Avoiding Meals. The patient will get up and wander away from the table shortly after beginning to eat; he or she may play with food but not eat it.

Possible Causes. In the later stages of dementing illness and in some acute psychiatric disorders, patients may be too restless to sit through a meal, attention span may be too short, and they may forget what it is they are supposed to be doing.

Intervention. Place snacks and finger foods where the patient will have access to them. Monitor weight. Decrease the amount of ceremony around a meal; keep it fast and simple. Feed several small meals a day. Provide a quiet place to eat. Feed the patient if needed.

Nocturnal Restlessness

Many elderly people suffer from sleep disturbances. Although universally distressing, not all sleep disturbances result in behavioral problems. Nocturnal restlessness associated with dementing illness, however, is a major problem in the home care setting when caregiving family members are deprived of their rest (Rabins, Mace, & Lucas, 1982).

Definition. Nocturnal wakefulness is a behavioral problem when patients, once awakened, behave inappropriately and by their behavior cause distress to others or real or potential harm to themselves.

Etiology. Patients with dementing illness, or those who are confused, are often temporally or spatially disoriented if they awaken in the middle of the night. Nondemented patients who manifest some of the other behavioral problems addressed in this chapter, particularly demanding and wandering, may exhibit their problematic behaviors when awakened. These behaviors are even more troublesome at night when the family is asleep, since these are hours when paid caregivers are less readily available. Therefore, those factors leading to nocturnal awakening will be briefly discussed.

A number of acute and chronic illnesses can lead to nocturnal wakefulness. In the later stages of dementing illness such as Alzheimer's disease, disturbances in the sleep-wake pattern are common. Dyspnea from congestive heart failure or chronic pulmonary disease and pain from arthritis are two common causes. Chronic use of sedatives, hypnotics, anxiolytics, alcohol, or caffeine and poor timing of administration of laxatives or diuretics are other potential contributors to interrupted sleep (Busse & Blazer, 1980; Norris, 1986). Boredom and lack of exercise during the day, long daytime naps, and too much activity near the time of sleep may cause nocturnal wakefulness. Hunger, cold, or overheating may cause disruptions in sleep.

Measures to correct the above causes of interrupted sleep may prevent these problems from occurring at night. The following section deals with the specific problem behaviors accompanying nocturnal restlessness.

Behavior—Nocturnal Panic. Once awake, the patient may be frightened, call out, panic, or attempt to leave.

Possible Causes. The patient may be demented or confused; he or she may awaken in the middle of the night and be temporally or spatially disoriented. The patient may not know what time of day it is or where he or she is. Nocturnal restlessness is particularly likely to occur if the demented patient is sleeping in a new or unfamiliar environment.

Intervention. Provide reassurance and reorientation. If the patient is able to read and comprehend, leave explanatory notes at the bedside; for example, "You are sleeping at your sister Ann's house and she is sleeping just across the hall." In institutions, it may be helpful to move the bed to the hallway or near the nurses' station, where the patient will have visual cues on awakening.

Behavior—Nocturnal Resumption of Daytime Activities. The patient may get dressed, turn on all the lights in the house, try to do chores, or try to go out. The patient may not be particularly distressed, just awake. He or she wants to wander about the house, rearrange belongings, engage in conversation with the caregiver.

Possible Causes. The patient may have a basic disturbance in diurnal rhythm as part of the later stages of Alzheimer's disease.

Intervention. Show the patient that it is dark outdoors. Be reassuring and calm. Put the patient gently but firmly back to bed. Try to determine and treat the causes for awakening.

Provide for physical exercise during the day and quiet activities before bedtime. Determine what helps the patient sleep, such as a warm bath or warm milk at bedtime, soft music, and dim lights. If the patient persists in awakening, provide a safe place for waking. If at home, be sure the room is free of hazards and install barriers to stairs, exits, and so on. A screen door installed on the bedroom that fastens on the outside is effective. Work with the family to help them accept this behavior without denying themselves adequate rest. In institutions, provide an illuminated seating area near the nurses' station and allow the patient to be awake.

Paranoid and Suspicious Behavior

Paranoid, suspicious behavior is a common feature of several mental illnesses of the elderly. Whatever the etiology, the behaviors that accompany paranoid and suspicious thinking, such as shunning others, physical assaults, or accusing others of theft or maltreatment, are distressing and painful to the family and others. The nature of these disorders and the attendant behaviors interfere with help-seeking behavior and make intervention difficult. Often what brings the patient to the attention of a helping professional is not the illness but the self-protective mechanisms that accompany it, such as not allowing the children into the home or repetitive calls to the police. These patients see no need for treatment, since they do not see themselves as ill, and in their view, it is others who are causing their suffering.

Paranoid and suspicious thinking is not a normal aspect of aging. When encountered, it should always be explored and, if possible, treated. If allowed to continue, the result may be further deterioration of the patient and a breakdown of the social support network.

Definition. Paranoid and suspicious thinking, as the term is used here, refers to unwarranted suspicions of others or the mistaken belief or misperception that one is an intended victim of harm.

Etiology. The major illnesses and conditions in which paranoid and suspicious thinking occurs are identified here with brief statements as to their etiology. Specific interventions are also briefly described.

Suspicious Personality. Paranoid, suspicious people may not be psychotic or demented. They may be showing exaggerated lifelong personality traits that stem from the belief and perception that they are neglected or mistreated. With aging, this turning against and blaming others may increase to the point that family members react by withdrawal, further reinforcing the elders' belief that they are being maligned and excluded (Verwoerdt, 1981). Generally, these behaviors are not severe enough to cause major problems in living, but rather it is the family caregivers who experience distress. Since patients seldom are motivated to change, interventions are best directed toward helping the family accept patients as they are, to learn not to react to their statements, and to continue to provide needed care and gain satisfaction from their own caregiving, independent of patients' response to them.

Paranoid State. Paranoid state, or atypical psychosis, refers to a psychosis that is a psychiatric illness characterized by a gradually developing delusional system of a persecutory nature in a person with otherwise unimpaired intellectual and occupational functioning (Leuchter, 1985). The delusions are often sexual in nature and may be accompanied by hallucinations. This illness occurs in old age in a person who has had no prior psychiatric history. Hospitalization is often not necessary and almost never is voluntarily sought (Epstein, 1980). Generally, low dose neuroleptics, such as Haldol, 1 to 2 mg BID, and environmental manipulation are sufficient for treatment.

Toxic Paranoid Psychosis—Drug-Induced. This psychosis is characterized by a sudden onset and may occur in someone who previously had a paranoid disorder or someone who was never mentally ill. Delusions of persecution are common. Anticholinergic medications such as amantadine may cause this psychosis, which is accompanied by confusion, a clouded sensorium, and hallucinations. Drugs used in the treatment of chronic obstructive pulmonary disease, such as Alupent inhalers or tolbutamide, may cause a paranoid thought disorder, which typically is manifest by an isolated delusion of persecution. L-dopa-induced psychosis is typically preceded by vivid nightmares (Klawans, 1978). The medical treatment for all of these iatrogenic paranoid disorders is the identification and discontinuation of the offending pharmaceutical agent.

Paranoia Associated with a Dementing Illness. In the early stages of dementing illness, accusing others of stealing, meddling in others' affairs, and playing tricks are compensatory mechanisms by which demented people attempt to deny or rationalize the cognitive deficits that are causing them difficulty in keeping track of their own affairs. These accusations are usually related to something they have misplaced or forgotten and are generally fleeting, as opposed to constant fixed delusions. In the later stages of the disease, people may develop actual delusions, which resemble a form of paranoid psychosis. In the first instance family education, reassurance of the patient, and interventions to minimize the chance for a lost object are sufficient treatment. People with full-blown delusions often require psychiatric and pharmacologic treatment.

Behavior—Inappropriate Accusations. The patient may hide things, not be able to find them, and accuse others of stealing them, or the patient may claim that he or she was burglarized.

Possible Causes. The paranoia may be an attempt to deal with the onset of memory loss in dementing illness. The sudden gaps in memory are frightening. In an attempt to maintain control and deny the illness, the patient may rationalize losing things by claiming that the family is stealing from him or that the home has been burglarized.

Intervention. Depersonalize the accusations. Respond with reassurance, not argument. Help to locate belongings. Reinforce a plan for keeping valuables in one place. Provide locks for drawers or purses and a safe place for storage. Try to organize belongings in a way that prevents loss.

Behavior—Fear. The patient may be fearful and confused or have obtunded sensorium. The patient may believe that he or she is in danger and may have frightening hallucinations.

Possible Causes. The patient may have a drug-induced paranoid psychosis associated with use of anticholinergic medications.

Intervention. Identify and remove offending medication from the drug regimen. Maintain a protected, quiet environment, free of sudden noise and overstimulation. The patient needs close observation because he or she may attempt to flee. If restraints are required, the patient should be under observation at all times.

Behavior—Suspicions of Intended Harm. The patient has a fixed idea that someone is intent on causing him or her harm. This may sound plausible or may be very fanciful. The patient generally (except in the case of dementia) does not have signs of mental disorder. The thoughts of persecution will remain unchanged over time.

Possible Causes. This may be a symptom of a paranoid state or a manifestation of dementing illness, usually in middle stages of the disease, or it may be associated with drug-induced psychosis associated with Alupent or tolbutamide. The patient may fear being poisoned and refuse to take medications or to eat.

Intervention. Do not try to convince the patient that he or she is wrong. Offer support by addressing the underlying fear. Control sudden changes in the environment; if these do occur, offer explanations. Recognize the potential for violence or attempts by the patient to escape the situation. For patients living in the community, try to elicit the cooperation and understanding of family, neighbors, police, and so forth, to protect and reassure, not confront, these patients.

In the case of medications: (1) be honest and tell the patient what the medication is; (2) reframe the reason for it, such as the medication will keep the patient strong to fight enemies; (3) there may be a need for involuntary treatment. Regarding food: allow the patient to select food, perhaps in sealed containers or from vending machines.

Assaultive Behavior

This section deals with assaultive behavior of elderly patients, which might be directed at family caretakers, other patients, or staff.

Definition. Assaultive behavior is defined as hitting, shoving, kicking, biting, being loudly verbally abusive, and making threatening gestures. Anger, a normal human emotion, is often an appropriate response to an environmental or interpersonal event. In assaultive behavior, however, anger escalates to an attempt to remove or harm a perceived threat.

Etiology. Assaultive behavior may be caused by one or a combination of the following factors:

1. Paranoid thinking may cause the patient to perceive threats or danger in benign situations through misinterpretation.

2. Dementia and confusion may cause misperception of people and their actions. Brain-damaged elderly often exhibit low frustration tolerance. This may be due to chronic pain, disorientation, or their own inability to communicate needs.

3. Rational elderly who are not confused may be responding to a perceived threat, loss, or disappointment of unmet expectations, which results in a sudden overwhelming sense of helplessness. This generates anxiety. The anxiety is countered by an aggressive act, which is an attempt to regain control and mastery over the situation. Threats and physical assault often occur in situations of high intensity, such as upon admission to a hospital or during an invasive procedure (Barile, 1982).

Staff members working in institutions for the elderly may themselves inadvertently provoke assaultive behavior by:

1. Approaching a patient in a group, rather than having one staff member approach the patient and explain what needs to be done

2. Allowing the patient to become increasingly restless and agitated without intervening

3. Allowing confused patients to wander and violate the personal space and possessions of others

4. Failing to detect painful physical problems (Felthous, 1984; Schuster & Greendyke, 1984)

5. Crowding patients into settings of high activity and noise, with few staff members, which has been linked to increased assaults (Jones, 1985)

The following principles apply to all situations wherein staff are dealing with patients with assaultive behavior:

1. Understand assaultive behavior as a provoked learned response to a perceived event

2. Determine the cause of the underlying distress

3. Determine precipitants to assaultive behavior

4. Respond in a way that prevents or minimizes the harm to the patient and others

Behavior—Striking Out. The patient may strike out suddenly at others, may address others by an inappropriate name, and may accuse them of planning to do him or her harm. The patient may seem not to recognize the person he or she is threatening. (One woman called her daughter "you other woman.")

Possible Causes. Assaultive behavior may be caused by a hallucinated threat or misperception of stimuli.

Intervention. Offer explanations, in simple terms, for environmental stimuli. If episodes occur at home with a single caretaker, the caretaker should avoid trying to subdue or reason with the patient, but should be coached to obtain outside help and protect himself or herself in this situation. If episodes occur in an institution, avoid trying to talk the patient down. Obtain sufficient staff to safely restrain the patient, even if outside help is needed. Appoint one, and only one, person to speak to the patient. Plan containment in advance, such as who will hold which arm, and so forth. Physically contain patients and move them to a quiet place, such as a single room or the empty dining room. Whoever speaks to the patient should use a firm but quiet tone, reassure the patient of safety, and remain with the patient until the patient is calm and no longer combative.

Behavior—Angry Actions. Agitation and anger may be directed at the person attempting to give care or at objects in the environment. The patient may throw things, spit, scream, kick out, pace rapidly, slam things, or demand to be left alone. A previously docile patient may suddenly become combative.

Possible Causes. Fatigue may be a cause. The patient may not be aware of being tired but will experience general discomfort. He or she may be reacting to physical discomfort caused by an undiagnosed illness. This should always be considered if a previously docile, pleasant patient suddenly becomes agitated. The patient may be experiencing loss of someone or something in the environment or may be feeling bullied, overwhelmed, and out of control.

Intervention. General: Learn to recognize warning signs: a sudden increase in activity, an expression, rocking, pacing, humming. At these times, avoid making demands on the patient or attempts to "jolly him out of it" by joking or teasing. Try to determine a precipitant event. Provide a quiet place away from stimulation. Caregivers may offer music or an oral treat. PRN medications may be effective. Plot time and frequency of agitated periods. If they recur, bring the patient to bed, provide quiet, use light restraints, soft music. Assess for constipation, impaction, abscessed teeth, painful corns, calluses, skin rash, urticaria, contact dermatitis. Consider a recent staff change, change in the caretaker or the caretaker's state of health. Provide nurturance, reassurance, and comfort. Examine the precipitant. Does this occur at the time for bathing, vital signs, institutional or home demands? If

so, modify demands, slow the pace, allow the patient as much control as feasible in the situation.

Inappropriate Sexual Behavior

Until recently our society has ascribed an asexual role to the elderly. Gurian (1986) theorizes that this asexuality myth may have its origins in the prevailing values of the 1930s and 1940s when sex was considered either secret or wrong. Parental sexuality was consequently denied by children who have grown up to be the health care professionals and adult child caregivers of today. Any overt sexual behavior on the part of frail, infirm, dependent elderly may evoke strong responses, such as avoidance, embarrassment, or criticism, in familial or professional caregivers (Kaas, 1978). Specific behaviors that will be dealt with in this chapter are suggestive personal questions and sexually explicit touching, public masturbation, and exhibitionism.

Definition. Cohen and Tannenbaum (1985) state two criteria for assessing patients' sexual behavior, which are useful in differentiating appropriate from inappropriate sexual behavior.

Is the behavior functional or dysfunctional? Functional behavior serves a useful, health-promoting purpose for the person performing the behavior.

Does this behavior fit within the norms of the setting in which it occurs (assuming that the norms are healthful)? Using this criterion, an elderly man in a nursing home may be performing a function behavior, gratifying sexual needs, but he is doing so inappropriately. Conversely, an elderly man in the community who forms sexual alliances with young men who then exploit and rob him may be acting appropriately, if he is discreet. His behavior, however, is dysfunctional if, as a result, he loses money he needs to meet his basic needs and loses his home. This section of the chapter deals only with inappropriate behaviors and related interventions.

Etiology. Normal sexual needs may be inappropriately expressed if the patient has impaired judgment as a result of chronic dementing or psychiatric illness. Disinhibition, the loss of ability to censure behavior in accordance with societal norms, may occur in dementing illness. It may also be produced iatrogenically by an adverse reaction to medications such as benzodiazepines. Disinhibition frequently occurs in advanced dementia and acute confusional state. In delirium and some highly agitated psychotic states clothing may be a tactile irritant and the patient will attempt to remove it.

Rare but severe behavioral disturbances, such as child molestation and bestiality, may be caused by a late onset personality disorder that occurs infrequently in old age in people without a prior psychiatric history but with a history of impotence (Pitt, 1982). These behaviors also may be associated with a dementing illness of the Alzheimer's type. Treatment of the former is directed primarily at protecting the community and may involve involuntary institutionalization of the patient. Treatment of inappropriate sexual behaviors that infrequently accompany dementing illness always involves extensive work with the family if the patient is still at home. Families need coaching to accept this behavior as a part of an illness beyond the patient's ability to control. Families can be taught to respond calmly and avoid those situations that may precipitate the behavior. Once family caretakers achieve some measure of comfort, they can explain the patient's behavior matter-of-factly to others, prepare others for it, and protect the patient from aversive responses. It is incumbent on the nursing specialist to exhibit a nonreactive, problem-solving approach to these disruptive behaviors.

Behavior—Suggestive Statements. The patient may ask suggestive personal questions.

Possible Causes. This may be an expression of sexual need or a need to affirm oneself as a sexual person, but it may be inappropriate to the place and situation. That is, this may be behavior that would be acceptable at a party or in a tavern but not in a hospital or nursing home.

Intervention. Do not answer in detail lest it trigger more suggestive questioning. State simply that the content of the question is out of place without cutting off communication.

Behavior—Intimate Touching. The patient may make physical overtures, such as touching another in an intimate or suggestive way.

Possible Causes. This behavior may be a result of a long-standing psychotic process in an institutionalized and regressed individual.

Intervention. Set limits clearly without reaction. Provide acceptable ways to validate the patient's sexuality within the norms of the institution, using compliments, advocating special attention to grooming and appearance, or providing a place for discussion of sexual feelings, such as a men's group led by a qualified person.

Behavior—Explicit Sexual Activity. Generally this is behavior that would be unacceptable in any situation—exposure, public masturbation, or touching others in a sexually explicit way.

Possible Causes. The behavior may be caused by a dementing illness with resulting disinhibition and loss of control.

Intervention. Be alert to environmental or behavioral antecedents to the behavior, such as new female staff or students arriving on the unit or increased pacing and restlessness. Use PRN medication, preferably before the behavior occurs. Encourage staff to express minimal response to behavior and when it occurs, give the patient "time out." Shape more appropriate behaviors. Protect others in the environment. Families may need special support in accepting the behavior as part of the illness. Be aware that certain medications such as antianxiety agents cause further disinhibition. Use specific behavioral programs, as outlined below. Avoid reprimands, labels such as "dirty old man," and judgmental phrases such as "loss of moral fiber."

Behavior—Fondling. Post–cerebrovascular accident (CVA) patients may fondle persons of the opposite sex.

Possible Causes. Behavior following a CVA may not be sexual but may be misinterpreted as sexual.

Intervention. Provide acceptable means of human contact or surrogate objects.

Behavior—Inappropriate Dressing. The patient may try to go out dressed only in underwear or may dress the top or bottom portions of the body only. The patient may remove clothes in public or may resist putting on clothes.

Possible Causes. Exhibitionism may be caused by loss of ability to select and put on proper clothing. Disrobing may be caused by hypersensitivity to heat or hyperirritability and irritation of clothing on skin.

Intervention. Be nonreactive. Simply guide the patient back to a private room and help him or her dress completely. Be alert to adverse medication effects that cause hypersensitivity. Observe skin for rashes or discoloration. Select loose-fitting garments such as sweatsuits or jumpsuits, and, if possible, put fasteners in the back. Use ties that are difficult for the patient to undo.

SUMMARY

The manifestation of a behavioral problem is not a normal response to aging or illness. While such problems frequently accompany the common illnesses of aging, particularly dementia, they should not be accepted with defeatism and resignation. Nurses, in their roles as direct care providers, patient and family advocates, and supervisors of those who provide care, are in a position to diagnose and ameliorate these problems. In so doing, they facilitate the process of caregiving and relieve the burdens of those who do the caring and those who require it. The process of behavioral management applies psychological theory to understanding and changing behavior of caregivers and patients. Its use enhances the nursing process of observation, analysis and intervention.

The diagnosis and treatment of the debilitating catastrophic illnesses of the elderly remain the province of medical practice. The management of a person's response to illness is the responsibility of the professional nurse.

References

Bandura, A (1969): *Principles of Behavior Modification.* New York, Holt, Rinehart & Winston.

Barile, L (1982): A model for teaching management of disturbed behavior. *J Psychosoc Nurs Ment Health Serv,* 20:9–11.

Burnside, IM (1980): Wandering behavior. *In* Burnside, IM(ed): *Psychosocial Nursing Care of the Aged* (ed 2). New York, McGraw-Hill, 298–309

Busse, EW, & Blazer, DG (1980): *Handbook of Geriatric Psychiatry.* New York, Van Nostrand Reinhold.

Cohen, D, & Tannenbaum, RL (1985): Sexuality education for staff in long-term care hospitals. *Hosp Community Psychiatry,* 36:187–188.

Epstein, L (1980): Paranoid illnesses of the elderly. *Consultant,* 20 (Sept): 65–71.

Felthous, A (1984): Preventing assault on a psychiatric inpatient ward. *Hosp Community Psychiatry,* 35:1223–1226.

Friesen, AJD (1983): Adverse drug reactions in the geriatric client. *In* Pagliaro, LA, & Pagliaro, AM (eds): *Pharmacologic Aspects of Aging.* St. Louis, CV Mosby, 257–293.

Gurian, NS (1986): The myth of the aged as asexual. *Hosp Community Psychiatry,* 37:345–346.

Hussian, RA (1981): *Geriatric Psychology: A Behavioral Perspective.* New York, Van Nostrand Reinhold.

Jenike, MA (1988): Psychoactive drugs in the elderly: Antipsychotics and anxiolytics. *Geriatrics,* 43:53–57, 61–62, 65.

Jones, M (1985): Patient violence: Report of 200 incidents. *J Psychosoc Nurs Ment Health Serv,* 23(6):12–17.

Kaas, MJ (1978): Sexual expression of the elderly in nursing homes. *Gerontologist,* 18:372–378.

Kane, RL, Ouslander, JG, & Abrass, IB (1984): *Essentials of Clinical Geriatrics.* New York, McGraw-Hill.

Klawans, H (1978): Levodopa-induced psychosis. *Psychiatric Ann,* 9(8):19–29.

Lawton, MP (1970): Ecology and aging. *In* Pastalan, LA, & Carson, DH (eds): *Spatial Behavior of Older People.* Ann Arbor, University of Michigan Press, 40–67

Leuchter, A (1985): Assessment and treatment of the late life psychosis. *Hosp Community Psychiatry,* 36:815–816.

Monsour, N, & Robb, S (1982): Wandering behavior in old age: A psychosocial study. *Social Work,* 27:411–416.

Norris, CM (1986): Restlessness: A disturbance in rhythmicity. *Geriatr Nurs,* 7:302–306.

Pagliaro, LA, & Pagliaro, AM (eds) (1983): *Pharmacologic Aspects of Aging.* St. Louis, CV Mosby.

Pitt, B (1982): *Psychogeriatrics: An Introduction to the Psychiatry of Old Age.* London, Churchill Livingstone.

Prehn, R (1982): Applied behavioral analysis for disturbed elderly patients. *J Gerontol Nurs,* 8:286–288.

Rabins, PV, Mace, NL, & Lucas, MJ (1982): The impact of dementia on the family. *JAMA,* 248:333–335.

Rader, J, Doan, J, & Schwab, M (1985): How to decrease wandering: A form of agenda behavior. *Geriatr Nurs,* 6:196–199.

Risse, SC, & Barnes, R (1986): Pharmacologic treatment of agitation associated with dementia. *J Am Geriatr Soc,* 34:368–376.

Salzman, C (1985): Geriatric psychopharmacology. *Annu Rev Med,* 36:217–228.

Salzman, C (1987): Treatment of the elderly agitated patient. *J Clin Psychiatry,* 48(5) (Suppl):19–22.

Salzman, C (1988): Treatment of the agitated demented

elderly patient. *Hosp Community Psychiatry*, 39:1143–1144.

Schuster, D, & Greendyke, R (1984): Assaultive behavior in brain damaged men. *Hosp Community Psychiatry*, 35:731.

Seligman, MWP (1975): *Helplessness: On Depression, Development and Death.* San Francisco, WH Freeman.

Snyder, LH, Rupprecht, P, Pyrek, J, et al. (1978): Wandering. *Gerontologist*, 18:272–280.

Thompson, TL, Moran, MG, & Nies, AS (1983a): Psycho-tropic drug use in the elderly—Part I. *N Engl J Med*, 308:134–138.

Thompson, TL, Moran, MG, & Nies, AS (1983b): Psycho-tropic drug use in the elderly—Part II. *N Engl J Med*, 308:194–199.

U'Ren, RC (1984): Organic disorders. *In* Cassell, CK, & Walsh, JR (eds): *Geriatric Medicine*, Vol. I. New York, Springer-Verlag, 553–576.

Verwoerdt, A (1981): *Clinical Geropsychiatry* (ed 2). Baltimore, Williams & Wilkins.

CHAPTER
22

Using Theory to Guide Nursing Interventions: A Case Study

W. CAROLE CHENITZ, R.N., Ed.D.

INTRODUCTION

When communication takes place a relationship is formed (Jackson, 1962). In order to understand the relationship, one must understand the behavior of participants in the relationship. To study behavior, one turns to the observable manifestations of the relationship, that is, communication. Communication in this sense is synonymous with behavior (Watzlawick, Beavin, & Jackson, 1967). This chapter presents a theory of communication and illustrates the usefulness of the theory to clinical practice by examining the application of communication theory to the case of a screaming nursing home resident.

COMMUNICATION THEORY

There are many theories that explain human communication. In the communication theory chosen here, communication is defined as "all those processes by which people influence one another" (Ruesch & Bateson, 1951). In other words, communication is synonymous with behavior and behavior is therefore synonymous with communication. If behavior is communication, then all behavior is meaningful. There can be no meaningless behavior, since behavior is communication (Ruesch & Bateson, 1951). Indeed, the individual's attempt to communicate may appear inappropriate or may not be very efficient or effective, but it is nevertheless an attempt to communicate. Within the context of this theory, it is the task of clinicians to understand the meaning of the behavior and the message the other person is trying to communicate (Watzlawick, Beavin, & Jackson, 1967).

423

In gerontological nursing, many clients are unable to communicate or have difficulty in communicating because of organic or functional impairments (Pimental, 1986). Therefore, it becomes critical for nurses to perform accurate assessment and intervention to understand the meaning in the behavior and the message the person is communicating. In order to do this, the behavior must be seen in context. In an effort to explain this point, the following story is recounted by Watzlawick and associates (1967):

> A man was seen by passersby in the garden of a French country home. He was dragging himself around, crouching down, walking in figures of eight, looking over his shoulder and quacking. The observers were horrified. The man, however, was Konrad Lorenz, and he had just completed one of his now famous imprinting experiments with ducklings. As he describes the situation,
>
> "I was congratulating myself on the obedience and exactitude with which my ducklings came waddling after me when I suddenly looked up and saw the garden fence framed by a row of dead white faces: a group of tourists was standing at the fence and staring horrified in my direction" (Lorenz, 1952, cited in Watzlawick, Beavin, & Jackson, 1967).

The ducklings were hidden from the tourists' view by tall grass. All the tourists saw was a man engaged in totally unexplained and apparently insane behavior. Unless the context of the situation were understood—that the man acting so crazy was really a scientist performing experiments with ducklings—the behavior would be interpreted incorrectly.

Basic Principles

The basic principles of communication theory are summarized in Table 22–1, and a detailed elaboration is contained in the following paragraphs.

The first principle of communication is that communication is essential; one is always communicating or receiving communication. As Watzlawick and associates state, "One cannot not communicate" (Watzlawick, Beavin, &

Table 22–1. PRINCIPLES OF COMMUNICATION THEORY

1. Communication is essential. One is always communicating and receiving communication.
2. Communication ability is developed within the individual as the result of a consistent series of experiences and relationships.
3. Communication establishes and defines all relationships.
4. Communication occurs at different levels of abstraction.

Jackson, 1967). The patient who is withdrawn and isolated and refuses to talk is communicating. Ruesch and Bateson explain that as human beings and members of society we are ". . . biologically compelled to communicate. Our sense organs are always on the alert and are registering the signals received, and inasmuch as our effector organs are never at rest, we are continually transmitting messages to the outside world" (Ruesch & Bateson, 1951). Biologically, humans are equipped with the ability to communicate via sense organs, which are the receivers; effector organs, which are the senders; the individual's communication center or the place of origin and destination of all messages; and the remaining parts of the body or the shelter of the communication machinery (Ruesch & Bateson, 1951).

In older persons, the machinery for communication may be impaired. For example, Laird (1979) writes of her experience in a hospital and later in a nursing home. After her surgery, she was given medication, which that night caused her to "lose contact with reality." She had a vivid dream and demanded to be let out of the hospital. She was then moved to a private room. She wrote, "There was no outside window in this room, and looking through an open doorway across the hall I saw, in the room opposite me, what to my nearsighted eyes appeared to be vertical bars. . . . I jumped to the conclusion that this was a place of confinement for potentially dangerous patients" (Laird, 1979).

Later, Mrs. Laird told her granddaughter that she was being held in the area of the hospital for dangerous cases. As it turned out, the bars were on a high crib in a children's room. Mrs. Laird's communication to her granddaughter was influenced by a perceptual problem, coupled with a nighttime move and medication, all of which created her belief about her situation. In order to understand what Mrs. Laird was really talking about we would need to go beyond the initial communication to her granddaughter to explore what created her understanding of her situation in the hospital.

This "machinery"—that is, the biological equipment for communication—enables the individual to make sense or to create patterns out of widely diverse events. These patterns are abstractions retained by the individual. As Ruesch and Bateson wrote, "In order to proceed with abstraction, the organism must be exposed to a sufficient number of events which contain the same factors. Only then is a person able to cope with the most frequent happenings he may encounter" (Ruesch & Bateson, 1951). The individual acquires patterns of communication.

The second principle of communication is that communication is developed within the individual as the result of a consistent series of experiences and relationships. Ruesch and Bateson (1951) delineate this series as " . . . through continuity and consistency of exposure to similar social events; it begins with the child's experiences with the mother, then with members of his family and later with contemporaries at school and on the playground." Throughout this period, a child is acquiring information about himself or herself as an individual, and about the relationships between an individual and a group, between groups and, as individuals, to a culture. The information an individual acquires forms patterns of communication and originates in the social behavior of other people and in the objects, plants, and animals that surround people. Gradually, from this information, an individual develops a pattern or style of communication. Ruesch & Bateson point out, " . . . the stimulus received and the response chosen become stylized, the stimulus shapes the response and once the response has been learned, the individual is conditioned to seek those stimuli which will elicit his learned responses. . . . Stimulus and response are thus welded into a unit; this unit we shall refer to as a value" (Ruesch & Bateson, 1951). Values, then, are preferred channels of communication or relatedness.

A third principle of communication holds that communication establishes and defines all relationships. Information about the values that people hold enables us to interpret their message and to influence their behavior. Values are not only characteristic of an individual but are also held by groups of people and by whole cultures. For example, in our culture (as in many cultures), a value held by families is that of nurturing and caring for family members. However, that cultural value can become problematic on an individual level as family members disregard their own health and welfare to care for a family member. For example, in the case of multigenerational families, the value of family caring often can become distorted. As Soyer points out, "It may be best for grandpa to remain with his family although he urinates on the floor, but it may be destructive to a teenage daughter" (Soyer, 1972).

A fourth principle suggests that communication occurs at different levels of abstraction. The levels of communication are intrapersonal or intrapsychic, that is, communication that occurs within the individual; interpersonal or between people; group communication or communication to a group of people, such as a class or a staff meeting; and mass communication to large numbers of people, often not on a face-to-face basis but through, perhaps, radio or television.

The individual interacts on multiple levels. The individual does not exist in a vacuum. Intrapsychic dynamics are not an important aspect of this theory. Individuals are seen as existing within meaningful relationships, inheriting a culture with its value system, within which they interact and define themselves and live within a certain time frame that presents stress and real-life human problems. For example, in a study of elders entering a nursing home for the first time, the author found in the analysis of data that the elders shared an ideology about independence and self-sufficiency, which meant to them that they would not be dependent upon their children or others for help and they would manage their own problems and affairs. A belief that these elders shared was that nursing homes were places where people go to die or places for the demented and senile who were placed by their families. Their ideology and beliefs about nursing homes were evidenced in their reactions to their admission to the nursing home (Chenitz, 1983). In order to understand their behavior in relation to admission to the nursing home, it was necessary to examine cultural ideologies and beliefs.

Summary

Communication theory, which defines communication as all behavior, is certainly all-encompassing. It enables clinicians to search out the meaning of behavior and to place that behavior in context. It allows us to work with and try to understand incomprehensible behavior within the system in which it occurs. Human emotions in this context play a minor role. Therefore, instead of focusing on intrapsychic dynamics—how a person is feeling—or insight into the intrapsychic realm, clinicians using this theory focus on what the person is doing, with what consequences, and, if necessary, how the behavior can be changed.

The following case study is presented to illustrate the use of communication theory applied to a problem patient. In this case, the behavior that made this patient a problem was screaming. However, this behavior could have been spitting, hitting, throwing things, leaving the facility, demanding, or others. Nursing interventions and methods for intervening are highlighted. The use of a case conference is presented to show how it helps to solve the staff's dilemmas of working with a difficult patient, as well as how it facilitates cooperation and consistent use of a plan for intervening in a problem behavior. The case conference with caregiving staff is an effective, efficient means for assessment and intervention.

COMMUNICATION THEORY APPLIED

Mrs. Gray: A Screaming Patient

Anna Gray is a 75-year-old Caucasian, married woman who had been living in a skilled nursing facility for 3 years at the time of this consultation. On her original admission, Mrs. Gray's diagnoses were hypertension and cerebrovascular accident (CVA) with aphasia and right-sided paresis. Treatment included antihypertensive drugs and admission to a skilled nursing facility for rehabilitation. If rehabilitation was not possible, then plans for long-term care in the facility were to be made, since Mrs. Gray's husband could not manage her disability at home.

Mrs. Gray's husband was an alcoholic who worked as a bartender in the tavern he owned. He visited the nursing home daily during mealtimes and fed Mrs. Gray during those visits. Her speech during the first few months in the nursing home was described as "garbled and loud." Over time, Mrs. Gray achieved her optimal level of functioning and her condition stabilized. Her speech remained the same, although staff were able to understand her and communicate with her. Mr. Gray continued to visit on an almost daily basis. He continued to drink during this period, but he did not appear intoxicated during visits to his wife. Two and one-half years after admission to the nursing home Mrs. Gray had another CVA.

The after-effect of this stroke was an increase in expressive aphasia. Mrs. Gray now became a screamer. She refused to feed herself or assist in dressing. She wanted to remain in bed and screamed periodically for extended periods. Her screams were loud, incessant, and disturbing to staff, other residents, and visitors. Her room was in the front of the facility, and the first thing one heard entering the building were her screams. The screaming had been intermittent but consistent for 6 months when consultation was requested by the staff.

Communication Theory and Mrs. Gray

In the following assessment, communication theory was used to direct the assessment and subsequent intervention. In order to be useful in directing nursing practice, the tenets of communication theory need to be applicable to a case such as Mrs. Gray's.

First, communication is essential; people are always giving or receiving communication. If this principle is accepted, then Mrs. Gray must be seen as acting, reacting, or interacting with her environment. In order to communicate, the organs for communication are essential. For Mrs. Gray, as well as for many older people, these organs are impaired. Several questions need to be raised during the assessment of her mode of communication. Since Mrs. Gray cannot talk, is she communicating by screaming? If so, what is she trying to tell us? Is she receiving communication immediately prior to screaming? If so, what is that communication?

Second, communication develops through a consistent series of experiences or relationships. Theoretically, Mrs. Gray's screaming is eliciting a reaction from others. Since she continues to scream, the reaction she elicits is meeting her needs. Screaming may not be the most effective, appropriate, or efficient way to communicate, but the assessment needs to account for the pattern of reaction to Mrs. Gray's screaming. What are the staff's reactions to her screaming? Does everyone on the staff respond in the same manner? Has there been a change in response over time? What does the staff do now in relation to Mrs. Gray's screaming?

Third, communication establishes and defines all relationships. Mrs. Gray's mode of communication is primitive and not socially acceptable. In terms of self-communication, that is, communication about the self, Mrs. Gray's mode of communication may indicate a state of internal chaos and distress. There are several reasons why people use culturally unapproved modes of communication. First, the person may be a member of a subcultural group that holds different values. For example, monks in a cloister do not speak for long periods of time. Second, the individual may be a member of another culture. Third, the individual may be unwilling or unable to comply with standard modes of communication. (An example is the sign language communication of people who are deaf.) Finally, the

individual may not wish to comply. The reason for adopting a culturally unacceptable mode of communication needs to be understood. In Mrs. Gray's situation, it was unclear why she screamed, since she still was able to speak, albeit in a garbled manner.

Finally, communication occurs at different levels of abstraction; in order to be understood, the communication must be seen in context. The application of this principle to Mrs. Gray means that her screaming must be understood in terms of her personal history, her interpersonal needs, and recent changes in her own and family life and her life within the nursing home. Questions that are raised are the following: Have her primary relationships changed? Have her relationships within the nursing home changed? Has her status in the nursing home changed?

Assessment Methods

The assessment included review of Mrs. Gray's medical records, an interview with the primary nursing staff, and interviews with Mrs. Gray, the director of nursing, the assistant director of nursing, the nursing student caring for Mrs. Gray, and the charge nurse on the unit. The interviews with many staff members provide background, context, history, and specific behaviors, interventions, and outcomes of intervention.

The immediate precipitating factors for the request for a consultation were: (1) Mrs. Gray's room was being changed and the staff anticipated an increase in the screaming; (2) Mrs. Gray's screaming had recently gotten worse; and (3) the staff were genuinely concerned about Mrs. Gray. A meeting with the primary staff of licensed practical (vocational) nurses and nurses' aides revealed that despite her aphasia, Mrs. Gray was understood by the more seasoned staff. They had cared for her intermittently over the past 3 years, and they had developed a relationship with her that consisted of concern and appreciation for her situation. Mrs. Gray had also negotiated a set of routines with these staff members—routines that they were aware of, adhered to, and which, when completed, seemed to make her happy. During the interview with the primary staff, the following questions were raised: How long has the screaming been going on? When did it start? Was there anything else, other than the CVA, that happened at that time?

The staff were in agreement about when Mrs. Gray started screaming. They also agreed that another significant event had occurred about that time—Mr. Gray stopped visiting on a daily basis. Staff reported several incidents of staff confrontations with an intoxicated Mr. Gray, who was loud and carried in liquor for his wife. Around this time, Mrs. Gray had the second stroke and was hospitalized briefly. After she returned from the hospital, her husband visited once or twice but did not assist her with eating, which had become even more difficult than before. He then stopped visiting on a regular basis.

Next, questions were raised about the specific conditions that might trigger the screaming. The staff all had ideas about those conditions that caused Mrs. Gray's screaming. Unknown to the others, members of the staff had each formed a hypothesis about the cause of her screaming. Given permission in staff conference to verbalize their hypotheses, a range of explanations about the cause of her screaming emerged. From these, agreement was reached about several conditions that seemed to trigger Mrs. Gray's screaming.

These specific conditions, as presented by the staff, were:

1. When a new staff member took care of her.
2. When she was not promptly put to bed after an activity.
3. When her husband visited, as he occasionally did.
4. When a staff member left the room without performing a part of Mrs. Gray's regular routine.
5. When she wanted attention, wanted to get something, or needed something.
6. When she could not reach something on her tray.
7. When she left the facility for any reason.

The staff also had hypotheses concerning the origins of the screaming. The central theme was that Mrs. Gray had suffered many serious losses. Her health and home were her first losses. She lost her ability to communicate easily and effectively. She lost her independence and needed staff to assist with functional tasks of daily living. Finally, she lost her husband's company and their relationship, since his behavior was unacceptable to the nursing home staff. It was agreed that the loss of her husband was her most difficult loss and that the screaming was related to this.

The concept of loss of control was presented to and accepted by the staff. Mrs. Gray had not only lost people, places, and things but had lost control over her life. Each of the specific conditions was examined with this in mind. They were all related to attempting to get staff to perform a behavior or to expressing frustration about a behavior she did not want to perform. The room change, anticipated to trigger an increase in screaming, surprisingly had occurred without any additional screaming.

The staff used a variety of tactics to control or stop Mrs. Gray when she started screaming. These tactics were (1) being firm and explaining that she would not get what she wanted by screaming; (2) letting her sit in her wheelchair on the patio when she screamed; (3) bargaining with her to get her to stop; and (4) issuing direct orders to stop the screaming. Each of these tactics worked briefly. Therefore, they were used again by the staff. However, subsequent use of these tactics was ineffective, and each time Mrs. Gray screamed the staff were required to attend to her. When viewed in terms of the outcome, Mrs. Gray's screaming was effective in getting attention and often gratification of her immediate needs.

The staff were questioned about their reactions to Mrs. Gray's screaming. They generally agreed that because of the noise and disturbance created by Mrs. Gray, each time she screamed they responded by trying to quiet her in some way. The important points for assessment were that staff felt they had responded, that they had to respond, and, indeed, that they did respond. Staff were frustrated with the situation, felt powerless to effectively meet Mrs. Gray's needs, and felt unable to decide on another acceptable course of action. But despite their efforts to assure Mrs. Gray that screaming would not get her what she wanted, the outcome was the opposite.

An interview with Mrs. Gray was framed positively by the consultant. The theme of the interview was that Mrs. Gray was especially liked by the staff and they wanted to do the best they could to make her comfortable. Her activities of daily living, eating and sleeping patterns, procedures for getting out of bed, and participation in activities were all reviewed with her. Mrs. Gray was requested to answer yes or no to the questions. A list of questions concerning these activities was informally presented to her.

In addition, woven throughout the interview were references to change and loss. Since the loss of her room was the most recent one, Mrs. Gray was asked how she liked the new room. Her behavior was immediate and reflexive. She bowed her head, grasped the interviewer's hand, and her shoulders shook in quiet sobs. This lasted for a moment, and Mrs. Gray began screaming. After a brief period the next question was posed and the screaming was ignored. Her anguish was acknowledged and her sorrow validated. Each time reference was made to a loss or to a change, such as participating in activities outside of the institution, Mrs. Gray's reaction was the same as described above and the screaming resumed.

This interview served several functions. It validated the concept of loss of control as a causative factor in her screaming. It verified the staff's hypothesis that Mrs. Gray could not cope with any more loss. It elaborated on the hypothesis that change meant to Mrs. Gray a new or unanticipated loss. It also showed the importance of the routines Mrs. Gray had been able to establish with the seasoned staff. In addition, by reviewing the activities of daily living, areas were identified wherein enrichments could be added to her daily life to offset her losses.

The key factor in Mrs. Gray's screaming was loss of control. Loss of control was precipitated by a series of losses and changes. At this point, all of Mrs. Gray's losses were enumerated, as well as her supports and strengths.

Using the factors of loss and change, it was decided that each aspect of daily life would be reviewed and Mrs. Gray's overall situation revised in terms of reducing loss, maintaining her daily routines, fostering no change, and slowly providing additions to her life.

Specific Assessment of Mrs. Gray

Communication. Mrs. Gray's screaming was an effective, though unpleasant, means to get attention or get her needs met. The screaming was related to interactional situations that had personal meaning to Mrs. Gray. She was understood by seasoned staff and did not usually scream if this staff took care of her or if a new member took care to carefully fill the requirements of her routine.

Food. Mrs. Gray did not like the food she was served. Food was pureed because Mrs. Gray had no teeth. Three attempts had been made by the staff to take her to the dentist, but each time she screamed through the whole experience or she refused to get in the van and go. She ate well but claimed she did not enjoy her meals.

Fluids. Mrs. Gray enjoyed coffee, apple juice, and alcoholic cocktails. She did not receive cocktails but was often given coffee and apple juice.

Sleep. Mrs. Gray did not sleep well but awakened often throughout the night. She wanted to sleep during the day because she felt tired.

Routines. Over time, Mrs. Gray had developed a set routine. Each time this routine was disturbed, she started screaming. Her routines were: having a washcloth in her hand at all times; going to bed right after lunch; and refusing to participate in activities, although she did go to exercise class and enjoyed it. She needed her glasses near her or on her at all times. She wanted the head of her bed up after being put to bed.

Visitors. Mrs. Gray's only visitor and her

primary significant relationship throughout her adult life had been her husband. His gradual reduction in visiting resulted in her isolation from any significant relationship. When her husband did visit, Mrs. Gray screamed. This further increased his reluctance to visit, and their relationship had deteriorated gradually over the previous 6 months.

Plan of Intervention

Problem. Loss with a behavioral manifestation of screaming precipitated by interactions that are stressful and upsetting for her.

Goal. Eliminate screaming by replacing it with more appropriate methods of communication and reducing stressful situations.

Short-Term Treatment Goals

1. Make no changes in Mrs. Gray's routine or environment.

2. Offset losses with gradual additions of activities.

3. Provide attention to emphasize her positive communication skills.

4. Reduce conditions that trigger screaming.

Nursing Care Plan for Mrs. Gray

Communication

1. Mrs. Gray would be cared for only by seasoned staff whom she knew. If that could not be done, orientation to her needs was given to the new staff member prior to assignment to Mrs. Gray.

2. A chart of her routines would be developed by Mrs. Gray, her favorite staff member, and the director of nursing. This chart would assure Mrs. Gray, with her input, that her routines were valid and respected by the staff. It would also assist the staff to remember her routines, thereby offsetting any unanticipated lapse in a routine that might trigger screaming.

3. Attention was focused on her more appropriate attempts to communicate. Use of a friendly visitor, who was already a regular visitor to the nursing home, was initiated. The visitor would check with Mrs. Gray each time

she came to the facility to chat briefly, and she would make routine errands to the store for Mrs. Gray's essential things, e.g., talcum powder.

4. Staff assigned to Mrs. Gray's unit would rotate checking on her every hour for 2 weeks. The purpose of these brief, unobtrusive checks would be to assure her of their concern and to assess whether she was comfortable.

5. Mrs. Gray would be given a bell for her use to notify the staff of her needs.

Diet

Mrs. Gray's right not to leave the facility was respected. Discussion of a dentist visiting her would be initiated. Mrs. Gray would be taken promptly to her room after meals, and this would be incorporated in her care plan.

Fluids

Mrs. Gray would be served decaffeinated coffee and apple juice regularly with her meals. Her physician had ordered wine, which Mrs. Gray did not enjoy. A discussion would be undertaken with the physician about substituting cocktails that she did enjoy.

Sleep

Mrs. Gray was currently taking Mellaril during the day. After discussion with her physician, the Mellaril was given at night.

Visitors

Mrs. Gray's husband would be contacted by the activity director. He would be notified that the facility wished to give her cocktails prior to dinner. His assistance with the cocktails would be requested in terms of bringing in the alcohol and mixer and helping the staff start her cocktail program. He was asked to assist in the program by monitoring the amount of alcohol available and ensuring that there was enough for a specific period of time. This program was to be initiated at the next upcoming holiday, which was Thanksgiving. Mr. Gray would be given 2 weeks' notice on the plan.

Evaluation

Several weeks after the plan was initiated, Mrs. Gray's screaming was no longer a problem. She occasionally screamed, but incidents became less frequent. The staff met regularly to discuss problems in the implementation of the plan and to revise the plan. Mrs. Gray's husband became a regular visitor in the nursing home and was extremely conscientious about fulfilling his role in Mrs. Gray's treatment. Overall, after several months, the plan was evaluated as a success.

Discussion

Mrs. Gray's case is not unique but illustrates the complexity of caring for older clients on a daily basis in all types of health care settings. Mrs. Gray's screaming was a noxious form of communication that produced stress and distress in staff, other residents, and visitors. In reviewing the reasons why this intervention plan was a success, several factors seem important to the outcome.

First, there was a concerned staff. This staff refused to accept that there was nothing they could do for Mrs. Gray. They intuitively knew that Mrs. Gray was communicating her pain by screaming, and they disliked the use of chemicals to change her behavior, particularly since the chemicals seemed ineffective. Second, members of the general administration and nursing administration of this nursing home were supportive of the staff and willing to be creative. Third, the use of a consultant may have been a factor in the success. The consultant was able to be objective and was removed from the day-to-day care needs of Mrs. Gray. The consultant, as a nurse, was familiar with institutional routines and nursing care practices. In addition, the consultant had the time and flexibility to interview those involved, explore possibilities, involve others, and call in other consultants and develop a plan for intervention. The consultant had knowledge of theories of human behavior and was able to assist the staff in analyzing Mrs. Gray's behavior and developing and implementing a plan of care for her. The consultant developed the care plan with the staff and involved them in specific methods for implementing the plan. A consultant may be given the authority by the administration to function

in this way. This case illustrates the usefulness of a consultant in the care of patients with very complex problematic patterns of behavior.

Finally, Mrs. Gray's case points out the role differentiation among nursing staff in the care of the aged. The primary staff provided the direct physical care for Mrs. Gray. However, they were neither qualified nor confident in intervening with her in relation to the problematic screaming behavior. This is the case whether the behavior is screaming, hitting, biting, withdrawing, or verbal abuse. The primary staff in nursing homes are nurses' aides, and they are not prepared to plan care for patients with complex problems. A registered nurse, manager, administrator, and consultant such as a clinical specialist are the critical decision-makers in the care of these patients.

Communication theory requires that prior to making a care plan in relation to a specific behavior, the behavior be understood in context. That is, the meaning of the behavior must be understood. This requires that care providers be reflective and not reactive. Indeed, this requires that a careful assessment precede intervention and that those involved in the patient's daily activities, including the client, be included in the assessment.

In Mrs. Gray's case, analysis of the case material revealed a significant series of losses. However, there were not many that could be reversed. Therefore, the losses that could be reversed were identified and interventions developed. A major loss and hence focus for intervention was the relationship between the Grays. The use of cocktails to draw Mr. Gray back into his wife's life was carefully thought out and discussed with the administration and the physician. While no care providers want to encourage an active alcoholic to drink, Mr. Gray never acknowledged alcoholism. It was felt that his withdrawal from his wife was due, in part, to staff censure of him and his behavior while he was intoxicated in the nursing home. It was decided that he not only needed an active role in his wife's life but also needed to be formally invited back into the nursing home via a mechanism that was comfortable and familiar to him.

Not everyone using communication theory would have arrived at the same conclusion. Indeed, it is recognized that the interventions described here may be a radical departure from existing practices in many situations. However, the interventions resulted from a careful analysis, and this analysis, as well as the plan, was carefully documented. In nursing homes, it is essential that registered nurses assume responsibility to place care based on client-specific analysis. This is particularly important with clients who exhibit problematic behaviors, such as Mrs. Gray. The use of nurse consultants to assist registered nurses in the assessment and care planning may be helpful.

An important issue not raised here is the use of communication theory with confused patients. Since communication theory requires that the meaning behind the behavior be understood, the theory requires that the cause of confusion be determined.

Communication theory is one of many theories that can be used to guide nursing practice. Communication theory as applied to Mrs. Gray was a useful tool around which to structure intervention. Nursing practice guided by such theories can assist nurses to demonstrate their creativity, often in the face of a grim reality. The mark of the professional nurse is the ability to translate theory into case analysis and interventions that reflect nursing knowledge and positively affect client care.

References

Chenitz, WC (1983): Entry into a nursing home as status passage: A theory to guide nursing practice. *Geriatr Nurs*, 4:92–97.

Jackson, D (1962): Interactional psychotherapy. *In* Stein, MI (ed): *Contemporary Psychotherapies*. Glencoe, IL, The Free Press, 256–271.

Laird, C (1979): *Limbo: A Memoir About Life in a Nursing Home by a Survivor*. Novato, CA, Chandler and Sharp.

Lorenz, KZ (1952): *King Solomon's Ring*. London, Methuen.

Pimental, PA (1986): Alterations in communication: Biopsychosocial aspects in aphasia, dysarthria and right hemisphere syndromes in the stroke patient. *Nurs Clin North Am*, 21:125–135.

Ruesch, J (1957): *Disturbed Communication*. New York, WW Norton & Co.

Ruesch, J (1961): *Therapeutic Communication*. New York, WW Norton & Co.

Ruesch, J, & Bateson, G (1951): *Communication: The Social Matrix of Society*. New York, WW Norton & Co.

Soyer, D (1972): The geriatric patient and his family: Helping the family live with itself. *J Geriatr Psychiatry*, 5:52–55.

Watzlawick, P, Beavin, JH, & Jackson, DD (1967): *Pragmatics of Human Communication*. New York, WW Norton & Co.

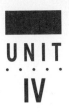

UNIT
IV

NURSING CARE FOR SELECTED HEALTH PROBLEMS IN THE OLDER ADULT

CHAPTER
23

Depression

SALLY A. SALISBURY, R.N.C.S., M.S.

INTRODUCTION

In our culture, with its emphasis on self-awareness and interpersonal understanding, the word "depression" has become a colloquial expression. As such, it is used to refer to a transient feeling of sadness, a prevailing mood of despondency, often in response to loss, as well as a clinical disorder. As a clinical disorder, the term "depression" is used to describe a symptom of abnormal mood, a syndrome or pattern of symptoms associated with an abnormal mood, or a specific disease, such as a dysthymic disorder or a major depression, characterized by a predictable course and accepted treatment (Gurland, 1980).

Depressive illnesses have a wide range of severity and morbidity. Dysthymic disorders are common sequelae to bereavement or loss and may resolve without treatment. Untreated major depressions may result in severe functional disability or suicide. Psychotic depressions are always potentially life threatening, due to the severity of the symptoms and the potential for suicide. The elderly are particularly vulnerable to depression in all of its

435

manifestations. This chapter presents an overview of the incidence and severity of depression in the elderly and establishes the relevance of a knowledge of depression for the gerontological nurse. Grief and loss, normal bereavement, and the major depressive illnesses are briefly discussed in terms of their characteristic presentations. Theories of causation and treatment for each of the depressions will be defined. The final section of this chapter addresses specific clinical considerations for diagnosing and treating an elderly depressed patient. In the summary, a case study is used to illustrate successful treatment of an elderly depressed patient.

Incidence and Severity of Depression in the Elderly

Community-based elderly in this country have an incidence of clinical depression as high as 13% (Gurland & Cross, 1982). Nonhospitalized elderly are more likely to report depressive symptoms if they reside in low status areas than if their residence is in middle status areas (Goldsmith, Kramer, Brenner, et al., 1986) or if they are experiencing social stressors such as poor physical health, bereavement, or isolation (Blazer, Hughes, & George, 1987).

The presence of depression is highly correlated with physical illness, and the highest severity of depression is found in those individuals who are both pervasively depressed and physically ill (Gurland, Golden, Lantagua, et al., 1984). In a study of outpatients of a medical clinic treating chronic illness, Borson and associates (1986) found a significant correlation between depression and functional disability, defined as the inability to work because of chronic disease. Cardiovascular disease, arthritis, Parkinson's disease, and diabetes all occur with increasing frequency in the elderly. These illnesses are often associated with depression (Fry, 1986). Verwoerdt (1976) relates the severity of accompanying depression to the severity of the primary physical illness, the organ system involved, and the duration and rate of progression of the dis-

ease. Depression is reported as more severe at the onset of both cardiac disease and Parkinson's disease, with decreasing severity as adaptation to the primary illness occurs. Depression is also associated with familial caregiving for the chronically physically or mentally ill (Gallagher & Thompson, 1983; Zarit, Orr, & Zarit, 1985). Without addressing issues of causality, it is clear that a relationship exists between depression and the presence of illness, disability, and social stressors, all of which are common in the elderly (Dohrenwend & Dohrenwend, 1981; Epstein, 1976; Pitt, 1982).

Relevance of Depression to the Practice of Gerontological Nursing

Although depression occurs frequently in the elderly, it is often not recognized by them as a treatable condition, and it may be accepted as a fact of life or a naturally occurring response to life's events. One patient recovering from a cerebrovascular accident (CVA) expressed this eloquently when he responded, "I'm not *depressed*, that's a head sickness. I got *real troubles*. I can't walk, my wife is sick, and she has to put me in a home. Naturally I can't sleep and I don't care for nothing, but I have misery, not depression." Underutilization of mental health services by the elderly is well documented (Cohen, 1982; Gaitz, 1974; Lasoski, 1986). Those surveyed elderly who acknowledge depressive symptoms indicate that if they chose to seek treatment, they would do so with primary care physicians, rather than mental health professionals (Waxman, Carner, & Klein, 1984; Goldstrom, Burns, Kessler, et al., 1987). These facts have implications for the practice of gerontological nursing.

The nurse may be the first health care provider to assess depression in an elderly patient or the patient's primary caregiver. Working with the elderly in a variety of health care settings and focusing on the patient's response to illness and treatment, the nurse is in a position to identify depression early in its development and to arrange for appropriate diagnosis and treatment. Patients who may be reluctant to report depressive symptoms to physicians may be more comfortable in describing their feelings to a nurse. It is incumbent on the gerontological nurse, therefore, to have an understanding of depression in its many manifestations and to be able to distinguish a depressive illness from a transient and appropriate response to a life event.

CLINICAL MANIFESTATIONS OF DEPRESSION

Grief and Bereavement

Bereavement is the normal response to loss of a loved one. It is characterized by the same signs that signify depression: dysphoric (painfully depressed) mood, poor appetite, weight loss, insomnia, guilt, and thoughts of death (Diagnostic and Statistical Manual of Mental Disorders [DSM III-R], 1987). The process of recovery generally occurs over a year's time. During this time the bereaved person is more likely than the nonbereaved to experience illness, hospitalization, increased alcohol consumption, social difficulties, and emotional distress (Parkes & Weiss, 1983). Morbid preoccupation with worthlessness, marked functional impairment, and psychomotor retardation, particularly if these occur 3 months or longer after the loss, are indicative of a major depression and are not a normal part of bereavement (DSM III-R, 1987). The tasks of grieving involve coming to accept the loss and arriving at a new identity, for example, that of widow or widower. For those elderly who see their remaining years and resources as limited, a significant loss may be generalized to represent multiple losses, anticipation of further grief, and hopelessness (Blazer, 1982). One 74-year-old man, hospitalized for depression following the loss of his lover, remarked to the author, "At your age, if you lose a lover, you can always hope to meet someone around the next corner. At my age there are no more corners to turn." Protracted grief and pervasive despondency and hopelessness require the treatment of specialists in mental health.

Depressive Illness

The clinical manifestations of depressive illness in the elderly population are not markedly different from those in the young. Confusion arises because some of the symptoms of depression—loss of energy, difficulty concentrating and sleeping—are mistakenly assumed to be normal aging changes or concomitant with a physical illness (Fry, 1986; Shamoian, 1985). Many of today's elderly first developed symptoms of depressive illness in the earlier part of this century, when less attention was paid to psychological health. They and their families may have not considered chronic or episodic mood disturbances as illness and may have simply accepted them as a personal characteristic or trait.

Dysthymia-Depressive Neurosis. DSM III-R defines this illness as "a chronic disturbance of mood involving depressed mood, for most of the day, more days than not, for at least two years." Accompanying signs and symptoms are poor appetite, insomnia or excessive sleeping, fatigue, disorders of attention and concentration, and feelings of hopelessness. This common disorder has no marked precipitating event. This disease may follow a familial course, and it often goes untreated because of the chronic nature and low level of severity of symptoms, which seldom markedly impair function. A person with a depressive neurosis, however, may be less able than others to adapt to life's stresses, may have less psychological resilience, and may be prone to major depression in the event of catastrophic life events.

Major Depression. The following is a summary of the DSM III-R definition of a major depressive episode.

1. At least five of the following symptoms will have been present for at least 2 weeks and represent a change from previous functioning; depressed mood; loss of interest or pleasure in most activities (one of the preceding two must be present); weight loss or gain; insomnia, particularly early morning wakening; psychomotor retardation or agitation; fatigue; feelings of worthlessness or guilt; decreased concentration or ability to make

decisions; recurrent thoughts of death, including suicidal ideation or attempts.

2. These symptoms are not attributable to an organic factor and are not accompanied by delusions or hallucinations.

Major depressive episodes are more common in people with a familial history of depression. During the course of the illness, functioning is markedly impaired. If untreated the disease may resolve within 6 months, but the individual may develop recurrent episodes of increasing frequency with age. Unresolved bereavement may evolve into a major depression. The most serious sequela of an undiagnosed and untreated major depression is suicide. Younger patients may be more likely than the elderly to receive prompt diagnosis and treatment for this disorder, simply because their decrease in function is readily noted by their families, peers, and co-workers. Among the elderly, particularly those who live alone, symptoms may go undetected for long periods of time. The physical manifestations of this disease—weight loss, malnutrition, exhaustion—may seriously or fatally compromise a preexisting physical illness. The author recently received a referral for an elderly male living in a single-room occupancy hotel who had been suffering from an undiagnosed major depression and chronic obstructive pulmonary disease (COPD). When brought to the clinic by his concerned friend, the patient weighed 80 pounds and required immediate hospitalization for correction of severe electrolyte imbalance and malnutrition.

Psychotic Depression. A major depression is classified as psychotic when it is characterized by faulty reality testing and impaired function. Delusions or hallucinations are often present, accompanied by disorders of affect or mood. Psychomotor retardation or agitation may be profound. If agitated, the patient may pace, continually wringing his or her hands and mutter phrases like "help me, help me" over and over. Delusions often express themes of guilt, shame, and doom in the context of physical disease. Examples are a belief that one cannot swallow, a belief that one is infected with syphilis and is contaminating everyone, a belief that one's insides are rotting

and emitting a putrid odor. Paranoid thinking may be present. This serious illness, which constitutes a medical psychiatric emergency, is frequently seen in the elderly. Delusions are more common when the first episode of depression occurs at age 60 years or beyond (Meyers, 1987).

Bipolar Disorder (Manic-Depressive Illness). The essential feature of bipolar disorder is the presence of one or more manic episodes, usually with a history of intervening depressive episodes (DSM III-R, 1987). During a manic episode, the patient's mood is euphoric, to the extent that it is noticeably inappropriate to the situation and circumstance in which it occurs. Irritability may be present. The patient is hyperactive and may not sleep for days. Dress may be flamboyant or inappropriate for age and occasion. The patient may be delusional, grossly exaggerating his or her abilities and wealth. Sudden expenditures of large sums of money, real or fictitious, may be the behavior that brings the patient's disturbance to the attention of others. One elderly man, who lived on a disability income in a single-room occupancy hotel, grandly wrote a bad check for $5,000 and drove a new truck off the lot. These episodes are interspersed with periods of remission and depressive episodes. Bipolar disorders typically have their onset in early adulthood, but episodes of both depression and mania may occur throughout life, with depression being the form more common in the elderly. The first manic episode, however, can occur after age 60 years (Lehman, 1982). Sometimes in the elderly, early-life manic or depressive episodes passed undiagnosed and untreated and only a careful history will reveal them. One such case involved a 64-year-old man, hospitalized following a serious suicide attempt. His wife related that he had periods of being "moody" throughout their 45-year marriage. She then related what she called "an up time." Shortly after his retirement at age 50 years, this man had volunteered to help his brother-in-law with the family hardware store. His wife recalled that he singlehandedly remodeled the store, going without sleep for days on end. He began waiting on customers wearing shorts and Hawaiian shirts in their midwestern conservative town. The family had just assumed it was a stage he was going through, and the episode was passed over. Careful evaluation of any marked mood disturbance in the elderly is always necessary to rule out the presence of this illness, which is a major psychiatric disorder and one that is amenable to treatment.

Suicide. People over the age of 65 years comprise approximately 10% of the population of this country, yet they account for one-fifth to one-quarter of all successful suicides (Templer & Cappelletty, 1986). Rates and prevalence of suicide in the elderly show changes that correspond with population shifts. In the years preceding 1976 the highest suicide rates occurred in white males over the age of 75 years (Stenback, 1980). The fastest growing segment of our population is that of people over 85 years. Suicide rates of the old-old and of nonwhite men show corresponding increases (Manton, Blazer, & Woodbury, 1987). The suicide rate of men over the age of 85 is five times that of the population at large (Bromberg & Cassel, 1983). Whereas suicide attempts in younger persons often are an expression of hostility to others or a cry for help, older persons who attempt suicide most often fully intend to die. The rate of suicide attempts in young people is much higher than the rate of successful suicide, but in older persons the rates of suicide attempts compares nearly equally to the rate of successful suicides (Pfeiffer, 1977). Variables that have been linked to suicide in the elderly are the presence of depression, bereavement, isolation, living alone, and chronic illness (Bromberg & Cassel, 1983; Pfeiffer, 1977).

Suicide, as the term is used here, refers to the willful taking of one's own life by a self-destructive action. It is generally accepted to be a product of disturbed thinking. Suicidal thinking or attempted suicide is defined both by standards of medical practice and civil law as an indication that a person is not competent and requires medical intervention. Recently, some practitioners who work with the elderly and the elderly themselves have raised issues that call these basic tenets into question. Issues

of the right to self-determination and control of one's own destiny have surfaced, giving rise to living wills and right-to-die laws. The right to refuse or curtail medical treatment to prolong life is generally thought of as passive suicide. Ethical norms regarding how much control over the course of treatment should rest with the patient, the physician, family, or the institution delivering care vary widely, with individuals, institutions, and state legislators involved in the discourse. It is incumbent on gerontological nurses to be clear in their own ethical beliefs and cognizant of those of both colleagues and patients (Roth, 1983b).

No less a problem is an individual's choice to end life by active means or to refuse treatment for a terminal illness. In attempting to resolve the dilemma of how and when to intervene, health care professionals are often caught between two powerful but conflicting ethical principles, beneficence versus respect for autonomy (Bromberg & Cassel, 1983). There are no easy solutions. Some practitioners of geriatric psychiatry advocate that if the decision to end one's life is made in the absence of a depressive illness, thought disorder, or crisis state, it should be respected. For some elderly, and even for some young people, faced with a certain prognosis of slow and painful death, knowing that they are without human succor or sufficient material resources to ensure basic comforts, death may be the preferred alternative.

THEORIES OF THE CAUSE OF DEPRESSION

For purposes of discussion, theories of depression can be divided simply into those that arise from the medical model and those that have been generated by the social and behavioral sciences. Theories of causation are used to explain observed phenomena in a specific population, and, in the case of depression, they may determine the treatment approach selected. This section will present a brief overview of the major medically derived and social-behavioral science theories of depression. The reader who desires more than a general knowledge of depression theory is urged to study further the direct sources.

Medical Psychiatric Theories

While no definitive relationship between physiology and depression has been established, researchers are examining biochemical correlates in depression. Affective disorders are thought to be linked to a deficiency in the neurotransmitter catecholamines, norepinephrine or serotonin (Small & Jarvik, 1982) or an imbalance in the two (Zarit, 1980). Since these neurotransmitters modulate the secretion of hypothalamic neuroendocrine cells, deficiencies of hormonal response are anticipated. It is known that a number of depressed patients secrete large quantities of cortisol (St. Pierre, Craven, & Bruno, 1985). There is some evidence that the activities of the thyroid and pituitary may be associated with onset and recovery from depression (Zarit, 1980). Aging changes may contribute to the incidence of depression, since in aging there is a general decline in the overall function of hormones and receptors (St. Pierre, et al., 1985). With aging, levels of monoamine oxidase (MAO), which destroys norepinephrine at neuron ends, increase (Zarit, 1980).

Psychodynamic theory holds that depression is the result of introjected hostility, that is, rage and anger are turned inward toward the self (Verwoerdt, 1976). Feelings of ambivalence, guilt, and self-loathing interfere with the ability to form and maintain relationships and result in isolation and apathy. Depressed persons indirectly express their anger toward significant others by their passivity and pervasive gloom.

Family systems theorists believe that interaction between people affects behavior. In durable relationships such as families, patterns of interaction develop and are maintained and may provoke and sustain problem behaviors in one or more family members. Signs and symptoms of a mental illness such as depression are seen as one outcome of family interaction, and the family as a unit is seen as the patient (Herr & Weakland, 1979).

Social and Behavioral Science Theories

Cognitive theory holds that every dysphoric mood or emotional state is accompanied by a corresponding mental set that consists of ideas and beliefs occurring at the time the negative mood is experienced. In depressed individuals, these thoughts and beliefs center around themes of worthlessness, hopelessness, and sometimes suicide (Burns & Beck, 1980). Depressed people associate all negative events in their lives with their own real or imagined shortcomings, and they form associative links from past failures to present events and to future disappointments. According to this theory, the depressed person interprets many situations incorrectly, and what a person thinks about what is happening influences how that person feels (Beck & Greenberg, 1974).

Self-efficacy, the belief that one is capable of mediating life events and acting upon others and the environment to one's benefit, is linked to an internal locus of control. An external locus of control, the belief that one is powerless to influence events, has been linked to learned helplessness, decreased self-efficacy, and an increased vulnerability to depression (Becker, 1977; Holahan & Holahan, 1987).

The occurrence of depression has been related to stressful life events such as bereavement, loss of job, moving, major illness, and change in financial status (Brown, Harris, & Peto, 1973; Paykel & Meyers, 1969). Recent thinking on the relationship of stressful life events and depression is moving from an examination of stressful events as isolated variables to a consideration of stressors in the context of the individual's life experience, circumstance, and role performance (Stuart, 1981). An individual who is experiencing stress associated with the fulfillment of assigned role expectations is said to be experiencing role strain. Role strain, or difficulty in carrying out one's role, is thought to be causally linked to depression. Thus, whether isolated stressors are harbingers of depression is now thought to be determined by the amount of difficulty they cause a person in engaging in daily activities of life, meeting responsibilities, and attending to tasks at hand (Lieberman, 1983). This broader view argues for a holistic, comprehensive understanding of people and the world in which they live.

These theories of the cause of depression are not mutually exclusive. Depression is a complex illness, and an individual's susceptibility to it may be mitigated by many complex, interrelated variables. In clinicians' attempts to isolate and codify complex human phenomena, there is a danger of oversimplification. A rigid adherence to one theory may result in overlooking significant psychosocial or physiologic events. Theories of causation relate to taxonomy, which may in itself lead to further fragmentation and oversimplification of human response. In one small descriptive study, Thomas, Sanger, and Whitney (1986) identified 12 nursing diagnoses in six depressed subjects, with five of the 12 diagnoses occurring more than once. Williams and Skodol-Wilson (1982) advocate that psychiatric nurses focus on further developing axes IV and V of the DSM III, Severity of Psychosocial Stressors and Global Assessment of Functioning, rather than develop another isolated nosology. These axes, which are within the domain of nursing, could be used by nurses to relate their expertise to the practice of psychiatry, in conjunction with psychiatrists and psychologists. As of this writing, it is unclear how psychiatric nurses will elect to link their practice to clinical psychiatry. Those who work with the elderly also must choose a common language for articulating their assessment and interventions with the elderly depressed patient.

TREATMENT OF DEPRESSION

The treatment of depression receives much attention in our culture. A perusal of the popular printed and broadcast media reveals a wide array of available services, such as self-help groups, holistic and folk medicine techniques, and various therapies. Ironically, the disease of depression, in the young and in the old alike, is often underdiagnosed and undertreated. When correctly treated, many depressive illnesses are resolved. For this reason, it is important that gerontological nurses be aware of available and appropiate treatment resources and utilize them either in practice or in referral to those qualified to treat them. Depression, no less than heart disease or diabetes, is an illness that requires skilled treatment.

Psychopharmacologic Treatment

Tricyclic antidepressants (TCAs) are the basic pharmacologic agents used to treat depression. These drugs act to block serotonin or norepinephrine uptake, or they alter the binding or sensitivity of neurotransmitter receptors. Imipramine, doxepin, nortriptyline and desipramine are frequently used TCAs. Newer medications, such as Trazodone and amoxapine, have slightly different, reputedly more selective mechanisms of action (Prien, Blaine, & Levine, 1985). Monamine oxidase inhibitors (MAOIs) have fewer anticholinergic effects than the TCAs but require the patient to adhere to dietary restrictions. For this reason, they are seldom the first drug of choice. MAOIs do have a different mechanism of action than the TCAs and are used in the treatment of TCA-resistant depression, either alone or in combination with TCAs (White & Simpson, 1987). The anxiolytics, benzodiazepines such as Librium, do not target the chief symptoms of depression but may be used in combination with TCAs to relieve agitation. Lithium is used specifically in the treatment of bipolar disorders and occasionally in combination with TCAs in treatment-resistant depression. Thyroid hormones are infrequently used, also as an adjunct to TCAs. The above comments refer to the treatment of nonpsychotic depression without delusions. For psychotic depression with delusions, antidepressants alone are seldom effective. The preferred treatment is a combination of neuroleptics and antidepressants (White & Simpson, 1987). Attempts to treat elderly psychotically depressed patients with higher than average dosages of tricyclics without adjunctive neuroleptic drug therapy have been successful in only a small number of documented cases (Brown, Kocsis, Glick, et al., 1984). Mechanism of action and side effects of the more common antidepressant medications are summarized in Table 23–1.

A word of caution must be interjected regarding the proper use of antidepressant medications. Often they are prescribed by nonpsychiatrists as an adjunct to medical treatment of another disorder. While many geriatricians and internists have a thorough working knowledge of these medications, the selection and titration of antidepressants are complex. Patients who do not respond to one may respond well to another. Often several medications must be tried before the maximal therapeutic effect with minimal side effects is found. Because the therapeutic effects of TCAs are often not seen for 4 to 6 weeks after starting the medication, many patients discontinue

dosage too soon or do not progress to therapeutic dosage. Abruptly stopping TCAs may result in a sudden catastrophic relapse. Often patients need to remain on antidepressant medication, with dose monitoring, for prolonged periods of time, often longer than 1 year. When discontinued, the dosage must be tapered slowly, with careful observation for the return of symptoms (Risse, Bertman, & Brinkley, 1985).

In summary, patients with severe depressive symptomatology deserve a methodical, complete trial of antidepressant therapy, which is best provided by a specialist in mental health care. (See Tables 23–2 and 23–3.)

Electroconvulsive Therapy

Electroconvulsive therapy, once widely used, has fallen into disrepute as a legitimate

Table 23–1. ANTIDEPRESSANTS—ACTION AND SIDE EFFECTS

Drug Type and Action	Side Effects	Drug Type and Action	Side Effects
Tricyclic Antidepressants **Tertiary Amines**		**Drugs Similar in Efficacy to** **Tricyclics**	
amitriptyline (Elavil): blocks serotonin reuptake	High sedative effect High anticholinergic effect	trazodone (Desyrel): selectively blocks serotonin uptake	Little anticholinergic effect, sedating, may interact with digoxin, elevate digoxin level
doxepin (Sinequan, Adapin): blocks serotonin reuptake	Moderate anticholinergic effect High sedative effect	amoxapine (Ascendin): inhibits reuptake of both serotonin and	Extrapyramidal effects, may cause tardive dyskinesia
imipramine (Tofranil): blocks serotonin and norepinephrine reuptake	Moderate anticholinergic effect Moderate sedative effect	norepinephrine, blocks dopamine receptors **Tetracyclic** **Antidepressants**	
Secondary Amines		maprotiline (Ludiomil)	Little anticholinergic effect, low incidence of
desipramine (Norpramin): blocks norepinephrine reuptake	Low anticholinergic effect Low sedative effect	**MAO Inhibitors**	cardiovascular effects
nortriptyline (Aventyl): blocks norepinephrine and serotonin reuptake	Moderate anticholinergic effect Moderate sedative effect	phenelzine (Nardil) and tranylcypromine (Parnate): cause increased concentration of catecholamines and indolamines due to their decreased metabolism by MAO	Very low anticholinergic effects, less sedating, more stimulating than tricyclics, may cause orthostatic hypotension and insomnia
Possible Side Effects of All Tricyclics		**Special Precautions**	
Orthostatic hypotension Dry mouth Blurred vision Accommodation paralysis Urinary retention Arrhythmia	Delayed ejaculation Parkinsonism Tremors Fasciculations Hyperreflexia Ataxia	Patients on MAO inhibitors must be on a low tyramine diet and must avoid over-the-counter cold medications that contain ephedrine. MAO inhibitors have a toxic reaction with meperidine.	

(Data from Jenike, 1985; Knoben & Anderson, 1982; Verwoerdt, 1976.)

Table 23–2. SPECIAL CONSIDERATIONS FOR ELDERLY PEOPLE ON ANTIDEPRESSANTS

Illness	Effect
Possible Interaction Between Antidepressants and Medical Illness	
Cardiovascular illness	
Arrhythmias	Increase
Congestive heart failure	Worsens
Angina	Worsens
Seizure disorder	Lower seizure threshold
Hyperthyroidism	May exacerbate arrhythmias and tachycardia
Liver disease	Decreases metabolism of antidepressants
Renal failure	
Prostatic hypertrophy	Urinary retention
Angle-closure glaucoma	Glaucoma
Medications That Cause Increased Plasma Levels of Antidepressants	
phenytoin	
allopurinol	
sulfonamides	
chloramphenicol	
cimetidine	
Medications That May Have Diminished Therapeutic Effect if Given with Antidepressants	
propranolol	
antihypertensive agents	

(Data from Fava & Sonino, 1987.)

therapeutic modality in recent years. The efforts of patient rights advocacy groups and negative portrayals of this treatment in theater and literature resulted in severe legal and ethical repercussions with subsequent curtailment in the administration of what was popularly called "shock treatment." Patients who had received electroshock treatment often complained of subsequent memory loss and amnesia. With the advent of antidepressants and rise in negative public opinion, its use has declined. The technique of administration of electroconvulsive therapy has markedly changed, however. The current method involves administering a low-dose, rapid-acting general anesthetic before treatment. Succinylcholine, a curariform, is administered to block convulsive motor activity. A brief electric current is applied for 0.5 to 2 seconds via two electrodes that are placed on the nondominant cerebral hemisphere (Blaine, 1986). When administered in this way, electroconvulsive therapy is found to have minimal cognitive dysfunctional side effects and is therapeutically effective. Electroconvulsive therapy is used primarily for those patients who are severely depressed and for those patients who either cannot tolerate or do not respond to pharmacologic treatment.

Psychotherapeutic Treatment

The style and method of psychotherapy of the depressed patient is dependent on the training, theoretical orientation, and skill of the therapist. Psychodynamically oriented therapists use the mechanisms of transference and countertransference to bring about insight in their patients. Insight refers to an awareness of how one's feelings and reactions in the present are governed by past events. Cognitive therapists strive to alter the way in which their patients think in certain situations and during certain emotional states. Family systems therapists treat the family as a unit, rather than focusing on the identified patient, and work to bring about more positive adaptive patterns of behavior and interaction in the family. These are but a few of the theoretical and methodological approaches to psychotherapy and only brief definitions are presented here. Therapists often use one or a combination of methods and may vary their choice of method according to the goals of treatment, the time available for treatment, and the mental status of the patient. Psychotherapy can be used alone or in conjunction with medications and may be practiced individually, in groups, or with families and couples. What then is the relationship of the gerontological nurse to psychotherapy?

Gerontological nurses who are not specially trained in psychotherapy have an important role in referring patients needing treatment to appropriate resources. Before a referral is made, the nurse should have an awareness of the patient's mental state, cultural and educational background, and the severity of the depressive illness. An isolated elderly patient with coronary artery disease who lives in a retirement home and is psychotically de-

Table 23–3. PATIENT TEACHING GUIDELINES FOR ELDERLY PEOPLE
ON ANTIDEPRESSANT MEDICATIONS

General Considerations

The severely depressed patient has decreased concentration ability and a decreased learning curve. Instruction should be given to the patient and to a primary caregiver. It is important that medication be given as ordered, especially in the initial treatment of acute depression. Responsibility for ensuring this is best assigned to someone other than the patient.

Key Points

1. The onset of maximal therapeutic effect may be from 2 to 6 weeks. Unpleasant untoward effects may be noticed by the patient before symptom relief. Many patients and their families become discouraged and stop the medication before an adequate trial is completed.

   Patients and caregivers should be advised to contact the prescribing physician to report the onset of the following:
   a. Dizziness
   b. Blurred vision
   c. Staggering gait
   d. Inability to empty the bladder
   e. Racing pulse, pounding heart
   f. Sudden mood changes
   g. Excess sleepiness or insomnia
2. If the patient is being treated for any other illness by another physician, the physician prescribing the antidepressants must communicate with the other physician before antidepressants are started and before any medication change is made.
3. Patients should contact their physician before using any over-the-counter medication.
4. Antidepressants must never be abruptly discontinued but should be gradually withdrawn. Patients need to be advised that an even more severe depression may occur if the drug is withdrawn suddenly.

5. Unpleasant side effects can be mitigated. Patients can be cautioned to rise slowly from a sitting position and to sit on the edge of the bed before standing to decrease the effect of postural hypotension. Increasing fluid and fiber intake can decrease constipation. The sedating effect, which is often the first noticed, lessens in time as the patient accommodates to the medication.
6. Patients who are suicidal before antidepressant treatment is begun may be at increased risk for suicide as they become more energized from the medication. Such patients must be under psychiatric care and closely observed during the initial treatment phase, until their suicidal ideation is no longer present.
7. Patients on MAO inhibitors must be on special tyramine-free diets. They need to avoid the following foods:
   a. All cheese and foods containing cheese
   b. Sour cream
   c. All fermented or aged foods
   d. Liver of any animal
   e. Liverwurst
   f. Broad bean pods
   g. Meat or yeast extracts
   h. Dried fruit
   i. Red wine
   j. Cognac
   k. Sherry
   l. Vermouth
   m. Beer and ale

(Date from Jenike, 1985.)

pressed needs prompt referral to an expert in geriatric psychopharmacology. A retired lawyer, a sophisticated and articulate woman who is showing a protracted bereavement characterized by indecisiveness and a mild sleep disturbance may be effectively treated by a nonmedical therapist, but she may require one who is acceptable to her social standards. Patients who do not work effectively with one therapist may find that they are more comfortable with another. As with medications, the selection of a therapist may involve trial and error. Initial treatment failures should not be interpreted as a patient's inability to respond to treatment. The fit between patient

and therapist is no less important or difficult with the old than with the young.

SPECIAL CONSIDERATIONS OF DEPRESSION IN THE ELDERLY

The remainder of this chapter focuses on the characteristics of the elderly patient that affect depression in this population. Special attention is paid to the developmental tasks of the elderly that may relate to depression. The occurrence of depression in the elderly is examined in relation to physical and dementing illness. Special treatment considerations are addressed. Finally, a case study is used to illustrate the course and prognosis of depression in an elderly patient.

Developmental Tasks of the Elderly in Relation to Depression

Even well elderly are theoretically nearer to death than the young. For the chronically or terminally ill, the closeness to death is undeniable. The developmental task of the elderly is to bring about closure to one's life and prepare for death. How well a person does this is dependent on many theorized variables: family constellation, overall health, resources and place of dwelling, religious belief, to name a few (Roth, 1983a). Butler (1963), writing from a psychodynamic perspective on individuals arriving at closure of life, used the term "life review" to describe the process of remembering the past and reintegrating it, with the goal of arriving at resolution of conflict and acceptance. He postulates that for some people, those who were heavily future oriented or those who were willfully cruel or prideful, this naturally occurring developmental event might give rise to depression.

Health care providers who concern themselves with the maintenance and prolongation of life may have difficulty hearing the themes of death awareness their older patients express and so may miss valuable opportunities for assessment and intervention. In one such case, an end-stage COPD patient with a diagnosis of bipolar disorder was hospitalized on a psychiatric unit. He continually sabotaged his respiratory treatment or engaged in provocative acts such as urinating on staff. The result was that he had frequent transfers to the medical intensive care ward. These stays were always short and he would return to the psychiatric unit for another brief stay. Finally a nurse calmly explored his behavior with him in a nonjudgmental way. He admitted that he knew he was dying but was afraid to die alone. He wanted to remain on the medical intensive care unit, which was more heavily staffed than the psychiatric unit, particularly at night. He then spoke at great length about his past life

and thoughts of the afterlife. When his concerns were shared with the staff, staffing was altered to ensure attention to the patient on both units. He died 3 days later, calmly and at peace.

Often, elderly spouses of ill or dependent partners need help in planning for the continued care of their infirm spouse while they are still able to do so. Knowing that things are in order can be comforting to an elderly person, because anxiety about unfinished business can interfere with day-to-day coping. The role of psychotherapy in helping a person prepare for death is addressed in works by Fry (1986), Roth (1983a), and Blazer (1982).

Earlier in this chapter the relationship of life events to depression was discussed. For the elderly, life events may have different significance than for the young. Though research findings are not consistent, of particular interest is a study by Keith (1987). She demonstrated that although life events correlated with depressive symptoms differently in the young and in the old, dissatisfaction with one's marital partner and oneself was significantly correlated with depression in all ages. Thus the "cute old couple" who have been married 50 years may be demonstrating endurance, not life satisfaction. Depressive symptoms are often of an interpersonal nature over the lifespan. Clinicians need awareness of this fact when considering treatment options, such as placement of one member of a couple or choosing family therapy as a treatment modality.

Relationship of Depression to Physical Illness

The link between physical illness and depression was established earlier in this chapter. In this section, the complex nature of the link between physical illness and depression will be developed further. This relationship has importance for the gerontological nurse, since it can be anticipated that many patients have one or more chronic illnesses. The relationship between physical illness and depressive symptoms is most difficult to evaluate when both are found together, as is often the case. In this instance, the depression may be thought mistakenly to be a manifestation of the physical illness and may go untreated.

Certain physical illnesses are known to be likely to cause depression. Cardiovascular disease in its early stages can cause depression. The symptoms of depression, fatigue, insomnia, exhaustion, and difficulty breathing may be mistaken for manifestations of cardiac insufficiency (Fry, 1986). Other diseases that may cause depression are: Parkinson's disease; neoplasms, particularly primary cerebral tumors or metastases or pancreatic tumors; hypo- or hyperthyroidism; adrenal cortex dysfunction; electrolyte imbalance; malnutrition; and folate deficiency (Field, 1985; Lehman, 1982). Medications used regularly in the treatment of chronic illness may also produce depression. In these instances, a danger exists that the depressive symptoms will be seen as a manifestation of the primary medical problem and not a drug side effect. Medications that have been linked to depression are: antihypertensives, propranolol and clonidine, steroids, and antiparkinsonism agents (Field, 1985; Klerman, 1983). Thus, both physical illness and its treatment play a role in the etiology of depression in the elderly.

The issue is further complicated by the fact that in the elderly somatic symptoms are often the primary manifestation of depression. Somatic symptoms may occur in either the presence or absence of a physical illness. Gurland and associates (1984) reported the highest incidence of somatic complaints and more severe depression in those who were both depressed and chronically ill. Waxman (1985), however, found that depressed individuals reported more somatic complaints than nondepressed people, whether or not they had a chronic physical illness. Somatic complaints have been reported to be higher in depressed women than in depressed men (Berry, Storandt, & Coyne, 1984). Patients who first experience depressive episodes in later life have been reported to show more somatic symptoms and agitation than those who had early life depressive episodes, even when early and late groups were matched for current age (Brown,

Sweeney, Loutsch, et al., 1984). Somatic complaints, which may take the form of anxiety about one's health or vague symptoms of constipation, flatulence, insomnia, and agitation, may be mistaken for signs of normal aging. An older person may be using physical symptoms to both mask depression and ask for help. Elderly people may not realize that they are depressed and may be aware only of vague feelings of fatigue, physical discomfort, and restlessness. Not all patients who experience depression are able to identify dysphoric moods. A lack of interest in activities that formerly were pleasurable may be attributed to a physical condition. Clinicians who work in nonpsychiatric settings need to be alert to patients who suddenly begin to make frequent clinic appointments for treatment of nonurgent physical complaints, since this may be the only clue to the presence of a depressive illness. A careful history may uncover a masked depression and should result in a referral for successful treatment.

Relationship of Depression to Dementing Illness

The term "pseudodementia" has been used to describe depression that is the primary cause of cognitive difficulty (Reding, Haycox, & Blaiss, 1985). This descriptive term is applied to patients with minimal neurologic deficits and those who are profoundly depressed. In clinical practice, it is often difficult to distinguish a true case from a pseudodementia, particularly when the patient with the presenting symptoms has preexisting cognitive deficits. Generally, pseudodementia is characterized by a clear time of onset, rapid progression of symptoms, and a depressed mood (Frances & Teusink, 1984). A depressed patient complains of decreased memory function and gives frequent "I don't know" responses to questions. Impairment in social functioning and regressed behavior often are present (Wells, 1979). One study (Keith, 1987) found that complaints about memory correlated more closely with depression than with actual cognitive function. The pattern of errors in cognitive testing by those who are primarily depressed is usually different from errors of those who are demented. Demented patients often give a high number of false positive responses and show substantial disorganization of secondary (delayed) memory. Depressed individuals are more cautious in responding and have a pattern characterized by "I don't know" responses or nearly correct answers, rather than intrusions of irrelevant material or confabulations (LaRue, 1982).

In the latter stages of dementing illness, patients often are unaware of their deficits and deny difficulties. This is not true, however, in the early stages of a progressive dementing illness, such as Alzheimer's disease, multi-infarct dementia or Parkinson's disease. The patient may be aware of cognitive difficulty before deficits are apparent to others. This may precipitate depression. The presence of a depressive illness in a patient with mild cognitive deficits will impair cognitive functioning beyond what would be expected for either disorder alone (Reifler, Larson, Teri, et al., 1986; Spar, Fora, & Liston, 1980; Teri, 1984). If the presence of a dementing illness is known, the cognitive deficits may be wrongly attributed to it and the diagnosis of depression may be missed. Error can be made in the other direction, by underdiagnosing dementia and attributing symptoms solely to depression. Reding, Haycox, and Blaiss (1985) found a high percentage of patients initially diagnosed as depressed to be demented on followup examination. The diagnoses on followup were senile dementia of the Alzheimer's type, Parkinson's disease, multi-infarct dementia, as well as the uncommon supranuclear palsy.

Thus, depression in the elderly is seen as a complex issue and may exist as an isolated illness, as a secondary effect of a medical illness, or even possibly as a prodromal sign of an impending vascular or neurologic dementia. Its presence in an elderly patient, particularly one without a prior psychiatric history, should never be taken lightly or dismissed as normal. Because the presentation of depression may be subtle or may mimic other disorders, its absence should never be assumed without careful evaluation. Various instruments have been developed that can assist the clinician in screening for depression in an elderly population.

Instruments for the Assessment of Depression

Geriatric Depression Scale. The Geriatric Depression Scale (GDS) was developed and tested with community-based elderly with no complaints of depression and with elderly people hospitalized for depression (Table 23–4). Items were specifically selected that would not be threatening to the elderly on a self-administered test, and care was taken not to include somatic symptoms that have been found to correlate poorly on total score on depression instruments. The GDS has been found to have a high degree of internal consistency, and total scores were found to be reliable over 1 week's time. The validity of this instrument is determined by comparison of total scores with the classification of patients as normal, mildly depressed, or severely depressed, according to the Research Diagnostic Criteria for Depression. The original 30-item test has been shortened to the GDS short form of 15 items. The GDS can be administered as a self-report test or as an interview and by individuals without special training (Yesavage, Brink, Rose, et al., 1983a). Although an effective screening tool, the GDS does not assay somatic symptoms that may be present in masked depression and does not correlate as closely to the Research Diagnostic Criteria as the Hamilton Rating Scale for Depression (HAM-D). It is not as sensitive to changes in the level of depression over time as the HAM-D (Yesavage, et al., 1983a). The major advantage of the GDS is the ease with which it is administered. Another advantage is that the GDS measures more variables specifically associated with depression in the elderly than other popular instruments (Weiss, Nagel, & Aronson, 1986).

Hamilton Rating Scale for Depression (HAM-D). The Hamilton Rating Scale for Depression was developed as an instrument to measure the severity of depression. It con-

Table 23–4. GERIATRIC DEPRESSION SCALE

1. Are you basically satisfied with your life?	Yes/No
2. Have you dropped many of your activities and interests?	Yes/No
3. Do you feel that your life is empty?	Yes/No
4. Do you often get bored?	Yes/No
5. Are you hopeful about the future?	Yes/No
6. Are you bothered by thoughts you can't get out of your head?	Yes/No
7. Are you in good spirits most of the time?	Yes/No
8. Are you afraid that something bad is going to happen to you?	Yes/No
9. Do you feel happy most of the time?	Yes/No
10. Do you often feel helpless?	Yes/No
11. Do you often get restless and fidgety?	Yes/No
12. Do you prefer to stay at home, rather than going out and doing new things?	Yes/No
13. Do you frequently worry about the future?	Yes/No
14. Do you feel you have more problems with memory than most?	Yes/No
15. Do you think it is wonderful to be alive now?	Yes/No
16. Do you often feel downhearted and blue?	Yes/No
17. Do you feel pretty worthless the way you are now?	Yes/No
18. Do you worry a lot about the past?	Yes/No
19. Do you find life very exciting?	Yes/No
20. Is it hard for you to get started on new projects?	Yes/No
21. Do you feel full of energy?	Yes/No
22. Do you feel that your situation is hopeless?	Yes/No
23. Do you think that most people are better off than you are?	Yes/No
24. Do you frequently get upset over little things?	Yes/No
25. Do you frequently feel like crying?	Yes/No
26. Do you have trouble concentrating?	Yes/No
27. Do you enjoy getting up in the morning?	Yes/No
28. Do you prefer to avoid social gatherings?	Yes/No
29. Is it easy for you to make decisions?	Yes/No
30. Is your mind as clear as it used to be?	Yes/No

(From Yesavage, J, Brink, TL, Rose, T, et al. [1983]: Development and validation of a geriatric depression screening scale: A Preliminary Report. *J Psychiatr Res* 17:37–49. Reprinted with permission.)

sists of 21 items that are rated by the interviewer on a range of scores from 2 to 4. The structured interview takes approximately 30 minutes to administer and the interviewer requires special training and a high level of interviewing skill. This instrument was not intended to be used as a screening tool, but rather was intended to measure the severity and change in depression in a patient already diagnosed as having an affective disorder. Its reliability is dependent on the skill of the interviewer (Hamilton, 1960). Interrater reliability and validity have been established, and the HAM-D effectively measures change over time and response to treatment (Hedlund & Vieweg, 1979). Although not developed specifically for use with the elderly, recent studies have shown that the HAM-D does have reliability and validity with an elderly population (Yesavage, et al., 1983a).

Beck Depression Inventory (BDI). The Beck Depression Inventory is widely used and cited in psychiatric literature. It is a self-administered, self-report instrument. Twenty-one and 13-item instruments are available, and in each the patient selects one of four response choices for each item. Categories covered are sadness, pessimism, sense of failure, dissatisfaction, guilt, self-dislike, self-harm, social withdrawal, indecisiveness, negative self-image, work difficulties, fatigue, appetite disturbance (Gallagher, 1986). Published data are available concerning the use of this instrument with the elderly as a screening tool and as a measure of response to treatment (Thompson & Gallagher, 1984).

When items on the long form of the BDI were examined for their ability to determine the severity of depression in psychiatric and medical samples, using a latent trait analysis, only the core symptoms of dissatisfaction, loss of social interest, indecision, sense of failure, sense of punishment, and suicidal thoughts were found to discriminate depressed from nondepressed patients in both populations (Clark, Cavanaugh, & Gibbons, 1983). This suggests that the use of this instrument may be problematic with medically ill elders, unless there is careful analysis of individual items.

Zung Self-Rating Depression Scale. Like

the BDI, the Zung Self-Rating Depression Scale (SDS) is a short, self-report instrument (Table 23–5). The SDS is the most widely cited of all the depression instruments. Its reliability and validity have been established with all age groups and across cultures. It has been used with elderly community samples as a screening tool and has been found to discriminate such subpopulations as recently widowed from nonwidowed and mildly cognitively impaired from nonimpaired (Zung & Zung, 1986). It has been used to measure treatment effectiveness and as a program evaluation measure (Zung & Zung, 1986). Because the SDS contains a number of somatic items that may be factors of normal aging, mean scores have been established for different age groups (Zung & Zung, 1986). When compared to the HAM-D, the BDI, and the GDS, the SDS was able to measure the most variables consistent with the DSM III criteria for depression and characteristic of depression in the elderly (Weiss, et al., 1986). The SDS is copyrighted and can be obtained by writing to Dr. William

Table 23–5. ZUNG SELF-RATING DEPRESSION SCALE

For each item the respondent rates the statement as "a little of the time," "some of the time," "a good part of the time," "most of the time."
 1. I feel downhearted and blue.
 2. Morning is when I feel the best.
 3. I have crying spells or feel like it.
 4. I have trouble sleeping at night.
 5. I can eat as much as I used to.
 6. I still enjoy sex.
 7. I notice that I am losing weight.
 8. I have trouble with constipation.
 9. My heart beats faster than usual.
10. I get tired for no reason.
11. My mind is as clear as it used to be.
12. I find it easy to do the things I used to.
13. I am restless and can't keep still.
14. I feel hopeful about the future.
15. I am more irritable than usual.
16. I find it easy to make decisions.
17. I feel that I am useful and needed.
18. My life is pretty full.
19. I feel that others would be better off if I were dead.
20. I still enjoy the things I used to do.

(From Zung WK [1965]: A self-rating depression scale. *Arch Gen Psychiatry*, 12:63–70. Reprinted with permission. Copyright 1962, 1965, 1974, William Zung. All rights reserved.)

Zung, Veterans Administration Medical Center, Durham, NC 27705.

In selecting instruments to measure depression in the elderly, clinicians need to be clear on what it is they want to measure, what level of sensitivity is desired, who the population is that will be tested, the time required and level of training needed to complete the instrument, and the level of acceptance of the instrument in published research and clinical practice. If screening instruments are used, what use will be made of the information that is obtained? Ideally, using prevalence studies done in a clinical setting is a method of case-finding. Patients who demonstrate the presence of depression on a self-report or screening instrument should be further evaluated by a psychiatric interview, with appropriate treatment offered. If the clinician wants to measure response to treatment or intervention, care must be taken to select an instrument that has proved to be sensitive to measuring change in level of severity. The preceding section has addressed some of these issues.

These instruments are only a few of the available resources that the gerontological nurse can draw on to improve diagnostic acuity and to monitor the cause of illness and the response to treatment. Instrument rating scores are not intended to be used as a substitute for direct clinical assessment and documented observations.

Treatment of Depression in the Elderly

As with the young, treatment with antidepressants has been demonstrated to be effective in elderly depressed patients free of organic illness and memory deficits (Georgotus, McCue, Hapiworth, et al., 1982). Patients with pseudodementia have demonstrated improvement in cognitive testing after treatment with antidepressants (Sternberg & Jarvik, 1976). Patients with a presumed diagnosis of primary degenerative dementia have been shown to have a higher incidence of depression than age-matched normal controls (Lazarus, Newton, Cohlers, et al., 1987). While making a diagnosis of depression in this population is difficult because the symptoms of depression, psychomotor retardation, sleep disturbance, and memory loss are also characteristic of dementia, patients with dementia and depression do respond to antidepressant therapy (Winograd & Jarvik, 1986). The patients' mood and motivation may show improvement in the absence of cognitive improvement, but this change may make a significant difference in the quality of life and response to caregiving.

While proved to be efficacious, treatment of a depressed elderly person with psychopharmacology is more complicated than treatment of a young, physically well patient. The elderly are more susceptible to the anticholinergic side effects of the TCAs, particularly the tertiary amines, imipramine and amitriptyline. These medications are more likely to produce orthostatic hypotension, which may lead to falls and injury (Georgotas, et al., 1986). Other side effects such as dry mouth and constipation may be tolerated less well by the elderly. Secondary amines such as desipramine have fewer anticholinergic effects. When available, blood levels should be obtained to ensure proper absorption, especially if no response is shown after 4 to 6 weeks of treatment. If tricyclics are ineffective, they may be boosted by concurrent treatment with lithium or thyroid extract. A more conservative course of treatment is to taper the dosage of the tricyclic and substitute an MAOI. Demented patients are thought to be particularly responsive to MAOI therapy, since they have a higher MAO level than age-matched controls (Georgotas, et al., 1986). However, because of their memory problems, these patients may not be able to adhere to the dietary restrictions required, and care must be taken that medication administration and dietary supervision be provided by a reliable caregiver.

Antidepressants are contraindicated in the treatment of cardiovascular disease because of their potential for producing arrhythmias. Patients with a history of cardiovascular disease who have arrhythmias, conduction defects, or heart failure should not be given TCAs (Fava & Sonino, 1987). All elderly depressed patients should have a careful evaluation, including an electrocardiogram, before antidepressant therapy is started. The anticholinergic effects of the antidepressants may exacerbate such preexisting conditions as glaucoma, prostatic hypertrophy, hyperthyroidism, and impaired renal function. Medically ill elderly people may be taking other medications that will potentiate the side effects of antidepressants or interfere with their absorption. In addition, community-based elderly may be taking over-the-counter preparations that produce the same results. Some over-the-counter sleep and antihistamine drugs, for example, potentiate the anticholinergic effects of TCAs or neuroleptics (Salzman, 1982). A careful and exhaustive drug history must be obtained before treatment is started (refer to Table 23–1).

Electroconvulsive therapy is often faster and safer to use than medications in treating the elderly depressed patient. It may be the treatment of choice if the patient has medical problems, provided particular attention is paid to pretreatment evaluation, pretreatment oxygenation, and adequate muscle relaxation during treatment (Salzman, 1982). It is also often the treatment of choice in severely psychotically depressed elderly who have somatic delusions, especially if their response to the delusions results in life-threatening fasting or suicide attempts.

With the elderly, as with the young, the preferred treatment is a combination of pharmacologic intervention and psychotherapy. The elderly have been shown to be responsive to psychotherapy (Gallagher & Thompson, 1983; Stever, Mintz, Hammen, et al., 1984). They often do not seek therapy on their own as readily as younger patients and may require specially trained therapists who are sensitive to issues of aging and the impact of culture and generation on communication styles. The therapist may need to be more actively engaged than therapists for the young, serving as a source of nurturance and comfort, as well as therapy, but the elderly, once engaged, respond to treatment at least as well as their younger depressed counterparts. An elderly person who is depressed may need to be taught that his or her dysphoric mood, agitation, and somatic symptoms are indications of a real treatable illness. Again, the gerontological nurse, in any practice setting, may be the health care professional most likely to be in a position to provide this information and refer the patient for treatment.

SUMMARY

THE CASE OF GERALD M

Mr. M, a widowed Caucasian male, age 93 years, felt very out of place at his first community meeting on the psychiatric ward, surrounded as he was by young, acting out, and disorganized patients. Moreover, he was feeling shame that, as he put it, "I should come to this, a psycho ward, after all I have lived through." His admission to a psychiatric unit had been arranged for him involuntarily. He was made a legal ward for danger to self after he had overdosed on his antihypertensives. His nephew had discovered him unconscious at home and called the ambulance. For the first few meetings, during mandatory group therapy sessions and individual treatment sessions with his therapist, Mr. M sat mute and embittered. Gradually, he shared with the group the events that had led to his suicide attempt, although he continued to deny that he had an illness and insisted that his life was over and in attempting to take his own life he was merely "finishing what nature forgot."

Mr. M had been married for 71 years, had no children, and had been a successful businessman until he retired at age 81. His wife died 4 years earlier. By this time, all of the couple's friends had also died, as had most of their extended family. Mr. M, at the encouragement of his nephew, had sold his home and moved into a retirement community. He later recalled that this had been a "mistake." In his home at least, Mr. M recalled, "I had memories of my wife and our life in every room—in the retirement home I had nothing, I was a fish out of water." Mr. M's wife had been the affect-bearer and social contact of the couple and without her Mr. M did not know or care to learn how to connect with people or make friends. After a period of despondency, Mr. M contacted his other remaining relative, a brother in New Hampshire, who was a year older. The brother, with whom Mr. M had had little contact since his move to the West Coast 60 years before, encouraged Mr. M to return to New Hampshire. The two brothers could live out their remaining years together on the ancestral New England family farm. Mr. M kept his retire-

ment residence but packed most of his belongings and moved east. Four months after his arrival at the family farm, his older brother married a neighbor woman who was then 79 years old. Mr. M felt that he "would be a third leg, I would be in the way of their honeymoon." So he returned to his retirement apartment, where he became increasingly depressed, finally deciding that he had outlived his usefulness and purpose.

Since Mr. M had no major physical illnesses, except for mild hypertension, he was started on antidepressants after a thorough medical workup. Slowly, as the medication began to take effect, he was able to respond to the psychotherapy of the milieu and his individual treatment. He began to believe that he still had value as a person and was tentatively able to form new bonds with people, particularly his therapist and a few of the younger patients on the ward. He was discharged with a plan that he continue as an outpatient with his therapist and remain on medications. One year after hospitalization, he was doing well and had come to be more connected with his nephew and nephew's family. He continued to believe that his longevity was an accident of nature, but he no longer felt despondent or alone. As of this writing he was volunteering 1 day a week at an outpatient clinic as a clerk.

This case has been selected to illustrate that depression is a treatable illness, with an optimistic prognosis at any age.

References

Beck, AT, & Greenberg, RL (1974): *Coping with Depression.* New York, Institute for Rational-Emotive Therapy.

Becker, J (1977): *Affective Disorders.* Morristown, NJ, General Learning Press.

Berry, JM, Storandt, M, & Coyne, A (1984): Age and sex differences in somatic complaints associated with depression. *J Geront,* 39:465–467.

Blaine, JD (1986): Electroconvulsive therapy and cognitive function. *Hosp Community Psychiatry,* 37:15–16.

Blazer, DG (1982): *Depression in Late Life.* St. Louis, CV Mosby.

Blazer, D, Hughes, DC, & George, LK (1987): The epidemiology of depression in an elderly community population. *Gerontologist,* 27:281–286.

Borson, S, Barnes, RA, Kukull, WA, et al. (1986): Symptomatic depression in elderly medical outpatients. 1. Prevalence, demography, and health service utilization. *J Am Geriatr Soc,* 34:341–347.

Bromberg, S, & Cassel, CK (1983): Suicide in the elderly: The limits of paternalism. *J Am Geriatr Soc,* 31:698–703.

Brown, G, Harris, T, & Peto, J (1973): Life events and

psychiatric disorders. Part 2. Nature of causal link. *Psychol Med*, 3:159–176.

Brown, RP, Sweeney, J, Loutsch, E, et al. (1984): Involutional melancholia revisited. *Am J Psychiatry*, 141:24–28.

Brown, RP, Kocsis, JH, Glick, ID, et al. (1984): Efficacy and feasiblity of high dose tricyclic antidepressant treatment in elderly delusional depressives. *J Clin Psychopharmacol*, 4:311–314.

Burns, DD, & Beck, A (1980): Cognitive behavior modification of mood disorders. *In* Forest, JP, and Kathjen, DP (eds): *Cognitive Behavior Therapy Research and Application*. New York, Plenum Press.

Butler, R (1963): The life review: An interpretation of reminiscence in the aged. *Psychiatry*, 26(1):65–76.

Clark, DC, Cavanaugh, SJ, & Gibbons, RD (1983): The core symptoms of depression in medical and psychiatric patients. *J Nerv Ment Dis*, 171:705–713.

Cohen, GD (1982): The older person, the older patient, and the mental health system. *Hosp Community Psychiatry*, 33:101–104.

Diagnostic and Statistical Manual of Mental Disorders (DSM III-R) (1987): Washington, DC, American Psychiatric Association.

Dohrenwend, B, & Dohrenwend, BP (1981): Socioeconomic factors, stress, and psychopathology. *Am J Community Psychol*, 9:128–164.

Epstein, L (1976): Depression in the elderly. *J Gerontol*, 31:278–282.

Fava, GA, & Sonino, N (1987): The use of antidepressants in the medically ill. *Psychiatric Ann*, 17:42–44.

Field, WE, Jr (1985): Physical causes of depression. *J Psychosoc Nurs*, 23:7–11.

Frances, A, & Teusink, P (1984): Elderly patients' confusion confounds diagnoses and treatment of depression. *Hosp Community Psychiatry*, 35:1091–1093.

Fry, PS (1986): *Depression, Stress, and Adaptations in the Elderly: Psychological Assessment and Intervention*. Rockville, MD, Aspen.

Gaitz, CM (1974): Barriers to the delivery of psychiatric services to the elderly. *Gerontologist*, 14:210–214.

Gallagher, DG (1986): The Beck Depression Inventory and older adults: Review of its development and utility. *Clin Gerontol*, 5:149–161.

Gallagher, DE, & Thompson, LW (1983): Effectiveness of psychotherapy for both endogenous and non-endogenous depression in older adult outpatients. *J Gerontol*, 38:707–711.

Georgotas, A, McCue, RE, Hapiworth, BF, et al. (1982): Comparative efficacy and safety of MAOIs versus TCAs in treating depression in the elderly. *Biol Psychiatry*, 21:1155–1166.

Goldsmith, HF, Kramer, M, Brenner, B, et al. (1986): Strategies for investigating effects of residential context. A study of depressed mood and major depression. *Res Aging*, 8:609–633.

Goldstrom, ID, Burns, BJ, Kessler, LG, et al. (1987): Mental health services use by elderly adults in a primary care setting. *J Gerontol*, 42:147–153.

Gurland, BJ (1980): The assessment of the mental health status of older adults. *In* Birren, JE, & Sloane, RB (eds): *Handbook of Mental Health and Aging*. Englewood Cliffs, NJ, Prentice-Hall.

Gurland, BJ, & Cross, P (1982): The epidemiology of psychopathology in old age: Some clinical implications. *Psychiatr Clin North Am*, 5:11–26.

Gurland, BJ, Golden, R, Lantagua, R, et al. (1984): The overlap between physical conditions and depression in the elderly: A key to improvement in service delivery. *In* Aronowitz, E, & Bromberg, EM: *Mental Health and Long-Term Physical Illness*. New York, Prodist.

Hamilton, M (1960): A rating scale for depression. *J Neurol Neurosurg Psychiatry*, 23:56–62.

Hedlund, JL, & Vieweg, BW (1979): The Hamilton Rating Scale for Depression: A comprehensive review. *J Operational Psychiatry*, 10:149–165.

Herr, JJ, & Weakland, JH (1979): *Counseling Elders and Their Families*. New York, Springer, 45–59.

Holahan, CK, & Holahan, CJ (1987): Self-efficacy, social support and depression in aging: A longitudinal view. *J Gerontol*, 42:65–68.

Jenike, MA (1985): *Handbook of Geriatric Psychopharmacology*. Littleton, MA, PSG, 51–67.

Keith PI (1987): Depressive symptoms among younger and older couples. *Gerontologist*, 27:605–610.

Klerman, GL (1983): Problems in the definition and diagnosis of depression. *In* Lawrence, B, & Haug, M (eds): *Depression and Aging: Causes, Care and Consequences*. New York, Springer.

Knoben, JE, & Anderson, PO (eds) (1982): *Handbook of Clinical Drug Data*. Hamilton, IL, Drug Intelligence Publications, 482–488.

LaRue, A (1982): Memory loss and aging distinguishing dementia from benign senescent forgetfulness and depressive pseudodementia. *Psychiatr Clin North Am*, 5:89–103.

Lasoski, MC (1986): Reasons for low utilization of mental health services by the elderly. *Clin Gerontol*, 5:1–18.

Lazarus, LW, Newton, N, Cohler, B, et al. (1987): Frequency and presentation of depressive symptoms in patients with primary degenerative dementia. *Am J Psychiatry*, 144:41–45.

Lehman, HE (1982): Affective disorders in the aged. *Psychiatr Clin North Am*, 5:27–41.

Lieberman, ML (1983): Social contexts of depression. *In* Lawrence, B, & Haug, M (eds): *Depression and Aging: Causes, Care and Consequences*. New York, Springer.

Manton, KG, Blazer, DM, & Woodbury, MA (1987): Suicide in middle age and later life: Sex and specific life tables and cohort analysis. *J Gerontol*, 42:219–227.

Meyers, BS (1987): Late-life depression and delusions. *Hosp Community Psychiatry*, 38:573–574.

Parkes, CM, & Weiss, RS (1983): *Recovery from Bereavement*. New York, Basic Books.

Paykel, E, & Meyers, J (1969): Life events and depression. *Arch Gen Psychiatry*, 21:753–760.

Pfeiffer, E (1977): Psychopathology and social pathology. *In* Birren, JE, & Schaie, K (eds): *Handbook of the Psychology of Aging*. New York, Van Nostrand Reinhold.

Pitt, B (1982): *Psychogeriatrics: An Introduction to the Psychiatry of Old Age*. London, Churchill Livingstone.

Prien, RF, Blaine, JD, & Levine, J (1985): Antidepressant drug therapy: The role of the new antidepressants. *Hosp Community Psychiatry*, 36:513–516.

Reding, M, Haycox, J, & Blaiss, J (1985): Depression in

patients referred to a dementia clinic. *Arch Neurol, 42*:894–896.

Reifler, BV, Larson, E, Teri, L, et al: (1986): Dementia of the Alzheimer's type and depression. *J Am Geriatr Soc, 34*:855–859.

Risse, SC, Bertman, BD, & Brinkley, JR (1985): Evaluation of long-term use of antidepressant medication. *Hosp Community Psychiatry, 36*:1215–1216.

Roth, PA (1983a): Aging and death: Psychosocial perspectives. *In* Hall, B (ed): *Mental Health and the Elderly.* New York, Grune & Stratton.

Roth, PA (1983b): Aging and death: Ethical perspectives. *In* Hall, B (ed): *Mental Health and the Elderly.* New York, Grune & Stratton.

St. Pierre, J, Craven, RF, & Bruno, P (1985): Late life depression: A guide for assessment. *J Gerontol Nurs, 12*:5–10.

Salzman, C (1982): Key concepts in geriatric psychopharmacology. *Psychiatr Clin North Am, 5*:181–188.

Shamoian, CA (1985): Assessing depression in elderly patients. *Hosp Community Psychiatry, 36*:338–339.

Small, GW, & Jarvik, LF (1982): Depression in the aged: A commentary. *Psychiatr Clin North Am, 5*:45–66.

Spar, JE, Fora, CV, & Liston, EH (1980): Hospital treatment of elderly neuropsychiatric patients: eleven statistical profiles of the first 122 patients in a new teaching ward. *J Am Geriatr Soc, 29*:539–543.

Stenback, A (1980): Depression and suicidal behavior in old age. *In* Birren, JE, & Sloan, B (eds): *Handbook of Mental Health and Aging.* Englewood Cliffs, NJ, Prentice-Hall.

Sternberg, DE, & Jarvik, M (1976): Memory functions in depression. *Arch Gen Psychiatry, 33*:219–224.

Stever, JL, Mintz, J, Hammen, C, et al. (1984): Cognitive-behavioral and psychodynamic group psychotherapy in treatment of geriatric depression. *J Consult Clin Psychol, 52*:180–189.

Stuart, GW (1981): Role strain and depression: A causal inquiry. *J Psychosoc Nurs Ment Health Serv, 19*:20–28.

Templer, DI, & Cappelletty, GG (1986): Suicide in the elderly: Assessment and intervention. *Clin Gerontol, 5*:475–485.

Teri, L (1984): Assessing depression in patients with senile dementia of the Alzheimer's type. Paper presented at the 35th Annual Scientific Meeting of the Gerontological Society of America, New Orleans.

Thomas, MD, Sanger, E, & Whitney, JD (1986): Nursing approach of depression. *J Psychosoc Nurs Ment Health Serv, 24*:6–12.

Thompson, LW, & Gallagher, DG (1984): Efficacy of psychotherapy in late life depression. *Adv Behav Res Ther, 6*:127–139.

Verwoerdt, A (1976): *Clinical Geropsychiatry.* Baltimore, Waverly Press, 189–191.

Waxman, HM, McCreary, G, Weiniet, RM, et al. (1985): A comparison of somatic complaints among depressed and non-depressed older persons. *Gerontologist, 25*:507–510.

Waxman, HM, Carner, EA, & Klein, M (1984): Under-utilization of mental health professions by community elderly. *Gerontologist, 24*:23–30.

Weiss, IK, Nagel, CL, & Aronson, MR (1986): Applicability of depression scales in the old person. *J Am Geriatr Soc, 34*:215–218.

Wells, CE (1979): Pseudodementia. *Am J Psychiatry, 136*:895–900.

White, K, & Simpson, G (1987): Treatment-resistant depression. *Psychiatr Ann, 17*:274–278.

Williams, JB, & Skodol-Wilson, H (1982): A psychiatric nursing perspective on DSM-III. *J Psychosoc Nurs Ment Health Serv, 20*:14–20.

Winograd, CH, & Jarvik, LF (1986): Physician management of the demented patient. *J Am Geriatr Soc 34*:295–308.

Yesavage, J, Brink, TL, Rose, T, et al. (1983a). The geriatric depression rating scale: Comparison with other self-report and psychiatric rating scales. *In* Crook, T, Ferris, S, & Barties, R (eds): *Assessment in Geriatric Psychopharmacology.* New Canaan, CT, Mark Powley.

Yesavage, JA, Brink, TL, Rose, T, et al. (1983b): Development and validation of a geriatric depression screening scale: A preliminary report. *J Psychiatr Res 17*:37–49.

Zarit, SH, Orr, NK, & Zarit, JM (1985): *The Hidden Victims of Alzheimer's Disease.* New York, New York University Press.

Zarit, SH (1980): Aging and mental disorders: Psychological approaches to assessment and treatment. New York, Free Press.

Zung, WK (1965): A self rating depression scale. *Arch Gen Psychiatry, 12*:63–70.

Zung, WK, & Zung, EM (1986): The use of the Zung Self-Rating Depression Scale in the elderly. *Clin Gerontol, 5*:137–148.

CHAPTER
24

Dementia and Delirium

HELEN D. DAVIES, R.N.C.S., M.S.

INTRODUCTION

Clinicians have long recognized that dementia is a common symptom of the elderly, but only recently has the condition been the subject of intensive systematic study (Schoenberg, 1986). A recent study by the United States Congress Office of Technology Assessment (Alzheimer's Research Review, 1987) projects that by the year 2040, an estimated 7.4 million people will be afflicted with some form of dementia. Similar trends are expected for many developed countries (Schoenberg, 1986; Rocca, Amaducci, Schoenberg, et al., 1986).

Dementia can be caused by more than 60 disorders (Katzman, 1986). Recognizing dementia is only the first step toward a plan for care. To care for the patient means also understanding the impact of the symptoms on the family and the environment. This chapter examines dementia as both a diagnostic and psychosocial entity involving the patient and family.

DEMENTIA: WHAT IT IS AND WHAT IT IS NOT

Dementia is a symptom complex characterized by intellectual deterioration occurring in the presence of a clear state of consciousness, which is severe enough to interfere with social or occupational function (Katzman, 1986). Dementia involves progressive deficits not only in memory but also in other cognitive areas,

455

such as language, perception, praxis, and learning, problem-solving, abstract thinking, and judgment. Personality characteristics are maintained or exaggerated in some patients and may be otherwise altered in others. Social withdrawal, fearfulness, and anxiety are common features. Paranoid symptoms and delusions can sometimes occur. Irritability, agitation, and verbal and physical aggression toward family members may develop as the dementia progresses and the individual experiences an increasing loss of control of the environment (Katzman, 1986; American Psychiatric Association [APA], 1980). A clear state of consciousness is an essential feature in establishing the diagnosis of dementia. Differentiating dementia from delirium, an acute condition in which the level of awareness fluctuates, is of vital importance (Albert, 1981; Sullivan & Fogel, 1986).

Prevalence

The prevalence of dementia increases with age. Community surveys demonstrate that 4.6% of individuals over 65 years of age have severe dementia and 10% have mild to moderate dementia, but the rates are quite different between the ages of 65 and 85 years. Severe dementia is thought to be present in less than 1% of those who are 65 years of age but in more than 15% of those who are over 85 years. In the age range of 75 to 85 years, severe dementia occurs as frequently as myocardial infarction (Katzman, 1986; Oxman, 1987). Documenting the onset of dementia, as is required for studies of incidence or survival, is difficult due to the slowly progressive nature of the condition. Mortality tabulations do not provide a reliable estimate, since deaths among demented individuals are often attributed to other underlying causes. Despite the prevalence of dementia in the elderly, the diagnosis is frequently missed (U'Ren, 1987). One study (McCartney & Palmateer, 1985) demonstrated that in patients over 65 years admitted to medical and surgical units, examining physicians missed diagnosing 79% of cognitive deficits. Since many patients in the early stages

of dementia may not be seen by a physician or are not diagnosed, the true magnitude of the problem may be underreported (U'Ren, 1987).

Typology of Dementias

Dementia can occur from a multitude of causes and is broadly classified into two main categories: reversible and irreversible. Table 24–1 shows the most common forms of dementia under those categories.

Within this framework some causes of dementia symptoms can be cured, others ameliorated, and others, given our current state of knowledge, are irreversible (Beck, Benson, Scheibel, et al., 1982). Data from studies of 406 hospitalized patients with a clinical presentation of dementia show that 80% were found to have irreversible forms of dementia, and 20% had potentially reversible forms (Smith, 1981; Wells, 1978). More than two-thirds of those with potentially reversible dementias showed improvement when treated. (See the section on progressive dementias for prognosis of specific dementias.)

Major Dementias in the Elderly

Currently it is estimated that there are more than 60 disorders causing dementia, with ac-

Table 24–1. REVERSIBLE AND IRREVERSIBLE CAUSES OF DEMENTIA

Potentially Reversible Causes	Probably Irreversible Causes
Depression ("pseudodementia")	Alzheimer's disease
Drug toxicity (including ETOH)	Pick's disease
Normal pressure hydrocephalus	Huntington's chorea
Resectable mass lesions	Multiple infarcts
Metabolic-endocrine derangements	Creutzfeldt-Jakob disease
Deficiency states (B_{12}, folate)	Associated immune disease syndrome
Brain disorders (infection, subdural hematoma, meningitis)	Amyotrophic lateral sclerosis (ALS)
Cardiopulmonary disorders	Marchiagava-Bignami disease
Generalized infections	Alcoholism
	Cerebrocerebellar degenerations

(Data from Beck, Benson, Scheibel, et al., 1982.)

quired immune deficiency syndrome being the latest cause identified. Alzheimer's disease (AD) accounts for approximately 50% to 60% of the cases, and vascular disease for approximately 10% to 20%; some patients may have both disorders. Intracranial masses cause an estimated 5%, alcoholic dementia an estimated 5% to 10%, normal pressure hydrocephaly (NPH) an estimated 6%, Huntington's chorea accounts for approximately 3%, and in 5% of the cases the cause remains unknown (Katzman, 1986; Cohen & Eisdorfer, 1986). Patients with depression may also appear demented on mental status examination, and it is important to rule out depression in establishing the cause of the dementia. Table 24–2 illustrates the relative incidence of various dementia-related diseases.

The most common dementias seen in the elderly are those associated with AD, multi-infarct disease (MID), and dementias secondary to drug toxicity and metabolic endocrine derangements.

The Progressive Dementias: Alzheimer's Disease, Multi-infarct Dementia, and Alcoholic Dementias

Alzheimer's Disease

Alzheimer's disease, named after Alois Alzheimer, who first described its neuropathology in 1907, is a neurologic disorder of the brain that occurs primarily in middle or late life, although it may occur earlier. Its primary characteristic is a progressive dementia. The pa-

Table 24–2. RELATIVE INCIDENCE OF DEMENTIA IN ASSOCIATED DISEASES

Cause	Percentage Having Dementia
Alzheimer's and related disorders	50%–60%
Multi-infarct dementia	10%–20%
Alcohol-related	5%–10%
Normal pressure hydrocephalus	6%
Tumor	5%
Huntington's chorea	3%
Unknown	5%

(Data from Katzman, 1986, and Cohen & Eisdorfer, 1986.)

thology includes degeneration and loss of nerve cells (neurons), particularly in those regions essential for memory and cognition, and the presence of neuritic plaques and neurofibrillary tangles. Aggregates of amyloid protein can be seen adjacent to and within blood vessels (Wurtman, 1985).

Alterations occur in the neurotransmitter levels, especially in the cholinergic system and frequently in the somatostatinergic and noradrenergic systems (Katzman, 1984; Constantinidis, 1984; Beck, et al., 1982; Lumpkin, Negro-Vilar, & McCann, 1981; Bondareff, 1984). Currently a definitive diagnosis of AD can be made only by examination of brain tissue obtained during either postmortem examination or brain biopsy. In the majority of cases the risks of brain biopsy far outweigh the benefits. Therefore, the diagnosis is made by exclusion, that is, systematically excluding all other possible causes of dementia. If the symptoms are progressive, follow a pattern over time, and are attributable to no other cause, a clinical diagnosis of probable AD is made. In patients with an atypical presentation, a diagnosis of possible AD may be made and the patient followed at regular intervals to assist in clarifying the diagnosis.

Incidence. The incidence of AD increases with age. Approximately 1% of persons over 65 years develop the disease each year (Sagar & Sullivan, 1988; Mortimer, Schuman, & French, 1981).

Theories of Causation. The cause of AD remains unknown. Several theories have been proposed and form the basis for current research.

Slow Virus Theory. The causes of most degenerative diseases are unknown. However, in three degenerative diseases of the central nervous system (CNS)—kuru, Creutzfeldt-Jakob disease, and the Gerstmann syndrome—transmissibility to animals has been demonstrated. These findings indicate that the cause must be an infectious agent, presumably a virus. The incubation period, roughly one-fourth of the affected individual's normal lifespan from time of exposure to the first appearance of clinical symptoms, has led to these viruses being labeled "slow viruses" (Wurtman, 1985; Pruisner, 1984). Researchers have further defined these agents as prions. In highly purified preparations of prions that contain the infectious agent, numerous rods have been observed. Because of the ultrastructural similarities between prion rods and purified amyloid, researchers speculate that a connection exists between these and AD. Collections of amyloid protein in the form of plaques have been observed in the brains of patients dying of kuru, Creutzfeldt-Jakob disease, and Gerstmann syndrome. One line of research involves exploring scrapie, a fatal, slowly progressive brain disease in sheep and goats. Amyloid plaques have been found in infected animals and the causative virus has been transmitted to other animals. Amyloid plaques are a constant feature in the brains of AD patients, but attempts to transmit the disease to animals have been unsuccessful. Several possibilities have been suggested for the lack of transmissibility: (1) the infectious agent does not replicate in animals; (2) the infectious agent is not transmissible to animals within the incubation times studied; (3) the infectious agent is not involved in the pathogenesis of AD.

Aluminum Theory. Some investigators have theorized that aluminum may contribute to the development of AD. Aluminum salts are present not only in aluminum cans and utensils but also in drinking water, medications, many processed foods, and the general environment. Injection of aluminum salts can generate neurofibrillary tangles in the brains of certain animals (Terry & Pena, 1965; Deary & Whalley, 1988). Aluminum has also been found to accumulate preferentially in human neurons with neurofibrillary tangles. Kidney dialysis patients who have had repeated dialysis treatments with solutions high in aluminum have developed irreversible dementia and have been found to have elevated brain aluminum levels. It is known that certain brain enzymes can be inhibited by aluminum. High aluminum levels have also been found in the brains of dementia patients in certain communities in Guam. The drinking water in these communities is known to have a lack of calcium, which seems to enhance the body's absorption of aluminum. Despite these findings, the evidence is inconclusive. It is unclear whether the association between aluminum and neurofibrillary tangles is causative or whether the neurofibrillary tangles, once formed, happen to have an affinity for aluminum. Tangles induced in animals have only one filament, unlike the paired helical filaments found in Alzheimer's patients. It is possible that aluminum in itself may not be responsible for the disease but its presence may contribute to the disease process in individuals predisposed to the disease or exposed to other causative factors (Deary & Whalley, 1988).

Cholinergic Theory. In 1976, two groups of researchers reported the first clear biochemical abnormality associated with AD. Levels of choline acetyltransferase (CAT) were reduced by as much as 90% in the hippocampus and cerebral cortex of Alzheimer's patients. CAT acts as a catalyst in the synthesis of acetylcholine. The loss of CAT activity reflects the loss of cholinergic, or acetylcholine-releasing, nerve terminals in these areas of the brain. The cholinergic terminals in the hippocampus are vital in the formation of memory, thus accounting for one of the primary symptoms of the disease. Alterations have also been found in 15 other neurotransmitters, including norepinephrine, serotonin, and somatostatin. These findings have suggested possibilities for therapy. Drugs that can restore the acetylcholine levels in Alzheimer's patients may be effective in the same way as L-dopa has been in the management of Parkinson's disease. Attempts to treat patients with supplemental choline or with purified lecithin have so far been unsuccessful in improving behaviors associated with AD or in slowing the rate of progression of the disease (Wurtman, 1985).

Autoimmune Theory. AD is clearly associated with abnormal protein structures. The pathologic findings of neurofibrillary tangles and amyloid plaques reflect an accumulation of protein not normally found in the brain. Investigators have reported success in producing antibodies to these abnormal proteins in the brain. One mechanism proposed for explaining the pathologic changes found in this disease is a kind of autocannibalism, in which the body destroys its own neuronal tissues. Immune response theories suggest that the resistance of brain cells to degeneration is destroyed, allowing a selective loss of cells in regions of the brain that control memory for recent events. Genetic explanations suggest that some individuals carry an increased liability for this selective degeneration in their chromosomes, which in later life may fail to regulate the production of vital substances in these brain cells (Wurtman, 1985).

Trauma Theory. Several studies have investigated the role of trauma in the development of dementia (Heyman, Wilkinson, Stafford, et al., 1984; French, Schuman, Mortimer, et al., 1985; Mortimer, French, Hutton, et al., 1985). It has long been known that boxers develop a form of dementia known as dementia pugilistica. Researchers have reported a higher incidence of AD in individuals with a history of head trauma sufficient to cause loss of consciousness. Individuals with head trauma sustained 30 years before had a 30% higher incidence of AD than those without a history of head trauma. One suggestion has been that the trauma may have caused microscopic damage to the blood-brain barrier, which then leaves the individual vulnerable to either penetration by a slow virus or environmental toxins. Further investigation is necessary before this theory can be assigned a definite role in the development of AD.

Genetic Theory. Patients with Down's syndrome who live past the age of 40 years almost always show changes similar to those of individuals with AD. The presence of plaques, tangles, loss of CAT, and abnormal amyloid protein found in the neocortex and hippocampus of these patients has led to the speculation that genetic and chromosomal factors play a role in the development of AD. Lending evidence to this theory is the presence of an apparently autosomal-dominant pattern of inheritance in a small percentage of families with AD. The heritability of AD has been studied by investigators in many countries. The results show an unmistakable connection, demonstrating that some first-degree relatives of Alzheimer's patients show a higher incidence of

the disorder than would be expected in the general population.

Other forms of hereditary transmission are not as high in frequency, nor do they affect each generation in a predictable autosomal-dominant pattern. Nevertheless, a number of researchers feel that genetic factors possibly play a significant role in over one-half of the individuals who eventually develop the disease. The variations in the pattern of transmissibility point to a strong probability that there are several different modes of genetic transmission or even subtypes of the disease itself (Bondareff, Mountjoy, Roth, et al., 1987). Other theorists believe that the susceptibility for the disease is inherited, but the actual development depends on other factors. It may require an interaction between the gene for the disease and other factors or chance events, such as gene copying errors, infectious agents, ionizing radiation, nutritional deficiencies, exogenous toxins, or exposure to toxic metabolites over time, to produce clinical manifestations. While many researchers believe that age and heritability are the two most closely associated risk factors in the development of AD, neither definitive markers nor abnormal chromosomes have yet been identified. The search for a genetic marker continues to be a primary focus for many researchers.

Clinical Presentation of Alzheimer's Disease

Progression of the Disease. AD is a progressive neurologic disorder that has an insidious onset and progresses over time, leaving the individual in a vegetative state. The progression of the disease involves personality changes, mental status changes, social role dysfunction, difficulty with activities of daily living, speech deterioration, visual perceptual deficits, incontinence, and gait disorders.

AD has an insidious onset with gradual progression of a wide variety of symptoms. Lapses of recent memory, decreased ability to learn, altered attention span, agnosia, and lack of spontaneity are among the most typical initial changes. Delusions have been reported in 13% to 53% of AD patients. These tend to be primarily paranoid in nature, involving misbeliefs about infidelity or theft (Cummings

& Benson, 1983; 1984). In approximately 10% of patients there may be an atypical presentation. For these patients, the first presenting symptoms may be difficulty with word finding, agnosia, visuospatial deficits, apraxia, personality changes, and pure memory loss (Katzman, 1986; Shuttleworth, 1984; Crystal, Horoupian, Katzman, et al., 1982). These focal symptoms may occur many years prior to the typical generalized progression seen in most AD patients. The rate of deterioration differs among patients and within patients over time. The Global Deterioration Scale (GDS) developed by Reisberg (Reisberg, Ferris, & de Leon, 1982) is useful for measuring the changes and identifying the stage of the disease (Table 24–3).

Interview Behaviors in Alzheimer's Disease. The patients with AD make continuous attempts to answer questions, whereas patients with depression complain of memory deficits and inability to recall but, if encouraged, may do well on testing. Patients with early dementia are often aware of and frightened by their deficits. They frequently try hard to minimize or rationalize their errors in testing. Denial, confabulation, perseveration, and avoidance of questions are typical interview behaviors of the patient in the later stages of AD.

Prognosis in Alzheimer's Disease. Patients with AD have a reduced life expectancy (Chandra, Bharucha, & Schoenberg, 1986; Schoenberg, Okazaki, & Kokmen, 1981). The disease may have a course as short as 18 months or as long as 27 years, but the average duration of illness is about 10 to 12 years (McLachlan, Dalton, Galin, et al., 1984). The leading cause of death in patients with AD has been reported to be respiratory conditions or bronchopneumonia. Chandra and associates (1986) reported that patients with AD are at greater risk for infections, trauma, nutritional deficiency, Parkinson's disease, and epilepsy.

While there is no cure for AD at this time there seem to be many preventable and treatable conditions that could, with appropriate management, extend the life-span and improve the quality of life in this population (Chandra, et al., 1986).

Multi-infarct Dementia

Definition. Dementia resulting from vascular diseases that cause multiple small or large cerebral infarcts is labeled multi-infarct dementia (MID). Multiple cerebral infarcts can produce a condition in which dementia can be the dominant symptom. The onset is generally acute. Clinicians report focal neurologic deficits, a stepwise deterioration, and, frequently, hypertension (Erkinjuntti, 1987; Read & Jarvik, 1984; Albert, 1981).

Incidence and Prevalence. As with most causes of dementia, the incidence of cerebrovascular disease increases with age. Neuropathologic studies show that approximately 12.5% of dementias in the elderly are caused by MID and 13.6% by a combination of both MID and AD or a mixed dementia (MIX) (Meyer, Judd, Tamaklna, et al., 1986).

Theories of Causation. Atherosclerosis is related to the pathogenesis of cerebral infarcts (Hachinski, Lassen, & Marshall, 1974). Cerebral aneurysms or arteriovenous malformation (AVM) are more likely than dementia to result in a focal syndrome (Read & Jarvik, 1984).

Lacunar State. A small focal infarct resulting from occlusion of a branch artery that penetrates the brain is called a lacuna. The basal ganglia, thalamus, pons, and internal capsule are particularly vulnerable to these infarcts. Lacunae are frequently too small to be seen on computed tomography (CT), but an accumulation of these lesions can cause progressive mental deterioration, similar to the process of MID. When the infarcts are limited only to subcortical white matter, the condition is referred to as Binswanger's disease. Hypertension is thought to be the major cause for both the lacunar state and Binswanger's disease (Read & Jarvik, 1984).

Multi-emboli. Although any vessel may yield emboli, studies indicate that extracranial arteries and the heart are most likely to produce the widely distributed lesions that produce MID (Hachinski, et al., 1974; Barnett, 1983).

Vasculitis. This may be infectious, idiopathic, granulomatous, or the result of toxins or immune complex disease. Lupus erythematosus is one of the most frequent causes of vascular lesions (Read & Jarvik, 1984).

Table 24–3. GLOBAL DETERIORATION SCALE (GDS) FOR AGE-ASSOCIATED COGNITIVE DECLINE AND ALZHEIMER'S DISEASE

GDS Stage	Clinical Phase	Clinical Characteristics	Diagnosis
1 = No cognitive decline	Normal	No subjective complaints of memory deficit. No memory deficit evident on clinical interview.	Normal
2 = Very mild cognitive decline	Forgetfulness	Subjective complaints of memory deficits. No objective deficits in employment or social situations. Appropriate concern with respect to symptomatology.	Normal aged
3 = Mild cognitive decline	Early confusional	Earliest clear-cut deficits. Decreased performance in demanding employment and social settings. Objective evidence of memory deficit obtained only with an intensive interview. Mild to moderate anxiety accompanies symptoms.	Compatible with incipient Alzheimer's disease
4 = Moderate cognitive decline	Late confusional	Clear-cut deficit on careful interview. Inability to perform complex tasks. Denial is dominant defense mechanism. Flattening of affect and withdrawal from challenging situations occur.	Mild Alzheimer's disease
5 = Moderately severe cognitive decline	Early dementia	Patients can no longer survive without some assistance. Patients are unable during interview to recall a major relevant aspect of their current lives. Persons at this stage retain knowledge of many major facts regarding themselves and others. They invariably know their own names and generally know their spouse's and children's names. They require no assistance with toileting or eating but may have some difficulty choosing the proper clothing to wear.	Moderate Alzheimer's disease
6 = Severe cognitive decline	Middle dementia	May occasionally forget the name of the spouse upon whom they are entirely dependent for survival. Will be largely unaware of all recent events and experiences in their lives. Will require some assistance with activities of daily living. Personality and emotional changes occur.	Moderately severe Alzheimer's disease
7 = Very severe cognitive decline	Late dementia	All verbal abilities are lost. Frequently there is no speech at all—only grunting. Incontinent of urine; requires assistance toileting and feeding. Loses basic psychomotor skills (e.g., ability to walk).	Severe Alzheimer's disease

(From Reisberg, B, Ferris, SH, de Leon, MJ, et al. (1982): The global deterioration scale for assessment of primary dementia. *Am J Psychiatry, 139*:1136–1139. Copyright 1982 by the American Psychiatric Association. Reprinted by permission.)

Blood Dyscrasias. These are uncommon but have been known to cause vascular lesions (Read & Jarvik, 1984).

Hypoperfusion. Hypoperfusion of the brain, from systemic hypotension or occlusion of a major vessel, can cause damage to those areas of the brain perfused by the most distal vessels (Read & Jarvik, 1984).

Anoxic Episodes. Anoxic episodes resulting from cardiac arrest, anesthesia, or other similar causes can result in neuronal loss leading to dementia, but without the presence of infarcts (Read & Jarvik, 1984).

Table 24–4 lists theories of causation in MID.

Cerebral aneurysms or AVM, which are other causes of stroke, are more likely to result in a focal syndrome rather than dementia (Read & Jarvik, 1984).

Clinical Presentation. Patients with MID have a stepwise decline with a fluctuating clinical course. The onset tends to be acute with focal neurologic signs and symptoms. A

Table 24–4. MULTI-INFARCT DEMENTIA: THEORIES OF CAUSATION

Cause	Theory
Lacunae	Small focal infarcts resulting from occlusion of branch arteries that penetrate the brain. Accumulation of these lesions can cause progressive mental deterioration.
Binswanger's disease	Infarcts are limited to the subcortical white matter. Hypertension is thought to be major cause.
Multiemboli	Any vessel can cause emboli but extracranial arteries and the heart are most likely to produce the widely distributed lesions that produce MID.
Vasculitis	May be idiopathic, infectious, granulomatous, or the result of toxins or immune complex. Lupus erythematosus is one of the most frequent causes.
Blood dyscrasias	Uncommon, but have been known to cause vascular lesions.
Hypoperfusion	Systemic hypotension, or occlusion of a major vessel, can cause damage to areas of the brain perfused by the most distal vessels.
Anoxic episodes	Caused by cardiac arrest, anesthesia, or other similar causes resulting in neuronal loss leading to dementia without the presence of infarctions.

(Data from Read & Jarvik, 1984.)

history of transient ischemic attacks (TIAs), hypertension, strokes, diabetes mellitus, vasculitis, and cardiac arrhythmias is frequently associated with MID. Family history of stroke or cardiovascular disease may be present (Read & Jarvik, 1984).

Emotional lability, depression, and crying spells are often seen. Delusions may occur. Recent studies have found delusions in up to 40% of MID patients (Cummings, Miller, Hill, et al., 1987). Mental status examination is very important in delineating patchy deficits. Dysarthria, hemi-neglect of visual space, movement disorders, or a subtle paresis may be evident. Inability to distinguish left from right, to reproduce two-dimensional drawings, and to identify letters traced on the hand may exist. Focal slowing may be seen on the electroencephalogram (EEG) in patients with infarcts too small to be visible on CT (Read & Jarvik, 1984; Benson, Cummings, & Tsai, 1982). The Hachinski Ischemia Rating is a useful tool in differentiating AD from MID. A score of 4 or below is considered indicative of AD, whereas a score of 4 or above is an indication of MID or possibly a combination of both, MIX (see Table 24–5).

Course of the Disease. The course of MID can be intermittent and fluctuating, punctuated by episodes of clouded sensorium. Patients may maintain a plateau for long periods of time. Hypertension is the most important risk factor for stroke in patients with MID. Specific cardiovascular diagnosis and management are the key to arresting progression and reducing mortality (Read & Jarvik, 1984; Hachinski, et al., 1974). When deterioration proceeds rapidly following a single cerebrovascular accident (CVA), it is probable that there has been slowly advancing subclinical change, now potentiated by infarction, which has served to push the neuronal damage beyond the threshold point.

Prognosis. Chances of social survival are better in patients with MID and MIX than in those with AD. Treatment of the underlying illness and the secondary psychiatric and medical conditions can substantially improve the prognosis (Read & Jarvik, 1984). Some people with MID may benefit from anticoagulation therapy or surgery. Some cases of MID are remediable and, occasionally, reversible (Meyer, et al., 1986).

Alcoholic Dementia

Definition. Alcohol abuse gives rise to a large and diverse group of mental disorders. The effects of alcohol on the brain range from acute reversible conditions, such as acute intoxication, alcoholic hallucinosis, and pathologic intoxication, to withdrawal states, such as delirium tremens and withdrawal seizures, to chronic, largely irreversible conditions reflecting a long-term derangement of metabo-

Table 24–5. HACHINSKI ISCHEMIC RATING

Instructions: Record the presence or absence of the clinical features of dementia listed below and add the point values assigned each feature (value in parenthesis) whenever "Present" is checked. Summation of points produces an Ischemic Score. Scores of < + 4 indicate patients with pure primary degenerative dementia (Alzheimer's type dementia). Scores of > 4 indicate patients with multi-infarct dementia (MID).

Feature	Absent	Present	Point Value
1. Abrupt feature	_____	_____	2
2. Stepwise deterioration	_____	_____	1
3. Fluctuating course	_____	_____	2
4. Nocturnal confusion	_____	_____	1
5. Relative preservation of personality	_____	_____	1
6. Depression	_____	_____	1
7. Somatic concern	_____	_____	1
8. Emotional incontinence	_____	_____	1
9. History of hypertension	_____	_____	1
10. History of strokes	_____	_____	2
11. History of associated atherosclerosis	_____	_____	1
12. Focal neurological symptoms	_____	_____	2
13. Focal neurological signs	_____	_____	2

(From Hachinski, VC, Iliff, LD, Zilhka, E, et al. (1975): Cerebral blood flow in dementia. *Arch Neurol*, 32:632–637. Copyright 1975, American Medical Association.)

lism, as seen in Wernicke-Korsakoff's syndrome, alcoholic pellagra, and hepatic encephalopathy. This latter group of conditions can result in a form of dementia with impaired memory, language disorders, confusion and disorganization, and general decline in social and occupational functioning (Victor & Banker, 1978).

The role of alcohol is considered to be secondary in the pathogenesis of these dementias. The adverse effects on the nervous system are the result of nutritional and liver diseases that are engendered by chronic abuse of alcohol. Alcoholic dementias are thought to differ in this respect from other pathologic intoxication states that are due directly to the effect of alcohol on the central nervous system or result from withdrawal of alcohol following a period of chronic intoxication (Victor & Banker, 1978). Wernicke-Korsakoff's syndrome (amnesic or amnestic confabulatory psychosis), alcoholic pellagra, and hepatic encephalopathy constitute a small percentage of the alcohol-induced dementias, but they have a high mortality rate and are capable of producing chronic crippling effects.

Wernicke-Korsakoff's Psychosis: Etiology. Thiamine deficiency is the specific nutritional factor thought to be responsible for this condition. The lesions responsible for memory loss are structural rather than biochemical. Korsakoff's psychosis is most often associated with alcohol but may be a symptom of various other disorders as well (i.e., lesions, tumors, herpes simplex encephalitis). A transient version can occur in patients with temporal lobe epilepsy, concussion, and transient global amnesia.

Clinical Presentation. In the alcoholic patient, Korsakoff's syndrome (or Korsakoff's disease) usually begins with an acute attack of Wernicke's disease (global confusion, apathy combined with ataxia, and ocular abnormalities). With adequate diet and thiamine, patients become increasingly alert, responsive, and gradually less confused, with the major remaining impairment being a decreased retentive memory.

Korsakoff's and Wernicke's are not separate diseases but are instead stages of one syndrome. The syndrome is diagnosed as Wernicke's with or without Korsakoff's or Wernicke-Korsakoff's, if both components are present. Korsakoff's disease is unique and is characterized by two abnormalities that always occur together—retrograde amnesia (losing information acquired in the past) and anterograde amnesia (decreased ability to acquire new information). Confabulation is not consistently present and is not required for diagnosis.

Retentive memory is impaired out of proportion to other cognitive functions in an otherwise alert and responsive patient. Other cognitive functions (those not memory-dependent) may be impaired but to a lesser degree. Limited insight, apathetic behavior, inertia, and indifference to persons and events may also be present.

Neuropathologic findings include lesions in the thalamus, hypothalmus, midbrain, pons, and medulla, with symmetrical and paraventricular distribution. Advanced lesions are characterized by virtually complete necrosis of tissue. Hemorrhages are present in only a small proportion of cases (Victor & Banker, 1978).

Course of the Disease. Improvement begins anywhere from a few weeks to 3 months after treatment, and the maximum degree of recovery may not be obtained for a year or longer. Recovery proceeds very slowly and is governed by the inherent slowness of recovery of damaged brain tissue and the extent of damage present.

Prognosis. Once Korsakoff's disease symptoms are established, complete or almost complete recovery occurs in approximately 20% of patients. A few patients show no recovery. The majority fall somewhere between slight and almost complete recovery (Victor & Banker, 1978). The syndrome is preventable.

Alcohol-induced Pellagra. Pellagra affects the skin, nervous system, and hematopoietic system, but its major symptoms are in the cerebral area, causing a dementia syndrome.

Theories of Causation. Pellagra is caused by a deficiency of niacin or tryptophan, an amino acid precursor. In the alcoholic patient it is the result of poor nutritional status over time.

Clinical Presentation. Insomnia, fatigue, nervousness, depression, apathy, and memory impairment are the presenting symptoms. In some cases acute confusional psychosis dominates the clinical picture. These neurologic disturbances are the result of brain lesions.

Course of the Disease. Left untreated, the condition can be fatal. Aggressive treatment can produce considerable improvement. Neurologic disturbances resulting from brain lesions may be resistant to treatment (Victor & Banker, 1978).

Prognosis. The degree of improvement is dependent on the severity of the brain lesions.

Hepatic Encephalitis. The most common of all cerebral lesions producing a dementia syndrome in alcoholic patients are those induced by hepatic failure. Hepatic encephalopathy can be either acute or chronic.

Theories of Causation. Chronic abuse of alcohol, resulting in liver disease, with decreased liver metabolism and resultant increased ammonemia, is the cause of this condition.

Clinical Presentation. In the acute phase, there is derangement of consciousness, presenting first as confusion, with either decreased or increased psychomotor activity leading to progressive drowsiness, stupor, and eventually coma. The confusional state is frequently combined with intermittent periods of sustained motor contractions resulting in an irregular flapping movement of the outstretched hands, known as asterixis. EEG activity is abnormal, with paroxysms of bilaterally synchronous slow waves in the delta range.

Course of the Disease. Symptoms evolve over a period of days or weeks, are often fatal, or, after reaching a certain stage, can sometimes regress completely. In some patients symptoms may stop short of coma and in others they may become chronic in nature, resulting in mood, personality, and intellectual changes over months or years.

Prognosis. Symptoms are essentially reversible if treatment is aggressive and timely. Patients who survive an episode of hepatic coma are occasionally left with residual neurologic abnormalities, such as tremors of the head or arms, asterixis, grimacing ataxia, or decreased intellectual function. Symptoms may worsen with repeated comas.

Table 24–6 lists the alcoholic dementias.

Table 24–6. ALCOHOLIC DEMENTIAS

Disease	Cause	Treatment	Progression	Prognosis
Wernicke-Korsakoff's	Thiamine deficiency	Thiamine, adequate diet	With treatment improvement begins in a few weeks to 3 months. Recovery is slow, 1 year or longer.	Varies. Complete or almost complete recovery in about 20%. Small percentage show no recovery. Majority fall in between.
Alcohol-induced pellagra	Poor nutrition over time. Deficiency of niacin or tryptophan	Niacin, adequate diet	Degree of improvement depends on severity of brain lesions.	Aggressive treatment can produce considerable improvement. Fatal if untreated.
Hepatic encephalitis	Chronic alcoholism resulting in liver disease, leading to increased ammonemia	Treat liver disease	Symptoms evolve over days or weeks. Coma may occur. Symptoms may regress completely, become chronic, or worsen with repeated comas.	Symptoms are reversible if treatment is timely. Fatal if untreated.

The Dementia Workup

The workup for establishing a diagnosis of dementia consists of a history, physical and neurologic examinations, CT or magnetic resonance imaging (MRI), biochemical studies to rule out other causes of dementia, psychiatric assessment, and a full mental status examination (Katzman, 1981). Even with this extensive workup, it may not be possible to make a definitive diagnosis, and followup examinations of mental status may be required. A period of several months should be allowed between these evaluations to detect progression and emergence of symptoms.

Taking a History

In the early stages of a dementing illness, many patients maintain their social skills and conversational abilities. Patients may be unaware of symptoms or deny that there is a problem. It is essential when taking a history to have someone present who knows the patient well to verify the patient's responses and supply additional information. If possible, it is best to interview the patient with a family member present and also to see each separately. This gives the advantage of revealing the interactions between the patient and the family and also provides each with the opportunity to discuss information and concerns that they may be reluctant to divulge in the other's presence.

Interview Style. In working with this population it is of the utmost importance to be empathic, patient, and observant. Interviewers must wait for the patient's response to questions. Interviewers must *look as well as listen*, noting whether the patient is easily distracted, whether he or she can comprehend the question but is having difficulty with expressive speech. Does the person look depressed or restless and unable to sit still? Are there myoclonic movements, tremors, or gait disturbances?

Medications have long been known to cause fatigue, apathy, mental slowing, and confusion in the elderly (U'Ren, 1987). Many older individuals take multiple medications prescribed by several physicians and may also take several over-the-counter medications and large doses of vitamins. Compounding the problem may be forgetfulness for whether they have taken their medications and repeated inappropriate dosing with previously prescribed drugs. Taking a detailed inventory of medications is essential, but care must be taken to *ask both what prescribed medications the patient is taking, and also what other over-the-counter medications and vitamins he or she uses*. Many do not consider these preparations medications and will not report taking them unless specifically asked. Not only what is taken but how and when drugs are taken must be ascertained. A detailed medical and family history and review of systems is the basis for recognizing the presence of dementia and establishing its cause.

Questions for the History. Is there a history of hypertension, TIAs, syncopal episodes, strokes, or cardiovascular disease? Has the individual ever suffered a head injury? Was there a loss of consciousness associated with the injury, and if there was, how long did it last, was there a medical assessment done, a CT scan or MRI? Were there any long-term effects (amnesia, confusion, headaches, dizziness)? If living alone, is there any supervision? Have friends or neighbors expressed any concerns or noted any changes?

Is there a family history of dementia, depression, psychiatric illness, or other neurologic disorders? Many psychiatric illnesses, including depression and anxiety disorders, tend to run in families (U'Ren, 1987; Winokur, 1981). Individuals with a family history of Alzheimer's disease are at greater risk for developing the disease by age 85 years than are individuals without a family history (Heston, Mastri, Anderson, et al., 1981). A survey of psychiatric signs and symptoms should include an evaluation for depressive symptoms, a sad mood or affect, lack of energy, loss of interest in and inability to enjoy everyday activities and former interests, changes in sleep patterns, loss of appetite, and weight loss not attributable to a physiologic cause. Is there a past history of depression or other psychiatric disorders? If there is, what are the details regarding the diagnosis, treatment, and outcome? Most psychiatric disorders follow a pattern in the presenting symptoms, repetition of episodes, and response to treatment in an individual with a particular disorder. Obtaining this information will assist in clarifying the diagnosis and choice of therapeutic interventions.

Has the individual experienced any recent major losses, environmental changes, or traumas? Many individuals with early dementia manage to cover up their deficits until such time as there is a sudden change in their environment. Loss of a spouse, financial resources, or physical health can add a heavy emotional burden and heighten fears of dependency and loss of autonomy to already stressed and impaired people, pushing them into obvious confusion and bringing the existing symptoms to the family's attention (U'Ren, 1987).

Have there been any changes in memory, intellect, or personality? Memory deficit is one of the earliest signs of dementia, manifesting itself in the form of difficulty remembering dates, names, appointments, and the location of familiar household objects and personal effects. Changes in intellect and cognition can be seen in the decline of an individual's level of functioning. Inability to write a check, balance a bank statement, or manage finances may be seen in a formerly competent individual, as may difficulty cooking a full meal, doing the shopping, and managing everyday household affairs in a previously efficient homemaker. Changes in productivity, making inaccurate reports, and inability to solve problems or make appropriate decisions in a previously highly functioning employee are all early manifestations of cognitive decline. Social withdrawal and apathy are the most common early personality changes. Irritability, angry outbursts, suspiciousness, and lapses in judgment are also frequently seen in individuals with dementia (U'Ren, 1987; Katzman, 1986). Information about the individual's personality before the onset of illness should be obtained from family or close friends; patients are not always aware of these changes and cannot always give an accurate assessment.

When and where were the symptoms first noted? Establishing the date of onset of symptoms may be difficult. Patients are often not aware of the changes and family members may not note the early deficits or changes until the symptoms become more pronounced. Nevertheless, it is important to establish the date of onset as closely as possible with specific questions, especially when there may be more than one condition present. Did the memory loss come before the depression? Did the personality changes occur before or after the stroke? Asking the question, "Knowing what you now know about the individual's problems, think back and try to remember when you first may have seen changes but didn't think they were serious" is a good way to assist families in establishing a date of onset. Table 24–7 outlines some of the key questions asked in the dementia assessment.

Mental Status Examination

The mental status examination plays a key role in the diagnosis of dementia. It is especially important in the very early stages of impairment. Patients in the very early stages of cognitive decline may be able to carry on a normal conversation and answer questions about their personal history during an interview but show cognitive deficits on mental status examination (Sagar & Sullivan, 1988).

The main components of the mental status examination include orientation, memory, calculation, information and speech comprehension, concentration, and constructional ability. The goal is not only to identify the presence of cognitive deficits but also to measure the changes and establish a baseline against which to measure further changes over time. The basic strategy of the mental status examination

Table 24–7. QUESTIONS FOR ASSESSING DEMENTIA

Ask not only what medications the individual is taking, but also what over-the-counter preparations and vitamins are used.
Is there a history of hypertension, TIAs, syncopal episodes, strokes, or cardiovascular disease?
Is there a family history of dementia, depression, psychiatric illness, or other neurologic disorders?
Psychiatric signs and symptoms: Is there evidence of depressive symptoms, a sad mood or affect, lack of energy, loss of interest and enjoyment in former activities, changes in sleep patterns, loss of weight, loss of appetite?
Is there a past history of depression or psychiatric disorders?
Has the individual experienced any recent major losses, environmental changes, or traumas?
Have there been any changes in memory, intellect, or personality?
Did the memory loss come before the depression?
Did the personality changes occur before or after the stroke?

is to start with very simple questions and advance to more complex questions that test the patient's basic cognitive abilities (Katzman, 1981).

Short-term memory and concentration are usually the first areas to be affected in individuals with dementia, with other symptoms increasing in severity and number as the condition progresses. It is important to note that in the very early stages of dementia some highly trained individuals with IQs in the above-average range before illness can continue to score well on a mental status examination. Impairment in one area by itself does not indicate presence of dementia. Decline from a premorbid level of function over time is more indicative of a progressive dementing illness than of an isolated deficit. There are many reliable and well-validated mental status examinations available, ranging from the simple to the complex. The Folstein Mini-Mental State Examination is one frequently used by both clinicians and researchers (Folstein, Folstein, & McHugh, 1975; U'Ren, 1987).

Neuropsychological Testing

Neuropsychological testing and mental status examinations are essential components of the dementia workup. Brief cognitive tests such as the Folstein Mini-Mental State Examination are screening instruments used to detect cognitive impairment. Neuropsychological testing clarifies and refines the presence of cognitive impairment and provides additional information in the differential diagnosis of dementia. In addition, neuropsychological tests, because of their increasing complexity, are used to identify less severely impaired individuals. Patients may score normally on a mini-mental status examination but may show widespread cognitive impairment when tested by detailed neuropsychological examinations (Sagar & Sullivan, 1988). Utilized in longitudinal assessment, neuropsychological testing can measure the progression of the disease by comparison with the individual's previous performance on the same test measures. Correlations between clinical changes, test performance, and findings of scanning or imaging

Table 24–8. NEUROPSYCHOLOGICAL EVALUATION*

Cognitive Area	Test
Orientation	Folstein Mini-Mental State Examination (Folstein, Folstein, & McHugh, 1975)
Attention	Continuous-Performance Test (Hooper, 1958)
	Attentional Focusing (Nissen, Corkin, & Growdon, 1982)
	Reaction Time Task (Benton, 1977)
Memory	Brown Peterson Distractor Test (Brown, 1958; Peterson & Peterson, 1959)
	Free recall test of concrete nouns
	Recognition Span Test (Moss, 1984)
	Wechsler Memory Scale (Wechsler, 1945)
Language	Boston Naming Test (Kaplan, Goodglass, & Weintraub, 1978)
	Boston Diagnostic Aphasia Examination (Goodglass & Kaplan, 1972)
	The Western Aphasia Test (Kertesz, 1979)
Visual perception	Gollin Incomplete Pictures Test (Gollin, 1960)
	Hooper Test (Hooper, 1958)
Praxis	Tests in which the patient copies a drawing (cube, cross, clock, or house)
	Block design subtest of the Wechsler Adult Intelligence Scale (Wechsler, 1981)
	Matchsticks Test (Benson & Barton, 1970; Butters & Barton, 1970)
Problem-solving skills	Wisconsin Card Sorting Test (Grant & Berg, 1948; Milner, 1963)
	The Poisoned Food Problem Task of Arenberg (Arenberg, 1968; 1974)
Social function, activities of daily living, and instrumental activities of daily living	Philadelphia Geriatrics Center Forms (Lawton, Moss, Fulcomer, et al., 1982)
Psychiatric evaluation	Tests of the conditions that affect memory, such as depression, should be included, to rule out pseudodementia.

*The major cognitive processes evaluated in a dementia workup, with examples of the kinds of tests used to assess these functions.

(Adapted from McKhann, G, Drachman, D, Folstein, M, et al. (1984): Clinical diagnosis of Alzheimer's disease: Report of the NINCDSADRDA work group under the auspices of Department of Health and Human Services Task Force on Alzheimer's Disease. *Neurology*, 34:939–944.)

procedures are helpful in further identifying areas of deficit and establishing a diagnosis in cases of atypical presentation of symptoms (McKhann, Drachman, Folstein, et al., 1984). Memory and cognition are processes that depend on specific anatomic loci or neuronal networks. Depending on the site and nature of the pathology, diseases of the brain can disrupt these processes selectively. This enables clinicians to recognize different patterns in differing disorders and to obtain quantitative and qualitative measures of these differences by means of neuropsychological and clinical assessments (Sagar & Sullivan, 1988).

Neuropsychological Battery. Neuropsychological testing consists of a comprehensive battery of tests measuring various specific aspects of cognition, memory, language, sensory perception, motor function, visual spatial performance, and psychiatric evaluation. Table 24–8 illustrates the areas most commonly covered in neuropsychological assessments (McKhann, et al., 1984).

A wide variety of test measures is available, the Wechsler Adult Intelligence Scale (WAIS) and memory test and the Luria-Nebraska test battery being among the most commonly known. The Minnesota Multiphasic Assessment is frequently used for psychiatric evaluation purposes. (For more detailed information and standardized method summaries, refer to specific references, such as Lezak, 1983, and Kolb & Whishaw, 1985.) In recent years the development of computerized test batteries has increased, and now computerized measures are often included in the neuropsychological assessment package. Computerized testing has a number of advantages. Because the computer controls stimulus presentation and response time can be more precisely measured and recorded, test reliability is increased. Recent studies have also shown that automated testing is more acceptable to older individuals than standard paper and pencil methods. The refusal rate is lower and subjects report finding the video displays more interesting (Watts, Braddeley, & Williams, 1982; Henderson & Huppert, 1984).

In progressive dementias such as AD the range of deficits extends from a mild memory impairment to global brain failure virtually incompatible with life. This creates an additional problem in testing patients over time and at different stages of the disease process, making the use of a single clinical tool over the entire course of the illness difficult. A new rating instrument, the Alzheimer's disease assessment scale (ADAS) was developed specifically to evaluate the severity of cognitive and noncognitive behavioral dysfunctions characteristic of individuals with AD (Rosen, Mohs, & Davis, 1984). This standardized instrument, specific to this disease, may become a standard for use in reporting AD research. Since the symptoms of AD and other dementias have some overlapping of areas, the ADAS may also be applicable to other dementias (Rosen, et al., 1984). Table 24–9 shows areas covered by the ADAS.

Physical Examination

A detailed medical, social, and family history, as well as a review of systems to identify infectious, metabolic, cardiovascular, and nutritional problems, is essential in the dementia workup. The physical examination should include a neurologic assessment to evaluate the presence or absence of focal neurologic signs and symptoms and to assist in defining the cause of the dementia.

Neurologic Assessment. The neurologic assessment should include examination of the sensory and motor systems, including cranial nerves, gait, coordination, tone, reflexes, and proprioception. Patients in the early stages of

Table 24–9. THE ALZHEIMER'S DISEASE ASSESSMENT SCALE

Cognitive Items	Noncognitive Items
Spoken language ability	Tearful
Comprehension of spoken language	Depressed mood
	Concentration distractabilty
Recall test instructions	Uncooperative to testing
Word-finding difficulty	Delusions
Following commands	Pacing
Naming: objects, fingers	Motor activity: increase
Constructions: drawing	Tremors
Ideational praxis	Appetite change
Orientation	
Word recall	
Word recognition	

(From McDonald, 1986. Adapted from Rosen, Mohs, & Davis, 1984. Copyright 1984 by the American Psychiatric Association. Reprinted by permission.)

AD are comparatively free of neurologic changes, with the exception of the occasional presence of snout reflex, rigidity, and myoclonus. These symptoms may also be seen in nondemented elderly people (McKhann, et al., 1984). As the disease progresses, myoclonic movements and rigidity increase and patients in the later stages may develop seizures. MID patients show a higher frequency of focal neurologic signs and symptoms and higher scores on the Hachinski ischemic scale (Hachinski, et al., 1974).

Laboratory Examinations

Laboratory examinations should include a complete blood cell count, metabolic screen, and VDRL test. Table 24–10 shows a standard

Table 24–10. DEMENTIA WORKUP

SMA 20
Complete blood count with differential and platelets
FTA-ABS (fluorescent treponemal antibody absorption)
B_{12} levels
Serum folate
Free T_4 and thyroid-stimulating hormone
Sedimentation rate
Urinalysis
EKG electrocardiogram
Chest x-ray—PA and lateral
CT/MRI
Electroencephalogram (optional)
Spinal tap (optional)

laboratory workup for dementia. Blood chemistry tests are obtained to identify abnormalities that could be contributing to or are the cause of the dementia. Elevated calcium levels and abnormal liver and kidney function can cause memory deficits. Blood counts and sedimentation rates are utilized to identify infections or tumors. Abnormal thyroid function can contribute to memory loss and confusion. Correcting the abnormality may clear or improve the patient's difficulties. In the past, syphilitic dementia was a more common problem, but it is still important to rule out the possibility of syphilitic infection. Obtaining cerebrospinal fluid by means of a spinal tap is included by some physicians as a routine part of the dementia workup, whereas others examine cerebrospinal fluid only in cases where there may be some question of infection, malignancy, or toxic substances contributing to the dementia (McKhann, et al., 1984).

Specific Findings

Age-Associated Memory Impairment. Performance on neuropsychological tests declines with aging (Birren & Schaie, 1985; Sagar & Sullivan, 1988). Individuals who do not meet standardized criteria for dementia but who score outside the age-matched normal range are sometimes defined as having age-associated memory impairment (AAMI). In these cases, longitudinal followup is needed to see if the condition remains stable or marks the very early stages of a progressive, severe dementia such as AD.

Alzheimer's Disease. Individuals with AD show dramatic evidence of deterioration in short-term memory; learning; disorientation in time, place, and person; and, in the later phases of the disease, apraxias, aphasias, visual perceptual deficits, and motor difficulties. In general, psychometric testing shows that memory is impaired before psychomotor performance and that language performance is least involved in the early stages of AD. Scores on the Wechsler Adult Intelligence test decline at varying rates, but changes of 8 to 10 IQ points may be seen over a period of a year. In some cases, the disease presents with a strong focal onset. Aphasia without generalized dementia has been described in some cases (Wechsler, 1977; Mesulam, 1982). Dementia in AD is progressive, but the rate of progression and deterioration differs between patients as well as within patients.

Patients with AD have impaired ability in both verbal and nonverbal learning. They show short-term forgetfulness of both verbal and nonverbal material much more readily than normal subjects. Clinically, these patients show relatively good preservation of the ability to recall remote events, and they tend to more readily recall incidents that are associated with important life events, such as births, marriages, and wars (Sagar, Sullivan, Cohen, et al., 1987; Sagar & Sullivan, 1988). Sentence structure is not usually affected in earlier stages, and there may be little or no evidence of a deficit in casual conversation. Language disturbance is common in moderate or severe AD. Work fluency and naming deficits may be noted on careful evaluation in even relatively mild cases. Visuospatial function involves a number of processes relating to visual perception and spatial relationships. Visuospatial deficits are frequently found in cases with right hemisphere pathology. Drawing ability, personal spatial orientation, and construction of three-dimensional figures is affected in AD patients. Drawings are small and cramped, key features tend to be omitted, and patients may "close in" on figures (draw figures on top of the existing ones). Difficulties in this area can also result in spatial disorientation, reading difficulties, and anomia when objects are presented visually (Cogan, 1979; Huff, Corkin, & Growdon, 1986). Figure 24–1 shows examples of constructional apraxias.

Rigidity of the extrapyramidal type occurs in 60% to 80% of people with AD (Sagar & Sullivan, 1988; Pearce, 1974; Molsa, Marttila, & Rinne, 1984). Balance and gait disturbances are fairly frequent. Decreased arm swing, reduced stride length, and postural instability are the most frequent abnormalities seen. Dyskinesia and myoclonus are common. Myoclonic jerks and generalized seizures may occur in the later stages of the disease. One study reports aphasia and apraxia as the most

Original Figure   Closing In   Cramped Figures   Leaving Out Details

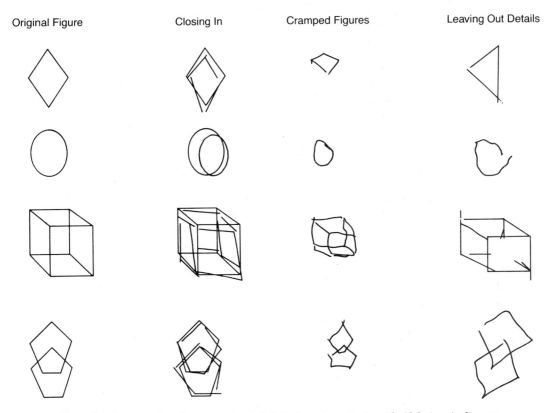

Figure 24–1. Examples of constructional deficits seen in patients with Alzheimer's disease.

common clinical features of AD (Huff, Growdon, Corkin, et al., 1987). Oculomotor function is impaired. There may be deficits in upward gaze with perseveration of downward gaze. Severely impaired and demented patients show gaze perseveration. Disorders of mood are common and contribute to cognitive dysfunction (Sagar & Sullivan, 1988). Changes in affect and impulse control, as well as motivation and general interest, are frequently found.

Multi-infarct Dementias. The extent and type of cognitive dysfunction found in MID patients depend on the location and size of the lesions. Small bilateral infarcts in the hippocampus or thalamus may produce considerable dysfunction in recent memory, while the same size infarcts in the optic radiation may produce only minor visual field limitations. Some studies have found that at times multiple infarcts do not produce any cognitive

dysfunction (Fisher, 1965; Heyman, 1978; Kase, 1986). Patients with MID tend to have a more severe drop in motor functions than do patients with AD (Erkinjuntti, Laaksonen, Sulkava, et al., 1986; Erkinjuntti, Ketonen, Sulkava, et al., 1987). The most telling clinical features are abrupt onset, stepwise deterioration, fluctuating course, history of stroke and hypertension, and focal neurologic signs. Hemi-neglect of visual space, subtle paresis, and inability to distinguish right from left are also seen in these patients (Read & Jarvik, 1984). Studies have reported much greater variability on subtests of the WAIS than that seen in patients with AD (Perez, Rivera, Meyer, et al., 1975). Reports of specific cognitive function changes in MID are scarce, probably because the nature of the deficit is so closely dependent on the location and size of the infarcts. They vary widely between cases. To compound the difficulty in measuring dysfunction, a certain percentage of patients is afflicted with both AD and MID. The cognitive deficits of the two conditions may be additive, so that higher cerebral dysfunction may be seen following a stroke in patients who already have AD changes in the brain (Sagar & Sullivan, 1988).

Korsakoff's Disease. Recent memory is impaired in patients with Korsakoff's disease (KD). In contrast to AD patients, those with KD fail to learn and remember new information, despite the fact that they can effectively retrieve and use previously acquired knowledge. Patients are frequently able to learn and perform complex skills and procedures but are unable to recall the context in which these procedures were learned. There is dissociation between knowing how to do something and recalling that something was learned (Tariot & Weingartner, 1986). Patients with KD frequently lack motivation or initiative and appear apathetic. Central nervous system functions other than memory are usually normal (Sagar & Sullivan, 1988).

Depression. Depressed patients frequently complain of deficits in concentration, memory, learning, and attention. In some cases the picture presented may resemble that of AD but careful analysis indicates qualitative differences. Chapter 23 offers more detailed information on depression.

Huntington's Disease. Intellectual deterioration is a key component in the diagnosis of Huntington's disease (HD). In the advanced stages of the disease, memory, intelligence, and verbal fluency are all impaired. In the earlier stages severe deficits are seen primarily in learning ability, whereas verbal fluency is only mildly impaired. Intelligence is within normal range, with the exception of selective deficits as seen on the picture arrangement and digit symbol subtests of the WAIS. Memory is more impaired in recognition tasks than it is in recall tasks. Long-term memory is impaired, as is the ability to learn skills. Language function is usually relatively well preserved. Visuospatial capacity is impaired but differs from that in AD. Patients with HD show deficits in personal orientation in space but usually not in their ability to copy draw-

ings. Sequencing is impaired, as is evident in the picture arrangement subtest of the WAIS (Sagar & Sullivan, 1988; Butters, Sax, Montgomery, et al., 1978). General chorea is the classic presentation, with severity correlating with the severity of the cognitive deficits. Choreiform movements are generally mild in the earlier stages, increasing in severity as the disease progresses. Oculomotor disturbances are seen, the most striking being the absence of rapid eye movements.

Parkinson's Disease. Approximately 20% to 30% of patients with Parkinson's disease show clinical evidence of dementia (Mortimer, Christensen, & Webster, 1985; Sagar & Sullivan, 1988). A detailed discussion of the dementia seen in these patients can be found in Chapter 25 on Parkinson's disease.

Electroencephalogram

The electroencephalogram (EEG) is useful in establishing a diagnosis of dementia in cases with atypical presentations and in clarifying the cause of the dementia. Patients with AD show a general decrease in alpha rhythms, which are replaced by diffuse theta and delta waves of moderate amplitude (Obrist, 1978). Approximately 80% of AD patients show a characteristic slowing of basic frequencies as the disease progresses (Katzman, 1981). In cases of cerebrovascular disease the background rhythms, although slow, are generally well preserved, and there is an increased incidence of focal (as opposed to diffuse) slow activity (Obrist, 1978). Studies utilizing evoked potentials (EP), such as P300, which is thought to reflect speed of cognition, indicate that there is an increased latency of P300 in approximately 50% to 80% of AD patients, whereas P300 remains normal in depressive syndromes. This may assist in differentiating AD dementia from that of depression (McKhann, et al., 1984). Individuals with epilepsy may have subtle seizures that are not readily apparent and may present as a dementia syndrome. The EEG is particularly useful in identifying the presence of seizure activity. In some cases it may require more than one EEG to document the problem.

Functional Assessment

In assessing the patient, three areas are crucial: cognitive state, ability to perform activities of daily living, and frequency and quality of emotional symptoms and behaviors. Patients' strengths as well as their weaknesses must be sought and used to assist them in compensating for their deficits. Patients need to maintain some power over their lives. Cognitive dysfunction does not mean lack of feeling, and patients should be allowed to do as much as possible for as long as possible. Table 24–11 illustrates specific areas of functional ability that should be included in assessment.

Since the patient with a dementing illness increasingly relies on family support and assistance, assessment must of necessity include the family. Table 24–12 illustrates the five most critical areas to be covered when performing a family assessment. It is essential to refocus thinking away from purely custodial care to perceive the patient as having functional capabilities. The goal should be to maintain the patient and the caregiver in as independent and functional roles as possible and to keep the patient in the community for as long as is therapeutic for both the patient and the family (Eisdorfer & Cohen, 1981).

Imaging

Computed Tomography. The advent of computed tomography (CT) has dramatically

Table 24–11. FUNCTIONAL ACTIVITIES ASSESSMENT

Writing checks, paying bills, keeping records
Assembling tax records, making out business and insurance papers
Shopping alone for clothes, groceries, and household necessities
Playing a game of skill, such as bridge, other card games, or chess
Heating water for coffee or tea and turning off the stove
Preparing a balanced meal
Keeping track of current events
Paying attention to and understanding a TV program, book, or magazine
Remembering appointments, family occasions, and medications
Traveling away from the neighborhood

Table 24–12. FAMILY ASSESSMENT

Who is the family?
Who is the primary caregiver?
What is the family history?
What are the family coping styles?
What is the meaning of the illness and its symptoms?

increased understanding of the human brain, the changes that occur with normal aging, and various pathologic processes leading to dementia. Penetrating the body with thin, fan-shaped x-ray beams, CT scanners produce a cross-sectional view of the tissues within, enabling clinicians to visualize the intracranial contents in a way that was not previously possible. By revolving the x-ray tube around the patient, the scanner can view a slice of the brain from many angles. Detectors on the opposite side record the images, and a computer compares the views and produces a single video picture (Forsyth & Miller, 1987). The rapid technical advances made since the advent of the original scanners have provided increased resolution in the visualization of normal structures (i.e., white and gray matter) and spaces (i.e., sulci, cisterns, and ventricles) (Jacobs, Kinkel, Painter, et al., 1978).

CT scans have been used with and without contrast media in ruling out or locating infarcts, aneurysms, neoplasms, and normal pressure hydrocephaly (NPH) and in establishing the diagnosis and causes of dementia. A single CT scan is not diagnostic of AD; it is merely exclusionary for other factors. Mere atrophy is not diagnostic; at least two scans are needed over time to detect progressive atrophy. AD and vascular dementia are the two most common types of dementia. CT scans have not always been able to differentiate adequately between these two types, especially in the cases of more discrete white matter changes (Erkinjuntti, et al., 1987).

Magnetic Resonance Imaging. Magnetic resonance imaging (MRI), a more recent scanning technique that avoids ionizing radiation, offers flexibility and unprecedented spatial range, making it increasingly popular and widely accepted as a diagnostic tool. MRI scanners surround the body with powerful electromagnets. Supercooled by liquid helium, they create a strong magnetic field. This has a profound effect on protons, the nuclei of hydrogen atoms. By manipulating these protons, radio signals are given off. Computers translate these signals into images of the area of the brain being scanned (Forsyth & Miller, 1987). MRI has proved to be very sensitive to subtle changes in the brain parenchyma and is widely used in screening for a variety of neurologic disorders (Awad, Spetzler, Hodak, et al., 1987). MRI is used in place of or in conjunction with CT to detect abnormalities not normally visualized by CT alone. The extreme sensitivity of MRI has identified a large number of incidental and at times unexpected lesions in which prevalence and clinical significance are not clearly understood. In a study conducted by Awad and associates (1987), it was found that incidental lesions correlated significantly with age and risk factors for cerebrovascular disease. They concluded that deep hemispheric lesions are frequently found in the elderly and may represent an index of chronic cerebrovascular disease in this population. These lesions may have different significance in varying age groups. Further research is needed to clearly define, clarify, and understand their clinical significance. At present, clinicians utilizing MRI for screening must continue to take into consideration the current lack of specificity regarding these lesions when establishing a diagnosis.

Positron Emission Tomography. Positron emission tomography (PET) utilizes short-lived radionuclides requiring the availability of a cyclotron- or positron-emitter generator system. It enables clinicians to study the physiologic activity of the brain in vivo. With the use of tracers capable of measuring regional cerebral blood flow and glucose metabolism in the brain, it has been used in the study of dementia. Studies utilizing PET have demonstrated specific abnormalities in patients with AD. In particular, they have shown the deficits in glucose metabolism to be most severe in the temporoparietal cortex (Matsui & Hirano, 1978). This pattern has been considered to be of diagnostic significance in differentiating between AD, normal aging, normal pressure

hydrocephaly, and Pick's disease. Cerebral blood flow (CBF) has been shown to be reduced in both MID and AD. Table 24–13 shows differences between the two conditions (Rogers, Meyer, Mortel, et al., 1986).

PET used to examine the integrity of the blood-brain barrier in patients with AD and in controls demonstrated no evidence of blood-brain barrier breakdown in patients with AD (Schlageter, Carson, & Rapoport, 1987). Due to the need for a cyclotron- or positron-emitter generator system and the expense involved, the use of PET is limited to specific centers and is not currently available for widespread clinical application.

Single Photon Emission Computed Tomography. Single photon emission computed tomography (SPECT), utilizing radionuclides that are part of routine nuclear medicine studies, is a more practical modality for studying physiologic cerebral activity. Single photon-emitting radiopharmaceuticals that are capable of measuring cerebral function have been recently developed and are commercially available. Studies have shown that SPECT is effective in demonstrating the same temporoparietal deficits that had been seen with PET, and it is useful in differentiating among patients with varying degrees of clinical dementia, patients with multi-infarct dementia, and normal controls (Jagust, Budinger, & Reed, 1987). CT and MRI remain the most commonly used screening tools in establishing a diagnosis of dementia. PET and SPECT add important data to our understanding of the pathophysiology of dementia and assist in the differential diagnosis of the more atypical presentations, but expense and lack of availa-

Table 24–13. CEREBRAL BLOOD FLOW (CBF) IN ALZHEIMER'S DISEASE AND MULTI-INFARCT DEMENTIA

Alzheimer's Disease	Multi-infarct Dementia
Symmetrical decrease in cerebral blood flow	Focal/patchy cerebral blood flow reductions
Cerebral blood flow normal until symptoms of dementia appear; thereafter cerebral blood flow decreases rapidly	Decreased cerebral blood flow evident approximately 2 years before onset of symptoms

bility prevent their wide clinical application at this time. Table 24–14 illustrates the changes in understanding of AD resulting from new imaging techniques. The ability to measure physiologic changes in the brain over time by the use of these measures will prove invaluable in the development of treatment approaches in the future.

Treatment Approaches

Management of dementia resulting from MID or alcohol abuse is focused primarily on treating the underlying condition and eliminating those factors that predispose or directly lead to the problem. For patients with MID, controlling hypertension, stabilizing the cardiovascular system, and treating secondary medical conditions or psychiatric disorders improve the prognosis and the quality of life for the patient (Read & Jarvik, 1984). Anticoagulation therapy and vascular surgery may benefit some patients with MID.

Shunts are sometimes the treatment of choice for patients with normal pressure hydrocephaly, although statistics show that the success rate for improvement is low (Beck, et al., 1982). In patients with alcohol-related dementias, eliminating alcohol use, improving nutrition, stabilizing the patient's medical status, and utilizing high doses of thiamin, niacin, and B_{12} are the standard treatments of choice (Victor & Banker, 1978). The management of secondary symptoms and behaviors is discussed in greater depth in the section covering treatment and management of AD.

Alternative Treatment Approaches

Chelation therapy and megavitamin therapy have been promoted as alternative approaches

Table 24–14. CHANGES IN CONCEPTS ABOUT ALZHEIMER'S DISEASE

1965	1988
Rare	Common
Diffuse	Multifocal
Neuroanatomical	Physiologic/neurochemical
Severe neuronal loss	Moderate neuronal loss

in the treatment of dementias. Statistics have not shown any basis for their therapeutic claims; in fact, the use of megavitamins may cause more difficulties and adverse reactions than improvement (Funkenstein, Hicks, Dysken, et al., 1981; Thal, 1988). Some preliminary studies (Gold & Stone, 1988; Hall, Gonder-Frederick, Chewning, et al., 1989) have shown that circulating glucose may control acetylcholine synthesis and enhance memory in older individuals. Many AD patients develop cravings for sweets, and PET and SPECT data show deficits in glucose metabolism in the brains of these patients. Better control of blood glucose levels achieved through dietary control or medications might help alleviate age-related memory deficits in some elderly individuals, but as yet the mechanisms for doing this are still to be developed. High intake of glucose on a regular basis has not been effective, and there is no evidence that this would be beneficial in AD. Maintaining a balanced nutritional status is important for the patient, and families should be taught to do so.

Treatment Approaches: Alzheimer's Disease

At this time there are no known cures for Alzheimer's disease. Drug treatment approaches are divided into two types—symptomatic, which concerns the management of emerging symptoms, and specific, which focuses on the presumed cause of the basic disorder (Hollister, 1985).

Symptomatic Treatment. Medications in this category are utilized to achieve either simple control or symptomatic relief.

Behaviors Treated by Medication to Achieve Simple Control. Behaviors treated by medication to achieve simple control include aggression, agitation, restlessness, hyperboisterousness, hyperactivity, verbal hostility, and insomnia.

Medication Utilized to Provide Symptomatic Relief. Antipsychotic medications are utilized to provide symptomatic relief in anxiety, depression, regressed behavior, hallucinations, and delusions (see Table 24–15).

Medication Principles. Patients with AD are

Table 24–15. MEDICATIONS USED TO PROVIDE SYMPTOM RELIEF

Drug (Generic)	Drug (Brand Name)	Daily Dosage
Antidepressants		
amitriptyline	Amitril	25–150 mg
	Elavil	
desipramine	Norpramin	25–150 mg
doxepin	Adapin	25–150 mg
	Sinequan	
imipramine	Tofranil	25–150 mg
	Antipress	
maprotiline	Ludiomil	25–150 mg
nortriptyline	Aventyl	10–50 mg
	Pamelor	
protriptyline	Vivactil	5–30 mg
trazodone	Desyrel	50–300 mg
Sedative/Hypnotics		
chloral hydrate	Cohidrate	500 mg–1 gm
	Noctec	
triazolam	Halcion	0.125–0.5 mg
temazepam	Restoril	15–30 mg
flurazepam	Dalmane	15–30 mg
Antipsychotics		
haloperidol	Haldol	0.5–2 mg BID
thiothixene	Navane	2–5 mg BID or TID
chlorpromazine	Thorazine	25–50 mg BID
thioridazine	Mellaril	25–50 mg BID
trifluoperazine	Stelazine	2–5 mg BID
fluphenazine	Permitil	1–5 mg BID
	Prolixin	
molindone	Moban	25–50 mg BID
loxapine	Loxitane	25–50 mg BID
Antianxiety agents		
diazepam	Valium	2 mg QD–BID
chlordiazepoxide	Librium	5 mg BID–QID
clorazepate	Tranxene	7.5–15 mg QD
lorazepam	Ativan	0.5–1 mg BID
triazolam	Halcion	0.125 mg QD
oxazepam	Serax	10 mg TID
alprazolam	Xanax	0.25 mg BID–TID

(Data on antidepressants and sedative/hypnotics adapted from Cohen & Eisdorfer, 1986, by permission. Data on antipsychotics and antianxiety agents adapted from Maletta, 1985.)

acutely sensitive to central nervous system (CNS) neurotransmitter alteration; small changes can have significant effects. Many AD patients have idiosyncratic reactions to medications (Thornton, Davies, & Tinklenberg, 1986). Medications must be initiated at very low doses and carefully titrated. Less emphasis should be placed on dosage and more on the individual patient's clinical response (Maletta, 1985). Some behaviors can be managed or decreased by means of behavioral and environmental changes. It is always recom-

mended that these approaches be tried first, before medications.

Before beginning medications, a concomitant medical illness or use of contraindicated drugs must be determined. It is important to ask whether the patient had these behavioral problems in the past and whether any medications were effective or any side effects developed. Haldol (haloperidol) is frequently used to control behavioral problems in patients with Alzheimer's disease. In very small doses, Haldol can be effective, but some patients respond by becoming increasingly agitated, with dosage increases only escalating the problem. Parkinsonian symptoms can become marked after Haldol, and the patient can rapidly become severely dysfunctional (Maletta, 1985). In these situations, the dosage must be appreciably decreased or sometimes discontinued. A rule of thumb in drug therapy with these patients is to use the smallest possible dose and temporarily discontinue the drug on a regular basis to evaluate response (Yesavage & Hollister, 1978).

Specific Drug Therapies. Specific drugs for Alzheimer's disease are intended to treat the disease itself. Table 24–16 lists specific strategies and medications utilized in the treatment of AD. The majority of these treatment approaches are tried as clinical drug studies following strictly regulated research protocols. While some findings have reported small changes in attention, mood, and concentration, unfortunately there have not been any major revelations. Most drug trials are based on animal studies, and although some drugs appear promising in animal trials the results have not been duplicated in humans.

Management Approaches. Dementia is a multifaceted problem. Integrated management focuses not only on the individual but on the family, the environment, and the community. Assessment and planning must begin early. Planning, implementation, and evaluation should be concurrent and longitudinal. Because of the complexity of the problem there is a need for a multidisciplinary approach to provide diagnosis, pharmacologic management, nursing management, and resource management. In working with this population a commitment to a long-term relationship between the patient, the family, the staff, and health professionals is essential. Learning to live with a dementing illness is also learning to live with uncertainty. The course of the disease may be unpredictable and varies among individual patients. Questions families frequently ask are: How long will the individual live? How soon will changes take place? Will the patient become assaultive? Will the patient wander? Will he or she hallucinate? Will our children get the disease? Unfortu-

nately there are no firm answers. While the outcome of AD is known, there are many factors and variations that influence its progression. Some patients have a more gradual decline with plateau periods, whereas others have a more rapid rate of decline with more severe behavioral changes.

The responsibilities of the nurse are threefold, including assessment, planning, and coordination. Plans must be realistic, tailored to the individual, consistent with the psychosocial environment, and financially feasible. Because of the progressive nature of the disease, planning should anticipate and accommodate the patient's decline, with the support system increasingly activated to the escalating need for assistance (Eisdorfer & Cohen, 1981).

Behavioral Management. There are no magic tricks for dealing with problem behaviors. Dementia patients are extremely sensitive to nonverbal cues and tend to mirror the affective behavior of those around them. Nurses serve as role models to help soothe the patient. Patience, gentleness, and calmness can be very effective. See Table 24–17 for effective communication techniques. *The 36-Hour Day* (Mace and Rabins, 1981) and *Understanding Alzheimer's Disease* (Aronson, 1988) are excellent sources for general strategies. Eisdorfer and Cohen (1981) and Steele, Lucas, and Tune (1982) also provide useful information. Supportive psychotherapy may be helpful in disrupting a cycle of frustration, anger, anxiety, and rage in patients with mild to moderate dementia (Verwoerdt, 1981).

Environmental Safety Issues. Individuals with a dementing illness have changes not only in memory and learning but also in visuoperceptual areas, smell and taste, balance, and gait disturbances. Dysphagia is frequently a problem. Table 24–18 notes areas of safety that must be assessed and considered when caring for these patients.

Caregiver Education and Support. Families must be taught to respond to their loved ones' catastrophic and massive emotional overresponse to minor stress by remaining calm and removing the patient from any threatening situations. Caregivers must learn to work on specific solvable problems within a general

Table 24–16. SPECIFIC DRUG THERAPIES IN ALZHEIMER'S DISEASE

Strategy	Treatment
Improve cerebral circulation and blood oxygenation	
Blood oxygenation	hyperbaric oxygen
Vasodilation	papaverine
	Cyclospasmol
	Vasodilan
	betahistine
Anticoagulation	bishydroxycoumarin
Reduce blood viscosity	pentoxifylline
Vasodilation and metabolic activation	dihydroergotoxine
	Nafronyl
	pyritinol
Metabolic activation	pyrithioxin
	piracetam
	oxiracetam
	pramiracetam
Neuropeptides	ACTH-4-10
	ORG 2766 (ACTH 4-9 analog)
	1-Desamino-8-d-argine vasopressin (DDAVP)
	Lysine vasopressin
Nutritional supplements	Niacin-pentylenetetrazol combination
	Vitamin B_{12}
	Folate and B_{12}
	B complex and C vitamins
	Glutamate, B vitamin, iron
	Dried bakers' yeast
	RNA
	Zinc sulfate
Reduce aluminum levels	
Chelation therapy	Tetracycline
Alter CNS neurotransmitters: "the cholinergic hypothesis"	
Precursor loading	choline chloride
	lecithin
	deanol
Enhance transmitter release	4-aminopyridine
Inhibit acetylcholinesterase	Oral physostigmine
	IV physostigmine
	Tetrahydroaminoacridine
Receptor stimulation	arecoline
	bethanechol chloride (continuous intracranial infusion)
	pilocarpine
Psychostimulation	methylphenidate
	pentylenetetrazol
Dopamine precursor loading	levodopa
Dopamine receptor stimulation	bromocriptine
Opioid antagonism	naloxone
	naltrexone
Serotonin precursor loading	L-tryptophan
Inhibit serotonin re-uptake	alaproclate
Correct monoamine neurotransmitter deficits	amitriptyline

(Adapted from Bagne, C, Pomara, N, Crook, T, et al. (1986): Treatment development strategies for Alzheimer's disease. *In* Crook, T, Bartus, R, Ferris, S, et al. (eds): *Treatment Development Strategies for Alzheimer's Disease.* New Canaan, CT, Mark Powley, 586–589.)

Table 24–17. COMMUNICATION TECHNIQUES

Avoid arguments
Dementia patients reason by a different set of rules and arguments, usually resulting in aggravation for both parties.

Use distractors
The patient's memory deficits can frequently be used to advantage to distract and redirect attention.

Communicate nonverbally
By touching or holding hands.

Praise desired behavior
And make it emotionally meaningful.

Ignore undesired behaviors
But only if it is safe.

(Data from Thornton, Davies, & Tinklenberg, 1986.)

framework. By developing a strategy for dealing with problems in advance, caregivers gain a measure of control and do not need to approach each problem behavior as a crisis. This also helps stabilize the environment for the patient. Teaching families to remain calm and improve nonverbal communication often helps reduce behavioral disturbances in the patient (Thornton, et al., 1986; Bartol, 1979). Responding to feelings rather than expressed content is an important lesson for caregivers and families and an effective way of dealing with the frequent repetition of questions.

Fear and uncertainty cause caregivers to dread the future. Learning about the disease, how to handle specific contingencies as they arise, to break down dilemmas into smaller, solvable problems, and, most important, to take care of themselves by allowing others to provide support for the patient, are all measures that allow families to accept uncertainty and stand prepared for emergencies. Learning that a family member has AD or a related dementing illness is shocking, but once families have made the appropriate legal and financial adjustments they should be encouraged to focus not on the disease and its disabilities but on positive experiences. With early diagnosis and supportive therapies, patients are capable of enjoying many family activities and intimacies for a considerable period of time. It is tragic when fear and anxiety in both the patient and the family are allowed to deprive them of those years. Counselors and support groups should be made available to all patients and their families. There is nothing worse than to tell patients and their families that "there is nothing to be done," and leave them without any additional support. Families are often tremendously relieved and helped by meeting others who are sharing the same experiences and problems. There are a number of nationally and regionally organized groups that provide information, assistance, and regularly held support meetings throughout the country. One of the most helpful things that the clinician can do for patients and families is to put them in contact with these groups. Table 24–19 lists

Table 24–18. ENVIRONMENTAL SAFETY CHECKS

Keep environment simple. Remove knickknacks or clutter that may distract or confuse.
Remove items that can prove dangerous: car keys, iron, power tools, matches, cleaning solvents, knives.
Keep all medications out of reach and under lock and key.
Install gates on stairs. Check handrails.
Install grab bars.
Reduce temperature on water heater.
Remove rugs that slip.
Remove glass tables, unsteady or delicate furniture.
If possible, arrange an outside area that is safe and accessible where the patient can walk or sit.
Put bright reflector tape on steps.

(Data from Mace & Rabins, 1981.)

Table 24–19. SUPPORT GROUPS FOR ALZHEIMER'S DISEASE PATIENTS AND FAMILIES

Categories
Informational/networking
Supportive/therapeutic
Transitional
Target populations

Currently Available Groups
Caregiver groups
Men's groups
Adolescent and young adult children of AD parents groups
Couples groups
Sexuality and sexual adjustment groups
Young grandchildren of AD patients groups
Spouses of institutionalized AD patients groups
Life satisfaction groups
Daughters of AD patients groups
Problem-solving groups

the types of support groups currently available. More than one group is frequently required as patients and their families move along the various stages of the disease process. The Alzheimer's Disease and Related Disorders Association (ADRDA), a national organization for people with Alzheimer's disease with chapters in most major areas of the country, is an excellent resource for information regarding support groups and services.*

Impact of a Diagnosis of Dementia for the Patient and Family

The person who has a dementing illness must cope simultaneously with associated psychopathological states, such as depression, anxiety, and paranoia, as well as a number of losses. Loss of memory, loss of a job, loss of a role as head of a household or breadwinner, and loss of a future are only a few of the losses experienced by these individuals. In addition, they must cope with the reactions of others toward them, perhaps by overprotective spouses or distant children and friends. They may feel embarrassment and shame.

The nuclear family experiences fear, anger, helplessness, and hopelessness. Feelings of abandonment and isolation are frequent. Criticism by relatives is a common occurrence, wherein they have difficulty accepting the diagnosis and try to rationalize the patient's symptoms in the earlier stages of the disease by attributing blame to family members. The patient may deal with fears and anxiety by becoming verbally and physically abusive toward family members.

Spouses are in social limbo; they cannot mourn decently because the patient is still alive and frequently shows few outward signs of change. They cannot divorce with dignity, even if they wished to do so, and are left with no acceptable outlets for their sexual frustrations and emotional needs.

Young children living in the home are fre-

quently ignored by the patient and neglected by the caregiver who is mentally and physically drained in attempting to cope with the meaning of the diagnosis and the changes in the patient. The patient may bully the children or vie for attention with them. This is more often seen in fathers whose teenaged sons try to assume that parent's role and are viewed as a "threat" by the patient. Younger children frequently incorporate and misinterpret the family's frustrations, fears, and self-recriminations (Lezak, 1978).

Older children living away from home must cope with feelings of guilt, fear, and loss. Torn between conflicting needs, they may become actively involved or they may distance themselves from the parent and the disease. As the disease progresses in the parent the adolescent and young adult children engage in a socio-psychological process with distinct stages and phases (Davis, Ingram, Priddy, & Tinklenberg, manuscript in preparation). The stages of this process of sequential resolving are: awareness, in which the children come to realize that something is truly wrong; exploration, in which they seek a reason for the parent's behavior and deal with the physical and psychosocial consequences of the diagnosis; and definition, in which they separate the patient that *is* from the parent that *was*. Factors that influence the adjustment process are the child's age, developmental stage, personal coping style, and family dynamics.

Compounding the difficulties, the disease can affect insight, judgment, and decision-making abilities. Attempts by caregivers and professionals to deal with evolving deficits may be viewed by the patient as obstructive, interfering, and manipulative (Lezak, 1978).

Family Stages After Diagnosis

A diagnosis of dementia in a family member results in many changes in the family system. Roles, family expectations, and alliances are altered. In order to cope, families must learn to deal with many new demands. In the author's clinical practice, we have identified several stages that families must move through

---

*To contact ADRDA, write to ADRDA National Headquarters, 70 East Lake Street, Chicago, IL 60601. Or telephone 1-800-621-0379; in Illinois 1-800-572-6037.

following diagnosis. Table 24–20 illustrates these stages.

Institutionalization as a Family Crisis

The decision to seek nursing home placement frequently presents a crisis in the family. Family members often disagree as to the need and timing for placement. Feelings of anger and guilt and a sense of self-recrimination and failure are common. Most people, particularly older people, have a fear and deep aversion to nursing homes, and patients often extract promises from their spouses and families that these family members will never put them in a nursing home. Clinicians thus are often faced with a situation where a patient's care needs far exceed the resources of the caregiver or family, and yet a spouse may insist on caring for the patient at home, even if in reality it is against both the patient's and family's best interests (Meier & Cassel, 1986). A scarcity of resources, other financial issues, and the clinician's own biases and feelings may compound the problem, which, for the family is highly complex. The sense of guilt and personal responsibility felt when contemplating nursing home placement can be devastating, especially if there is disagreement within the family as to what should be done. The clinician should be aware of all these factors when assisting families in making the decision to institutionalize. Important questions to be considered are the patients' needs and (if known) their preferences, the caregivers' needs, and the needs of the overburdened family. Have all other alternatives been thoroughly explored? Emotional support, reassurance, and assistance in evaluating existing resources are

Table 24–20. FAMILY STAGES AFTER DIAGNOSIS OF DEMENTIA

Coping with diagnosis
Beginning to look at management
What do we do?
Coping maximally
Transition to institutionalization
Making the decision
Acting on it

essential at this time. Letting the patient and the family know that they will not be cut adrift from their previous support systems is very helpful. Ideally, working with the patient and family on the issue of possible future placement should be discussed early in the disease process when the patient may be able to voice concerns and preferences and designate a surrogate decision-maker.

Conclusion

Dementia is a devastating problem for everyone concerned. Prolonging patients' stay in the community and providing social support systems for the family add to the quality of life for both the individual and the family. But prolonging the inevitable is not enough. Additional research is needed for effective treatment and, someday, prevention methods for the underlying causes of the disorder may be found.

Future Trends in Research

Clinical and research interest in dementia and its causes has greatly increased in recent years. Researchers have begun studying a broad spectrum of areas associated with the problem. It is still uncertain whether AD is an infectious process, a toxic disorder, a biochemical deficiency, or an exaggeration and acceleration of the normal aging process with dementia appearing when the neural reserves are exhausted and compensatory mechanisms fail (Khachaturian, 1985).

One of the most important research issues in AD is accurate diagnosis. Past studies (National Institute on Aging Task Force, 1980) have charged that incorrect diagnosis was made in the range of 10% to 30% of cases. Early and accurate diagnosis is essential to the progress of research on AD and other dementing disorders. Recently, criteria have been developed that in turn have led to broader epidemiologic studies being conducted. To advance research on the diagnosis of Alzheimer's disease, longitudinal studies are necessary and are currently being undertaken. Researchers in this area are collecting detailed information on individuals with the disease as well as normal aging populations to identify premorbid events and conditions that may predispose some individuals to develop the disease and to gain a better understanding of the normal aging process. One of the major difficulties in diagnosing AD involves the variations in presentation and the need to understand the relationships among neuropsychological, neuropathologic, and neuroradiologic findings. Neuroimaging techniques and the development of more precise neuropsychological tests are a high priority. The role of environmental factors is another central research theme. For many years memory loss had been considered a normal consequence of aging. The process of normal aging has not been clearly understood, and until a better knowledge is gained in this area the diagnosis of AD will continue to be a difficult and somewhat imprecise process. For some time now, it has been clearly established that there is a serious defect in the cholinergic system of patients with AD. This finding has continued to generate a tremendous amount of interest. Research in this area has focused on several factors: understanding the cause and effect of the defect and looking for pharmacologic approaches to treat, prevent, or stop the disease process. Along with pharmacologic studies there is an interest in developing new ways of dispensing medications, for example by pumps and skin patches, which will be useful not only in AD but in many other disorders as well.

It is not yet determined why brain cells die in AD. Many researchers are studying the chemistry of the neurofibrillary plaques and tangles found in the brains of AD patients. Others are studying the membrane structures and how membrane changes influence transport and homeostasis of essential ions. Pedigree studies investigating the familial genetic aspects of AD are essential in understanding the disease and in helping predict those who are at risk for the disease. Identifying genetic markers and biologic correlates of AD is a high priority in current research. Recent data from a longitudinal study of aging twins suggest a possibility of genetic factors in vascular dementia (Matsuyama & Jarvik, unpublished data; Jarvik, et al., 1980). Recent animal studies have shown that nerve growth factor (NGF) can promote survival of central nervous neurons in adult life. Work is being done in looking for therapeutic approaches utilizing this information.

Finally, the current success of tissue transplants in Parkinson's disease is providing the basis for studies that may evaluate this procedure in AD and other disorders in the near future.

DELIRIUM

Definition

DSM III-R defines delirium as an organic brain syndrome that has as an essential feature a clouded state of consciousness manifested by difficulty in sustaining attention to both external and internal stimuli, sensory misperception, and a disordered stream of thought. In addition, disturbances of sleep-wakefulness and psychomotor activity are present. Onset is relatively rapid and the course typically fluctuates. The total duration is usually brief. Delirium is especially prominent in infants and the elderly. Delirium is to the elderly what fever is to the young. The majority of individuals presenting with delirium suffer from a specific physical illness. Theoretically, progressive cerebral disease can first declare itself as an acute delirious or confusional state. However, unless there is evidence of a focal neurologic lesion, this is rare (Roth, 1978). Delirium may occur during the course of a dementing illness due to the development of a new medical condition, such as an acute infection, which may evolve "silently" without a fever or other physical signs (Roth, 1978).

Incidence

Exact figures on the epidemiology of delirium are not available because this disorder is often undiagnosed, there is a failure to use consistent diagnostic criteria, terms are used inconsistently, and varying methods of case finding are used by researchers (Lipowski, 1984). Studies of acute confusion among acute-care hospital admission patients report between 10% and 40% of the elderly have acute confusion on admission (Levkoff, Besdine, & Wetle, 1986). In examining the incidence of postoperative confusion in the elderly, researchers report a wide range of occurrence, from 9% to 14% (Levkoff, et al., 1986). Williams and associates (1985a) found a 51% incidence of confusion in elderly patients with hip fractures.

Causation

Causes of delirium can be classified under the heading of predisposing and precipitating factors. Age itself is a predisposing factor. Delirium can occur at any age but is most often seen in the very young and the elderly. Thus, anything that affects brain function in the elderly can exacerbate the predisposition to delirium (Zisook & Braff, 1986). At high risk are individuals with cardiac disorders, alcohol and drug abusers, and elderly patients who have cognitive or memory disorders and have undergone trauma, surgery, or sudden environmental changes. Oncology patients are at risk from metabolic and nutritional imbalances, metastases, and infections. Patients with known neurologic disturbances, strokes, head trauma, and brain tumors, and those with fever and dehydration are also at high risk. Studies have indicated that postoperative delirium is a frequent occurrence. Patients recovering from vascular and cardiac surgery may have prolonged periods of delirium (Sullivan & Fogel, 1986). Williams and associates (1985b) followed 237 subjects ages 60 years or over from the time of admission to the fifth postoperative day. All of the subjects had traumatic hip fractures and none had a preexisting history of chronic mental impairment. They found that the most significant variables related to the development of postoperative confusion were age, increased errors on admission mental status examination, and low preinjury physical activity. In an expanded study, Campbell, Williams, and Mlynarczyk (1986) found the above variables to be related to postoperative confusion but added variables of urinary problems, slow postoperative mobilization, and pain. Table 24–21 shows some of the most frequent causes of delirium.

Presenting Signs and Symptoms

The individual suffering from delirium has a decreased ability to attend to environmental stimuli and often shows highly disruptive and variable behavior. The onset of delirium is acute, ranging from a few hours to a few weeks. Delirium is usually worse at night, and patients with delirium may have lucid intervals during which it is difficult to detect any disorder. Patients with delirium may present with a range of psychopathologic symptoms, including delusions, hallucinations, irritability, and impulsive behaviors (Lipowski, 1980). Clouding of consciousness, disorientation, memory impairment, incoherent speech, and perceptual disturbances—all characteristic features of delirium—give rise to behavior that appears confused. Performing frequent assessments of mental status in high-risk patients at the first signs of inappropriate or labile behavior is essential in early recognition and treatment of delirium. Evidence of disturbance in attention and arousal as well as disorientation and abnormal behavior is essential in establishing the presence of delirium (Zisook & Braff, 1986). Sullivan and Fogel (1986) caution against overemphasis of disorientation as a presenting sign for the diagnosis of delirium. They describe four early cases of delirium that masqueraded as a violent personality disorder, a factitious illness, and an uncooperative and psychotic suicidal idea.

Differentiating Delirium from Dementia

Dementia must be ruled out in the differential diagnosis of delirium. Dementia usually follows a relatively stable course of impair-

Table 24–21. SYSTEMIC AND CENTRAL NERVOUS SYSTEM CAUSES OF DELIRIUM

Systemic Causes

Cardiovascular disease
  Congestive heart failure
  Arrhythmias
  Cardiac infarction
  Hypovolemia
  Aortic stenosis

Infections
  Pneumonia
  Urinary tract infection
  Bacteremia
  Septicemia

Medications
  Analgesics
  Anticholinergics
  Antidepressants
  Antihistamines
  Antiparkinsonian agents
  Cimetidine
  Digitalis glycosides
  Diuretics
  Neuroleptics
  Sedative/hypnotics

Metabolic
  Electrolyte and fluid
    imbalance
  Hepatic, renal, or
    pulmonary failure
  Diabetes, hyper- or
    hypothroidism, and
    other endocrinopathies
  Nutritional deficiencies
  Hypothermia and heat
    stroke

Neoplasm

Postoperative state

Substance abuse and
  poisons
  Alcohol
  Amphetamines
  Sedative/hypnotics
  Heavy metals
  Solvents
  Pesticides
  Carbon monoxide

Trauma
  Head injury
  Burns
  Hip fracture

Central Nervous System Causes

Infection
  Meningitis
  Encephalitis
  Septic emboli
  Neurosyphilis
  Brain abscess

Neoplasm
  Primary intracranial
  Metastatic (bronchogenic,
    breast)

Trauma
  Subdural hematoma
  Extradural hematoma
  Contusion

Vascular disorder
  Transient ischemic
    episodes
  Stroke
  Chronic subdural
    hematoma
  Vasculitis
  Arteriosclerosis
  Hypertensive
    encephalopathy
  Subarachnoid
    hemorrhage

Seizure
  Ictal and postictal states

(From Zisook, S, & Braff, DL (1986): Delirium: Recognition and management in the older patient. *Geriatrics, 41*(6):67–78. Reprinted by permission.)

ment, whereas delirium is often a variable waxing and waning syndrome (Roth, 1978).

treat the syndrome provisionally as delirium (Zisook & Braff, 1986). It is important to remember that dementia patients may become delirious, but when delirium clears the dementia remains. Table 24–22 shows the differences between delirium and dementia.

Treatment and Its Importance in Delirium

Delirium can present a life-threatening situation and must be recognized and treated promptly. Determining and treating the underlying medical causes and providing supportive care are essential. When treated promptly delirium is usually completely reversible. If the underlying factor is not reversed, delirium can lead to chronic organic brain impairment and death. Delirium itself is not the cause of death, but the underlying medical condition may be. Delirium should always be treated as a medical emergency.

Treatment efforts are geared toward determining and treating the cause or causes responsible for the delirium and maintaining physiologic balance with hydration, nutrition, oxygen supply, and electrolyte balance. All unnecessary medications should be discontinued until the problem is resolved. The use of a low-dose neuroleptic such as haloperidol, 0.5 to 2.0 mg BID, may be necessary if the patient is agitated, but it should be discontinued as soon as the patient has recovered. Due to the fluctuating course of delirium, patients must be deemed stable for 48 hours before recovery can be considered certain (Zisook & Braff, 1986).

Nursing Management

Nursing intervention in delirium may include prevention, detection, and intervention.

Using knowledge of the predisposing factors as a guide, the nurse can anticipate delirium and institute preventive measures. The follow-

Table 24–22. CLINICAL FEATURES IN DELIRIUM AND DEMENTIA

	Delirium	Dementia
Duration	Few weeks to 3 months	In progress at least 1 to 2 years
Paranoid states	Prominent while cognitive impairment is mild or variable	More consistent with degree of impairment; less prominent paranoia
Fluctuations	Marked contrasts in levels of awareness	Not seen in such contrast Progressive decline
Persecutory delusions	Ordered and cohesive	Vague, random, contradictory
General intellectual powers	Preserved during lucid intervals	Consistent loss and decline
Affect	Intermittent fear, perplexity, or bewilderment	Flat or indifferent affect
Perceptual disturbances	Hallucinations are often disturbing and very clearly defined	Hallucinations vague, fleeting, ill-defined, and in many cases it is difficult to make a clear judgment that they exist.

(Data from Roth, 1978.)

ing specific measures will benefit an elderly patient who is hospitalized with a preexisting dementia or one whose cerebral function is compromised. If the patient is being hospitalized for scheduled elective surgery, family members can be encouraged to have a familiar person stay with the patient around the clock for the first few postoperative days. A familiar person can provide reality feedback, comfort, and a sense of continuity with the patient's life before hospitalization. Analgesic medications predispose a patient to delirium. Therefore, attention should be paid to nonpharmaceutical comfort measures. Proper positioning, massage, maintaining comfortable temperature, and allowing maximum mobility may decrease the patient's reliance on medication. Decreasing unnecessary noise, explaining all actions, providing orienting sensory input with brief but frequent contacts, and using staffing patterns that allow for continuity of care all contribute to the patient's orientation and alertness (Campbell, et al., 1986). Carefully monitoring intake, output, skin turgor, and laboratory test results will decrease the incidence of dehydration or electrolyte imbalance.

Patients in the community are equally susceptible to delirium. Particularly at risk are those who are frail, impaired, and living alone and those with one or more chronic illnesses. Nurses may take an active role in caregiver education, teaching caregivers to be alert to subtle changes and to seek medical attention promptly for any sudden appearance of agitation, hallucinations, lethargy, somnolence, or sleep disturbance, even in a patient with a preexisting dementia. The latter are particularly likely to have an undiagnosed delirium because the sudden change is interpreted simply as worsening of the existing dementia. Public health and home care nurses need to monitor routinely for adequate nutrition and hydration, alcohol use, or misuse of medications in frail, community-dwelling elderly. The same interventions are applicable for patients in long-term care settings.

Because nurses have continual contact with elderly in many settings, they are often the first to detect delirium. The appearance of signs and symptoms that might indicate delirium, specifically difficulty thinking, remembering, and perceiving with disorientation, disordered attention, and somnolence or night wakefulness, all of which fluctuate, should lead to further investigation immediately. Vital signs should be taken and compared to baseline values. Assessment includes neurologic status, cardiovascular status, respiratory status, and a review of current medications. The patient is screened for fluid volume deficit and hypo- or hyperglycemia. Laboratory studies, including complete blood count with differential, blood urea nitrogen, creatinine, electrolytes, and glucose, should be done. If there are physical findings of respiratory insufficiency, a specimen for arterial blood gases should be drawn (Foreman, 1984). The presence of signs of delirium and positive findings in any of the above tests indicate that delirium is a likely diagnosis.

The first step in the treatment of delirium is to find and treat or remove the causative factor. This process involves time. In the interval, nursing care of the patient with delirium presents a challenge. Primary nursing goals are to provide for patient safety and comfort and intervene to mitigate psychiatric symptoms. Patients with delirium require hospitalization. If possible, they should be in a private room, with continual supervision. The immediate environment should be quiet and as uncluttered and simple as possible. Patients with delirium are highly excitable and irritable and are prone to misinterpret stimuli. The presence of familiar objects, such as a large calendar and clock, are important. Ideally the room should have a view to provide cues to time and place. Lighting should be soft and diffuse to avoid sharp contrasts and shadows that can be misperceived. Patients who normally use hearing aids or glasses should be allowed to keep them (Levkoff, Besdine, & Wetle, 1986).

Interactions with the patient should be kept to the minimum during periods of agitation. Medication may be used to treat symptoms of sleep-wake disturbance, hallucinations, and illusions present during agitated periods. Liston (1984) recommends avoiding phenothiazines, which may increase confusion due to their anticholinergic effects. He suggests butyrophenones such as haldoperidol to control disturbances of thought and hallucinations and short half-life benzodiazepines such as temazepam to correct disturbed sleep-wake cycles. Because a patient with delirium is already impaired, care should be taken to use the lowest effective dose. As a rule of thumb, the starting dose should be one-third the usual adult dose of any of the drugs mentioned. Needed nursing care, attending to hygiene, hydration, and nutritional needs, should be given during periods of relative calm and lucidity. At these times the nurse can provide corrective sensory input while administering

care. The patient may need frequent reorientation to the surroundings and situation. Patients with delirium may not remember where or why they are hospitalized and may need to be retold the location and duration of the hospital stay and the events leading up to it. This can be done in a gently reassuring manner, emphasizing the positive aspects. Small improvements, such as the change from parenteral to oral nutrition, ambulating for greater distances, or taking a shower independently can be praised in a way that encourages the patient. A conversational tone and style by the nurse conveys respect and concern without being condescending.

The successful management of delirium depends on close cooperation between nurse and physician. Monitoring and reporting the patient's condition and providing protection, support, and basic physical needs are the functions in successful nursing management of delirium.

References

Albert, MS (1981): Geriatric neuropsychology. *J Consult Clin Psychol*, 49:835–850.

Alzheimer's Research Review (Summer, 1987). Published by Alzheimer's Disease Research, Rockville, MD.

American Psychiatric Association (APA) (1980): *Diagnostic and Statistical Manual of Mental Disorders* (ed 3). Washington, DC.

Arenberg, D (1968): Concept problem solving in young and old adults. *J Gerontol*, 9:90–100.

Arenberg, D (1974): A longitudinal study of problem solving in adults. *J Gerontol*, 29:650–658.

Aronson, MK (1988): Caring for the dementia patient. *In* Aronson, MK (ed): *Understanding Alzheimer's Disease.* New York, Macmillan, 95–127.

Awad, IA, Spetzler, RF, Hodak, JA, et al. (1987): Incidental lesions noted on magnetic resonance imaging of the brain: Prevalence and clinical significance in various age groups. *Neurosurgery*, 20(2):223–227.

Bagne, C, Pomara, N, Crook, T, et al. (1986): Treatment development strategies for Alzheimer's disease. *In* Crook, T, Bartus, R, Ferris, S, et al. (eds): *Treatment Development Strategies for Alzheimer's Disease.* New Canaan, CT, Mark Powley, 586–589.

Bartol, MA (1979): Nonverbal communication in patients with Alzheimer's disease. *J Gerontol Nurs*, 5:21–31.

Barnett, HM (1983): Heart in ischemic stroke—a changing emphasis. *Neurol Clin*, 1:291–316.

Beck, JC, Benson, DF, Scheibel, AB, et al. (1982): Dementia

in the elderly: The silent epidemic. *Ann Intern Med*, 97:231–241.

Benson, DF, & Barton, MI (1970): Disturbances in constructional ability. *Cortex*, 6:19–46.

Benson, DF, Cummings, JF, & Tsai, SY (1982): Angular gyrus syndrome simulating Alzheimer's disease. *Arch Neurol*, 39:616–620.

Birren, JE, & Schaie, KW (1985): *Handbook of the Psychology of Aging*, ed 2. New York, Van Nostrand Reinhold.

Bondareff, W (1984): Neurobiology of Alzheimer's disease. *Psychiatr Ann*, 14(3):179–185.

Bondareff, W, Mountjoy, CQ, Roth, M, et al. (1987): Age and histopathologic heterogeneity in Alzheimer's disease. *Arch Gen Psychiatry*, 44:412–417.

Brown, J (1958): Some tests of the decay theory of immediate memory. *Q J Exp Psychol*, 10:12–21.

Butters, N, & Barton, M (1970): Effects of parietal lobe damage on the performance of reversible operations in space. *Neuropsychologica*, 8:205–214.

Butters, N, Sax, D, Montgomery, K, et al. (1978): Comparison of the neuropsychological deficits associated with early and advanced Huntington's disease. *Arch Neurol*, 35:585–589.

Campbell, EB, Williams, MA, & Mlynarczyk, SM (1986): After the fall, confusion. *Am J Nurs*, 86(2):151–154.

Chandra, V, Bharucha, NE, & Schoenberg, BS (1986): Conditions associated with Alzheimer's disease at death: Case control study. *Neurology*, 36:209–211.

Cogan, D (1979): Visuospatial dysgnosia. *Am J Ophthalmol*, 88:361–368.

Cohen, D, & Eisdorfer, C (1986): The diagnosis of dementia. *In The Loss of Self: A Family Resource for the Care of Alzheimer's Disease and Related Disorders*. New York, New American Library, 33–57.

Constantinidis, J (1984): Acetylcholine, glutamate, GABA and neuropeptides in senile dementia of Alzheimer type. *In Wertheimer, J, & Marois, M (eds): Senile Dementia: Outlook for the Future*. New York, Alan R. Liss, 55–68.

Crystal, HA, Horoupian, DS, Katzman, R, et al. (1982): Biopsy-proved Alzheimer disease presenting as a right parietal lobe syndrome. *Ann Neurol*, 12:186–188.

Cummings, JL, & Benson, DF (1983): *Dementia: A Clinical Approach*. Woburn, MA, Butterworth.

Cummings, JL, & Benson, DF (1984): Subcortical dementia: Review of an emerging concept. *Arch Neurol*, 41:874–879.

Cummings, JL, Miller, B, Hill, MA, et al. (1987): Neuropsychiatric aspects of multi-infarct dementia and dementia of the Alzheimer's type. *Arch Neurol*, 44:389–393.

Davies, HD, Ingram, L, Priddy, JM, & Tinklenberg, JR: Responding to the loss of a parent over time: Experiences of young adult children of Alzheimer patients. *Manuscript in preparation*.

Deary, IJ, & Whalley, LJ (1988): Recent research on the causes of Alzheimer's disease. *Br Med J*, 297:807–810.

Eisdorfer, C, & Cohen, D (1981): Management of the patient and family coping with dementing illness. *J Fam Pract*, 12:831–837.

Erkinjuntti, T (1987): Differential diagnosis between Alzheimer's disease and vascular dementia: Evaluation of common clinical methods. *Acta Neurol Scand*, 76:433–442.

Erkinjuntti, T, Ketonen, L, Sulkava, R, et al. (1987): Do white matter changes on MRI and CT differentiate vascular dementia from Alzheimer's disease? *J Neurol Neurosurg Psychiatry*, 50:37–42.

Erkinjuntti, T, Laaksonen, R, Sulkava, R, et al. (1986): Neuropsychological differentiation between normal aging. Alzheimer's disease and vascular dementia. *Acta Neurol Scand*, 74:393–403.

Fisher, CM (1965): Lacunes: Small deep cerebral infarcts. *Neurology*, 15:774–784.

Folstein, MF, Folstein, SE, & McHugh, PR (1975): Mini-mental state: A practical method for grading the cognitive state of patients for the clinician. *J Psychiatr Res*, 12:189–198.

Foreman, M (1984): Acute confusional states in the elderly: An algorithm. *Dim Crit Care Nurs*, 3(4):207–215.

Forsyth, P, & Miller, J (1987): Inner vision. *UCSF Magazine*, 10:(1), (University of California, San Francisco). UCSF Department of News and Public Information Services, 3–9.

French, LR, Schuman, LM, Mortimer, JA, et al. (1985): A case-control study of dementia of the Alzheimer's type. *Am J Epidemiol*, 121:414–421.

Funkenstein, HH, Hicks, R, Dysken, MW, et al. (1981): Drug treatment of cognitive impairment in Alzheimer's disease and the late life dementias. *In Miller, NE, & Cohen, GD (eds): Clinical Aspects of Alzheimer's Disease and Senile Dementia* (Vol 15). New York, Raven Press, 139–160.

Gold, PE, & Stone, WS (1988): Neuroendocrine effects on memory in aged rodents and humans. *Neurobiol Aging*, 9:709–717.

Gollin, ES (1960): Developmental studies of visual recognition of incomplete objects. *Percept Mot Skills*, 11:289–298.

Goodglass, H, & Kaplan, E (1972): *The Assessment of Aphasia, and Related Disorders*. Philadelphia, Lea & Febiger.

Grant, DA, & Berg EA (1948): A behavioral analysis of degree of reinforcement and ease of shifting to new responses in a Weigl-type card-sorting problem. *J Exp Psychol*, 38:404–411.

Hachinski, VC, Iliff, LD, Zilhka, E, et al. (1975): Cerebral blood flow in dementia. *Arch Neurol*, 32:632–637.

Hachinski, VC, Lassen, NA, & Marshall, J (1974): Multi-infarct dementia: A cause of mental deterioration in the elderly. *Lancet*, 2:207–209.

Hall, JL, Gonder-Frederick, LA, Chewning, WW, et al. (1989): Glucose enhancement of memory in young and aged humans. *Neuropsychologia*, 27:1129–1138.

Henderson, AS, & Huppert, FA (1984): The problem of mild dementia. *Psychol Med*, 14:5–11.

Heston, LL, Mastri, AR, Anderson, VE, et al. (1981): Dementia of the Alzheimer type: Clinical genetics, natural history, and associated conditions. *Arch Gen Psychiatry*, 38:1085–1090.

Heyman, A (1978): Differentiation of Alzheimer's disease from multi-infarct dementia. *In Katzman, R, Terry, RD, & Bick, KL (eds): Alzheimer's Disease: Senile Dementia and*

Related Disorders. (Vol 7). New York, Raven Press, 109–110.

Heyman, A, Wilkinson, WE, Stafford, JA, et al. (1984): Alzheimer's disease: A study of the epidemiological aspects. *Ann Neurol*, 15:335–341.

Hollister, LE (1985): Alzheimer's disease. Is it worth treating? *Drugs*, 29(6):483–488.

Hooper, HE (1958): *The Hooper Visual Organization Test Manual*. Los Angeles Western Psychologic Services.

Huff, FJ, Corkin, S, & Growdon, JH (1986): Semantic impairment and anomia in Alzheimer's disease. *Brain Language*, 28:235–249.

Huff, FJ, Growdon, JH, Corkin, S, et al. (1987): Age at onset and rate of progression of Alzheimer's disease. *J Am Geriatr Soc*, 35:27–30.

Jacobs, TW, Kinkel, WR, Painter, F, et al. (1978): Computerized tomography in dementia with special reference to changes in size of normal ventricles during aging and normal pressure hydrocephalus. *In* Katzman, R, Terry, RD, & Bick, KL (eds): *Alzheimer's Disease: Senile Dementia and Related Disorders* (Vol 7). New York, Raven Press, 241–260.

Jagust, WJ, Budinger, RF, & Reed, BR (1987): The diagnosis of dementia with single photon emission computed tomography. *Arch Neurol*, 44:258–262.

Jarvik, LF, Ruth, V, & Matsuyama, SS (1980): Organic brain syndrome and aging: A six-year follow-up of surviving twins. *Arch Gen Psychiatry*, 37:280–286.

Kaplan, E, Goodglass, H, & Weintraub, S (1978): *The Boston Naming Test*. Boston, Kaplan & Goodglass.

Kase, CS (1986): Multi-infarct dementia. A real entity? *J Am Geriatr Soc*, 34:482–484.

Katzman, R (1981): Early detection of senile dementia. *Hosp Pract*, 6:61–76.

Katzman, R (1984): Dementia. *In* Apple, SH (ed): *Current Neurology* (Vol 5). New York, John Wiley & Sons, 91–110.

Katzman, R (1986): Alzheimer's disease. *N Engl J Med*, 4:964–972.

Khachaturian, ZS (1985): Progress of research on Alzheimer's disease. *Am Psychol*, 40:11, 1251–1255.

Kolb, B, & Whishaw, IQ (1985): *Fundamentals of Human Neuropsychology* (ed 2). New York, WW Freeman.

Lawton, MP, Moss, M, Fulcomer, M, et al. (1982): A research and service oriented multilevel assessment instrument. *J Gerontol*, 37:91–99.

Levkoff, SE, Besdine, RW, & Wetle, I (1986): Acute confusional states in hospitalized elderly. *In* Eisdorfer, C (ed): *Annual Review of Gerontology and Geriatrics*, 6. New York, Springer.

Lezak, MD (1978): Living with the characterologically altered brain injured patient. *J Clin Psychiatry*, 39:592–598.

Lezak, MD (1983): *Neuropsychological Assessment* (ed 2). New York, Oxford University Press.

Lipowski, ZJ (1980): *Delirium: Acute Brain Failure in Man*. Springfield, IL, Charles C Thomas.

Lipowski, ZJ (1984): Acute confusion states in the elderly. *In* Albert, ML (ed): *Clinical Neurology of Aging*. New York, Oxford University Press, 279–297.

Liston, E (1984): Diagnosis and management of delirium in the elderly patient. *Psychiatr Ann*, 14(2):109–117.

Lumpkin, MD, Negro-Vilar, A, & McCann, SM (1981): Paradoxical elevation of growth hormone by intraventricular somatostatin: Possible ultrashort-loop feedback. *Science*, 211:1072–1074.

Mace, NL, & Rabins, PV (1981): *The 36-Hour Day*. Baltimore, MD, Johns Hopkins University Press.

Maletta, GJ (1985): Medications to modify at home behavior of Alzheimer's disease patients. *Geriatrics*, 40(12):31–42.

Matsui, T, & Hirano, A (1978): *An Atlas of the Human Brain for Computerized Tomography*. New York, Igaku-Shoin.

McCartney, JR, & Palmateer, LM (1985): Assessment of cognitive deficit in geriatric patients: A study of physician behavior. *J Am Geriatr Soc*, 33:467–471.

McDonald, RS (1986): Assessing treatment effects: Behavior rating scales. *In* Poon, LW, Crook, T, Davis, KL, et al. (eds): *Handbook for Clinical Memory Assessment of Older Adults*. Washington, DC, American Psychological Association, 129–138.

McKhann, G, Drachman, D, Folstein, M, et al. (1984): Clinical diagnosis of Alzheimer's disease: Report of the NINCDS-ADRDA work group under the auspices of Department of Health and Human Services Task Force on Alzheimer's Disease. *Neurology*, 34:939–944.

McLachlan, DR, Dalton, AJ, Galin, H, et al. (1984): Alzheimer's disease: Clinical course and cognitive disturbances. *Acta Neurol Scand*, 99:83–89.

Meier, DE, & Cassel, CK (1986): Nurisng home placement and the demented patient. *Ann Intern Med*, 104:98–105.

Mesulam, MM (1982): Slowly progressive aphasia without generalized dementia. *Ann Neurol*, 11:592–598.

Meyer, JS, Judd, BW, Tawakina, T, et al. (1986): Improved cognition after control of risk factors for multi-infarct dementia. *JAMA*, 256:2203–2209.

Milner, B (1963): Effects of different brain lesions on card sorting. *Arch Neurol*, 9:90–100.

Molsa, PK, Marttila, RJ, & Rinne, UK (1984): Extrapyramidal signs in Alzheimer's disease. *Neurology*, 34:1114–1116.

Mortimer, JA, Christensen, KJ, & Webster, DD (1985): Parkinsonian dementia. *In* Vinken, PJ, Broyn, GW, Klawans, HL (eds): *Handbook of Clinical Neurology*, 2(46). Amsterdam, Elsevier, 371–384.

Mortimer, JA, French, LR, Hutton, JT, et al. (1985): Head injury as a risk factor for Alzheimer's disease. *Neurology (NY)*, 35:264–267.

Mortimer, JA, Schuman, LM, & French, LR (1981): Epidemiology of dementing illness. *In* Mortimer, JA, & Schuman, LM (eds): *The Epidemiology of Dementia*. New York, Oxford University Press, 3–23.

Moss, MB (1984): Assessment of memory in amnesic and dementia patients: Adaptation of behavioral tests used with non-human primates. Presented at the 12th Annual Meeting of the International Neuropsychological Society, Houston, TX.

National Institute on Aging Task Force (1980): Senility reconsidered. Treatment possibilities for mental impairment in the elderly. *JAMA*, 244:259–263.

Nissen, MJ, Corkin, S, & Growdon, JH (1982): Attentional

focusing in amnesia and Alzheimer's disease. (Unpublished manuscript).

Obrist, WD (1978): Electroencephalography in aging and dementia. *In* Katzman, R, Terry, RD, & Bick, KL (eds): *Alzheimer's Disease: Senile Dementia and Related Disorders.* New York, Raven Press, 227–232.

Oxman, TE (1987): Alzheimer's dementia: Molecular biology, society treatment. *Psychiatric News,* July 3.

Pearce, J (1974): The extrapyramidal disorder of Alzheimer's disease. *Eur Neurol, 12:*94–103.

Perez, FI, Rivera, VM, Meyer, JS, et al. (1975): Analysis of intellectual and cognitive performance in patients with multi-infarct dementia, vertebrobasilar insufficiency with dementia, and Alzheimer's disease. *J Neurol Neurosurg Psychiatry, 38:*533–40.

Peterson, LR, & Peterson, MJ (1959): Short-term retention of individual verbal items. *J Exp Psychol, 58:*193–198.

Pruisner, SB (1984): Some speculations about prions, amyloid and Alzheimer's disease. *N Engl J Med, 310:*661–663.

Read, SL, & Jarvik, LF (1984): Cerebrovascular disease in the differential diagnosis of dementia. *Psychiatr Ann, 14*(2):100–108.

Reisberg, B, Ferris, SH, & de Leon, MJ (1982): The global deterioration scale for assessment of primary degenerative dementia. *Am J Psychiatry, 139:*1136–1139.

Rocca, WA, Amaducci, LA, & Schoenberg, BS (1986): Epidemiology of clinically diagnosed Alzheimer's disease. *Ann Neurol, 19:*415–424.

Rogers, RL, Meyer, JS, Mortel, KF, et al. (1986): Decreased cerebral blood flow precedes multi-infarct dementia, but follows senile dementia of Alzheimer's type. *Neurology, 36:*1–6.

Rosen, WG, Mohs, RC, & Davis, KL (1984): A new rating scale for Alzheimer's disease. *Am J Psychiatry, 141*(11):1356–1364.

Roth, M (1978): Diagnosis of senile and related forms of dementia. *In* Katzman, R, Terry, RD, & Bick, KL (eds): *Alzheimer's Disease: Senile Dementia and Related Disorders* (Vol 7). New York, Raven Press, 71–85.

Sagar, HF, & Sullivan, EV (1988): Patterns of cognitive impairment in dementia. *In* Kennard, C (ed): *Recent Advances in Clinical Neurology, 5:*47–86.

Sagar, HJ, Sullivan, EV, Cohen, NJ, et al. (1987): Autobiographical memory in normal aging and dementia. *J Clin Exp Neuropsychol, 9:*16.

Schlageter, NL, Carson, RE, & Rapoport, SI (1987): Examination of blood-brain barrier permeability in dementia of the Alzheimer's type with [68 Ga] EDTA and positron emission tomography. *J Cerebral Blood Flow Metab, 7:*1–8.

Schoenberg, BS (1986): Epidemiology of Alzheimer's disease and other dementing illnesses. *J Chron Dis, 39*(12):1095–1104.

Schoenberg, BS, Okazaki, H, & Kokmen, E (1981): Reduced survival in patients with dementia: A population study. *Trans Am Neurol Assoc, 106:*306–308.

Shuttleworth, EC (1984): Atypical presentations of dementia of the Alzheimer type. *J Am Geriatr Soc, 32:*485–490.

Smith, JS (1981): The investigation of dementia: Results in 200 consecutive admissions. *Lancet, 1:*824–827.

Steele, C, Lucas, MJ, & Tune, LE (1982): An approach to the management of dementia syndromes. *Johns Hopkins Med J, 151:*362–368.

Sullivan, N, & Fogel, B (1986): Could this be delirium? *Am J Nurs, 12:*1359–1363.

Tariot, PN, & Weingartner, H (1986): A psychobiologic analysis of cognitive failures. *Arch Gen Psychiatr, 43:*1183–1188.

Terry, R, & Pena, C (1965): Experimental production of neurofibrillary degeneration. *J Neuropathol Exp Neurol, 24:*200–210.

Thal, LJ (1988): Treatment strategies: Present and future. *In* Aronson, MK (ed): *Understanding Alzheimer's Disease.* New York, Charles Scribner's Sons, 55–60.

Thornton, JE, Davies HD, & Tinklenberg, JR (1986): Alzheimer's disease syndrome. *J Psychosoc Nurs Ment Health Serv, 24*(5):16–22.

U'Ren, RC (1987): Testing older patients' mental status: Practical office-based approach. *Geriatrics, 42*(3):49–56.

Verwoerdt, A (1981): Individual psychotherapy in senile dementia. *In* Miller, NE, & Cohen, GE (eds): *Clinical Aspects of Alzheimer's Disease and Senile Dementia.* New York, Raven Press, 187–208.

Victor, M, & Banker, BO (1978): Alcohol and dementia. *In* Katzman, R, Terry, RD, & Brick, KL (eds): *Alzheimer's Disease: Senile Dementia and Related Disorders* (Vol 7). New York, Raven Press, 149–170.

Watts, K, Braddeley, A, & Williams, M (1982): Automated tailored testing using Raven's matrices and the Nill Hill vocabulary tests: A comparison with manual administration. *Int J Man-Machine Studies, 17:*331–344.

Wechsler, AF (1977): Presenile dementia presenting as aphasia. *J Neurol Neurosurg Psychiatry, 40:*303–305.

Wechsler, DA (1945): A standardized memory scale for clinical use. *J Psychol, 19:*87–95.

Wechsler, D (1981): *The Weschsler Adult Intelligence Scale—Revised Manual.* New York, The Psychological Corporation.

Wells, CE (1978): Chronic brain disease. An overview. *Am J Psychiatry, 135:*1–12.

Williams, MA, Campbell, EB, Raynor, WJ, et al. (1985a): Reducing acute confusional states in elderly patients with hip fractures. *Res Nurs Health, 8*(4):329–337.

Williams, M, Campbell, E, Raynor, W, et al. (1985b): Predictors of confusional states in hospitalized elderly patients. *Res Nurs Health, 8*(1):31–40.

Winokur, GD (1981): Depression: The facts. Oxford, Oxford University Press.

Wurtman, RJ (1985): Alzheimer's disease. *Sci Am, 252*(1):62–74.

Yesavage, JA, & Hollister, LE (1978): The treatment of senile dementia. *Ration Drug Ther, 12*(8):1–6.

Zisook, S, & Braff, DL (1986): Delirium: Recognition and management in the older patient. *Geriatrics, 41*(6):67–78.

CHAPTER
25

Parkinson's Disease

JEANIE S. KAYSER-JONES, R.N., Ph.D., F.A.A.N.
THEODORE H.D. JONES, Ph.D.

DEFINITION AND CLASSIFICATION

Parkinson's disease (PD) is a degenerative, neurologic condition that is due to progressive death of specific subpopulations of neurons in the brain. It affects primarily the elderly and leads to muscle tremor, muscle rigidity, akinesia, and neuropsychological difficulties. The course of the disease is unpredictable, there is great variation in individual disabilities and needs, and responses to medication are both variable and somewhat unpredictable. In some patients, with appropriate drug therapy, the disease is well controlled for long periods of time and may never progress to invalidism. In other cases, however, patients can become severely rigid, dysarthric, and nearly immobile (Mastrian, 1984). Most cases can be classified

491

as one of several distinct types of PD. These are shown in Table 25–1.

This chapter will describe the essential characteristics of PD and apply this knowledge to the nursing care of patients with PD.

PREVALENCE

About 15% of all cases of PD are first observed in people aged 30 to 49 years and 75% in people aged 50 to 65 years. About 1% of the population over age 50 is affected (Boller, 1985; Schoenberg, 1987), so that in the United States there are more than 1 million cases; as the population ages, this figure will increase significantly. Since the early signs of the disease may be overlooked, mild or late-onset cases can go unreported and the true frequency of PD may be higher.

THEORIES OF CAUSATION

Genetics

Studies of monozygotic twins show that there is no strongly dominant genetic factor in determining susceptibility to or onset of PD (Ward, Duvoisin, Ince, et al., 1983). Some investigators have identified specific subtypes of Parkinson's disease, a tremor-associated form and a juvenile form, in which there is a weak familial association. Responses to environmental chemicals, a possible cause of idiopathic PD, do show genetic variation in human populations. Patients with drug-induced parkinsonism characteristically have lower amounts of the liver enzymes that detoxify foreign compounds than do normal subjects (Barbeau, Cloutier, Roy, et al., 1985).

Biologic Factors

The symptoms of PD can be greatly intensified by emotional stress, but there is no

Table 25–1. CLASSIFICATION OF PARKINSON'S DISEASE

Type	Frequency (%) of All Cases	Pathology	Specific Characteristics
Idiopathic	66–75	Death of neurons in substantia nigra	Progressive; other brain ganglia are normal in size and weight
Degenerative	15–20	Death of neurons in multiple regions of the brain	Includes senile parkinsonism (a late-onset [about 80 years of age] condition with dementia, possibly related to Alzheimer's disease) and Parkinson dementia complex (common in Guam)
Vascular	6	Tissue damage in basal ganglia of brain due to multiple infarcts in cerebral arteries	Not progressive, may improve with time
Postencephalitic	4		Only in patients infected with viral encephalitis in 1916–1928 epidemic; frequency decreasing as these subjects die
Symptomatic	3	Damage to basal ganglia from brain tumors, Creutzfeldt-Jacob disease, neurolipidoses, etc.	
Posttraumatic	1	Damage to basal ganglia from traumatic injuries	Includes boxing injuries (dementia pugilistica)
Toxin- or drug-induced	1	Tissue damage from environmental chemicals and pharmaceuticals	Associated with carbon monoxide, carbon disulfide, manganese, and neuroleptic drugs
Unclassified	2		

evidence to show that stress itself is the cause of the condition. PD is observed more often in individuals with subdued personality or long-term depression, but this association may simply reflect a common cause (Poewe, Gerstenhand, Ransmayr, et al., 1983). Chronic depression can be the result of a decrease in the amount of dopamine in the central nervous system, which is also the essential defect in PD.

Vascular and Traumatic Injury

In a small percentage of cases, parkinsonism is the result of vascular damage occurring in the brain or of traumatic injury to the head.

Toxins

Positive correlations have been reported between the incidence of PD and the use of pesticides in communities (Lewin, 1985). The fact that PD was first described in 1817 (Critchley, 1955), as the Industrial Revolution was beginning, supports the idea that PD may be caused by chronic exposure to environmental toxins (Langston, 1986; Spencer, Nunn, Hugon, et al., 1987).

Aging

The only risk factor that is unequivocally associated with PD is increasing age. As individuals age, there are significant changes in the basal ganglia that may be responsible for the movement disorders characteristic of the healthy elderly: slower movement, greater difficulty in coordination, and decreased ability to perform finely controlled movements. Changes in the basal ganglia with age are implicated in the development of PD (Finch, Randall, & Marshall, 1981; Jellinger, 1986). In normal aging individuals the substantia nigra (SN) loses 30% to 50% of its neurons. The concentrations of dopamine, the neurotransmitter in SN cells, show parallel decreases. In PD the SN loses 80% to 99% of its cells, so the

normal loss of cells during aging, while leading to some slowing in motor activities (a possible pre-Parkinson state), would not alone be sufficient to result in PD. Variations in the normal rate of loss and in the threshold percentage loss at which PD symptoms appear will result in varying, genetically determined individual susceptibilities. The probability of PD developing thus clearly increases in all individuals as they age but at different rates.

Therapeutic Drugs

Drugs that interfere with dopaminergic function, e.g., antipsychotics, or that stimulate cholinergic function, e.g., cholinergic agonists, can cause drug-induced parkinsonism or exacerbate a parkinsonism condition already present.

NATURE OF THE LESION

Dopaminergic cells function as inhibitory nerve fibers in the central nervous system. In PD the massive death of the SN dopaminergic cells, whose axons form synapses with the neostriatal cholinergic cells, removes some of the activity that normally modulates impulses leaving the striatum (Finch, Randall, & Marshall, 1981). This decrease in input to the striatum and resulting imbalance in dopaminergic and cholinergic activity are the important defects in PD and produce the motor abnormalities. Striatal signals, unmodified by inhibitory input from the SN, are transmitted through the ventral thalamus to the motor cortex and spinal motor neurons and result in oscillating electrical signals that produce the involuntary rhythmic muscular movements (tremor), muscle rigidity, and bradykinesia, which are the three classic symptoms of PD.

CLINICAL SYMPTOMS

PD shows three characteristic symptoms affecting motor activity: an involuntary shaking of the limbs (tremor), resistance of the muscles to stretching (rigidity), and slowness or absence of movement (bradykinesia or akinesia) (Birkmayer & Riederer, 1983).

Tremor

This is the most obvious symptom of PD and therefore is often the one that first indicates the onset of the disease. The resting tremor is usually seen as a rhythmic, involuntary movement of the thumb and fingers in a rocking motion called "pill rolling," but it may also occur in the feet, head, jaw, or lips; it may be unilateral or bilateral. This movement results in little energy drain on the body and can therefore be maintained all day without the patient requiring rest. Parkinsonian tremor cannot be controlled by cognitive effort. Restriction of tremor in one limb will transfer it to another limb. Emotional stress, such as self-consciousness or interpersonal conflict, exacerbates the tremor. The tremor is very similar to basic motor rhythms seen in organisms with simpler brain structure, which suggests that the defect in PD results in the expression of activities of the more primitive regions of the brain.

Rigidity

This condition is present in nearly all cases of PD and can be detected by moving the patient's joints so as to stretch the skeletal muscles. Passive resistance to this stretching is felt during the movement, often together with jerky, intermittent resistance called "cogwheel rigidity." When the muscle spindles are stretched, abnormal contraction of the main muscle is developed and sustained, producing tension in major muscle groups, especially in the antigravity muscles affecting the shoulders, trunk, and pelvis. Continuous muscle tension leads frequently to pain in the joints, which may be misdiagnosed as rheumatism or arthritis.

The essential motor deficit in rigidity is the inability to activate or relax muscles selectively for a particular movement (Lannon, Thomas, Bratton, et al., 1986).

Bradykinesia and Akinesia

Bradykinesia (slowness of movement) and akinesia (inability to move) are the most incapacitating of all the disabilities encountered in PD (Stern & Lees, 1982). These symptoms result from a deficiency in the ability to convert the will to move into actual motion. As with tremor and rigidity, akinesia may be symmetric or asymmetric, in which case the patient tends to turn toward the freer side and so balance is disturbed. Akinesia is independent of muscle rigidity and tremor (Birkmayer & Riederer, 1983), but together they produce major changes in overall appearance and behavior. The severity of the akinesia is, like tremor, influenced by mood and greatly increased by emotional stress.

Autonomic Disturbances

Changes in the function of the autonomic nervous system may cause hyperthermia, seborrhea, loss of appetite, and profuse perspiration, all of which indicate a disturbance of brain stem function. Episodes of profuse diaphoresis may occur, for example, even in cold weather and may be severe enough to drench the patient's clothing. This is due partly to anticholinergic medications as well as to an impaired temperature regulatory mechanism and perspiration control.

Neuropsychological Symptoms

Impaired visuospatial perception, dementia, and depression are conditions commonly found among patients with PD (Boller, 1985). Virtually all patients with idiopathic PD are impaired in visuospatial perception, having more difficulty in identifying accurately the relative position of objects in space, in orienting objects or body parts in specific directions, and in performing other mental tasks involving spatial relationships. Patients with PD have been found to have difficulty in shifting from one type of perceptual organization to another, which results in an inability to perform sequential or predictive voluntary movements. Studies suggest that perceptual motor impairment in PD may result from an inability to use incoming sensory information to generate the spatial precept necessary for expected movements (Mayeux & Rosen, 1983). Oculomotor problems may contribute to visuoperceptive spatial and constructional problems. Patients may find it difficult to perceive objects in the peripheral field of vision.

Dementia

Progressive generalized dementia occurs with different degrees of severity in about 30% to 80% of PD patients, about 20% to 30% of PD patients having cognitive impairment severe enough to cause serious difficulty in their lives (Mayeux & Stern, 1983). Specific cognitive deficits associated with PD are an inability to encode, comprehend, and analyze new material; remember recent events; follow instructions; and shift behavior to meet new task requirements (Cools, Van Den Bercken, Horstink, et al., 1984). Bradyphrenia, a slowing of thinking processes, is the most commonly reported cognitive impairment. Long-term memory, social judgment, social manners, verbal fluency, object recognition, auditory attention, and rhythmic pattern discrimination remain intact (Loranger, Goodell, McDowell, et al., 1972; Matthews & Haaland, 1979; Pirozzolo, Hansch, Mortimer, et al., 1982; Talland, 1962).

Recent studies of PD patients with dementia have shown the additional presence of cortical atrophy, cell loss in the nucleus basalis, plaques and Alzheimer-type tangles, and decreased concentrations of the acetylcholine-synthesizing enzyme choline acetyltransferase. These findings, together with the observation that the patterns of cognitive deficits in PD and Alzheimer's disease show many similarities, suggest that these are not two separate conditions but rather may be part of a clinical and pathologic continuum ranging from predominant dementia with motor dysfunction in Alzheimer's disease, to predominant motor dysfunction with dementia in PD (Boller, 1985). Clinically recognizable Alzheimer's disease and PD occur together in patients at rates much higher than could be expected from their individual incidences.

Depression

Most studies report that between 30% and 40% of all PD patients are clinically depressed (Celesia & Wanamaker, 1972; Damasio, Lobo-Antunes, & Macedo, 1970; Goodwin, 1971; Lieberman, Dziatolowski, Kupersmith, et al., 1979; Mayeux, Stern, Cote, et al., 1984). The diagnosis of depression in PD is difficult because some of the symptoms of depression are similar to the behavioral manifestations of the disease. Some studies have found that patients with PD were significantly more depressed than other chronically ill patients, such as patients with cancer, multiple sclerosis, and stroke. These findings are especially significant since the patients in the comparison groups were more disabled physically than the Parkinson's patients (Dakof & Mendelsohn, 1986). There is evidence that for some chronically ill patients, the psychological disturbance is usually greatest in the early stages of illness (Cassileth, Lusk, Strouse, et al., 1984; Meyerowitz, 1980). Singer (1974) found that the longer Parkinson's patients had the disease, the more stoically they accepted its symptoms.

IMAGING AND DIAGNOSIS

As with many degenerative, neurologic diseases that involve gradual deterioration in motor and behavioral activities, it is often difficult to identify the onset of PD or to be aware of the condition in its early stages. There is currently no laboratory test that specifically identifies the preclinical condition. The recent development of positron emission tomography (PET) may provide a method for the early diagnosis and measurement of the severity of the disease, as well as furthering research into the neurochemistry of the condition (Phelps & Mazziotta, 1985). Using these techniques, it has now become possible to observe dopaminergic defects directly in the living human brain, which should improve our understanding of the nature and course of the disease and, possibly, provide a reliable method of early detection (Garnett, Firnau, Lang, et al., 1986).

PHARMACOLOGIC TREATMENT

The treatment of PD, today, is almost exclusively pharmacologic, along with supportive medical and nursing care. The pharmacologic approach is aimed at reestablishing a normal relationship between dopamine and acetylcholine. The patient usually receives some combination of drugs, which may include antihistamines, anticholinergics, amantadine, levodopa, and carbidopa (Table 25–2).

Long-term management of the treatment regimen is challenging and requires excellent communication between patients, their families, and health care providers. Drug toxicity to L-dopa and anticholinergics may occur, with confusion, loss of drug effectiveness, hallucinations, nightmares, dyskinesias, dystonia, and a reversal of sleep-wake patterns. A reduction in dosage may lead to improvement of symptoms, but a period of complete cessation of medication, a "drug holiday," may be necessary. The drug holiday should take place in an inpatient setting where appropriate cardiac monitoring and supportive care are available (Todd, 1985).There is no general consensus as to the ideal duration of a drug holiday. Aminoff (1987) recommends a 10-day respite from antiparkinsonian medication. A drug holiday may be complicated by venous thrombosis, pulmonary embolism, aspiration pneumonia, and depression. The drug holiday is effective about 60% of the time. That is, responsiveness to the medication is improved for at least 6 months afterward and benefit occurs with a lower dosage (Aminoff, 1987). The effectiveness of L-dopa may tend to wear off after a period of 3 to 5 years. Patients may note that they get only 2 to 3 hours of symptom relief from each dose of medication. In addition to the wearing-off effect, long-term L-dopa therapy may result in abnormal involuntary movement (AIMs). AIMs, or dyskinesias, typically occur either at the time of peak drug action (usually 1½ to 2 hours after taking the drug) or at the end of the period of drug action (about 3 to 4 hours after ingestion). (See Lannon, Thomas, Bratton, et al., 1986, for detailed guidelines for patients on a drug holiday.)

Another complication of long-term therapy is the "on/off" phenomenon in which periods of total functional ability (often accompanied by AIMs) are suddenly interrupted by akinetic spells during which the patient is immobilized. These vacillations can occur many times each day and are the most difficult problem encountered in treating PD patients (Lannon, et al., 1986).

The autonomic and neuropsychological symptoms of PD may be treated with specific drugs. Dysfunction of heat-regulating mechanisms, which results in profuse sweats and hyperthermia, is probably due to disturbance of the serotonin system and can be controlled by administering L-tryptophan, the amino acid precursor of serotonin. Depression can be ameliorated with standard antidepressant therapy.

All of the pharmaceuticals used in the treatment of PD affect only the symptoms of the disease. None of them stops or reverses the progressive degeneration of the SN cells, and therefore such chemotherapy does not cure the condition. Indeed, long-term administration of L-dopa may contribute to the atrophy of the nigrostriatal system. Use of substitution chemotherapy, however, has improved the quality of life and raised the life expectancy of patients with PD.

NURSING CARE RELATED TO PHARMACOLOGIC TREATMENT

To achieve the ideal therapeutic range, continuous monitoring of medications is neces-

Table 25–2. DRUG THERAPY IN PARKINSON'S DISEASE

Drug	Mode of Action	Effect	Use	Side Effects
Anticholinergics atropine	Inhibits cholinergic function, no effect on dopamine function; improves cholinergic-dopaminergic balance	Improves tremor and rigidity; no effect on akinesia	Especially useful when patient is receiving neuroleptic drugs	Digestion, hormone secretion, heart rhythm can be affected. Newer synthetic anticholinergics have fewer side effects.
L-dopa	Is a precursor of dopamine; is inactivated by L-dopa decarboxylase inhibitors, especially carbidopa	Improves all physical and cognitive symptoms for 1–5 days; excessive dose causes hyperkinesia	Sinemet is a 10:1, by weight, mixture of L-dopa and carbidopa. Long-term use results in shorter benefit and in periods refractory to the drug ("off-periods"). Initiation of L-dopa therapy should therefore be delayed as long as possible.	High doses can affect gastrointestinal and cardiovascular systems. Patients may develop anxiety, paranoia, and disorientation.
amantadine	Uncertain but appears to bind to dopamine receptors	Effective for only a few months	Often combined with anticholinergics or L-dopa to delay use of higher doses of L-dopa	Few side effects. May disturb sleep or cause visual disturbances or psychoses.
Monamine Oxidase B Inhibitors deprenyl	Inhibits MAO B, the principal enzyme that degrades dopamine in the brain	General improvement lasting several hours; effective for many years	Permits the use of smaller doses of L-dopa, delaying the onset of unresponsiveness to L-dopa	Occasionally dopa psychosis is observed. Foods containing biogenic amines or MAO inhibitors, e.g., certain types of cheese, cause serious side effects. Should not be taken with anticholinergics.
Dopamine Agonists bromocriptine	Mimics dopamine action by binding to dopamine receptors	General improvement, but effectiveness decreases after 1 year	Less effective than L-dopa, so higher doses are required; often given with L-dopa	Nausea, vomiting, hypotension, and confusion may occur.
pergolide, lisuride, lergotrile	Currently being evaluated			

sary. Nursing care related to pharmacologic treatment centers on educating the patient in regard to the side effects of medications, drug interactions, and dietary restrictions. The patient needs specific written information as to the dosage, frequency, possible side effects, and expected outcome of medications.

Certain drugs should be avoided when taking levodopa. Phenytoin (Dilantin) and the phenothiazine derivatives block dopamine receptors. Pyridoxine (vitamin B$_6$) is a cofactor of dopa decarboxylase and reduces the amount of levodopa available for conversion in the brain. The amount of pyridoxine content of a normal diet should not interfere with levodopa therapy; only excess pyridoxine (more than 10 mg per day), such as that in vitamin supplements or fortified cereals, must be avoided (Mastrian, 1984; Todd, 1985). Levodopa is an amino acid; dietary habits can therefore affect its action. A high protein diet can block the effects of levodopa. This blocking can occur whether levodopa is given alone or in combination with an inhibitor like carbidopa. Patients receiving the inhibitor, however, are less susceptible. Whereas a reduction of protein in the diet would be advantageous, in Western culture a high protein diet is considered necessary and indicative of economic success. Low protein diets are considered dangerous and are usually resisted. Thus, rather than having patients adopt a low protein diet, they should be advised to decrease foods high in protein (e.g., meat, milk, fish, poultry, cheese, eggs, nuts, whole grains, and soy bean products) and to take small amounts of protein throughout the day (Garrett, 1982). Caffeine may contribute to the development of AIMs, probably because of its acidity, which speeds the absorption of dopa into the system (Langan & Cotzias, 1976). Also, alkaline products, such as antacids and milk, slow the absorption of drugs; patients may therefore experience a delay between taking their medication and noticing an improvement in symptoms (Garrett, 1982).

Alcohol, in large amounts, can antagonize the effects of levodopa. Patients on L-dopa should be advised to drink no more than two cocktails per evening, to take only a small amount of wine at dinner, to avoid all alcohol during the day, and never to drink while alone (Garrett, 1982).

Obesity may complicate the regulation of L-dopa, since the drug appears to be absorbed into fat depots and to become sequestered erratically. Patients who are overweight should, therefore, be encouraged to lose weight.

SURGERY

Recent technological advances have now greatly improved the practice of stereotactic surgery (Tasker, 1987). Very precise stereotactic localization is possible using new imaging methods, physiologic correlations, stereotactic atlases, computer-controlled microelectrode probes, and intraoperative computer graphics that permit the surgeon, by electrical stimulation with a microprobe, to identify single human neurons and locate those populations of neurons that control tremor. Microlesions then may be produced to reduce or abolish tremor in those patients for whom this is the major impairment. In one such study, 82% of carefully chosen patients treated by this procedure were free of tremor 2 years later (Tasker, Siqueira, Hawrylyshyn, et al., 1983).

Adrenal implants in human patients immobilized by PD have resulted in rapid and significant recovery of mobility (Madrazo, Drucker-Colin, Diaz, et al., 1987; Lewin, 1987), allowing some patients to return to work. Implants of fetal nigral cells into humans with PD are now being performed. All of these results are preliminary and many questions are unanswered: Is the improvement due simply to nonspecific stimulation of the SN by the surgery? What is the long-term fate of the implants? Could fetal implants become tumors? It is being suggested that a multicenter clinical trial be initiated by the National Institutes of Health to determine with absolute certainty that the promise offered by this research is real (Moore, 1987).

NURSING CARE OF PATIENTS WITH PARKINSON'S DISEASE

Nurses may encounter PD patients in the home, in day care centers, in outpatient clinics, in acute-care hospitals, and, in the later stages of the illness, in skilled nursing facilities (nursing homes). The nurse, working collaboratively with physicians and other health care providers, can plan and coordinate the care of patients in these multiple settings. The major components of nursing care for PD patients fall into four categories: (1) assessment of patient and family needs and patient and family education; (2) promotion and maintenance of autonomy and independence; (3) consideration of the psychosocial needs of patients and families; and, (4) prevention of complications. These catetgories will be discussed separately, but it must be noted that they are interrelated and that addressing a problem in one area may achieve a positive outcome in another. For example, providing patients with assistive devices so that they can remain mobile contributes to autonomy and independence, but it also improves morale, thus promoting psychological well-being. Further, exercise such as walking improves muscle tone, thus preventing or at least delaying immobility, which may occur in advanced PD.

Assessment and Education of Patient and Family

Patients with PD and their families are faced with a new, unknown, and somewhat frightening situation. A nurse can be instrumental in helping them to accept the reality of PD and in helping them to realize that with adaptation, planning, treatment, and supportive services, they can live meaningful lives (Caine, 1984). Initially, it is important to assess the level of knowledge about the disease process and the treatment regimen and to provide patients and their families with accurate information regarding treatment and the nature of the disease. It is also important, early in the course of the disease, to assess the patient's and caregiver's abilities to cope with PD and to anticipate how they will be able to manage the progressive disability that occurs. A home visit is valuable in assessing the family's knowledge of the disease process, their support of the patient, and their awareness of supportive community services. During the home visit, the nurse can evaluate the patient's understanding of the medical regimen, inquire about any over-the-counter drugs in the home, discuss the danger of self-medication, and evaluate the home to determine if any changes are necessary to provide a safe environment.

Drug therapy can bring about a dramatic improvement in the patient's condition; drug therapy, however, is complex and must be monitored carefully to achieve maximal benefits. If possible, the patient should be allowed to take medications independently. It must be recognized, however, that forgetfulness, depression, or dementia may contribute to medication errors. Therefore, the spouse or other responsible family member should be included when instructing patients about their treatment regimen.

As new drugs become available, treatment regimens change. Further, drug therapy is tailored to each patient, and patients may respond differently to medications. It is therefore necessary for a nurse to develop a specific teaching plan for each patient. Some general principles, however, apply to all patients. Patients should be advised, for example, that medication doses must not be omitted or altered without first checking with their physician. Over-the-counter drugs should not be taken unless recommended by the physician, and periodic evaluation of the treatment regimen by the physician or nurse is essential.

A teaching plan that includes a complete written and verbal explanation of the treatment regimen, possible side effects, and recommendations for accurate administration of medications is essential. The nurse may suggest, for example, that medications for each day be placed in medication cups or envelopes in the morning so that a dose is not duplicated or forgotten. Explaining the therapeutic effects of each drug and the possible side effects, and making recommendations to counter the adverse effects of the drug are extremely helpful to patients and their families and give them some control in managing the disease.

Last, patient and family education cannot be achieved without good communication skills on the part of all those involved in the patient's care. Appraising the ability of patients to understand, assessing their readiness for learning, and allowing time to repeat the information at a later time are important principles to follow when teaching patients and their families.

Promotion and Maintenance of Autonomy and Independence

Although we are all dependent to some degree on others during our lives, our society places a high value on autonomy and independence. Clark and Anderson (1967) found that the elderly feared dependency and would endure great hardships in order to remain independent. When a chronic illness such as PD begins to erode independence, it can have a devastating effect on the patient's morale. Due to the clinical symptoms of tremor, rigidity, bradykinesia and akinesia, independence, and autonomy begin to decline as patients experience difficulty in walking, talking, eating, dressing, bathing, and performing other activities of daily living. The nurse provides a tremendous service to patients by helping them to identify their remaining strengths and resources and by adapting the environment to prolong independence. For example, rigidity of the trunk muscles contributes to the inability to roll over in bed or to rise to a sitting position. Some patients find that satin sheets facilitate movement in bed and that maneuvering a rope tied to the foot of the bed assists them in turning and getting out of bed independently (Caine, 1984). Further, gentle range-of-motion exercises for 10 minutes four times a day will help to maintain full range of motion and prevent rigidity and contractures. Tremor can make it difficult for patients to eat independently. Assistive devices such as utensils with large handles facilitate eating (the handles of cutlery can be enlarged with foam rubber secured with tape), and providing patients with straws and cups designed to prevent spillage enables them to drink without assistance. Food should be prepared and served so that the patient can eat as independently as possible, for example, by cutting meat before serving and by slicing fruit into small pieces. Rigidity of the facial and pharyngeal muscles contributes to difficulty with mastication and swallowing; the rate of swallowing is decreased and eating may become slower and assume a deliberate quality. As the disease progresses, eating may become increasingly difficult. Both liquids and solids are difficult to swallow, while soft foods are swallowed more easily. Pureed foods should be avoided unless absolutely necessary. Patients should be instructed to take small bites, to chew thoroughly, and to swallow slowly, and they should be allowed as much time as necessary to eat (Mastrian, 1984).

Communication may become a problem for patients with PD. The patient's voice may become low and speech sometimes slurred, making it difficult to understand what is being said. Patience, listening carefully, and assigning the same nurse to the patient for a period of time will facilitate nurse-patient communication.

Physical exercise prevents muscle atrophy and helps to prevent contractures, and it also improves patients' morale. In general, it is wise for patients to be as active as possible without becoming unduly fatigued. Walking is perhaps the most beneficial activity. Frequent and regular short walks in a quiet park or neighborhood are preferable to long, irregular walks on a crowded, noisy street. The physical symptoms of PD may discourage independent physical activities. If, however, patients anticipate situations that are likely to cause an episode of akinesia (freezing), they can plan accordingly and have some sense of control over the situation. Akinesia occurs because of the inability to convert the will to move into actual motion. The mechanisms that underlie the execution of normal movement can be prodded by visual and auditory cues. Attention to lines on a carpet or cracks in the pavement, for example, can facilitate the initiation and maintenance of rhythmic stride and prevent freezing episodes. Some patients have found that counting while walking helps, and others report that listening to marching music on a small headset stereo is helpful. When freezing occurs, another technique is to take a small step either backwards or sideways to initiate rhythmical movement. If the patient is walking with a companion, it may be helpful to have the companion place one foot in front of the patient's and ask the patient to step over the obstacle. Families should be advised against attempting to pull the person forward, since this only increases the problem and may result in a fall (Stern & Lees, 1982).

Tremor, rigidity, and bradykinesia interfere with the normal performance of activities of daily living; given enough time, however, patients can often successfully dress, bathe, and feed themselves. Simple modifications help the person with PD to be independent. Velcro closures, elastic shoelaces, and loose-fitting clothing make dressing a manageable activity; handrails in the bathroom, raised toilet seats, and shower chairs are also helpful (Mastrian, 1984).

Dependency may be fostered by staff or family caregivers who, perhaps unconsciously, motivated by their role as caregiver, do things for patients rather than allowing them to care for themselves. Frequently, nurses and families have a tendency to help as they watch a person struggle to accomplish these tasks. It is important to withhold unnecessary help; this approach contributes immeasurably to patients' self-esteem. Medical treatment is most effective when patients remain active physically and strive for independence in their daily routine (Lannon, Thomas, Bratton, et al., 1986).

Psychosocial Care

The physical and psychological symptoms of PD are interdependent; it must be recognized that symptoms such as tremor, drooling, masked facies, and impaired visuoperceptual and motor coordination can lead to psychological problems. In turn, psychological problems such as depression, along with difficulty in swallowing, can contribute to malnutrition and weight loss, and malnutrition can precipitate respiratory infections. Again, the interrelationship of the problems surrounding patient care is apparent.

Emotional support is a major need for patients with PD; as the disease progresses, the body image changes, and the patient needs an understanding, supportive person to help deal with these alterations. Many of the symptoms of PD, such as tremor, drooling, loss of facial expression, and shuffling gait, may cause embarrassment and discourage patients from engaging in social activities. Tremor, for example, is rarely a physically disabling symptom; it can, however, have serious psychological consequences. If people stare at this involuntary movement, it may be embarrassing and stressful to the patient, and embarrassment along with the fear of spilling food or drink may deter PD patients from attending social gatherings. Further, discomfort in a social gathering may be stressful to the person with PD, and as mentioned above, the tremor is aggravated when an individual is nervous or fearful. Stress exacerbates the tremor; yet, it is important for the patient to be active socially. The nurse must, therefore, work with patients and their families to reduce stress and encourage them to attend social functions despite fear of embarrassment. Encouraging attendance at parties where finger foods are served and straws can be used, for example, may prevent embarrassing spills and enable the person to remain independent.

It is important for people with PD to be active socially for as long as possible. If a person with PD tends to withdraw from social engagements, the spouse also tends to socialize less at a time when social support is necessary. Social activities may need to be planned around the energy level of the patient. People with PD tend to become very tired at the end of the day. In order to maintain an active social life, activities such as brunch, luncheons, or movies can be planned early in the day, before fatigue begins.

Eating is a social activity, and the family should be encouraged to have their meals with the patient and to reduce embarrassment by providing tissues to wipe saliva and to provide enough time for the patient to eat comfortably. In an institutional setting, the patient should also be encouraged to eat in the company of others, and again the nurse should provide assistive devices that facilitate independent eating. A bib should not be used during meals unless absolutely necessary. The use of a bib emphasizes the patient's difficulty in eating, is a source of embarrassment, and reduces the patient's self-esteem.

An accurate assessment of the psychological and cognitive status of the patient is essential. Developing a plan of care that maintains and strengthens the patient's remaining abilities is an important goal.

The etiology of depression is controversial; the nurse, however, can be instrumental in relieving some of the symptoms and in helping patients cope with the cognitive deficits found in PD. As mentioned earlier, some of the physical symptoms of PD are similar to the neuropsychological symptoms. Unfortunately, nursing staff may tend to withdraw from patients who are cognitively impaired and depressed. It is important for nurses to spend quality time with the patient. Sitting at the bedside and engaging the patient in conversation demonstrate acceptance, and acceptance is a primary need (Fischbach, 1978). Most patients enjoy talking about earlier life experiences, and since long-term memory is not usually impaired, this can be a meaningful experience for them. If patients are no longer able to walk, it is important to take them out of their room at least once a day to a pleasant environment where they can observe other people, outdoor scenery, or engage in enjoyable social activities.

Promoting autonomy, treating patients with dignity and respect, and helping them to maintain a strong sense of individuality and identity will strengthen their remaining abilities and help to prevent depression (Kayser-Jones, 1984). Recently, while conducting research in a nursing home, one of us (JKJ) observed that a man with PD who had been a pianist in a fashionable urban hotel was lying in his bed for hours without access to music. Providing him with a radio with headphones pleasantly filled long hours when his wife could not be with him. Enabling him to listen to music at will gave him a sense of autonomy and helped to diminish the feeling of helplessness that can contribute to depression. Further, a sense of identity derives from a belief that an individual possesses unique characteristics that set one apart; a sense of identity is an important aspect of psychological health (Kayser-Jones, 1984). Music was an integral part of this man's identity, and providing him with music helped to maintain his identity and individuality.

As the disease progresses, patients also need a great deal of help with physical activities. Most of the burden for providing this support and care falls upon the primary caregiver who is often a spouse or a daughter. Meeting the dependency needs of a person whose physical and cognitive status continues to decline is physically and psychologically demanding, and a caregiver realizes that the demands for care will increase as the disease progresses. As the burden for providing care increases, social isolation becomes a problem for the caregiver as well as for the patient. Sensitivity to the needs of caregivers, counseling them in regard to their needs, assessing their emotional status to determine if outside supportive services are necessary, and directing them to agencies in the community that provide these services is an important role for the nurse. For a thorough discussion of caregiver burden, see Chapter 29.

Prevention of Complications

Preventing complications is an important aspect in the management of PD. Infections, gastrointestinal problems, and falls are the most commonly occurring complications.

Infections. Upper respiratory infections are among the most dangerous complications of PD; bronchopneumonia is the second leading cause of death in advanced PD. Dysphagia or choking, due to poor muscle tone and rigidity of the pharyngeal muscles, contributes to aspiration of food and fluids, which can result in aspiration pneumonia. In advanced PD a nasogastric tube may be inserted for feeding; aspiration pneumonia is a complication that commonly occurs when nasogastric tubes are in place. The use of tube feeding is a controversial issue, but if tube feedings are indicated a gastrostomy tube causes fewer complications, is more comfortable, and is psychologically more acceptable to the patient and family. When dysphagia occurs, the physician should be consulted regarding the need for diagnostic studies, such as laryngoscopy, to rule out the possibility of an obstruction. Providing the patient with soft and semisoft foods diminishes the risk of aspiration. Respiratory function must be carefully assessed on an ongoing basis, and patients must be observed and monitored for signs of respiratory infections. Nursing measures such as deep breathing exercises, getting the patient out of bed regularly, and changing the position of the bedfast patient all decrease the risk of respiratory infections. Breathing exercises, consisting of deep inspirations with maximal chest expansion, stretch the chest wall and carry oxygen to poorly aerated parts of the lung. Personnel with respiratory infections should not care for the patient, and family and friends with respiratory infections should be discouraged from visiting. The nurse should advise the patient's family that a low-grade fever may not necessarily be an indication of infection, but if the patient develops a fever, the family should be instructed to notify the nurse or doctor so that the source of infection can be determined.

Urinary tract infections (UTIs) are common. Anticholinergic drugs may cause urinary retention, and urinary retention and urinary stasis contribute to UTIs. A lack of mobility and insufficient fluid intake may also precipitate UTIs (Robinson, 1974). Fluids should be readily available and offered frequently. Tremor may make drinking difficult, but patients can usually manage to drink with the use of a flexible drinking straw. Further, foods high in water content such as fresh fruits (e.g., melons and apples) are a good source of water and may be easier for the patient to swallow.

Seborrhea is commonly found in patients with PD and may contribute to the incidence of external eye infections. Frequent showers and hair washing with antidandruff shampoos are necessary, and the patient should be taught good eye hygiene. Gently washing the eyelids, eyelid margins, and eye lashes with a small amount of a "no tears" shampoo on a moist cotton ball and then rinsing the eyes with warm water help to prevent eye problems. Vigorous cleaning must be avoided so as not to cause a mechanical conjunctivitis.

Gastrointestinal Complications. Gastrointestinal motility is slowed as a result of PD and antiparkinsonian agents (Hahn, 1982). Decreased motility of the gastrointestinal tract, a lack of saliva in the gastrointestinal tract (lost through drooling), and dehydration contribute to constipation. Providing a diet high in fiber, encouraging fluids and daily exercise, and adding bulking agents and stool softeners all help to prevent constipation.

Anorexia, nausea, and vomiting are common side effects of drugs such as Sinemet and L-dopa, and this problem combined with dysphagia may result in severe weight loss. Patients should be weighed periodically; high-caloric supplemental feeding may be necessary to prevent weight loss.

Falls. Postural instability with falling affects about 25% of patients with PD, and serious injury along with fractures occurs in about 15% of patients (Hahn, 1982). Falling is most likely to occur when turning, backing up, reaching for an object, getting out of chairs, and when attempting to move unassisted from one location to another.

Many falls can be prevented by encouraging the patient to use a cane, tripod, or walker, by teaching the patient how to ambulate safely, and by providing assistive devices such as handrails in the bathroom. The environment at home and in institutional settings should be carefully assessed to prevent falls. Rubber mats in the tub and shower are mandatory, small throw rugs should be removed, and electrical cords and telephone cords should be eliminated in any area where the patient may be walking.

Long-term management of PD requires the cooperative efforts of a multidisciplinary team. The nurse working collaboratively with the physician can plan and coordinate the services of all health care providers. A physical therapist, for example, is essential in designing a specific program of exercise and mobility training to help reduce the symptoms of PD and to encourage functional independence. An occupational therapist can assess skills such as bathing, dressing, feeding, and swallowing, and can work closely with the family to suggest adaptive equipment and devices. A speech therapist evaluates the communication status of the patient, and a social worker assesses the psychosocial situation of the patient and family and makes appropriate suggestions. A social worker, for example, may suggest individual counseling sessions or support group meetings with patients and their families (Lannon, et al., 1986). It is important for health care providers to know that the American Parkinson's Disease Association (APDA) provides funds for research, subsidizes information and referral centers, and provides counseling to patients and their families. Information on all services provided can be obtained by contacting the national organization: The American Parkinson's Disease Association, 116 John Street, Suite 417, New York, NY 10038.

FUTURE POSSIBILITIES IN THE STUDY OF PARKINSON'S DISEASE

Despite the substantial improvement in the pharmacologic treatment of PD in the past two decades, it is painfully clear that L-dopa and the receptor agonists provide only limited ameliorative treatment. The course of the disease, for most patients, is still one of inexorably progressive disability, regardless of therapy (Moore, 1987), but recent studies provide reason to hope that further progress in the prevention, treatment, and cure of the disease may soon be made. Intense effort is currently being focused on identifying environmental toxins that may exacerbate or cause PD, on testing new drug regimens of Deprenyl with antioxidants like tocopherol, on refining stereotactic surgery, and on developing procedures for successful brain transplants. Success with any one of these approaches could make the debilitating effects of this disease a thing of the past.

References

Aminoff, MJ (1987): Parkinson's disease in the elderly: Current management strategies. *Geriatrics,* 42(7):31–37.

Barbeau, A, Cloutier, T, Roy, M, et al. (1985): Ecogenetics of Parkinson's disease: 6-hydroxylation of debrisoquine. *Lancet,* 2(8466):1213–1215.

Birkmayer, W, & Riederer, P (1983): *Parkinson's Disease.* New York, Springer-Verlag.

Boller, F (1985): Parkinson's disease and Alzheimer's disease: Are they associated? *In* Hutton, JT, & Kenny, AD (eds): Senile dementia of the Alzheimer type. *Neurology and Neurobiology,* Vol. 18. New York, Alan R. Liss.

Caine, S (1984): Parkinson's disease—helping the patient with a movement disorder. *Canadian Nurse,* 80(11):35–37.

Cassileth, BR, Lusk, EJ, Strouse, TB, et al. (1984): Psychosocial status in chronic illness—A comparative analysis of six diagnostic groups. *N Engl J Med,* 311(8):506–511.

Celesia, GG, & Wanamaker, WM (1972): Psychiatric disturbances in Parkinson's disease. *Dis Nerv Sys,* 33(9):577–583.

Clark, M, & Anderson, B (1967): *Culture and Aging: An Anthropological Study of Older Americans.* Springfield, IL, Charles C. Thomas.

Cools, AR, Van Den Bercken, JHL, Horstink, MWI, et al. (1984): Cognitive and motor shifting aptitude disorder in Parkinson's disease. *J Neurol Neurosurg Psychiatry,* 47:443–453.

Critchley, M (ed) (1955): *James Parkinson (1755—1824).* London, MacMillan.

Dakof, GA, & Mendelsohn, GA (1986): Parkinson's disease: The psychological aspects of a chronic illness. *Psychol Bull,* 99(3):375–387.

Damasio, AR, Lobo-Antunes, J, & Macedo, C (1970): L-dopa, parkinsonism and depression. *Lancet,* 2:611–612.

Finch, CE, Randall, PK, & Marshall, JF (1981): Aging and basal gangliar functions. *Annu Rev Gerontol Geriatr,* 2:49–87.

Fischbach, FT (1978): Easing adjustment to Parkinson's disease. *Am J Nurs,* 78(1):66–69.

Garnett, ES, Firnau, G, Lang, AE, et al. (1986): Imaging of dopamine in humans. *In* Fahn, S, Marsden, CD, Jenner, P, et al. (eds): *Recent Developments in Parkinson's Disease.* New York, Raven Press.

Garrett, E (1982): Parkinsonism: Forgotten considerations in medical treatment and nursing care. *J Neurosurg Nurs,* 14(1):13–17.

Goodwin, FK (1971): Psychiatric side effects of levodopa in man. *JAMA,* 218(13):1915–1920.

Hahn, K (1982): Management of Parkinson's disease. *Nurse Practitioner,* 7(1):13–25, 50.

Jellinger, K (1986): Pathology of parkinsonism. *In* Fahn, S, Marsden, CD, Jenner, P, et al. (eds): *Recent Developments in Parkinson's Disease.* New York, Raven Press.

Kayser-Jones, JS (1984): Psychosocial care of nursing home patients. *In* Hall, BA (ed): *Mental Health and the Elderly.* New York, Grune & Stratton.

Langan, RJ, & Cotzias, GC (1976): Do's and don'ts for the patient on levodopa therapy. *Am J Nurs,* 76(6):917–918.

Langston, JW (1986): MPTP-induced parkinsonism: How good a model is it? *In* Fahn, S, Marsden, CD, Jenner, P, et al. (eds): *Recent Developments in Parkinson's Disease.* New York, Raven Press.

Lannon, MC, Thomas, CA, Bratton, M, et al. (1986): Comprehensive care of the patient with Parkinson's disease. *J Neurosci Nurs,* 18(3):121–131.

Lewin, R (1985): Parkinson's disease: An environmental cause? *Science,* 229:257–258.

Lewin, R (1987): Dramatic results with brain grafts. *Science,* 237:245–247.

Lieberman, A, Dziatolowski, N, Kupersmith, M, et al.

(1979): Dementia in Parkinson's disease. *Ann Neurol,* 6(4):355–359.

Loranger, A, Goodell, H, McDowell, FH, et al. (1972): Intellectual impairment in Parkinson's syndrome. *Brain,* 95:402–412.

Madrazo, I, Drucker-Colin, R, Diaz, V, et al. (1987): Open microsurgical autograft of adrenal medulla to the right caudate nucleus in two patients with intractable Parkinson's disease. *N Engl J Med,* 316(4):831–834.

Mastrian, KG (1984): The patient with a degenerative disease of the nervous system. *In* Rudy, EB (ed): *Advanced Neurological and Neurosurgical Nursing.* St. Louis, CV Mosby, 265–287.

Matthews, CG, & Haaland, KY (1979): The effects of a symptom duration on cognitive and motor performance in parkinsonism. *Neurology,* 29:951–956.

Mayeux, R, & Rosen, WG (1983): The dementias. *In* Mayeux, R, & Rosen, WG (eds): *Advances in Neurology,* Vol 38. New York, Raven Press.

Mayeux, R, & Rosen, Y (1983): Intellectual dysfunction and dementia in Parkinson's disease. *In* Mayeux, R, & Rosen, WG (eds): *The Dementias.* New York, Raven Press, 211–227.

Mayeux, R, Stern, Y, Cote, L, et al. (1984): Altered serotonin metabolism in depressed patients with Parkinson's disease. *Neurology,* 34:642–646.

Meyerowitz, BE (1980): Psychosocial correlates of breast cancer and its treatment. *Psychol Bull,* 87:108–131.

Moore, RY (1987): Parkinson's disease—a new therapy. *N Engl J Med,* 316(14):872–873.

Phelps, ME, & Mazziotta, JC (1985): Positron emission tomography: Human brain function and biochemistry. *Science,* 228:799–809.

Pirozzolo, FJ, Hansch, EC, Mortimer, JA, et al. (1982): Dementia in Parkinson's disease: A neuropsychological analysis. *Brain Cogn,* 1:71–83.

Poewe, W, Gerstenhand, F, Ransmayr, G, et al. (1983): Premorbid personality of Parkinson patients. *J Neurol Transmission,* 19:215–224.

Robinson, MB (1974): Levodopa and parkinsonism. *Am J Nurs,* 74(4):656–661.

Schoenberg, BS (1987): Descriptive epidemiology of Parkinson's disease: Disease distribution and hypothesis formulation. *Adv Neurol,* 45:277–283.

Singer, E (1974): Premature social aging: The social-psychological consequences of a chronic illness. *Soc Sci Med,* 8(3):143–151.

Spencer, PS, Nunn, PB, Hugon, J, et al. (1987): Guam amyotrophic lateral sclerosis—Parkinsonism–dementia linked to a plant excitant neurotoxin. *Science,* 237:517–522.

Stern, G, & Lees, A (1982): *Parkinson's Disease: The Facts.* New York, Oxford University Press.

Talland, GA (1962): Cognitive functioning in Parkinson's disease. *J Nerv Ment Dis,* 135(3):196–205.

Tasker, RR (1987): Tremor of parkinsonism and stereotactic thalamotomy. *Mayo Clin Proc,* 62:736–739.

Tasker, RR, Siqueira, J, Hawrylyshyn, P, et al. (1983): What happened to VIM thalamotomy for Parkinson's disease? *Appl Neurophysiol,* 46:68–83.

Todd, B (1985): Drugs and the elderly—therapy for Parkinson's disease. *Geriatr Nurs,* 6(2)117–120.

Ward, CD, Duvoisin, RC, Ince, SE, et al. (1983): Parkinson's disease in 65 pairs of twins and in a set of quadruplets. *Neurology,* 33:815–824.

CHAPTER 26

Alcoholism in the Elderly

W. CAROLE CHENITZ, R.N., Ed.D.

"Since my release from the hospital, I have been back in there at least three times a week to attend meetings, I now go to lots of meetings and I have friends I never knew existed. My life since coming to A.A. has taken a dramatic turnaround ... I can truthfully say the last three years of my life have been the best of all my 81 years." (He joined AA at age 78.)

"The sober world isn't frightening at all, it's beautiful. It has so many rewards. The biggest is my second life on this earth ... my precious sobriety. I'm sorry it took so long. I'm glad it didn't take any longer." (Age 76 when he joined AA.)

From Alcoholics Anonymous, 1979

As these quotes from elderly members of Alcoholics Anonymous (AA) affirm, recovery from alcoholism is a valuable, lifesaving, and lifegiving experience regardless of age. Unfortunately, many older people who suffer from alcoholism never enter recovery programs. They are never identified as alcoholic and hence never face the disease of alcoholism and its effect on their lives. Many elders die without experiencing the joy of living in the later years. Alcoholism is a chronic, progressive, primary, and fatal disease that afflicts an estimated 10% of the population. Among those over 65 years, conservative estimates are that 3% to 10% of them suffer alcoholism and significant alcohol-related problems (National Council on Alcoholism [NCA], 1981). It is widely accepted that among the elderly, alcoholism is underdiagnosed and undertreated (Zimberg, 1979). There is also evidence that alcohol produces significant problems in the aged, despite the fact that they consume less alcohol (Chatham, 1983). In addition, alcoholism may present with different clinical manifestations in the aged than it does in the younger population. Compounding the problem are negative and conflicting attitudes toward both alcoholism and aging. Stereotypes of the alcoholic and the aged prevail among elders, their families, health professionals, and

507

the lay public. These factors make alcoholism a complex and serious problem in this age group.

In this chapter, the problem of alcoholism in the elderly is addressed, including a discussion of the types of elderly alcoholics and their clinical problems and manifestations of alcoholism. Assessment and treatment are presented, with a discussion on detoxification, treatment options, and resources.

THE DISEASE OF ALCOHOLISM

There are many different definitions of the alcoholic and alcoholism. Alcoholics Anonymous defines an alcoholic as a person who "has lost control. At a certain point in the drinking of every alcoholic, he passes into a state where even the most powerful desire to stop is of absolutely no avail" (AA, 1976). According to AA, alcoholism is a chronic, progressive illness characterized by a physical sensitivity (allergy) to alcohol and a mental obsession with drinking that cannot be stopped by use of self will power (AA, 1952; 1976).

The National Council on Alcoholism (NCA) defines alcoholism as a "chronic, progressive and potentially fatal disease characterized by tolerance and psychological and/or physical dependency. Generally, alcoholism is repeated drinking that causes trouble in the drinker's personal, professional or family life" (NCA, 1989). Once alcoholics begin drinking, they may not be able to stop, control how much they drink, or be able to predict what will happen or the consequences of drinking (NCA, 1989).

In 1987, the American Psychiatric Association (APA) defined alcohol abuse and alcohol dependence separately. "Alcohol abuse is a maladaptive pattern of the use of alcohol in spite of social, occupational, psychological or physical problems, or continued use in hazardous situations. For a diagnosis of abuse, symptoms must persist for at least 1 month or repeatedly over a longer period of time. Finally, the person exhibiting alcohol abuse

must not be able to meet criteria for dependence now or in the past" (APA, 1987).

Alcohol dependence is characterized by at least three of the following:
1. Increased amount of alcohol or increased time spent drinking
2. Loss of control over drinking with a desire and attempts made to stop
3. Increased time spent drinking or recovering from drinking
4. Frequent intoxication or withdrawal symptoms
5. Reduced or impaired social, occupational, or recreational activities
6. Continued use in spite of problems
7. Marked tolerance
8. Withdrawal symptoms
9. Continued use to avoid withdrawal

There are several patterns of pathologic use outlined by the American Psychiatric Association (1987). These are categorized as *continuous* (1) regular daily intake of large amounts, (2) regular heavy drinking limited to weekends, or *episodic*, which is (3) long periods of sobriety with binges of daily heavy drinking lasting for weeks or months (APA, 1987).

The cause of alcoholism remains unknown. There are several etiologic theories for alcoholism, but none has received the empirical support necessary to rule out others. The theory showing the greatest promise is the genetic theory, and there is general agreement among experts that at least one form of alcoholism is caused by inherited factors (Goldman, 1987–88, Gordis, 1987–88; Reich, 1987–88). Theories of the cause of alcoholism are presented in Table 26–1.

Tolerance, dependence, and withdrawal are key to understanding alcoholism. Tolerance is an increase in the amount of alcohol necessary to achieve the desired effect. Late in the disease, however, tolerance decreases. That is, the individual needs less alcohol to produce euphoria. Cross-tolerance also occurs. An individual with an addiction to alcohol can acquire a dependence to other central nervous system depressants rapidly, and vice versa (Hasselblad, 1984).

Dependence is the adaptation of the central nervous system to functioning with the seda-

Table 26–1. THEORIES OF THE CAUSE OF ALCOHOLISM

Genetic Theory

Inherited genetic personality traits influence susceptibility, control of the addictive process, protective factors, psychiatric disorders that may lead to alcoholism, and the predisposition toward medical complications.

Research is aimed at isolating genetic components related to inheritance of alcohol metabolism and linkage studies to identify genetic components in behavioral characteristics.

Personality Theory

Characteristics or clusters of traits predispose to alcoholism. Traits include exaggerated sensitivities, poor impulse control, low tolerance to frustration, dependency, weak ego, emotional and sexual immaturity, inability to delay gratification, and feelings of powerlessness.

Research cannot document causal relationship between personality traits and alcoholism. No single trait or cluster established for all alcoholics.

Transactional Therapy

Family communication patterns enable interactions in which member(s) can escape and/or avoid responsibility through alcoholism.

Behavioral/Learning Theory

Drinking is a learned behavior and produces psychological rewards to the individual. Rewards perpetuate the drinking and addiction follows.

Cultural Theory

Certain cultural groups have lower incidence and define specific ways in which alcohol in limited amounts can be used.

Social Theory

Alcoholism is the result of social deprivation, hopelessness, poverty, feelings of anomia and powerlessness. Alcohol is used as an antidote to negate negative social forces.

Multifocal/Multicausal Theory

No one theory explains alcoholism. The interaction between personality, genetics, social, and cultural forces produces alcoholism.

(Data from Denzin, 1987a & 1987b; Estes, Smith-DiJulio, & Heineman, 1980; Goldman, 1987–88; Hasselblad, 1984; Reich, 1987–88.)

tive effects of alcohol. Physiologic dependence means the person requires alcohol to function. Without alcohol, a person with physiologic dependence shows symptoms of withdrawal (Hasselblad, 1984; Strauss, 1983).

Psychological dependence also occurs and is manifested by feelings of craving and a sense of need. These feelings may be so strong as to interfere with the individual's ability to function (Strauss, 1983). Withdrawal occurs when alcohol intake is substantially decreased or stopped without substitution of other forms of sedation. Withdrawal from alcohol may be minor (mild) or major (severe) with delirium tremens. The severity of withdrawal depends upon general health, quantity of alcohol consumed, the duration of time of last drinking episode, and a history of severe withdrawal. Minor (mild) withdrawal begins several hours after the last drink, peaks in 24 hours, and then subsides rapidly. Major or severe withdrawal is called alcohol withdrawal delirium or delirium tremens and follows minor withdrawal. Delirium tremens occurs from 40 to 60 hours after alcohol intake is stopped or decreased, peaks after 80 to 90 hours, and lasts for approximately 3 days. Delirium tremens represents a medical emergency, and hospitalization is required. Key symptoms in delirium tremens are profound disorientation, disordered perception, and hallucinations (Hasselblad, 1984). The symptoms of minor and major withdrawal are presented in Table 26–2. Detoxification, the treatment for withdrawal, is discussed later in this chapter.

Alcoholism in the Elderly

Several studies on drinking patterns have demonstrated that with age comes a decline

Table 26–2. SYMPTOMS OF WITHDRAWAL

Minor	Severe
Tremor, insomnia	Gross tremor
Diaphoresis	Profuse diaphoresis
Anxiety	Extreme restlessness
Loss of appetite	Agitation
Alcohol withdrawal seizures	No seizures
Disturbed perception; benign	
Hallucinations	Frightening hallucinations
Brief minimal disorientation	Profound disorientation
Tachycardia	Tachycardia
Elevated blood pressure	Elevated blood pressure
Nausea and vomiting	
Diarrhea	
Generalized weakness	Fever

(Data from Hasselblad, 1984.)

in the consumption of alcohol and a decline in the incidence of alcoholism (Cahalan, Cisin, & Crossely, 1969; Moore, 1964; Mulford & Miller, 1963). In view of these studies, Drew (1968) postulated that alcoholism is a self-limiting disease and that alcoholics will spontaneously achieve remission with increasing age. A rival explanation for the decline in the incidence of alcoholism in old age is the selective survival hypothesis, which suggests that the incidence of alcoholism is lower in the aged because a significant number of alcoholics die before reaching the age of 65 years. Another explanation for the decreased incidence among the elderly is the cohort hypothesis, which suggests that heavy drinking is less likely to occur in the current cohort of elders because they lived during Prohibition and experienced the moral outrage that lead to prohibition. The latter two hypotheses may explain the lower incidence of alcoholism among the aged.

Mishara and Kastenbaum (1980) postulate that many older people decrease or eliminate their alcohol consumption because alcohol significantly affects performance of cognitive and motor tasks. Since the elderly have a gradual deterioration in these abilities as the result of the aging process, they may not wish to use alcohol because of its effect on these abilities. In addition, alcohol may affect the older person's reputation of competence (Mishara & Kastenbaum, 1980).

There are other explanations given for the decrease of alcohol consumption among the aged. Many older people report that they stop drinking because of a health problem or because alcohol has a negative effect on a health problem (Dunham, 1981). Others cite financial reasons for a decrease in alcohol consumption. That is, they simply cannot afford to drink on a pension or Social Security. Other reasons given are that older people do not go to social events where alcohol is served, and they have a loss of interest in drinking (Dunham, 1981).

Vestal, McGuire, Tobin, and associates (1977) speculated that there is a physiologic basis for the change in alcohol consumption with age. Since the usual dose of alcohol is based on body size, the increased effects in older persons may be due to increased blood levels resulting from changes in body composition rather than, or in addition to, alterations in the sensitivity of the brain or metabolism of alcohol (Vestal, et al., 1977). However, others believe that the diminished physical reserve of older people leads to a lowered ability to metabolize alcohol and other drugs, and hence small doses of alcohol will have a greater effect on an older person (Atkinson & Schuckit, 1981). While the exact mechanism remains unclear, it is widely accepted that the older alcoholic consumes less alcohol than the younger alcoholic and that the older person requires less alcohol than younger people to achieve similar blood alcohol levels.

The incidence of heavy drinking and alcoholism in the elderly has been the target of several studies. The National Institute of Alcohol Abuse and Alcoholism (NIAAA) estimates that approximately 10% of elderly males and 2% of elderly females are heavy or problem drinkers (Gomberg, 1982). The National Council on Alcoholism (NCA) estimated that based on the 1980 census, there are between 1 and 3 million elderly in this country who experience problem drinking or alcoholism, and this number is expected to increase as the absolute numbers of the aged increases (NCA, 1981). In a recent survey of outpatients in two urban Veterans Administration medical centers, Magruder-Habib, Saltz, and Barron (1986) found that 10.2% of those over 65 years were alcoholic.

Clinical Consequences of Alcoholism in the Elderly

Clinical problems that are also symptoms of alcoholism are social isolation, falls, malnutrition, general physical deterioration, and dementia (Rosin & Glatt, 1971). Other problems seen in the elderly alcoholic are self-neglect and aggravation of confusion (Glatt, Rosin, & Jauhar, 1978). These symptoms could be mistaken for effects of multiple chronic illnesses and advanced age (Rosin & Glatt, 1971). Table 26–3 presents problems associated with alco-

Table 26–3. PROBLEMS ASSOCIATED
WITH ALCOHOLISM

Social
Family problems
Problems with job, finances, the law, and personal
    relationships
Social isolation and withdrawal
Complaints about family, friends, relationships
Psychological/Emotional
Nervousness/anxiety
Depression/feelings of sadness/crying
Suicidal attempts/ideation
Resentful and jealous of others
Feelings of anger
No motivation
Use of sedatives, hypnotics
Amnesic periods or blackouts
Physical
Trauma, especially falls, head injuries, fractures,
    unexplained bruises or lacerations
Heavy smoking; burns on fingers, clothes, or furniture
Insomnia
Gastric distress
Chronic and/or frequent infections
History of withdrawal, seizures, pancreatitis, hepatitis,
    gastrointestinal bleeding
Diarrhea
Medical problems related to alcoholism

(Data from National Council on Alcoholism Criteria
Committee, 1972; Estes, Smith-DiJulio, & Heineman, 1980;
Hasselblad, 1984.)

holism that are often overlooked or can be explained away by other causes.

Miller (1979), in a study of geriatric suicides, found that "the prolonged use of alcohol was clearly related to the suicidal behavior of older men" in his sample (Miller, 1979). Survivors helped to identify approximately 27% of the total sample of older suicides as "alcoholic" and another 6% as "heavy or problem drinkers." The elderly alcoholics in this study had been drinking for many years. In addition, a significant number—two-thirds of the alcoholic suicides and 35% of all the suicides—were also drug-related. The drugs most commonly involved were analgesics, barbiturates, and soporifics. As Miller points out, "Valium was frequently mentioned by survivors and one man was said to have 'eaten aspirin like candy' " (Miller, 1979).

There are also medical problems that are related to alcoholism. Presence of these problems should alert the clinician to a diagnosis of alcoholism (Cohen, Kern, & Hassett, 1986). The medical problems related to alcoholism are presented in Table 26–4.

Profile of the Elderly Alcoholic

Blazer, George, Woodbury, and associates (1983) present a profile of the elderly alcoholic developed from an interview survey of 1,620 persons over age 60 years in five counties in North Carolina. They found that "current elderly alcoholics are more likely to fall into the 60–74 age range (the young old), to be male, to be non-white, to be separated or divorced, to have less than a high school education and to live with someone else" (Blazer, et al., 1983). Except for moderate to severe cognitive deficits, an elderly alcoholic does not exhibit other psychiatric disorders. Compared to younger alcoholics, elderly alcoholics in the study consumed less alcohol but were more likely to demonstrate alcohol dependence, that is, a need to drink in the morning. Elderly

Table 26–4. MEDICAL PROBLEMS RELATED
TO ALCOHOLISM

Gastrointestinal
Alcoholic hepatitis
Gastritis, acute and chronic
Laënnec's cirrhosis
Alcoholic pancreatitis
Mallory-Weiss syndrome
Esophageal varices
Neurologic/Neuropsychiatric
Withdrawal syndrome
Delirium tremens
Peripheral neuropathy
Seizures
Wernicke-Korsakoff syndrome
Organic brain syndrome (dementia)
Alcoholic cerebellar degeneration
Hematologic/Metabolic
Alcoholic thrombocytopenia
Folic acid, iron deficiency anemia
Thiamine, niacin, riboflavin deficiency
Cardiac
Alcoholic cardiomyopathy
Respiratory
Increased incidence of infections and pneumonia
    secondary to impairment of defense mechanisms in
    the lungs and immune system suppression

(Data from Cohen, Kern, & Hassett, 1986; National
Council on Alcoholism Criteria Committee, 1972; Hasselblad, 1984.)

alcoholics complained of more physical symptoms than their younger counterparts, such as chest pain, constipation, and fainting. Elderly alcoholics reported fewer blackouts but experienced "the shakes" more often than the younger alcoholics. In terms of medical treatment, the elderly alcoholics were more likely to have discussed their drinking with a physician and admitted that they wanted to stop but could not. They tended to use drug and alcohol clinics more than younger alcoholics but self-help groups less. Blazer and associates (1983) believe that the findings in this study suggest that alcohol dependence characterizes the elderly alcoholic.

Types of Elderly Alcoholics

It is now widely accepted that there are two types of elderly alcoholics: the chronic long-standing alcoholic and the late onset (also called reactive or newly incident) alcoholic (Magruder-Habib, et al., 1986). The chronic alcoholic comprises about two-thirds of elderly alcoholics (NCA, 1981).

Chronic, long-standing alcoholics are those whose drinking has persisted over time and into old age; they are young alcoholics grown old. These elderly alcoholics are survivors, since there is a higher mortality rate among alcoholics. It is estimated that 76% of older alcohol abusers are of this type (Dunham, 1981). Mr. G, for example, was an alcoholic of this type.

Mr. G was 72 years old when he was admitted to an acute-care medical center with confusion, incontinence, vomiting, and dehydration. He had a history of "heavy drinking" for the past 35 years. He accepted a referral to the alcohol rehabilitation unit and was transferred there when his acute confusion and medical crisis were over. On the alcohol unit, he remained by himself, needed to be called on to participate in community meetings and group sessions, and when he did participate, he gave only superficial attention. On psychological examination, Mr. G showed evidence of memory impairment and became irritable when questioned. He lived with his wife, who had brought him to the hospital emergency room for admission. According to Mrs. G, Mr. G had a problem with drinking for years. She had left him on several occasions, only to return when he promised to stop drinking. He would stop for a time, then resume his drinking again. He had been retired for 6 years and since then he drank all day, sitting in front of the television. However, he had never become so sick before, and Mrs. G was scared at the severity of his condition that brought them to the hospital. For the month that Mr. G was in the rehabilitation program he steadily improved physically, became more mentally alert and more able and willing to participate in the program. There was still memory loss. Both of the Gs had difficulty accepting that Mr. G was an alcoholic. Mrs. G felt that her husband had a problem but that he had always worked and therefore could not be an alcoholic. Mr. G believed that he could control his drinking, which he admitted had gotten out of hand. The major focus of treatment was to confront Mr. and Mrs. G's denial of alcoholism. A treatment program was worked out for Mr. G's aftercare that included daily attendance at AA and weekly groups at the hospital clinic. On his weekend pass from the alcohol rehabilitation unit, he was encouraged to attend AA meetings within walking distance of his house. Mrs. G was encouraged to but never did attend Al-Anon. She continued to feel hopeless about her husband's desire not to drink and felt that it was only a matter of time before he started again.

The Gs are an example of an older couple, with one member being an alcoholic for years, who has carried into old age a pathologic pattern of alcohol intake. Mr. G, as with many older alcoholics, came to a hospital in deteriorated physical and mental condition. These clients are difficult to evaluate upon initial assessment, since their condition will improve with abstinence from alcohol, an adequate diet, sleep, vitamin therapy, and medical control of other illnesses. It is difficult on the initial assessment to be able to determine how great an improvement an older, debilitated, seemingly demented client will make with several weeks of abstinence, medical supervision, and nursing care. The central questions in Mr. G's alcohol treatment were: (1) Will he regain enough memory to remember that he is not drinking and to attend meetings? (2) Can the intervention to confront the denial of his alcoholism produce a willingness to abstain? (3) Once in contact with AA, will he be willing to attend?

As the Gs illustrate, alcoholism is a family disease by which each member is affected (Chenitz & Granfors, 1988). Mrs. G was affected by her husband's alcoholism. Like many wives of chronic alcoholics, Mrs. G learned to live with an alcoholic spouse by adapting over time to accommodate changes caused by the disease. Also, like many wives of chronic alcoholics, Mrs. G could not make a decision regarding her own life and happiness, and hence she felt helpless to change the situation. She believed that her husband would not change and so felt hopeless about the future.

On the other hand, alcoholism is considered a family disease in that the family may, albeit unwittingly, assist the alcoholic to maintain the drinking. The process whereby family members are caught up in maintaining the alcoholism is called "enabling" (Johnson Institute, 1982). Family treatment is considered an essential part of alcohol rehabilitation and recovery. Another resource for the family is the Al-Anon family group, which is a peer support group and a recovery program for family and friends of alcoholics. Information about Al-Anon group meetings may be obtained from any local chapter of the National Council on Alcoholism or Al-Anon can be found in the telephone book.

A late onset alcoholic is a person whose pattern of moderate drinking changed during old age and often as the result of or in response to the losses associated with aging (Glatt, Rosin, & Jauhar, 1978). Brody (1982) believes there are several common conditions in later life that make the elderly susceptible to alcoholism. These are (1) retirement, which can produce boredom, loss of income, low self-esteem, and a change in role status; (2) death of family and friends; (3) poor health, discomfort, pain, and distress; and (4) loneliness. It is estimated that the late onset type represents approximately 30% of older alcoholics (Dunham, 1981).

Mr. A was a late life alcoholic who readily admitted that he was bored, angry, and lonely. Mr. A was a 70-year-old retired accountant who for 25 years drank 1 ounce of bourbon every evening after dinner. Shortly after his retirement, Mr. A developed diabetes and his drinking increased. "I had nothing else to do. I had big plans for my retirement and didn't want to do anything. I just started having a couple of drinks, then I drank earlier in the evening." Soon, Mr. A was drinking from the afternoon until bedtime. He never left his home and became unkempt and isolated. On a routine visit to his physician, Mr. A mentioned that he was not feeling well. His physician asked him about his drinking and Mr. A told him the truth. His physician wanted him admitted to the hospital for detoxification and recommended an inpatient rehabilitation program. He also put Mr. A in touch with another older recovering alcoholic he knew who was in AA. This recovering alcoholic became Mr. A's sponsor in AA and visited him throughout his hospitalization and rehabilitation. He took Mr. A to AA meetings and introduced him to people there. Mr. A attended the alcohol clinic and weekly group meetings upon discharge. He decided to have a roommate and chose one of the people he met in AA. Several months later, Mr. A relapsed and returned to drinking. His sponsor and roommate assisted him to return to the alcohol clinic and AA meetings, and provided emotional support while he stopped drinking. Six months after discharge from the rehabilitation program, Mr. A was sober.

Mr. A had several of the problems outlined by Brody that make an older person susceptible to alcoholism. As with many older alcoholics in need of treatment, Mr. A willingly mentioned it when asked by his doctor. Luckily for him, his physician was well versed in alcoholism and its treatment and readily connected him to both medical and social treatment for alcoholism. Again, like many recovering alcoholics, Mr. A stopped attending AA meetings and stopped his weekly group sessions and relapsed to drinking (Sheeren, 1988). Fortunately, his support system was available and, when activated, assisted him back into recovery. Mr. A's case points out the positive outcome of treatment for older alcoholics.

ASSESSMENT

The first step in treatment is discovering and uncovering an often hidden alcoholism

(Goodman, 1988). Assessment is critical. Despite social and medical problems associated with alcoholism, the condition in the elderly may be difficult to detect. Since the older person may be retired and avoids driving after dark, social and legal problems that call attention to alcoholism do not occur (Hinrichsen, 1984). In addition, many elders live alone and do not have daily contact with family and friends. Hence, indicators of problems with alcohol, such as depressed mood and poor grooming, may be overlooked (Hinrichsen, 1984). During interviews, the nurse must note several important points. First, an attitude of neutrality is maintained when asking questions about alcohol and related topics as part of a health history. Second, spouse, significant others, or a family member may be included in assessment for alcoholism and are often able to answer questions the alcoholic would not address. Family interviews may be more effective conducted separately (Estes, Smith-DiJulio, & Heineman, 1980; Hasselblad, 1984). Points or questions to include in the assessment are:

1. What is the person's drinking pattern? How often is there drinking? What is done during drinking? Has anything happened when drinking, such as accidents, falls, loss of memory (blackouts), or change in personality?

2. Has there been a change in the person's drinking pattern? If yes, what is the change? When did the change take place? What are the circumstances around the change?

3. Is there a history of alcoholism in the family? In the person's past? Is there a history of legal or illegal drug abuse in the past?

4. Has there been a change (over time) in self-care activities? In social activities?

5. What does the person do on a normal day? What activities, hobbies, work, or social relationships does the person engage in?

6. How does the person feel about himself or herself, his or her past life and life today, and about the family?

7. What is the person's affect? Is it sad or depressed? If yes, has the person ever thought about suicide? If yes, has the person ever considered suicide as an option? If yes, how would the person commit suicide (is there a plan)?

If the person is an alcoholic, the assessment will provide specific information about how the disease has affected the person's life. As mentioned, family members and significant others can be a source of assessment data and information the alcoholic client may deny, and these data are useful in confronting the alcoholic's denial of a problem. If, during the assessment, thoughts of suicide, especially those accompanied by a suicide plan, are revealed, the nurse must act immediately and refer the client to an appropriate mental health clinician or agency.

In addition to assessment interviews, there are several self-assessments available to aid in self-definition and recognition. A popular self-assessment called the NCA Self-Test developed by the National Council on Alcoholism (1989) is reprinted in Table 26–5. This assessment can be given to clients or family for their review.

The goal of treatment for alcoholism is recovery. Recovery is a state in which addicted individuals are at peace with themselves and others and experience a sense of an ever increasing quality of life. Sobriety—that is, complete abstinence from alcohol and mood-altering chemicals—is basic to recovery. Complete abstinence is necessary because there is a cross-tolerance between alcohol and other mood-altering drugs, such as the barbiturates and minor tranquilizers. It is not uncommon for an alcoholic to stop drinking and use other mood-altering drugs, both legal and illegal, to replace the alcohol. In this way, the individual stops the recovery process, which requires that the patient be willing to experience reality and discontinue altering it with chemicals.

The first step in the treatment of alcoholism is an admission that alcohol is a problem. This seemingly simple step is very difficult for an alcoholic. Denial is a central feature of the disease. Denial can be confronted by interventions aimed at establishing life problems associated with alcoholism—family problems, arrests for driving while intoxicated, and work-related problems, to name a few. In the elderly, these problems may not be obvious

Table 26–5. THE NCA SELF-TEST

What Are the Signs of Alcoholism?

Here is a self-test to help you review the role alcohol is playing in your life. These questions incorporate many of the common symptoms of alcoholism. This test is intended to help you determine if you or someone you know needs to find out more about alcoholism.

YES	NO	
☐	☐	1. Do you occasionally drink heavily after a disappointment, a quarrel, or when the boss gives you a hard time?
☐	☐	2. When you have trouble or feel under pressure, do you drink more heavily than usual?
☐	☐	3. Have you noticed that you are able to handle more alcohol than you did when you were first drinking?
☐	☐	4. Did you ever wake up on the "morning after" and discover that you could not remember part of the evening before, even though your friends tell you that you did not "pass out"?
☐	☐	5. When drinking with other people, do you try to have a few extra drinks when others will not know it?
☐	☐	6. Are there certain occasions when you feel uncomfortable if alcohol is not available?
☐	☐	7. Have you recently noticed that when you begin drinking you are in more of a hurry to get the first drink than you used to be?
☐	☐	8. Do you sometimes feel a little guilty about your drinking?
☐	☐	9. Are you secretly irritated when your family or friends discuss your drinking?
☐	☐	10. Have you recently noticed an increase in the frequency of your memory "blackouts"?
☐	☐	11. Do you often find that you wish to continue drinking after your friends say they have had enough?
☐	☐	12. Do you usually have a reason for the occasions when you drink heavily?
☐	☐	13. When you are sober, do you often regret things you have done or said while drinking?
☐	☐	14. Have you tried switching brands or following different plans for controlling your drinking?
☐	☐	15. Have you often failed to keep the promises you have made to yourself about controlling or cutting down on your drinking?
☐	☐	16. Have you ever tried to control your drinking by making a change in jobs, or moving to a new location?
☐	☐	17. Do you try to avoid family or close friends while you are drinking?
☐	☐	18. Are you having an increasing number of financial and work problems?
☐	☐	19. Do more people seem to be treating you unfairly without good reason?
☐	☐	20. Do you eat very little or irregularly when you are drinking?
☐	☐	21. Do you sometimes have the "shakes" in the morning and find that it helps to have a little drink?
☐	☐	22. Have you recently noticed that you cannot drink as much as you once did?
☐	☐	23. Do you sometimes stay drunk for several days at a time?
☐	☐	24. Do you sometimes feel very depressed and wonder whether life is worth living?
☐	☐	25. Sometimes after periods of drinking, do you see or hear things that aren't there?
☐	☐	26. Do you get terribly frightened after you have been drinking heavily?

Any "yes" answer indicates a probable symptom of alcoholism.
More than one "yes" answer indicates its presence.

To find out more, contact the National Council on Alcoholism in your area.

From National Council on Alcoholism, 1989. Reprinted with permission.

because the person may be more isolated, have fewer outside activities and responsibilities, and may not have close family and friends to notice the behavior. This can also affect the elderly alcoholic's recognition that alcohol is a problem (Schiff, 1988).

Nurses and other health care providers can facilitate an admission of alcoholism or they can foster denial. There are several myths about alcoholics that interfere with a nurse's ability to confront a patient's denial. The first myth is the belief that alcoholics are all skid row bums and, because the client is not a skid row bum, he or she cannot be an alcoholic. Skid row alcoholics constitute less than 5% of all alcoholics. While the common view of the alcoholic as a skid row bum has been challenged by famous people like Betty Ford who openly admit their alcoholism, the myth of the alcoholic as different from other persons and belonging to skid row continues to prevail.

Another myth is that alcoholics are hopeless. Why bother to do anything, since they will go back to drinking anyway? Alcoholism is a chronic disease and like other chronic diseases the individual may have acute exacerbations. However, because a disease is chronic does not mean that there are no means to treat it. In fact, in this country even terminal diseases are treated. Unfortunately personal experiences with alcoholics in the past may affect the way nurses and other health care providers interact with alcoholics in their practice. DiCiccio-Bloom, Space, and Zahourek (1986) describe an exercise in which nurses were asked to conjure up an image of an alcoholic and become aware of their feelings. The typical alcoholic they pictured was the skid row bum. These nurses felt anger, fear, repulsion, and a desire not to get involved. In addition, some expressed guilt about their feelings.

That alcoholism is merely a bad habit wherein the alcoholic needs to exercise willpower is another myth about alcoholism. This myth leads to what Bateson (1972) has described as the alcoholic's battle within himself to stop drinking. This is self against self in a hopeless battle that cannot be won, since a battle within oneself can have no victor. Alcoholism is a disease and not a moral problem. Unfortunately, the belief that alcoholism is the result of a weak will and defect in moral fiber continues to haunt us today. In fact, for the elderly who grew up during Prohibition when alcohol consumption was considered a moral disease of both individuals and society as a whole, many feel ashamed and guilty about their uncontrollable drinking. Some nurses and health care providers use the myth that alcoholism is a moral problem as an excuse to avoid becoming involved.

TREATMENT

Beginning Treatment

Few alcoholic programs are designed specifically for older clients. A barrier to treatment

for the older alcoholic may be an unrecognized ageism on the part of alcohol treatment staff. The operating myth may be "So what if they drink? If I were that age so would I." Another myth is "What else do they have to live for—let them drink!" Ageism may create therapeutic nihilism where the older client is concerned, as reflected in attitudes such as "They aren't going to change now—they're too old to change" (Walker & Kelly, 1981). Nurses' attitudes toward alcoholics are marked by ambivalence and negativity (Naegle, 1983). Research into nurses' attitudes has found that while nurses accept the disease concept, they also believed that the alcoholic can stop drinking if he really wants to. Yet, alcoholism is a disease that requires treatment (Burkhalter, 1975). Some reasons for nurses' attitudes are: feelings of frustration and discouragement during their first experiences with alcoholic clients; nurses' expectations of treatment; and nurses' personal values and beliefs combined with the chronic, relapsing nature of alcoholism and its behavioral manifestations (Burkhalter, 1975).

Another barrier to treatment may be medical problems that require medications. Alcohol treatment programs often have admission criteria that require no medications or concurrent illness. These criteria can serve as a barrier to treatment for the elderly alcoholic (Opstelten, 1982).

The older alcoholic may not enter treatment until there are serious medical problems. Often, the elderly alcoholic enters an alcohol treatment program from a general hospital or is referred by a primary care physician. Acute medical problems will, of course, have to be assessed, diagnosed, and treated. Medical problems that are nonacute or long-standing can be controlled but should not be the focus of treatment. Once in a treatment program, medical problems can interfere with the treatment for alcoholism in two ways. First, the problem can interfere with the elderly alcoholic's ability to participate in a treatment program. Second, the elderly alcoholic may focus on a medical problem as real while viewing alcoholism as a secondary issue. Since the elderly as a group may have a number of chronic medical problems, staff members expert in alcohol treatment but not familiar with gerontology may feel overwhelmed by medical problems and focus on them, unwittingly supporting the alcoholic's denial that alcoholism is the real problem. On the other hand, medical problems that potentially interfere with treatment cannot be ignored.

Mr. P was a 70-year-old alcoholic on the alcohol treatment unit who seemed to the staff to be indifferent to participating in the recovery program. In group therapy sessions, Mr. P was inattentive. He would not participate and, when called on by the therapist, was vague and did not answer questions. Mr. P was believed to have an organic mental disorder secondary to alcoholism and was scheduled for neuropsychological testing. While in group therapy, it was noted that Mr. P held his head to the side with his right ear toward the center of the group. After a session, Mr. P was asked whether he could hear while in the room, and it was found that he could not. Mr. P had lost his hearing aid while on a binge some time back. He was too embarrassed to mention it to anyone, particularly since he was the "old man" in the treatment unit. Mr. P was fitted for a new hearing aid and was able to become a full participant in the treatment program.

Detoxification

Since alcohol has serious physical effects, withdrawal from alcohol must be carefully planned, particularly in the elderly. Alcohol withdrawal includes symptoms such as anxiety; irritability; increases in pulse, blood pressure, and temperature; and sweating. Serious symptoms include hallucinations, convulsions, and delirium. These symptoms, which comprise delirium tremens, are avoided by the use of medications specifically for detoxification. Medications are carefully titrated with symptoms to assist the individual to withdraw smoothly from alcohol. The benzodiazepines have been demonstrated to be effective agents for detoxification. However, in the older person, a lower dose and careful monitoring of vital signs and level of alertness are important to prevent drug toxicity. Rest, nutrition, and vitamin therapy, particularly with thiamine,

are important components of a detoxification program (Atkinson & Schuckit, 1981).

Treatment for Alcoholism

Treatment for alcoholism can be achieved on an inpatient or outpatient basis. Generally, those alcoholics who have a history of relapse, who cannot stop drinking on their own, and who have complex medical or psychiatric problems require an inpatient program. Inpatient alcohol treatment programs are based on four models and are presented in Table 26–6. The comprehensive alcohol treatment model is the most common form of rehabilitation program. These programs offer close support, supervision, and therapeutic activities. In addition, comprehensive alcohol treatment programs commonly offer alcohol education, group and family therapy, individual counseling, and an introduction to Alcoholics Anonymous.

Finding Treatment. Many cities have alcohol programs designed specifically for the elderly alcoholic. However, this is still the exception, not the rule. Most treatment programs offering treatment to elderly alcoholics require varying states of health. Finding treatment once an elderly alcoholic is willing to stop drinking is important. Many alcoholics have successfully used the fellowship of Alcoholics Anonymous as a sole program for alcoholism treatment. The advantages of Alcoholics Anonymous are its ready availability in most communities, its no-charge policy, peer support, a program for recovery, and its extraordinary rate of success. Alcoholics Anonymous can be reached by telephone, with listings in most local telephone books. Some alcoholics may not be able to stay sober or may not wish to attend Alcoholics Anonymous. For these people, private or public alcohol programs can be used. As noted above, an inpatient program may be the treatment of choice, since it isolates the alcoholic from alcohol, at least for a time. Information on treatment programs can be obtained by calling the local affiliate of the National Coun-

Table 26–6. FOUR INPATIENT
TREATMENT MODELS

Detoxification

Assists clients to recover from acute alcohol intoxication
and withdrawal and is usually a precursor to other
treatment. Detoxification provides round-the-clock
supervised treatment, which includes:
  (1) Assessment of acute medical problems
  (2) Close supervision and treatment of intoxicated
      clients by nurses, medical, and paraprofessional
      staff
  (3) Assessment of psychosocial needs and
      development of a plan for continuing treatment
  (4) Transportation to medical and continuing
      alcoholism treatment. May be a social model,
      using no drugs, or a medical model, using drugs
      for detoxification. May be part of a hospital or a
      free-standing center.

Traditional Psychiatric Programs

May be the most common form of treatment for
alcoholics, since alcohol can mimic psychopathology.
Drinking is viewed as a symptom of a primary
psychiatric condition and as evidence of
maladaptation. Treatment focuses on the underlying
sources of the emotional problem or personality
defect. May use mood-altering drugs to relieve
symptoms and produce another dependence. Difficult
to keep the alcoholic in treatment.

Behavior Modification Therapy

Based on learning theory that drinking is a learned
behavior and tries to reverse the learned drinking
pattern with nondrinking or controlled drinking rather
than uncontrolled drinking. Treatment involves the
programmed manipulation of rewards or punishments
associated with drinking. Includes aversion therapy or
punishment such as Antabuse, a drug that produces
nausea, vomiting, and cardiovascular symptoms when
combined with alcohol in the body.

The Comprehensive Alcoholism Treatment Model

Alcoholism is viewed as a chronic, progressive,
multiphasic illness that can be arrested. Treatment is
focused on providing the essential needs of the
alcoholic and developing a comprehensive care plan.
May include other treatment approaches as needed,
such as psychiatric treatment.

(Data from Anderson, 1981.)

cil on Alcoholism or the NCA's national toll-free number, 1–800–NCA–CALL.

The Results of Treatment

There is a small but growing body of literature on the effects of treatment approaches for the older alcoholic. Schuckit (1977) found that older alcoholics are more likely to complete an alcohol treatment program than are younger alcoholics. Carstensen, Rychtarik, and Prue (1985) report that 50% of the elderly alcoholics they interviewed 2 to 3 years after treatment were abstinent, and an additional 12% significantly decreased their alcohol intake. Helzer, Carey, and Miller (1983) found no difference in outcome among treated alcoholics under 59 years followed for 6 to 10 years and those over 60 years. However, social isolation correlated strongly with continued alcoholism in the older group. Organic brain syndrome was associated with outcome in the older group.

Zimberg (1978), in a description of his clinical work with elderly alcoholics, cites his belief that treatment is most effective when offered through agencies already serving the elderly, such as senior programs and geriatric medical clinics. His experience shows that a large number of elderly alcoholics are not willing to go to alcohol programs and that treatment will be most successful if aimed at the stresses of aging. He supports the use of family and individual casework, group socialization, and treatment for medical and psychiatric problems, especially depression (Zimberg, 1978). Opstelten (1982), reporting the recommendation of a "think tank" of 100 leaders of alcohol treatment in California who met on the problem of alcoholism in the elderly, wrote that combining alcohol and aging agencies into a broad system for treatment of the elderly alcoholic is the best treatment alternative.

SUMMARY

Alcoholism is a devastating, progressive, and fatal disease that can fill the last stage of life with despair, isolation, and loneliness. In recent years, the growing number of aged people and society's heightened awareness of the problem of alcoholism and chemical dependency have forced recognition and treatment of alcoholism in the elderly. Many elderly alcoholics are able to live out their lives in the peace and happiness that freedom from alcohol addiction can bring.

References

Alcoholics Anonymous (1952): *44 Questions*. New York, Alcoholics Anonymous World Services.

Alcoholics Anonymous (1979): *Time to Start Living*. New York, Alcoholics Anonymous World Services.

Alcoholics Anonymous (1976): *Alcoholics Anonymous* (ed 3). New York, Alcoholics Anonymous World Services.

American Psychiatric Association (1987): *Diagnostic and Statistical Manual of Mental Disorders, DSM III-R* (rev ed 3). Washington, DC American Psychiatric Association.

Anderson, DJ (1981): *Perspectives on Treatment: The Minnesota Experience*. Center City, MN, Hazelden Educational Materials.

Atkinson, RM, & Kofoed, LL (1984): Alcohol and drug abuse. *In* Cassel, CK, & Walsh, JR (eds): *Geriatric Medicine*, Vol 2. New York, Springer-Verlag.

Atkinson, RM, & Schuckit, MA (1981): Alcoholism and over-the-counter prescription drug misuse in the elderly. *In* Eisdorfer, C (ed): *Annual Review of Gerontology and Geriatrics*. New York, Springer.

Bateson, G (1972): *Steps to an Ecology of Mind*. New York, Ballantine Books.

Blazer, D, George, L, Woodbury, M, et al. (1983): The elderly alcoholic: A profile. *In* National Institute on Alcohol Abuse and Alcoholism: *Nature and Extent of Alcohol Problems Among the Elderly*. Research Monograph No 14. Rockville, MD, US Department of Health and Human Services, NIAAA, 275–297.

Brody, JA (1982): Aging and alcohol abuse. *J Am Geriatr Soc*, 30:123–126.

Burkhalter, PK (1975). *Nursing Care of the Alcoholic and Drug Abuser*. New York, McGraw-Hill.

Cahalan, D, Cisin, IH, & Crossely, HM (1969): *American Drinking Practices: A national survey of American drinking behavior and attitude*. New Brunswick, NJ, Rutgers Center of Alcohol Studies.

Carstensen, LL, Rychtarik, RG, & Prue, DM (1985): Behavioral treatment of the geriatric alcohol abuser: A long-term follow-up study. *Addict Behav*, 10(3):307–311.

Chatham, LR (1983): Greetings from the National Institute on Alcohol Abuse and Alcoholism. *In* National Institute on Alcohol Abuse and Alcoholism (NIAAA): *Nature and Extent of Alcohol Problems Among the Elderly*. Research Monograph No 14. Rockville, MD, US Department of Health and Human Services (USDHHS).

Chenitz, WC, & Granfors, W (1988): Alcoholism and the family. *In* Gillis, CL, Highley, BL, Roberts, B, et al. (eds): *Toward a Science of Family Health Care*. Menlo Park, CA, Addison-Wesley.

Cohen, M, Kern, JC, & Hassett, C (1986): Identifying alcoholism in medical patients. *Hosp Community Psychiatry*, 37(4):398–400.

Denzin, NK (1987a): *The Alcoholic Self*. Newburg Park, CA, Sage Publications.

Denzin, NK (1987b): *Treating Alcoholism*. Newburg Park, CA, Sage Publications.

DiCiccio-Bloom, B, Space, S, & Zahourek, RP (1986): The homebound alcoholic. *Am J Nurs*, 86(2):167–169.

Drew, LRH (1968): Alcoholism as a self-limiting disease. *Q J Stud Alcohol*, 29:956–967.

Dunham, RG (1981): Aging and changing patterns of alcohol use. *J Psychoact Drugs*, 13:143–151.

Estes, NJ, Smith-DiJulio, K, & Heineman, ME (1980): *Nursing Diagnosis of the Alcoholic Patient*. St. Louis, CV Mosby.

Glatt, MM, Rosin, AJ, & Jauhar, P (1978): Alcoholic problems in the elderly. *Age Ageing*, 7:64–71.

Goldman, D (1987–88): Genetic studies on alcoholism at the NIAAA Intramural Laboratories. *Alcohol Health Res World*, 12(2):102–103.

Gomberg, EL (1982): Patterns of alcohol use and abuse among the elderly. *In* National Institute on Alcohol Abuse and Alcoholism: *Special Population Issues*. Rockville, MD, Alcohol & Health Monograph, No 4, 263–290.

Goodman, L (1988): Would your assessment spot a hidden alcoholic? *RN*, August, 56–60.

Gordis, E (1987–88): The genetic paradigm: Implications of research and treatment. *Alcohol, Health Res World*, 12(2):96–97.

Graham, K (1986): Identifying and measuring alcohol abuse among the elderly: Serious problems with existing instrumentation. *J Stud Alcohol*, 47:322–326.

Gulino, C & Kadin, M (1986): Aging and reactive alcoholism. *Geriatr Nurs*, 7(3):148–151.

Hasselblad, J (1984): *Alcohol Abuse Curriculum Guide for Nurse Practitioner Faculty*. Rockville, MD, USDHHS, NIAAA.

Helzer, JE, Carey, KE, & Miller, RH. (1983): Predictors and correlates of recovery in older versus younger alcoholics. *In* National Institute on Alcohol Abuse and Alcoholism: *Nature and Extent of Alcohol Problems Among the Elderly*. Res Monograph No 14. Rockville, MD, USDHHS, NIAAA, 83–99.

Hinrichsen, JT (1984): Toward improving treatment services for alcoholics of advanced age. *Alcohol, Health Res World*, 8(3):31–39.

Johnson Institute (1982): *The Family Enablers*. Minneapolis, MN, Johnson Institute.

Lasker, MN (1986): Aging alcoholics need nursing help. *J Gerontol Nurs*, 12(1):16–19.

Magruder-Habib, K, Saltz, CC, & Barron, PM (1986): Age-related patterns of alcoholism among veterans in ambulatory care. *Hosp Community Psychiatry*, 37:1251–1255.

Miller, M (1979): *Suicide After Sixty: The Deadly Alternative*. New York, Springer.

Mishara, B, & Kastenbaum, R (1980): *Alcoholism in Old Age*. New York, Grune & Stratton.

Moore, RA (1964): Alcoholism in Japan. *Q J Stud Alcohol*, 25:142–150.

Mulford, HA, & Miller, DE (1963): The prevalence and extent of drinking in Iowa, 1961: A replication and an evaluation of methods. *Q J Stud Alcohol*, 24:39–53.

Naegle, MA (1983): The nurse and the alcoholic: Redefining an historically ambivalent relationship. *J Psychosoc Nurs Ment Health Serv*, 21(6):17–23.

National Council on Alcoholism Criteria Committee (1972): Criteria for the diagnosis of alcoholism. *Am J Psychiatry*, 129:41–49.

National Council on Alcoholism (1981): Blue Ribbon Study Commission on Alcoholism and the Aging, *Report for the 1981 White House Conference on Aging*. Washington, DC, National Council on Alcoholism.

National Council on Alcoholism (1989): *What Are the Signs of Alcoholism?* The NCA self test, Washington, DC.

Opstelten, GE (1982): *Older Adults: A Unique Population at High Risk for Alcohol and Drug Abuse Problems.* Daly City, CA, Aging/Alcoholism Information Committee.

Reich, T (1987–88): Beyond the gene: Research directions in family transmission of susceptibility to alcoholism. *Alcohol, Health Res World, 12*(2):104–107.

Rosin, AJ, & Glatt, MM (1971): Alcohol excess in the elderly. *Q J Stud Alcohol, 32*:53–59.

Schiff, SM (1988): Treatment approaches for older alcoholics. *Generations, 12*(4):41–45.

Schuckit, MA (1977): Geriatric alcoholism and drug abuse. *Gerontologist, 17*:168–174.

Schuckit, MA, Atkinson, JH, Miller, PL, et al. (1980): A three-year follow-up of elderly alcoholics. *J Clin Psychiatry, 41*:412–416.

Shanley, C (1987): Nursing management of alcohol withdrawal. *Aust Nurs J, 16*(11):44–45, 62.

Sheeren, MHS (1988): The relationship between relapse and involvement in Alcoholics Anonymous. *J Stud Alcohol, 49*(1):104–106.

Simon, A, Epstein, LJ, & Reynolds, L (1968): Alcoholism in the geriatric mentally ill. *Geriatrics, 23*:125–131.

Strauss, R (1983): Alcohol problems among the elderly: The need for a biobehavioral perspective. *In* National Institute on Alcohol Abuse and Alcoholism: *Nature and Extent of Alcohol Problems Among the Elderly.* Research Monograph No 14. Rockville, MD, USDHHS, NIAAA, 9–27.

Vestal, RE, McGuire, EA, Tobin, JD, et al. (1977): Aging and external metabolism in man. *Clin Pharmacol Ther, 216*:343–354.

Walker, B, & Kelly, P (1981): *The Elderly: A guide for counselors.* Center City, MN, Hazelden Educational Materials.

Zimberg, S (1974): The elderly alcoholic. *Gerontologist, 14*:221–224.

Zimberg, S (1978): Treatment of the elderly alcoholic in the community and in an institutional setting. *Addict Dis 3*:417–427.

Zimberg, S (1979): Alcohol and the elderly. *In* Petersen, DM, Whittington, FJ, & Payne, BP (eds): *Drugs and Alcohol in the Elderly.* Springfield, IL, Charles C Thomas.

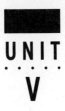

UNIT
V

THE CONTEXT OF NURSING CARE DELIVERY

CHAPTER
27

Environments for Nursing Care of the Older Client

JUDITH S. SCHAINEN, R.N.C., Ph.D.

INTRODUCTION

The social and physical environment significantly influences an older person's behavior and ability to function. On one hand, the environment can have positive effects by supporting function, activities, and competent behavior, enabling older persons to realize their full potential. On the other hand, it can create stress, discomfort, and confusion, and limit mobility, causing premature deterioration and disability. A basic fact is that as a person becomes less competent, there is greater dependency on the physical and social environment and increased sensitivity to environmental changes (Lawton, 1970). The environment should be considered a participant in the care of the elderly (Hiatt, 1982a).

This chapter examines the environments of care for older persons. The models of Lawton (1983) and Moos and Lemke (1985) on the nature of the environment and its relation to older people are presented. They provide the basis for assessment of the environment and planning, implementation, and evaluation of environmental interventions in the care of elderly persons. The use of these models by a nurse clinician in a number of settings (e.g., day care, respite, community and home care, and geriatric evaluation units) is discussed. Concluding the chapter is a description of some new environmental approaches to the care of the elderly and prospects for the future.

523

THE CONCEPT OF ENVIRONMENT

Lawton (1983) identified four determinants or sectors that comprise the "good life" for older people. These are behavioral competence, psychological well-being, perceived quality of life, and the objective environment (Figure 27–1). Within each of the four sectors, a hierarchy of measurable categories is established to facilitate the assessment of the older person's quality of life. These sectors, taken together, account for all of life, which includes all behavior, environment, and experiences (Lawton, 1983).

Behavioral competence is a person's capacity to function. Specific areas included in Lawton's concept of environment are bodily and functional health, cognition, use of time, and social behavior. Psychological well-being is a person's evaluation of the quality of his or her personal experience. This is a subjective evaluation, and the clinician can only estimate an older person's subjective state, determining affect, degree of happiness, and level of congruence between desired and attained goals. Perceived quality of life is the set of evaluations that a person makes about each domain of his or her life. These domains are housing and the neighborhood, the use of time, family,

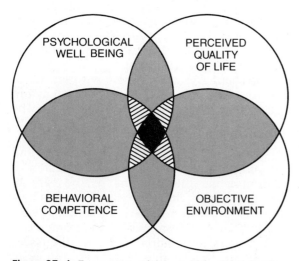

Figure 27–1. Four sectors of the good life. (From Lawton, MP: Other determinants of well being in older people. *Gerontologist*, 23:355, 1983. Reprinted with permission.)

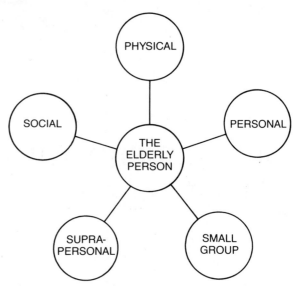

Figure 27–2. Diagrammatic presentation of Lawton's (1983) facets of the objective environment.

and friends. The objective environment consists of five facets:

1. The physical environment is the setting, composed of topography, climate, and buildings.

2. The personal environment includes significant other persons, such as family or friends.

3. The small group environment consists of those people with whom the elderly person has face-to-face contact.

4. The suprapersonal environment refers to the demographic and social characteristics of the group in proximity to the older person, such as age, socioeconomic status, and race.

5. The social environment is made up of all the social and cultural influences on the older person.

Figure 27–2 is a diagram representing the objective environment.

Lawton (1983) initially defined each of the four determinants of the good life as *separate* entities. Actually, *they are related*, albeit in varying degrees. A sense of well-being is one sector that may be reflected in one or more of the other sectors. For example, the basic elements of behavioral competence (health, cognition, and functional health) influence friends' interactions and time use, which in turn predict psychological well-being. However, Lawton (1983) also stated that lack of predictability from one sector of well-being to another is also normal for the human condition. This is why some people are able to maintain psychological well-being even when faced with physical illness.

Moos and Lemke (1985) describe a model that incorporates Lawton's four determinants of the good life in older people. Figure 27–3 depicts the interaction between the environmental system and the personal system to produce individual stability and change. The environmental system (panel I) includes the physical design and organizational structure of the setting and the overall characteristics and interpersonal relationships of the individuals involved. The personal system (panel II) encompasses an individual's sociodemographic and personal resources, such as health status, cognitive and functional ability, and self-esteem. The cognitive appraisal (panel III) and coping responses (panel IV) mediate the relationship between the environmental and personal systems and subsequent adaptation. That is, the individual's cognitive appraisal and coping responses determine the outcome

of the interaction between the environmental and personal systems (Moos & Lemke, 1985).

Efforts made by clients at adaptation influence well-being and level of functioning (panel V). The Moos and Lemke model acknowledges ongoing reciprocal interplay between individuals and their environment. Outcomes at a given point in time are inputs to future adaptation.

Moos and Lemke also indicate that for each person there is a degree of environmental demand that influences performance. Demands that deviate only slightly from a person's adaptive level will elicit a positive effect and adaptive behavior. Demands that vary greatly produce a negative effect and behavior that is maladaptive.

There are several advantages to using a model such as that of Moos and Lemke:

1. The use of a common conceptual framework permits the identification of similar processes occurring in man and his environments and allows the specification of environmental change experienced by a person when moving.

2. This framework postulates the influence of environment on health and adaptation.

3. This framework places emphasis on the

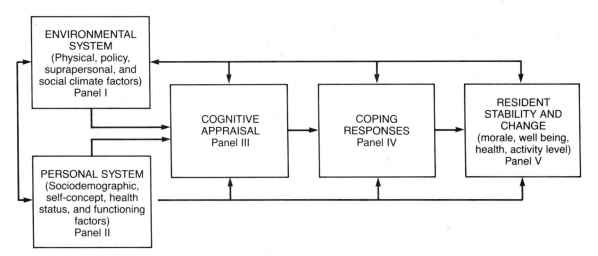

Figure 27–3. A model of the relationship between environmental and personal factors, producing resident stability and change. (From Moos, RH and Lemke, S: Specialized living environments for older people. *In* Birren, JE and Schaie, KW (eds). *Handbook of Psychology of Aging,* ed 2. New York, Van Nostrand Reinhold, 1985, p 867. Reprinted with permission.)

process between environmental and personal systems and the resulting stability and change in the individual.

THE ENVIRONMENT AND THE OLDER PERSON

The concept of the objective environment as developed by Lawton is a useful organizing framework to view the older person in relation to the environment.

Physical Environment

One of the earliest attempts to modify the environment for those with physical handicaps was made in 1961 by the President's Committee on the Employment of the Handicapped, the National Society for Crippled Children and Adults, and some other federal and private agencies (Costa & Sweet, 1976). These groups developed a set of 16 criteria for accessibility to structures. Eventually, all 50 states passed legislation to eliminate architectural barriers in buildings. In 1968, the Architectural Barrier Act (Public Law 90–480) was passed by the United States Congress. This law attempted to incorporate the American National Standards Institutes' Standards of Accessibility into buildings and facilities that were being constructed. Interventions now used to alter the physical environment in the community include public educational programs and political action lobbies to promote legislation for barrier-free design (Costa & Sweet, 1976).

Marcu (1983) points out that it is important to compensate for physical impairment, but not to the extent that people are made to feel helpless or crippled by their environment. People who are encouraged by their surroundings to perform as many tasks as possible can experience a strong sense of control over their environment.

In addition to the foregoing interventions, Marcu (1983) recommends the use of furniture and fixtures that reduce the need for bending and stooping. He suggests that toilets be close to beds, and door handles be placed at a level that permits opening by anyone. Because an older person requires more light than the young but is bothered by glare, lighting should be indirect and highly polished floors avoided.

Personal Environment

The personal environment includes significant others, such as friends and family. Staff members are also significant, primarily in the caregiver role. Substantial ambiguity exists in the subdivision of tasks between family and staff. This may hinder efforts to engage families as support resources in nursing care. Interventions to facilitate interaction between family and staff include (Montgomery, 1982):

1. Training sessions for all staff members, centered on the complexities of family-resident relationships
2. Staff training in communication skills
3. Inclusion of family members in the creation of the care plan
4. Provision for activities and meetings for family members only, as well as ones for residents and family members
5. Rules, regulations, and practices that connote welcome to the family, such as open visitation hours, refreshments for visitors, and direct invitations to the institution's events
6. Availability of key staff members, including the social worker and administrator, during peak visitation hours

The need of the elderly to have autonomy is an important factor for a health care provider to consider in institutions and the community. Lemke and Moos (1986) studied both the structure and process of care in 244 facilities throughout the United States. Their study included nursing homes, residential care facilities, and apartments. They observed that autonomy was uniformly low in nursing homes, high in apartments, and variable in residential facilities. Two reasons were given for these observations. First, in congregate settings, services are performed for a group rather than for individuals, and second, everything tends to be done for or to the patient, never with him or her (Coons, 1983). When individuals recognize that they have no control over their environment, they become apathetic, show a lack of response, and tend to become helpless. Interpersonal distance is created between health care providers and elderly persons as they assume the healer and sick roles, respectively (Solomon, 1982). The long-term outcome for the elderly tends to be decreased ability, resulting in increased emotional and physical costs to the provider.

A number of researchers have made some constructive suggestions to change this process. In institutions this can be accomplished by allowing self-care and choices in daily life to accommodate individual differences (Lichtenstein, Federspiel, & Schaffner, 1985). Measures that staff can use to contribute to an elderly person's sense of control over the environment include: (1) knocking on residents' doors before entering; (2) asking permission to speak with the resident; (3) returning at a more convenient time if requested to do so; (4) sitting down so as to bring the staff member to the same eye level as the person being visited; and (5) speaking slowly, avoiding jargon and medical terminology (Williams, C, 1985).

In any social interaction, the needs of all participants should be considered. Therefore, administrators should keep in mind the need of the staff as they relate to clients or residents. Staff and health care providers in the community all need recognition. When their interventions are completed, there may be no tangible or residual product that others can examine and evaluate. The residents whom they help are often unable to appreciate the quality of skill with which the interventions are performed. It is important, then, that staff be rewarded and their efforts acknowledged (Gordon, 1982).

Suprapersonal Environment

The suprapersonal component of the environment may be influenced by both social and cultural influences. For example, Chee and Kane (1983) reported attitude differences between black and Japanese-American elders. The latter tended to place more emphasis on all aspects of ethnic programming and on the homogeneity of patients and staff. Black elders tended to place greater emphasis on access to family rather than ethnicity. Culturally relevant adaptations in the design and provision of services could make the outlook on life of elderly residents more agreeable (Chee & Kane, 1983). Additional work needs to be done in this area to recognize and appreciate the culturally relevant needs of older people.

An interesting account of the impact of culture upon gerontological community nursing care is the recent report of Lewis, Messner, and McDowell (1985) describing the health care of elderly Appalachian residents. In this part of the United States, the elderly are cared for by family members who live considerable distances from health care centers. These people tend to value their privacy and prefer to be left alone. All of these factors, plus bad roads, make it difficult for patients to receive care. Health care staff, inpatient facilities, and services are limited in Appalachia. This forces nurses to work with little or no peer support. Doctors are often available only on a part-time basis or by phone. The elderly especially seek out the old "granny woman" or "herb doctor" for medications, even when they have been given a conventional medical treatment to follow. These people have an initial mistrust of strangers. For all of these reasons, nurses must take the time to establish rapport with this population, learn their culture, and even ask their advice, if they are to be effective health care givers.

Social Environment

The social environment refers to the social and cultural forces, such as norms and values, to which the elderly person is exposed. The following questions can be used to evaluate the social environment (Estes, Fox, & Mahoney, 1986; Koff, 1986; Longe, 1986):

1. What are the lifestyle habits of the elderly person?

2. How does the elderly person's culture affect the perceived need for health care?

3. What is the elderly client's status relative to some of the major changes in the social environment, such as retirement, threatening economic and social limitations, loss of social support systems, and loss of individual lifestyle?

Within institutions, the following questions are appropriate:

1. Are the residents allowed to modify the rules and regulations?

2. Is consideration given to the individuality of persons?

3. Are clients given opportunities for education, creativity, and the assumption of responsibility?

THE ENVIRONMENTS FOR CARE

A "setting" denotes a place for care of older persons, and is but one facet (e.g., physical) of a person's total environment (Lawton, 1983; Moos & Lemke, 1985). Within each setting, the person interacts with all facets of the objective environment; the physical, personal, small group, suprapersonal, and social. Combined, these create the environments for care.

Day Care for Clients with Alzheimer's Disease

Day care for the frail elderly began in 1974, and currently there are an estimated 800 to 1000 adult day care programs in the United States (Mace, 1984). These programs offer cognitively impaired persons a structured day outside their homes, which frees family caregivers to remain employed, to run errands, or simply to rest. Staff act to reinforce the client's activities of daily living and to monitor his or her general health. Rehabilitation therapies are offered by many centers, and physical exercise and good nutrition are emphasized (Panella, Lilliston, Brush, et al., 1984).

In the day care setting, the nurse is primarily concerned with the elderly client's objective environment, specifically with the physical domain of the environment (Lawton, 1983). The client is transported to and from the center, and orientation to person, time, and place is emphasized. The nurse tries to facilitate a client's independence for as long as possible. This may be reflected by activating a sense of autonomy (control over the environment), by providing space for exercise, and by convenient arrangement and choice of furniture. Broader nursing functions include health services, educating the community about the center's purpose, and providing health counseling. These broader nursing functions address the small group facet of the objective environment. Social workers deal with elderly persons' social environment by teaching families client-managing skills, offering short-term counseling, and assisting families in locating other services.

Respite Programs

The impetus for this service began in the late 1960s when deinstitutionalization of psychiatric and long-term care patients occurred. This meant discharging individuals from institutions or not sending them there in the first place (Warren & Cohen, 1985). Since many of these people were young and developmentally impaired, the burden for their care fell upon their families. It soon became apparent, however, that if deinstitutionalization was to work, these families required help. To some extent, this help has evolved. In the 1970s, statewide grass-roots movements began in support of respite care, especially in California, Washington, Maryland, and Massachusetts. In 1980, the federal government accepted a definition of respite care in Title XIX, or the Medicaid Home and Community-Based Waiver. During the 1980s, respite care became institution-based.

The burden of caregiving is expensive. There are significant psychiatric, physical, financial, and social costs of caring for a family member. Caregivers often suffer from chronic fatigue, declining physical health, financial hardship, family turmoil, and psychiatric symptoms, such as insomnia, depression, excessive irritability, and guilt. An especially difficult burden is being restricted in one's own home and unable to engage in outside activities (Warren & Cohen, 1985; Scharlach & Frenzel, 1986).

Analysis of the respite program in terms of Lawton's (1983) and Moos and Lemke's (1985) models reveals that interventions by health care providers again are directed toward improving clients' environments in several ways. In this case, relief is given to family members who care for the client. The nurse would therefore direct interventions at the personal and small group environments by, for example:

1. Facilitating or resolving problems of family dynamics
2. Encouraging self-care
3. Coordinating the involvement of other members of the medical team as the need arises, including doctors, dieticians, social workers, and psychologists
4. Providing relief for significant others to enhance clients' psychological well-being and perceived quality of life and to facilitate adaptation to their current status

Community Care

Most home-based aged persons have at least one chronic condition, and many suffer from multiple health problems. Therefore, community nursing care for the elderly involves facilitating health promotion. Nurses, too, are concerned with behavioral competence and the objective environment of clients.

Nurses work with elderly clients to assist them to manage their chronic illnesses and medical regimens, and provide information on health screening devices (e.g., cancer), home health and mobility aids, and a nutritious diet, to name a few functions (Ory, 1984; Clough, 1984; Mellilo, 1985; Minkler & Pasick, 1986; Longe, 1986).

Although many of these health education services are hospital- or clinic-based, Ory (1984) reports a gradual increase in community-based programs. For example, the Stanford Arthritis Center sponsors a self-management community education program for arthritis patients that uses lay people for pa-

tient education. In addition, many senior centers are also beginning to address the health and social needs of home-based elderly by offering individual and group-oriented health education programs, nutrition, and health promotion services.

The community nurse must be attentive to a client's social and suprapersonal environments. For example, the nurse must know if a client can afford a given medication or type of food before prescribing or recommending it. Elderly clients' cultural beliefs may not permit them to eat certain foods or attend an important appointment. Specific cultural input facilitates the plan of care for clients.

Home Care

There are several reasons for the current expansion in home health care. Hospitals are discharging patients earlier, in keeping with Medicare regulations, and are offering more outpatient services. This pattern of earlier discharge is encouraged by the fact that highly technical equipment, such as hyperalimentation, dialysis machines, and respirators, is being used in the home. Home care is less expensive. Medicare reimburses $39 per day for a home nursing visit and $350 per day for hospital care (Arbeiter, 1984). The terminally ill may prefer to die at home. In a recent survey, 60% of the patients sampled reported that they would rather die at home, especially if a nurse were available 24 hours a day (Putnam, McDonald, Miller, et al., 1980).

The principal benefits of home health care are that it allows older people to remain in their homes, continue to practice their individual cultural and spiritual beliefs, and retain their own values while receiving nursing services. In addition, the family may continue to be a major support group for these clients.

Geriatric Evaluation Units

Geriatric evaluations are designed to assess elderly clients' medical and psychological problems, to determine optimal placement, and to provide therapy and rehabilitation. Clients may be admitted from the emergency room, from outpatient clinics, or as scheduled admissions. Clients may also be transfers from other inpatient acute services (Saunders, Hickler, Hall, et al., 1983).

Staff in geriatric evaluation units (also called geriatric assessment units) report several benefits of these settings that enhance the behavioral competence of their clients.

Rubenstein, Abrass, and Kane (1981) reported several benefits derived by elderly clients who had been admitted to a geriatric evaluation unit. More thorough diagnoses occurred with each client, and the mean number of daily prescribed drugs was reduced by 32% per client. Placement following discharge was improved in nearly half the clients seen. Rubenstein, Rhee, and Kane (1982) also pointed out that geriatric evaluation units could be cost-effective if they were able to offset expenses by reducing the need for other services.

Saunders and associates (1983) have described modifications of the physical environment for the geriatric evaluation unit as follows:

Full length rails for beds
Call bells with long cords
Unit dose medications locked up in clients' rooms
Large print calendars by each client's bed
Hand-held showerheads permitting clients to operate showers while sitting
A communal dining room with adaptive feeding equipment
A free-standing whirlpool tub with hydraulic lift
A satellite occupational and physical therapy room
Alarm signals on stairway exit doors
A washer and dryer for clients' street clothes, which they are encouraged to wear rather than institutional garb or nightclothes

The effect of the suprapersonal environment on age-segregated geriatric evaluation units was addressed in a study by McAlpine and Wight (1982). After interviewing 100 cognitively intact patients admitted to a geriatric assessment unit, they found that those from upper social classes and those who lived alone tended to be upset by being admitted to an age-segregated unit, but the majority of patients felt that they were admitted to the right ward. One-quarter of all lucid patients, however, objected to the presence of confused patients on the unit.

NEW ENVIRONMENTAL APPROACHES TO ELDER CARE

Regardless of the setting, some new and exciting approaches to elder care have occurred over the past decade. Silverstone and Wynter (1975) reported on the integration of an all-male and all-female floor in a geriatric institution in order to provide a more natural climate for the elderly residents. Initial resistance to the change gave way to a more cheerful floor life. Significant improvements took place in the social behavior of the males. They appeared better groomed and used less profane language. The women also endorsed the presence of the men by expressing approval of the latter's behavior. Silverstone and Wynter (1975) underscored the need for heterosexual living spaces for institutionalized elderly in order to offset the shrinkage in their social life space.

Recently, the positive effects of full-time child care centers in long-term care facilities have been recognized. The advantages of such spring-winter relationships have been well documented. The older person can offer experiences, ideas, interests, skills, and craft ideas. The children learn and develop as they receive special attention from loving adults who have both the time and patience to listen to them (Tice, 1982). Other examples of this type of program are foster grandparents, retired senior volunteer programs, and teaching learning communities.

Pets have played an important role in alleviating the sense of loneliness experienced by the elderly. Frank (1984) pointed out that pets were first introduced in mental institutions in mid-eighteenth-century England. In 1944 to 1945, the Red Cross used dogs at a convalescent home in New York City. The animals served to distract people's attention from themselves and presented a responsibility for care and training (Levinson, 1972).

Animals have also been used as psychotherapeutic interventions to create healthier environments. Many gerontological psychologists believe that the institutional environment is directly responsible for the social withdrawal exhibited by residents. The key role of a pet is to provide opportunities for the projection and displacement of feelings. It also allows for direct expression of concern, care, anxiety, and fear, and it tests the person's capacities for power, authority, and influence. Finally, a pet can provide both an important link with the internalized past and an anchor in the security of something familiar. When an elderly person must leave home for a long-term care facility, a great void is experienced. A pet can possibly increase participation and interest in personal identity and continuity in the sense of self.

Another intervention used in nursing homes is plant therapy. Carroll, Mattson, Moss, and Moench (1978) have described the benefits of horticulture therapy to nursing home residents

as a means with which to mark the meaningful passage of time, to provide opportunities for gardening, and to create of a more home-like atmosphere by including plants in rooms.

The involvement of children and other community members in nursing home horticulture therapy programs has also been described in the literature. Both Martin (1981) and Hiatt (1982a) describe these interactions as being beneficial to all participants by encouraging the activities of learning and teaching, the feeling of being important to others, opportunity for regular exercise, and the sense of accomplishing something worthwhile.

In a similar program, residents at the Seattle Veterans Administration Medical Center/ Nursing Home Care Unit (SVAMC/NHCU), aided by nursing, recreational therapy staff members, and 4H children, have grown vegetables from seed in ground plots. They have also planted flowers in specially designed and built wheelchair-high planters, visited local nurseries, and heard gardening experts lecture at the unit. The benefits derived from this experience have been opportunities for reminiscence and a source of enjoyment and de-

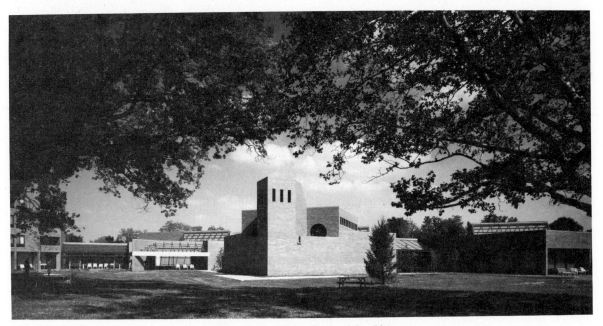

Maple Knoll Village, Springdale, Ohio.

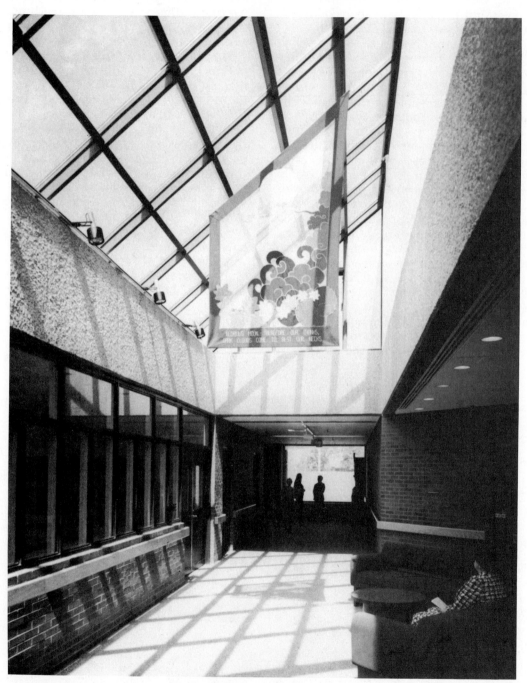

Maple Knoll Village, Springdale, Ohio.

light in being able to eat the vegetables and fruits (corn, radishes, tomatoes, beans, and strawberries) as they ripen.

Smart (1978) described the work of a group of architects in Springdale, Ohio, who sought to overcome the dehumanization generated by the institutionalization of the elderly. These architects, in conjunction with the local senior citizens group, planned Maple Knoll Village. This development enabled the elderly to live somewhat independent lives while receiving essential medical and nursing care. The village was built to preserve standing trees and to retain a grassy knoll that served as the town common. All buildings were linked by a broad skylit spine that included small intimate solaria well endowed with ficus and palms.

SUMMARY

The "environment" is a multifaceted concept involving physical, personal, small group, suprapersonal, and social environments. In this chapter, we examined the environments for care of the elderly and described existing alternative care settings.

References

Arbeiter, JS (November, 1984): The shift to home health care nursing. *RN*, 38–43.

Bartol, MA (1979): Nonverbal communication in patients with Alzheimer's disease. *J Gerontol Nurs*, 5(4):21–31.

Benefield, LE (1985): Trends in home health care. *In* Hogstel, MO (ed): *Home Nursing Care for the Elderly.* East Norwalk, CT, Appleton and Lange, 363–372.

Boling, TE (Spring, 1986): Alternative health care. *Prof Nurs Q*, 10.

Browning MA (1985): Home health care: The nurse's perspective. *In* Hogstel, MO (ed): *Home Nursing Care for the elderly.* East Norwalk, CT, Appleton and Lange, 85–105.

Butrin, J (1985): Day care: A new idea? *J Gerontol Nurs*, 11(4):19–22.

Cantor, MH (1983): Strain among caregivers: A study of experience in the United States. *Gerontologist*, 23(6):597–604.

Carroll, K, Mattson, LA, Moss, T, et al. (1978): *Therapeutic Activities Programming with the Elderly.* Minneapolis, Ebenezer Center for Aging and Human Development.

Chee, P, & Kane, R (1983): Cultural factors affecting nursing home care minorities: A study of Black American and Japanese-American groups. *J Am Geriatr Soc*, 31(2):109–112.

Christopher, MA (July, 1986): Home care for the elderly. *Nursing 86*, 16:50–55.

Clough, N (1984): A short answer to long-term care. *Nurs Times*, 80: 40–42.

Coons, DH (1983): The therapeutic milieu: Social-psychological aspects of treatment. *In* Reichel, W (ed): *Clinical Aspects of Aging.* Baltimore, Williams & Wilkins, 137–150.

Costa, FJ, & Sweet, M (1976): Barrier free environments for older Americans. *Gerontologist*, 16: 404–409.

Deutschman, M (1982): Environmental settings and environmental competence. *Gerontol Geriatr Educ*, 2(3):237–242.

Estes, CL, Fox, S, & Mahoney, CW (1986): Health care and social policy: Health promotion and the elderly. *In* Dychtwald, K (ed): *Wellness and Health Promotion for the Elderly.* Rockville, MD, Aspen, 55–70.

Flynn, PT, & Rich, AJ (1982): Photographic enlargement of printed music: Technique, application, and implications. *Gerontologist*, 22(6):540–543.

Fox, J (1985): Chronic respiratory patients: A new challenge for home health nursing. *Home Health Care Nurse*, 3(2):13–16.

Frank, SJ (1984): The touch of love. *J Gerontol Nurs*, 10(2):28–35.

Gordon, GK (1982): Developing a motivating environment. *J Nurs Admin*, 12: 11–16.

Hewner, SJ (1986): Bringing home the health care. *J Gerontol Nurs*, 12(2):29–30, 30–35.

Hiatt, LG (Spring, 1982a): The environment as a participant in health care. *J Long-Term Care Admin*, 10:1–17.

Hiatt, LG (1982b): The importance of the physical environment. *Nurs Homes*, 31:2–10.

Koff, TH (1986): Wellness and long-term care. *In* Dychtwald, K (ed): *Wellness and Health Promotion for the Elderly.* Rockville, MD, Aspen, 119–132.

Lawton, MP (1970): Ecology and aging. *In* Pastalan, LA, & Carson, DH (eds): *Spatial Behavior of Older People.* Ann Arbor, MI, University of Michigan Press, 40–67.

Lawton, MP (1983): Environments and other determinants of well being in older adults. *Gerontologist*, 23(4):349–357.

Lemke, S, & Moos, RH (1986): Quality of residential settings for elderly adults. *J Gerontol*, 41(2):268–276.

Levinson, BM (1972): The dog as a co-therapist. *Ment Hygiene*, 46(1):59–65.

Lewis, S, Messner, R, & McDowell, WA (1985): An unchanging culture. *J Gerontol Nurs*, 11(8):20–26.

Lichtenstein, MJ, Federspiel, CF, & Schaffner, W (1985): Factors associated with early demise in nursing home residents: A case control study. *J Am Geriatr Soc*, 33:315–319.

Longe, ME (1986): Hospitals and health promotion for older adults. *In* Dychtwald, K (ed): *Wellness and Health Promotion for the Elderly.* Rockville, MD, Aspen, 275–297.

Mace, N (1984): Day care for demented clients. *Hosp Community Psychiatry*, 35(10):979–980, 994.

Mace, NL, & Rabins, PV (1981): *The 36-Hour Day.* Baltimore, Johns Hopkins University Press.

Marcu, M (November, 1983): The living environment: Personal dignity through physical design. *J Am Health Care Assoc*, 8–11.

Martin, D (1981): Enjoyable activity for everyone. *Geriatr Nurs*, 2:210–213.

Masson, V (1986): How nursing happens in adult day care. *Geriatr Nurs*, 7:18–20.

McAlpine, CJ, & Wight, ZJ (1982): Attitudes and anxieties of elderly patients on admission to a geriatric assessment unit. *Age Ageing*, 11(1):35–41.

Mellilo, KD (1985): Who needs health maintenance? Teaching aged women to care about health prevention exams. *J Gerontol Nurs*, 11(2):18–21.

Minkler, M, & Pasick, RJ (1986): Health promotion and the elderly: A critical perspective on the past and future. *In* Dychtwald, K (ed): *Wellness and Health Promotion for the Elderly*. Rockville, MD, Aspen, 39–54.

Montgomery, RJV (1982): Impact of institutional care policies on family integration. *Gerontologist*, 22(1):54–58.

Moos, R (1979): Social-ecological perspectives on health. *In* Stone, G, Cohen, F, Adler, N, et al. (eds): *Health Psychology*. San Francisco, Jossey Bass.

Moos, RH, & Lemke, S (1985): Specialized environments for older people. *In* Birren, JE, & Schaie, KW (eds): *Handbook of the Psychology of Aging* (ed 2). New York, Van Nostrand Reinhold, 864–889.

Ory, MG (1984): Health promotional strategies for the aged. *J Gerontol Nurs*, 10(10):31–36.

Panella, JJ, Lilliston, BA, Brush, D, et al. (1984): Day care for dementia patients: An analysis of a four-year program. *J Am Geriatr Soc*, 32(12):883–886.

Pastalan, LA (1982): Design and application to the visual environment of the elderly. *Aging and Human Visual Function*. New York, Alan R Liss, 323–333.

Putnam, ST, McDonald, MM, Miller, MM, et al. (1980): Home as a place to die. *Am J Nurs*, 8: 1451–1453.

Robertson, CC (August 22, 1984): Old people in the community. Health visitors and preventive care. *Nurs Times*, 80:29–30.

Rubenstein, LZ, Abrass, IB, & Kane, RL (1981): Improved care for patients on a new Geriatric Evaluation Unit. *J Am Geriatr Soc*, 29(11):531–536.

Rubenstein, LZ, Rhee, L, & Kane, RL (1982): The role of geriatric assessment units in caring for the elderly: An analytic review. *J Gerontol*, 37(5):513–521.

Rubin, A, & Shuttleworth, GE (1983): Engaging families as support resources in the nursing home: Ambiguity in the subdivision of tasks. *Gerontologist*, 23:632–636.

Saunders, RH, Hickler, RB, Hall, SA, et al. (1983): A geriatric special care unit: Experience in a university hospital. *J Am Geriatr Soc*, 31(11):685–693.

Scharlach, A, & Frenzel, C (1986): An evaluation of institution-based respite care. *Gerontologist*, 15(1):83–87.

Silverstone, B, & Wynter, L (1975): The effects of introducing a heterosexual living space. *Gerontologist*, February, 83–87.

Smart, JD (1978): Landscaped campus site humanizes life for the elderly. *Hospitals/J Am Hosp Assoc*, 52:75–76, 78, 80.

Solomon, K (1982): Social antecedents of learned helplessness in the health care setting. *Gerontologist*, 22(3):282–287.

Sugarman, JG, & Brown, P (1983): Child care in long-term facilities. *Nurs Homes*, 341:4–7.

Tice, CH (1982): A gift from the older generation: Continuity. *Child Today*, 2–6.

Topf, M (1984): A framework for research on aversive physical aspects of the environment. *Res Nurs Health*, 7:35–42.

Warren, R, & Cohen, S (1985): Respite care. *Rehabil Lit*, 46(3–4):66–71.

Williams, C (1985): And this is home? *In* Schneider, EL (ed): *The Teaching Nursing Home*. New York, Raven Press, 137–144.

Williams, SD (1985): The role of the family in home care. *In* Hogstel, MO (ed): *Home Nursing Care for the Elderly*. East Norwalk, CT, Appleton and Lange, 45–65.

CHAPTER
28

Social Support of the Older Client

LINDA R. PHILLIPS, R.N., Ph.D., F.A.A.N.

INTRODUCTION

Belonging to a social structure that provides personal contact, affirmation of personhood, assistance in times of trouble, information and feedback, and opportunities for reciprocal in- timacy and affection is a human requirement, regardless of age. The appropriate definition of social support is controversial, as are the exact nature of social support and the role that social support plays in mediating stress and promoting health (Broadhead, Kaplan, James, et al., 1983; Brown, 1986; House, 1981; Wallston, Alagna, DeVillis, et al., 1983). However, there is little doubt that individual survival is nearly impossible without it. For elderly individuals who face an increasing threat of disability and chronic illness *and* loss of supporters with advancing age, the issue of social support assumes inordinate importance. As social support declines, so does the likelihood of independent functioning. The purpose of this chapter is to identify the structure of social support available to the elderly, including the types of social support and supporters and the organization of support services. In addition, the common difficulties encountered in providing social support and the essential components of a social support assessment for elderly individuals are presented.

STRUCTURE OF SOCIAL SUPPORTS FOR THE ELDERLY

Social supports for the aged can be seen as a matrix composed of subsystems, systems, and suprasystems crossed by formal and informal support mechanisms (Figure 28–1). The subsystems are composed of dyadic or triadic

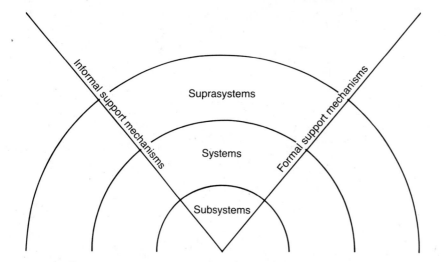

Figure 28–1. Social supports for the aged form a matrix composed of subsystems, systems, and suprasystems crossed by formal and informal support mechanisms.

relationships, which are characterized by intense mutual interdependence between the elderly person and significant others. The significant others do not necessarily have to be human; they can be, for example, companion animals. These subsystems are embedded in systems. Systems are composed of the interrelationships of the elderly persons and a more or less organized group, such as elderly persons and their family unit or an elderly person and a social service agency. Systems are embedded in suprasystems, which are composed of the interrelationships of the elderly and their social support systems within the context of the larger community. Examples of suprasystems include extended kinship systems, community-based outreach programs, and organized social service agencies.

Formal and informal support mechanisms are frequently cited in the gerontological literature. Formal support mechanisms are services provided by institutions, government agencies, or private organizations. Informal support mechanisms are those that are created by bonds of obligation or affection. These are not organized and do not necessarily involve the exchange of money. The support provided by family members, neighbors, and friends is considered to be informal.

Viewing social support from a matrix perspective is useful in gerontological nursing for a number of reasons. First, it helps to empha-size the inherent complexity of the notion of social support and permits the broadest possible range of supporters to be considered during assessment. Second, it provides the nurse with alternative views of social support when the elderly person appears to be totally devoid of interpersonal resources. Third, it assists the nurse to identify the range of supporters possible when the intervention strategy of choice is mobilization of social supports to prevent premature institutionalization or premature functional decline.

Components of Social Support

The components of social support vary, as described in the literature. In general, social support includes the provision of affirmation, affection, and aid (Kahn, 1979). Affirmation is evidenced by activities such as the provision of positive feedback (Barrera, 1981); validation behaviors (Caplan, 1974), such as encouragement, empathy, and recognition of competence (Cobb, 1976; Porrit, 1979); and the endorsement of a person's behaviors, perceptions, or expressed views (Kahn & Antonucci, 1981). Affection is characterized by intimate interaction (Barrera, 1981); sharing and reciprocity (Cobb, 1976); and expressing positive feelings (House, 1981). Aid can be symbolic, informational, or instrumental. Symbolic aid involves activities that assist the individual to mobilize personal resources and master emotional burdens (Caplan, 1974). Informational aid includes activities such as providing advice, information, suggestions, or directions (House, 1981). Instrumental aid involves the provision of physical assistance, money, time, skills, and labor (Caplan, 1974; Barrera, 1981; House, 1981; Kahn & Antonucci, 1981). Although everyone needs all of these types of support, it is not necessary nor is it always possible for any one supporter to provide all types. For most people, the total need for social support is met by the individuals in their social network. In this way the burden for total support is distributed among a number of individuals. The amount and type of support available are directly related to the total size of the social network, the support required, and the accumulated resources of the individual.

Effects of Aging on Informal Support Mechanisms

As an individual ages, the total number of individuals available to absorb the burden for support becomes smaller. In addition, with increasing age, the likelihood of disability and relative immobility increases. These changes have two important effects. First, the elderly person becomes progressively unable to independently replace losses within the social network. Relationships that represented long emotional ties cannot be replaced. Second, with increasing disability, a smaller social network must provide more direct aid. Consequently, there are fewer resources available to meet the need for affirmation and affection. Although formal mechanisms can supplement the losses within the social network, they focus on aid rather than affirmation and affection.

Caregiving is a major type of social support that is provided to the elderly. For the community-dwelling elderly, Bowers (1987) identified five categories of caregiving that family members provide to elderly relatives in the community:

1. Anticipatory caregiving—the support provided for potential needs of the elder
2. Preventive caregiving—the support provided for the purpose of preventing illness, injury, or physical and mental deterioration
3. Supervisory caregiving—the care management support described by Archbold (1980), which includes activities such as arranging for, setting up, and checking out
4. Instrumental caregiving—the provision of all types of actual care, including meal preparation, physical care, transportation, estate management, and provision of socialization opportunities
5. Protective caregiving—activities performed to protect the elder from threats to self-image and assaults to personal dignity

All of these qualify as social support because they meet an elderly person's need for affirmation, affection, and aid. Although a variety of individuals may be involved in providing support, it is often family members who assume the major responsibility (Table 28–1).

Types of Informal Support Mechanisms

In this country, most elderly individuals live their last years residing in the community (Mindel, 1979; Glick, 1979). While the chance of becoming institutionalized increases with each year of life (Mindel, 1979; Siegel, 1976), the vast majority (86% of all men and 73% of all women) over the age of 86 years remain community residents (Glick, 1979). Living in the community, however, cannot be assumed

Table 28–1. COMPONENTS OF INFORMAL SUPPORTS

Providers
Family members
Neighbors
Friends
Church associates
Companion animals
Services
Affirmation of personhood
Affection
Caregiving services
Financial assistance/management
Mobilization of social network

to be strongly correlated with functional independence. Among those over the age of 65 years, 80% have one or more chronic conditions (Rice & Feldman, 1983). Although the majority of the chronically ill elderly in the community are able to "get around," a substantial portion of these individuals require some form of personal assistance in order to survive. Shanas (1979) determined in a nationwide survey, for example, that approximately 3% of the elderly at home are bedfast and 10% are housebound. This accounts for over twice as many elderly individuals as the total number who are institutionalized at any given time. Social support is a chief variable in preventing premature institutionalization for community-dwelling elders.

Family members provide most of the home care and social support needed by the community-dwelling elderly (Bengston & Treas, 1980; Brody, 1981, 1985; Lang & Brody, 1981). Family members provide care to the elderly, regardless of the elder's health status or intensity of needs (Archbold, 1980, 1983) and the family members' other responsibilities (Lang & Brody, 1981; Cantor, 1983). Family caregiving is not substantially altered by: the family's ethnicity (Cantor, 1979; Jackson, 1980; Taylor, 1985; Markides, Boldt, & Ray, 1986); whether or not the elder lives alone (Moss, Moos, & Moles, 1985); whether or not the family receives support, instruction, or assistance from home care or social services agencies (Archbold, 1980, 1983; Shanas, 1979); and whether or not the elder has female relatives to assist with care (Horowitz, 1985). Although the types of support that male and female relatives provide to the elderly differ, the absence of a female relative does not mean that the elderly person will be devoid of support. While there are some differences in the types of services offered by family members who live geographically close compared to those who live at a distance, extreme geographic distance has not been shown to substantially interfere with family members assuming caregiving and social support roles (Brody, 1985; Horowitz, 1985; Moss, Moos, & Moles, 1985).

The patterns determining who provides support to elderly relatives is fairly predicta-

ble. If the individual is still married and the spouse is physically able, most caregiving is provided by the spouse, often with the assistance of children, other relatives, and neighbors. If the spouse is no longer available, responsibility for care is usually assumed by daughters, daughters-in-law, and granddaughters. Responsibility for financial assistance and management is usually assumed by sons, sons-in-law, or grandsons (Horowitz, 1985). In addition, Shanas (1979) showed that elders receive a substantial amount of social support from siblings, neighbors, friends, and church associates, if available. Companion animals serve as an important source of support for some elderly, including those who seem to have few humans remaining in their social networks.

Organization of Informal Supports

The organization of informal support mechanisms is also fairly predictable, with family members usually taking the initiative to mobilize and maintain the resources for an incapacitated elder. In a study (Glaser & Strauss, 1967) of 39 caregivers of the elderly, Phillips (1984) identified two types of organizational structures within families for meeting the social support needs of the elder. Both involved three distinctive roles taken by individuals within the caregiving constellation. These roles are usually filled by children of the elder and occasionally by spouses. In addition, these roles are enacted whether the elder is community-dwelling or institutionalized.

The first role is that of *designated caregiver*, which is given to the family member elected by the elder and other family members to assume the responsibility for organization and implementation of support services. In many families, the election is settled quite early, long before the question of caregiving is an issue and often while the designated caregiver (if a child of the elder) is still quite young. The responsibility of the designated caregiver is to monitor the elder's behavior and physical and emotional well-being in order to determine the type and amount of support services needed.

The designated caregiver is not required to provide for all the elder's needs, but is responsible for mobilizing the social network to ensure that the elder's needs are met. In addition, the designated caregiver acts as the family spokesperson in times of decision-making.

Abdicator is another family role identified by Phillips (1984). Abdicators are family members who are given the family's permission not to provide support for the elder. Often abdicators are "family ambassadors" who function to enhance the family's social status through their employment or other roles. The abdicator, rather than the designated caregiver, is often the elder's favorite. This can arouse a great deal of interpersonal conflict within the family.

The third role identified in the Phillips study is the *pretender*. Pretenders are relatives with potential for being designated caregivers. Often, pretenders feel that they are best prepared to assume the caregiving role, even though they are not the family's elected choice.

The two types of organizations identified in the Phillips (1984) study are differentiated by the degree to which decisions about the designated caregiver role are accepted by the family. In families with limited numbers of members for the designated caregiver role or in which the election result is uncontested, the major role of the designated caregiver is clear. These families are relatively conflict-free and interact quite well with health care professionals, when professionals acknowledge the authority of the designated caregiver and do not attempt to negotiate care decisions with others in the family unit.

The second type of organizational structure is found in families where there is more than one family member with potential for the designated caregiver position and where the election results are contested. These families are characterized by a great deal of interpersonal conflict within the unit, as individuals compete for the favored position of designated caregiver. Conflict is intensified during times of crisis. Even during times of relative calm, the pretenders tend to criticize the activities of both the designated caregiver and the abdicators. Often the conflict among family members results in long delays between the appearance of an elder's need for support and the mobilization of resources to meet the need.

The Phillips study shows that timing of support is one of the most troublesome problems encountered by designated caregivers, regardless of whether the role of designated caregiver is contested. Many of the caregivers interviewed in the study gave evidence of being immobilized in a vacillation cycle. The vacillation cycle was triggered by a change in the elder, signaling the possibility of a need for increased support. The caregiver then actively tested the elder's situation by sampling and observing the elder's behavior, seeking validation for opinions, and waiting. The cycle involved a great deal of time, effort, uncertainty, intrapsychic turmoil, and discomfort for the caregiver. Fearful of interfering with the elder's life or decreasing the elder's independence and reluctant to give up their view of the elder as competent and capable, caregivers caught in the vacillation cycle reported that they accurately saw the evidence for the need for increased support but were simply unable to act.

Vacillation was most commonly broken by some radical change in the elder's situation, for example, by a broken hip or death of a spouse, which spurred the caregiver to immediately mobilize support mechanisms. Unfortunately, such a "click" experience often occurred long after evidence of physical or mental deterioration of the elder was seen. Following a click experience, most caregivers reported a honeymoon period during which the elder was seen as vulnerable and frail and in need of increased nurturance. Sometimes, these clicks occurred in a cogwheel fashion, so that only part of the elder's needs for support was acknowledged. This came with a concomitant desensitization to the intensity of the rest of the elder's needs. For example, following the death of an elder's spouse, the caregiver might immediately act on the need for assistance with financial management but may be totally insensitive to the increased need for socialization. As a result, there can be long delays between the time when the elder's needs are evidenced and when the needs are met.

When elders become unable to maintain and organize their own social supports, family members with actual or acquired kinship ties most commonly assume these responsibilities. It is possible and not uncommon, however, for other individuals within the elder's social network to perform as designated caregiver. Many elders, in fact, prefer the support of lifelong friends, associates, or neighbors to the support of family when kinship ties are remote or family relations are strained. Often, these supportive relationships are assumed voluntarily. Sometimes, when the needs for support become intense, these roles are formalized by some form of payment for services or through the assignment of a legal role (e.g., conservator). A formal supporter on occasion becomes an informal supporter because of the intensity of the affective tie that has arisen from the intimacy of formal caregiving.

Formal Support Mechanisms

A wide variety of formal mechanisms exist in this country for providing social support to the elderly (Table 28–2). Communities vary in their ability to deliver resources and enlightened commitment to meeting the needs of the elderly. The three types of social support (affirmation, affection, and aid) are all provided to some degree by these formal mechanisms. Although most such mechanisms are primarily organized for the provision of aid, they often provide opportunities for affirmation and affection as well.

To a certain degree, the type of formal support mechanisms appropriate for an elderly individual depends on the degree of disability and available social resources. For example, when elders are well, mobile, and independent, they are able to utilize fairly unsophisticated formal mechanisms, such as churches and clubs, to meet their own needs for affirmation and affection. With slightly more disability, socialization and nutrition centers can provide the opportunity for affir-

Table 28–2. FORMAL SUPPORT MECHANISMS

In-Home
Social Services
  Socialization centers, e.g., senior centers
  Nutrition centers
  Transportation services
  Telephone reassurance
  Home delivery of meals

Serve to:
  Augment family support
  Provide alternatives to meet elder's need for support
  Prevent premature institutionalization

Home Health Agencies
  Chore services
  In-home environmental alteration services
  Instrumental services—shopping, transportation, laundry, meal preparation
  Personal care
  Supervisory services
  Respite services

Out-of-Home
  Case management
  Respite care
  Foster care
  Boarding homes
  Supervisory care homes
  Skilled nursing and extended care facilities
  Acute-care hospitals

mation and affection, while at the same time providing a hot meal daily. For some elders who attend socialization and nutrition centers, the services of the center must be supplemented by transportation services to accommodate decreased mobility. With increased disability, the services of community-based, short-term or long-term in-home services may be required, as provided by social service or home health agencies. Chore services, in-home environmental alteration services, and instrumental services such as shopping, transportation, laundry, and meal preparation are often required. If the elder lives alone, telephone reassurance and home-delivered meals can be major sources of social support. With prolonged disability and progressive deterioration, personal care and supervisory services are required. Respite care may be needed to relieve caregivers and permit them to tend to personal needs.

Out-of-home services are similarly graded on the basis of needs and amount of disability of the elder. Foster care, boarding homes, and supervisory care homes usually provide the least amount of physical care to the elder, but they do provide socialization, supervision, and meal preparation. Institutional care can range from personal care services and socialization only to total care provided in skilled nursing and extended care facilities. In many communities, formal social service systems exist to provide case management for elders and families. These agencies coordinate and organize necessary services, facilitate out-of-home placements, and coordinate reentry of the elder back into the community through discharge planning from acute and extended care facilities.

Regardless of whether the formal mechanisms provide in-home or out-of-home services, they serve several important purposes. Formal supporters supplement and augment the support provided by informal supporters and, in many cases, make it possible for families to continue to provide support despite other commitments and responsibilities. The relationship between formal and informal mechanisms is reciprocal. If it were not for the support provided by informal supporters to the elderly, the formal support mechanisms would be immobilized by the demand for services in a system that could not financially absorb the burden. Because of the presence of a variety of formal support mechanisms, elders and families have choices about the care mechanisms they can use. The presence of formal supporters helps many elders to remain at home despite progressive disability. In situations where the elderly person is geographically separated from informal supporters or is devoid of informal supporters, formal social support mechanisms help prevent premature institutionalization by providing alternative methods of delivering appropriate levels of support.

COMMON DIFFICULTIES ENCOUNTERED IN PROVIDING SOCIAL SUPPORT TO THE ELDERLY

Although there are multiple rewards to supporters for developing the intimate relationships involved in providing social support to the elderly, providing such support is not without problems. Aging alters the structure of social relationships as well as the context in which social support is offered. These alterations primarily affect the elderly individual and his or her supporters, particularly those supporters with the most intense responsibilities and intimate relationships with the elderly person.

Effects of Aging on the Structure of Social Supports

Reciprocity is a feature of social support that is affected by the aging process. Reciprocity refers to the exchange of goods, services, and sentiments within a relationship, and the degree to which these are distributed in a mutually satisfying manner (Homans, 1961). According to social exchange theory, as individuals interact over time, social norms dictate that each provides to the other an equitable distribution of rewards and reinforcements. Among the chief rewards and reinforcements exchanged is mutual support in the form of aid, affirmation, and affection. Regardless of the nature of the relationship (e.g., spousal, filial, casual, formal), individuals interact only as long as their investments into the relationship are perceived as more or less equal to their profits or returns. In young adulthood, under conditions of good health, individuals are able to exchange a full range of support. In addition, they are able to accumulate a store of credits on which they can draw when their bargaining assets are less numerous. The potential for the accumulation of credits is greater in some types of relationships (e.g., parents have the ability to accumulate large amounts of credits in their relationships with their children). Reciprocity, therefore, can be realized over long periods of time, with an unequal distribution of aid, affirmation, or affection in early years being rewarded many years later.

Dowd (1975) presents a succinct description of the effect of aging on social exchange. According to Dowd, as individuals age and disability becomes an issue, they become less able to reciprocate certain types of support while they are simultaneously requiring more and more support for themselves. Aid is the chief type of support that elders are unable to reciprocate. If financially able, they may be able to pay for the support they need or, if they have accumulated a large store of credits, they may be able to draw on previous relationship contributions. In either case, however, their bargaining position is severely hampered as they become progressively more dependent on those around them to fulfill their increasing need for support. The net result can be a reluctance on the part of elderly people to express their needs for all types of support and to accept the meeting of their needs for aid as sufficient for their survival but as inadequate to maintain their sense of well-being and life-satisfaction. For the supporters, the net result can be a sense of resentment at the unequal exchange, a sense of failure that the elderly person appears to need more than they can provide, and a sense of frustration that their efforts are not met by "appropriate" expressions of gratitude. Interestingly, the ability of the elder to exchange money for support may intensify rather than diminish the inequity in the exchange from the perspective of the supporter. When supporters perceive that the elder's only medium of exchange is money and that neither affirmation nor affection for the supporter is forthcoming, a great deal of resentment can be engendered. Neither formal nor informal supporters like the feeling of being bought. Expressions such as "I feel like her slave rather than her daughter" and "she acts like she is better than I am" are reflections of such resentments.

Effects of Aging on the Context in Which Social Support Is Offered

Social support is offered within a context characterized by some degree of intimacy and by rather stylized roles that have a structure, a history, and a set of role prescriptions. Because of the nature of social support, intimacy, among even comparative strangers, can rapidly deepen, sometimes before either individual is ready or willing for such close ties. Issues of power, control, autonomy, and independence are key to the comfortable continuation of the relationship.

In institutional situations where the dependent elderly person has little choice about the relationship, the elder's discomfort level with this forced intimacy may be high. The formal supporters, because of their monopoly on the distribution of good and services, are in a power position. For the elder, the necessary continuation of the relationship can become a negative form of social support rather than a positive one.

In homes, the same situation can occur, but elders at home usually have more access to the reciprocation of rewards than elders in institutions. As a result, power can vacillate between the elder and the caregiver in such a way that social support becomes a mutually negative force. Social support is negative for the informal supporter if the elder expresses needs that are beyond the supporters' capacities to fulfill. The elder may then use other sources of power (such as criticism of the supporter to other important people, threats of withdrawing financial support, or engendering guilt) to force the supporter's compliance. On the other hand, social support is negative for the elder when the supporter attempts to control the elder's access to other sources of power or uses threats of premature institutionalization to force the elder's compliance. In such situations, the net result is the establishment of negative reinforcement cycles that produce varying degrees of turbulence and conflict.

In families, the history of relationships is rich and complex. As a result, the nature of previous interactions and the degree to which these interactions have engendered mutual obligations can profoundly affect the nature of support offered in old age. Elders who have managed to build positive relationship credits without creating intense guilt or a crippling sense of obligation are the people most likely to be able to maintain mutually satisfactory social support systems despite progressive disability. Because of the effects of history on the different individuals who compose the elder's social network, supportive relationships are not always possible.

The types of roles enacted by the elder and his or her supporters and the flexibility of the role prescriptions can affect the degree to which relationships are supportive in old age. This is true regardless of whether the support mechanisms are formal or informal. Some elders relinquish roles of authority, such as the parent role or the role of boss, more slowly than is needed. In addition, some supporters assume roles of authority prematurely. As a result, conflict can arise, even among the most well-meaning supporters, when the types of support offered are not the types of support that are needed or wanted. Again, these types of situations present challenges for those who are attempting to reconcile the support needed with the support offered.

ESSENTIAL COMPONENTS OF A SOCIAL SUPPORT ASSESSMENT FOR THE ELDERLY

The support systems of elderly individuals are complex. Therefore, it is important that the information obtained during an assessment of social supports reflects the complexity that actually exists. The factors that should be considered as a part of a social support assessment are presented in Table 28–3.

Most social support systems for individual elders contain a combination of both formal and informal support mechanisms. Regardless of the number of formal supporters involved with an individual elder, for the majority of elders the family and other informal supporters are the primary source of social support. Assessment, therefore, should always focus on ways of capitalizing on the resources and organizational structures provided by informal supporters. The prerogatives, needs, and desires of the elder, the designated caregiver, and other informal supporters should be paramount in planning intervention strategies re-

Table 28–3. ESSENTIAL COMPONENTS OF A SOCIAL SUPPORT ASSESSMENT

The size, density, and diversity of the social network providing the social support, including the formal and informal mechanisms (remembering that not all social support is provided by humans)

The types of support offered and the individuals involved in providing each type of support

The types of support needs evidenced by the elderly person, the elderly person's and/or designated caregiver's desired goals for need fulfillment, and the requisites of the timing of need fulfillment

The degree to which existing supports actually meet the identified needs and goals

The potential social network available to the elderly individual

    Available formal and informal mechanisms not being currently used

    Mechanisms currently in use but could be used in different ways

The existing organizational structure of formal and informal support and the ways in which the organizational structure can be acknowledged and supported

The existing structure of the social relationships among the elder and individuals within the social network

    Distribution of rewards and reinforcements

    Past history of the relationship

    Type of roles enacted by members of the social network

    Flexibility of roles

lated to social support, even for elders in an institutional setting.

Although formal support mechanisms provide a certain amount of affirmation and affection, the primary purpose of these mechanisms is aid. Therefore, the simple existence of formal support mechanisms within an individual elder's social network in no way ensures that social needs other than those for aid are being met. Steele (1987) has demonstrated that developing new, intimate, and satisfying informal relationships is difficult for aging individuals. Observations in day care facilities, extended care facilities, and nutrition sites frequently demonstrate that elders tend to accept the aid offered by formal supporters. They solicit some affirmation and affection from the formal supporters but rarely initiate relationships or solicit affirmation or affection from other elders in the environment. The simple presence of other potential informal supporters in the environment does not guarantee that the need for affirmation and affection is being met. The elder's usual interaction patterns should be assessed to identify the type of intervention needed to facilitate the establishment of new informal supporters among the elder's peers.

Informal supporters tend to become consumed with satisfying the elder's needs for aid. The elder's social network often shrinks, and the individuals who used to provide affirmation and affection become unavailable. Past role structures may not have included the exchange of affirmation and affection between the elder and those who remain in the social network. The presence of a large and active informal social system does not guarantee that all of the elder's social support needs are being met. Therefore, the assessment of the elder's social supports should begin with the assumption that elders require affirmation and affection as well as aid.

SUMMARY

Social support is an essential feature in the existence of all human beings. In addition to making life pleasant and palatable for the frail elderly, the presence of social support is important for survival. With adequate social supports, the frail elderly can often maintain life in the community long after their physical care needs would require institutionalization. Without adequate social supports, frail elderly individuals face premature institutionalization. The organization of the social supports for elderly individuals is often complex, involving a variety of informal and formal supporters. The interactions between an elder and supporters can create turmoil and conflicts as well as intense burdens for the supporters who continue to remain within the often dwindling social network. In order to achieve the best possible outcomes for elderly individuals, the assessment of social supports should reflect the complexities of the support systems and the needs of all individuals within the support systems, as well as the complexity of social needs evidenced by the elder. Similarly, intervention strategies need to focus on up-

holding the existing structure of the support system and augmenting it by formulating care alternatives.

References

Archbold, PG (1980): The impact of parent caring on middle-aged offspring. *J Gerontol Nurs*, 6:79–85.

Archbold, PG (1983): Impact of parent-caring on women. *Fam Relat*, 32:39–45.

Barrera, M (1981): Social support in the adjustment of pregnant adolescents: Assessment issues. *In* Gottlief, BH (ed): *Social Networks and Social Support*. Beverly Hills, CA, Sage Publications, 69–96.

Bengston, VL, & Treas, J (1980): The changing family context of mental health. *In* Birren, J, & Sloan, R (eds): *Handbook of Aging and Mental Health*. Englewood Cliffs, NJ, Prentice-Hall.

Bowers, BJ (1987): Intergenerational caregiving: Adult caregivers and their aging parents. *Adv Nurs Sci*, 9:20–31.

Broadhead, WE, Kaplan, BH, James, SA, et al. (1983): The epidemiologic evidence for a relationship between social support and health. *Am J Epidemiol*, 117:521–537.

Brody, EM (1981): Women in the middle and family help to old people. *Gerontologist*, 21:471–480.

Brody, EM (1985): Parent care as a normative family stress. *Gerontologist*, 25:19–29.

Brown, MA (1986): Social support during pregnancy: A unidimensional or multidimensional construct? *Nurs Res*, 35:4–9.

Cantor, M (1979): The informal support system of New York's inner city elderly: Is ethnicity a factor? *In* Gelfand, E, & Kutzile, A (eds): *Aging and Ethnicity*. New York, Springer-Verlag, 153–174.

Cantor, M (1983): Strain among caregivers: A study of experiences in the United States. *Gerontologist*, 23:597–604.

Caplan, G (1974): *Support Systems and Community Mental Health*. New York, Behavioral Publications.

Cobb, S (1976): Social support as a moderator of life stress. *Psychosom Med*, 38:300–314.

Dowd, JJ (1975): Aging as exchange: A preface to theory. *J Gerontol*, 35:596–602.

Glaser, B, & Strauss, A (1967): *The Discovery of Grounded Theory: Strategies for Qualitative Research*. Hawthorne, NY, Aldine Publishing.

Glick, PC (1979): The future marital status and living arrangements of the elderly. *Gerontologist*, 19:301–309.

Homans, G (1961): *Social Behavior: Its Elementary Forms*. New York, Harcourt, Brace & World.

Horowitz, A (1985): Sons and daughters as caregivers to older parents: Differences in role performances and consequences. *Gerontologist*, 25:612–617.

House, J (1981): *Work, Stress, and Social Support*. Menlo Park, CA, Addison-Wesley.

Jackson, JJ (1980): *Minorities and Aging*. Belmont, CA, Wadsworth.

Kahn, RL (1979): Aging and social support. *In* Riley, MW (ed): *Aging from Birth to Death.* New York, Westview Press, 77–91.

Kahn, RL, & Antonucci, TC (1981): Convoys over the life course: Attachment, roles and social support. *In* Bales, PB, & Bream, O (eds): *Life Span Development and Behavior* (Vol 3). New York, Academic Press, 253–286.

Lang, A, & Brody, EM (1981): Patterns of family support to middle aged, older and very old women. Paper presented at the 33rd annual meeting of the Gerontological Society of America, San Diego, CA.

Markides, KS, Boldt, JS, & Ray, LA (1986): Sources of helping and intergenerational solidarity: A three-generations study of Mexican Americans. *J Gerontol,* 41:506–511.

Mindel, CH (1979): The multigenerational family households: Recent trends and implications for the future. *Gerontologist, 19:* 456–463.

Moss, MS, Moos, SZ, & Moles, EL (1985): The quality of relationships between elderly parents and their out-of-town children. *Gerontologist,* 25:134–140.

Phillips, LR (1984): On becoming a caregiver. Paper presented at the 13th annual Nursing Research Conference, University of Arizona, Tucson, AZ.

Porrit, D (1979): Social support in crisis: Quantity or quality? *Soc Sci Med, 13A:*715–721.

Rice, D, & Feldman, JJ (1983): Living longer in the United States: Demographic changes and health needs of the elderly. *Milbank Memorial Fund Quarterly—Health and Society,* 61:362–396.

Shanas, E (1979): The family as a social support system in old age. *Gerontologist,* 19:169–174.

Siegel, J (1976): Demographic aspects of aging and the older population in U.S. *Current Population Reports: Special Studies* (Series P-23, No 59). Washington, DC, US Government Printing Office.

Steele, EA (1987): Entrapment: Passage into despair in long-term care facilities. Unpublished master's thesis, University of Arizona, Tucson, AZ.

Taylor, RJ (1985): The extended family as a source of support to elderly blacks. *Gerontologist,* 25:488–495.

Wallston, BS, Alagna, SW, DeVillis, BM, et al. (1983): Social supports and physical health. *Health Psychol* 2:367–391.

CHAPTER
29

Balancing Resources: Demand Against Supply

JULIET CORBIN, R.N., D.N.Sc.

INTRODUCTION

Media sources have begun to paint a new picture of aging. They tell us that with proper nutrition, exercise, and mental stimulation, we can look forward to many productive years after the age of 65. This includes participation in activities such as sports and sex, and for some even the beginning of new careers.

It is true that there are many active men and women over the age of 65 years. However, one of the hazards of growing old is the increased risk of developing a chronic disease. Chronic illness is the major health problem of the aged, with many of the elderly having one or more chronic conditions (Estes, 1979; Vladeck & Firman, 1983; Strauss, Corbin, Fagerhaugh, et al., 1984). Eighty percent or more of the elderly are said to have some type of chronic disease (Vladeck & Firman, 1983). According to the National Center for Health Statistics (1981), 39.2% of those with chronic conditions have limitations in a major activity.

Staying active and productive in old age and having one or more chronic conditions seem contradictory. However, all of us know persons over the age of 65 years who remain actively engaged in life despite illness, just as we know those who have given in to despair. Some of the differences in how persons physiologically and psychologically respond to illness and aging can be accounted for by heredity. Other differences can be attributed to the nature of the illness, such as the type of disease, its severity, rate of progression, duration, and the degree to which it can be controlled by treatment regimens. Not all of the variation can be related to differences in the aging or illness processes; obviously personality and lifestyle factors are also important. In fact, these latter determine to a great extent the resources—finances, social support, motivation, energy, manpower, and so forth—that are available to persons who in their later years become chronically ill (Gerson, 1976).

This chapter explains how chronic illness can inexorably deplete the resources of the elderly—often already limited—and thus greatly affect the quality of their lives as well as their management of illness. Much of the data for this chapter comes from a grounded theory (Glaser & Strauss, 1967) study of how couples manage chronic illness at home. Sixty couples were interviewed, with each partner interviewed separately whenever possible. The interviews ranged from 2 to 3 hours in length. The majority of the couples participating in the study were over the age of 65 years, except for those with spinal cord injuries, who tended to be younger. A wide variety of illnesses were represented, including heart disease, stroke, Parkinson's disease, Alzheimer's disease, respiratory ailments, diabetes, and cancer. The interviews took place in the couples' homes and focused on problems that they had in trying to manage their illnesses and their lives.

AGING AND CHRONIC ILLNESS

Aging changes people's lives. So does illness. When the two are combined, the changes normally associated with aging can be accelerated and intensified. This creates an increased need for resources, paradoxically at a time when their actual availability may be low and decreasing *because* of illness or age.

Ordinarily, we take for granted the greatest resource of all: an unimpaired, properly functioning body. With it, we get things done by using hands, feet, and voice, and also by having that basic condition for getting things done—energy. Illness reduces some of the body's capacities. So does the aging process. Sometimes the reduction is drastic. Aging and illness together can undermine our taken-for-granted, primary resource. With this resource reduced, a person needs other resources—money, other people's manpower, and so on—to supplement or substitute for it. Yet, as will be discussed below, these may also be in short supply precisely because of resources having been depleted by these same two factors—illness and aging.

Aging

Aging is a progressive state, beginning with conception and ending with death. Associated with it are certain physical, social, and psychological changes. The exact age at which these changes occur varies among individuals. However, over time most persons experience many of the following: There is a decrease in visual acuity, hearing, muscle mass, skin and blood vessel elasticity, and body hair. Wrinkles appear, skin sags, energy wanes, and hair turns gray. There is an increased tendency toward arthritic joint changes, hypertension, osteoporosis, and other physical conditions (Kart, Metress, & Metress, 1978). The age of 62 years in women and 65 in men marks the beginning of full eligibility for Social Security and achievement of senior status. It brings with it the potential for retirement and freedom from the daily concerns of a job. On the other hand, retirement can mean living on a fixed income and, in some cases, in poverty (Estes, Newcomer, et al., 1983). As the years go by, children reach middle age and have problems of their own. Friends and kin begin to die. However, despite the changes associated with aging, the later years in life can be very happy and productive. All of this can suddenly change, though, with the advent of a chronic condition.

Chronic Illness

Chronic illnesses can develop at any age; however, the elderly make up the largest proportion of our country's chronically ill. The chronic illnesses that afflict the aged tend to be the slowly deteriorating types, such as emphysema, cardiovascular disease, diabetes, Parkinson's disease, Alzheimer's disease, and certain kinds of cancers (Strauss, et al., 1984). While any illness takes its toll, living with debilitating chronic conditions can be especially difficult. Having a deteriorating body can mean the end of one's dreams and plans for retirement. It can also mean increased output of money for medications, equipment, assistance, and home adaptations—money that often cannot be replaced because there is no longer a major source of income. Furthermore, debilitating chronic conditions often bring with them bodily changes, such as a loss of energy, crippling of hands and feet, shaking, mental confusion and memory losses, difficulty breathing, problems in maintaining balance, and pain (Cluff, 1981). Thus, tasks like dressing, cooking meals, cleaning, and balancing the checkbook become painful and time consuming; recreational and time-filling leisure activities like golf and traveling become impossible. With each downward step in the illness, limitations can increase, making activity even more difficult.

Complicating the picture further is multiple illness. Persons who became ill with a chronic condition early in their lives are likely with advancing age to develop complications and related diseases. For example, a person who was a childhood diabetic is likely to develop vascular complications leading to eye, heart, and kidney disease. In the later years of life, it is not uncommon for people to have two or more illnesses, often, but not always, related (Rice, 1986). Also, it is not unusual for both marital partners to be ill.

Thus, being elderly and chronically ill means having to cope with the physical and emotional signs of aging and the changes in lifestyle associated with retirement. In addition, this necessitates adjusting to limitations, managing symptoms, and living with the overarching threat of death (Feldman, 1974). A well spouse is not unaffected. He or she also must accommodate to the physical limitations of the ill mate, as well as adjust to the increased social isolation, the burden of caretaking, role reversals, and the possibility of a future as widow or widower, which are so often associated with chronic illness (Goldstein, Regnery, & Wellin, 1981).

Work and Resources Needed to Manage Illness and Life

The Work of Managing. Ordinarily, everyone engages in a great deal of work, whether explicit or implicit, in order to live through each day. This is true whether one is engaging in housework, earning a salary, preparing for a trip, throwing a party, or even "working out" a personal or marital problem. The ill and the elderly are not exceptions, except that they encounter special difficulties in carrying out life's activities. Also, when ill, they may have additional work to do that is associated with the illness itself. There are three major types of work to do to manage illness and keep life going. These are illness-related work, biographic-related work, and everyday life work (Corbin & Strauss, 1988).

Illness-Related Work. Illness-related work refers to the many tasks that are performed to keep an illness under control, manage symptoms and limitations, and prevent medical crises. It includes regimen work, which can range from taking a few pills daily to performance of highly complex and lengthy tasks, like those required for home dialysis. Another aspect of illness-related work is symptom monitoring and management. Though physicians and nurses can tell patients what symptoms they might expect and how to treat them, it is up to the patients to discover exactly what situations are likely to provoke symptoms and what to do to avoid or minimize their effects through regimens. For example, a cardiac patient must discover how far he or she can walk before exhaustion sets in or which situations are likely to bring on angina and which are not, and thus to take avoidance action. Also, the ill must learn how to administer their drugs and when taking them is most effective, how to use and maintain breathing machines and other equipment, and where to obtain and how to install helpful devices like handrails in bathrooms and hallways.

Biographic-Related Work. Biography refers to the many aspects of self (for example, husband, wage earner, friend, lover, parent, etc.) that make up our identity over time. Identity can be shaken and even shattered by illness, depending on the salience of those aspects of self that are lost due to limitations in performance ability. Biographic work, then, denotes the efforts that are necessary to let go of the past, come to terms with the present, and reconstitute identity around limitations and changed selves. Living with symptoms and limitations often brings about daily confrontation with loss and requires ongoing physical, emotional, and social adjustments. Finding the inner strength and adjusting to illness and aging can take a great deal of time and energy.

Everyday Life Work. Everyday life work refers to those tasks that are necessary to keep the person, family, and home ongoing. These include activities like dressing, housekeeping, paying bills, doing yard work, going to a job, and so forth. These tasks must go on despite illness and limitations. They also require the output of time, energy, manpower, knowledge, and money. Increased loss in performance ability can mean a change in normal household roles accompanied by new divisions of labor in which the well partner carries the burden of the work. For the well spouse (or other family members), having to juggle everyday life work with illness-related and biographic-related work can require intense effort and have considerable physical and emotional impact (Fengler & Goodrich, 1979; Brody, 1985; Corbin & Strauss, 1985).

Resource Need and Availability. The performance of each of these types of work necessitates obtaining, using, and maintaining such resources as time, knowledge, energy, manpower, equipment, and money. Yet, while the need for resources may be high, the actual supply available to meet the continued work demands is usually low. And those resources that are available often become depleted over time precisely because of the consequences associated with illness and aging.

Depletion of resources and resource availability may occur in several ways. (1) Physical limitations associated with aging and illness not only decrease performance ability but also increase the amount of time it takes to accomplish tasks. (2) Constricted social worlds may mean fewer friends and outside sources to provide help of various types, such as information gathering, driving, ill-person sitting, and running errands. (3) Middle-aged (or even aging) children often live out of town or are too busy handling problems in their own lives to be of much help to their parents. (An interesting finding of our study was that parents were very reluctant to call on their children for assistance because they did not want to burden them with their own problems.) (4) Living on a fixed income can mean that relatively little money is available to hire outside help or buy "Meals on Wheels" or other helpful services. (5) Finally, limited mobility makes it difficult to get out of the house to shop, go to the bank, obtain dental and other care, and socialize.

Considering the increased need for resources to perform all of the work associated with managing home, life, and illness and the limited ability of the chronically ill elderly to continually provide these year after year, it is no wonder that they become depressed and worn down, question the meaning of life, and eventually just give up. As one of the women interviewed for this study said: "I get very depressed. I ask myself why is all of this happening. Why does old age have to be this way?"

THE FARENTINOS: A CASE IN POINT

Obviously the constant demand for resources when the elderly become chronically ill can greatly affect their ability to carry out salient biographic activities and maintain quality of life. Even when a couple starts out relatively well prepared physically, emotionally, socially, and financially, resources dwindle because of constant demand and little opportunity to replenish them. The case presented below demonstrates what happens to couples when the workload is heavy and resources increasingly limited. The case follows a typical pattern. When the illness first appeared, the couple seemed to manage. But as time went on, managing became harder and harder. At the time of the interview, this couple, especially the caretaking spouse, was feeling the strain of what can be called a late phase of the "downward spiral of resource depletion."

ANNA AND GEORGIO FARENTINO

Georgio Farentino has Parkinson's disease. He has not responded well to the drug treatment, and therefore the rate at which his disease has progressed has been rapid. Before he became ill, Georgio owned a roofing business, which he ran with the help of his son. His symptoms were first noticed by his wife, Anna. She repeatedly asked her husband: "Why are you holding your arms like that? Why are you dragging your feet? Why are you walking that way?" He felt that she was criticizing him, and replied, "That is the way that I am." However, she thought he looked strange and urged him to see a doctor. He resisted until he began having difficulty driving and doing his work. The diagnosis was a blow to both of them. Anna said, "He was always such an active man. That is what is so heartbreaking about all of this."

Anna worked many years for a utility company. She hoped to work as long as possible. However, when her husband became too ill to care for himself, Anna retired. "I had to make a decision. I thought there is no way I can hire somebody to come in here to be with him. I didn't make that kind of money." As a consequence of her early retirement, Anna's pension is smaller than she had planned on. Before her husband became ill, the couple spent most of their holidays with her family, with whom they were very close. Anna also enjoyed the ballet, symphony, opera, and the companionship of her many friends. Anna said that they rarely had a vacation together over the years because of their different work schedules. Therefore, being able to vacation together was one of the main pleasures they anticipated in retirement. "We were planning on retiring and doing a few little things together. You plan and work and then bingo!"

In the beginning, Georgio was able to do much for himself. But his disease has progressed to a point where Anna must bathe, shave, and dress him. She has to lift him out of bed, bring him to the bathroom, and cut up all his food. She does all of this, in addition to handling the daily household problems and decisions and tidying up their home, which they own.

Frustrations and Concerns

Anna has back problems from all the heavy lifting. Her doctor has told her not to lift Georgio or pull him around in bed. "The doctors say you have to do it, but they don't ask how you are going to cope with all of this. They don't ask if you can afford to hire somebody, so that you don't have to do it."

Because she is the sole caretaker, Anna rarely has time to sit and rest. She says she is very organized and is used to working hard. However, she now feels her age and finds it difficult to do all that is required of her: "These things don't seem to happen until you are getting older too. When I was younger, this would have been pea soup for me. I had a good stomach and could stand to smell anything. But when you get older . . . I have a bad back and very bad arthritis. Sometimes when he calls me, I have to say wait a minute. He thinks I am being mean. I tell him it is not meanness but I too am in pain. I am frustrated because I can't be as fast as I used to be. Now my ribs started hurting and I wonder, what will happen to him if I have to go to the hospital?"

Anna also wonders what would happen if she could no longer do the caretaking, because she does not have the money to place Georgio in a nursing home or to hire outside help. Because the couple owns their own home, they are not eligible for assistance. "I just pray to God that I hold out."

Social Isolation and Constricted Social Worlds

Anna would like to go out more, both with and without her husband, but this is difficult because of Georgio's physical limitations. In order to go out, Anna has to dress him, lift him out of bed, and carry him down the stairs and into a car. Although their only son still lives at home, he works and cannot be there to help.

Anna doesn't like to leave her husband alone in the house because he is so helpless. "If I leave him here, I don't know what is going to happen. What if a fire breaks out? These are my fears, well-founded fears." Being confined to the house was especially hard on Anna when her father became ill and died. She wanted to be with her father but couldn't leave her husband. Another disappointment for her is that: "I wanted to go back to school and study a little music, but I can't find the time to do it. You just have to give up these things."

The Farentinos would not mind not being able to leave the house so much, if family would come to visit. "Sometimes I wish my sisters would come and spend the day with me, but they don't. They just go out and do what they want. I have nieces that I used to take care of but they don't even bother to call. They have just dropped out of sight."

The Burden of the Work and Lack of Resources

Anna does all of the work for the home and her husband without assistance. Many times she is unable to bathe and dress herself until later in the day. The only way she finds time for herself is if she lets some of the housework go, which she occasionally does when she is especially tired. "In a hospital, you have a person doing the meals and trays, a nurse doing something else, and someone else doing something else. In the home, you are doing the cooking, the serving, the trays, the housecleaning, and the wash, every day because he has accidents in the bed. You have to let yourself go, because you don't have the time."

Time is not the only reason Anna has had to let herself go. Money is also a problem for her. She needs dental work but is not able to go to the dentist at this time because she had a plumbing and a car problem. These cost her $2,000, the money she had set aside for dental care. While Medicare pays for many of the illness-related costs, it does not pay for her husband's medication, at $120.00 per bottle. Nor did it cover all of the costs for the hospital bed that Georgio needed. "Medicare only pays for 80%. What you could buy for that would be a piece of trash. The bed cost me $1,500." Furthermore, due to a mixup in the coverage with their private insurance, Georgio is not eligible for any extra funds from the private insurance either. "We really lost out on that deal."

Until his illness. Georgio did all the repairs around the house. Now that he can no longer do this, Anna has to hire someone or depend on one of her relatives. She doesn't like to bother her son with details because: "It is my responsibility, not my son's, even though he is part of the family. He helps some but he works and doesn't have a lot of time."

Anna does leave her husband alone long enough to go to the grocery store and to the bank. She manages to accomplish her chores quickly because she leaves the house early enough to be the first one in line and "runs fast."

Living with a chronically ill person can have its very humorous moments. Anna relates that one day her vacuum cleaner stopped working, so she got down on her hands and knees to look at it. Her husband, who was sitting nearby in his wheelchair, saw her trying to fix it, so he slipped out of the chair to see if he could help her. Just as she was about to get up, her knees gave out. So the two of them were stuck sitting on the floor. Both Anna and Georgio found the situation very amusing. They had a good laugh and eventually Anna was able to get herself and her husband up off the floor.

Anna said that whenever anyone in her family came upon hard times, she would give them money. Now she finds herself in a situation of need, but no one is willing to help her. "I wish someday to get a little help. I wish they could come up with something so that it wouldn't be so expensive to have someone come in and help out. When you are retired even $5 an hour is a lot of money, and think of how many hours it is going to be."

Contingencies of Life That Disrupt Routines

Anna has established routines for doing her work. "I am organized and always thinking in advance, now I have to cook, what am I going to do first. This can be going on while I am doing something else." However, as she has discovered: "No matter how you plan, it never works out quite like you would like it to. Your time has to be the patient's time. Like the other day, I was eating and he had to go to the bathroom immediately. I thought everything I ate was going to come up."

And you can't run a home like an institution: "He complains that things aren't quite right. Like in the hospital they feed you on time, but in the home you might be a little bit late. He bangs on the bed when he wants to eat. You can't run a home on a schedule like you can an institution. You have too much to do and think about. Then there are always interruptions, like to answer the doorbell and telephone. A few minutes here and there add up."

Sustaining Self and Others

Anna and Georgio sometimes play games or watch TV together. She buys juice and fruit that she knows he likes and he in turn calls her an "angel." "I am not an angel. Sometimes I feel ohhhhhh! and I have to sit down and talk to myself. I have to stand back and say there is always going to be rough times, does this outweigh that."

Anna wishes that she and Georgio could communicate better, maybe talk things out. She claims he was never very communicative but that the illness has it made it worse and she has no one else to talk to.

Illness-related Work

Georgio's medication has to be given every 6 hours. To do so, Anna must disrupt her sleep and get up in the middle of the night. She also monitors her husband for periods of muscle rigidity and then does things like put a towel under his chin so that he doesn't drool on himself and hand him his urinal, which he can't reach at these times. At the time of the interview, Mr. Farentino had some scrotal swelling. This concerned Anna and so she was watching the swelling carefully. Anna also monitors Georgio's fluid intake. Most of all Anna wishes that "medicine" could come up with something to stop her husband from deteriorating so quickly.

Synopsis

Mrs. Farentino is carrying a heavy physical and emotional burden of work. The qualities that she possesses that enable her to do so include her physical endurance, devotion, sense of duty to her husband, and ability to organize her time. However, throughout the interview Anna was crying. The burden of all of the work was getting her down. She described herself as being "burned out." She does not have the money to hire assistants or to take care of her own needs. Her aches and pains and constant fatigue are making it more difficult for her to continue the caretaking. Neither partner is actively engaged in activities that would enrich or make their lives easier, separately or together. The quality of life of both partners is suffering because they are caught in the downward spiral of resource depletion. Anna keeps giving for little reward in return. Her husband can do little to help. He could last many more years, yet it is

unlikely that Anna can continue to function at her present level unless she receives some help.

What kinds of help does Anna need? To list a few of the areas, Anna needs emotional support, someone who will listen to her and fill her "emotional bank." She needs knowledge about community resources that are specifically related to low-cost day care and dental services. She needs information about body mechanics and how to move her husband with the least amount of strain to her own body. Anna and her husband also need teaching about exercises that might help maintain some of his functional ability. Anna needs help in making arrangements to have a neighbor, relative, or volunteer come to the home on a regular basis so she can go out to do basic household chores like banking and grocery shopping and perhaps occasionally to socialize (Shanas, 1979). She needs assistance in finding and paying an attendant to come in during the week to help with Georgio's care, so that she might conserve her energy and have more time to devote to herself. The couple needs counseling to help them work through their respective feelings regarding his illness and the changes that it has brought to their lives. They also need help in learning to communicate with each other before communication becomes impossible.

ASSESSMENT AND INTERVENTION GUIDE

As this case illustrates, elderly couples in which one or both partners have a chronic condition need more than medical assistance to keep their illnesses managed and to maintain some quality of life. They need resources in the form of manpower, financial aid, information, helpful devices, and sociopsychological support (Brody, Poulshock, & Masciocchi, 1978; Hooyman, Gonyea, & Montgomery, 1985; Gallagher, 1985; Estes & Lee, 1986; Strauss & Corbin, 1988). Nurses are an important resource in coordinating aid. Much can be done by nurses to prevent, or at least slow down, the downward cycle of resource depletion by helping couples to extend, maintain, or replenish their resource supply (Cluff, 1981; Hewner, 1986; Rew, Fields, LeVee, et al., 1987). The use of the nursing process, with a focus on *resources*, is one means that nurses can use to reach this goal.

The first step is to identify resource need and then compare need against available supply. If resources are found to be low or limited, or if the potential exists for resource depletion over time because of the nature of the illness and biographic features of the couple's lives, intervention should be focused on helping a couple to obtain additional resources and to conserve the ones that they have. The evaluation component of the nursing process, using a resource focus, should take two forms. One would focus on monitoring resources over time in order to determine how well they are lasting, noting any potentially problematic areas. The second would be to assess for changes in well-being as related to specific interventions by the nurse. Below are a few suggestions on how nurses might use the ideas presented in this chapter in their practice.

Assessment

The first step of the nursing process is assessing. Questions that a nurse might use to assess a couple's need for resources include the following: What is the state of illness at this time: early, middle, late? Is the illness mild or severe? What limitations has it brought about? How do these limitations affect the individual's ability to carry out the tasks of daily living? What work is necessary to manage the illness? What is the couple's emotional status at this time? To what degree have they come to terms with the illness? To what degree is the well spouse involved in the management of the illness or in the caretaking of the ill partner? What physical problems or limitations does the well spouse have? What are the couple's strengths? In what areas do they seem to need assistance? Do they need knowledge, and if so, about what? How to carry out the

regimen? Time or energy management? Ways of simplifying the work? Would devices or equipment help make their work easier? Does the well spouse need time away, assistance with caretaking, more social outlets? If they are managing now, will they continue to do so, or is there something that can be done now that will help them in the future? (An example would be having a helper come for a few hours, two or three times a week, before the spouse wears out, in order to extend the spouse's caretaker abilities.)

Once the resource areas of need are identified, the next step is to assess a couple's resource supply, their lifestyle, and preferences. This is important because couples often fail to use resources that are offered. When asked why they failed to use available services, some of the reasons given by couples were too much pride to accept "charity," an unwillingness to admit that they need help, a desire to maintain their privacy, a belief that the service was too expensive, unawareness that services exist, a belief that obtaining and maintaining resources creates more problems than they are worth, or the notion that resources fail to fit in with their lifestyles.

Questions such as the following can help elicit this type of information. What types of help do you think would be most beneficial to you? Would it be helpful to you to talk to someone about managing your finances; anxiety or stress that you might be feeling; about sex; about ways to make the work easier? Do you need help in contacting agencies, such as day care programs, that might be helpful to you? Have you ever tried to use outside help? What problems did you encounter? How might it be worked out so that help would be more amenable to you? What can you afford to pay? Are you eligible for federal or state aid? Do you have private insurance? Have you ever asked a neighbor, friends, relatives, or church group if they could come once a week or month for a few hours so that you might get out? What do you know about services and support groups available to you in the nearby community?

Intervention

Once the nurse has a good understanding of (1) the type and amount of work to be done, (2) resources needed to do the work, and (3) an estimation of available resources, the next step is to use this information to work out a plan that will help to bring these resource demands and the available supplies into balance. The plan, of course, must be acceptable to the persons for whom it was designed and flexible enough to adapt to changes in either the workload or the couple's life, since either could affect resource need or availability.

The purpose of an intervention plan using a resource focus is to help a couple or individual use resources more creatively by (1) establishing routines for work performance (who will do what tasks, when, and how) with time set aside daily for sustaining self and other; (2) setting priorities on tasks by identifying what has to be done every day, what can be put off until every other day, every week, or every other week; (3) assisting a couple to locate and obtain community services appropriate to their need, lifestyle, and financial ability; (4) suggesting helpful aids and devices that conserve time and energy (like clothing that is easy to put on, take off, and wash); (5) helping a couple to develop a network of supportive family and friends; (6) providing a client with needed knowledge; and (7) making referrals for appropriate counseling.

Evaluation

Evaluation comes next. Questions that a nurse might ask to determine if a plan is effective include: Is the illness or condition being kept under control? Are there problems or complications? Have the involved persons adjusted to the illness and integrated it into their lives? Are routines for doing the everyday life work in place and working? Is anger, resentment, frustration, or fatigue expressed? Is important biographic work going on through the performance of social or recreational activities? What are these activities? Are arrangements for day care, housekeeping, and caretaking assistance in place and working? If not, why not? Are the needs of the well spouse being taken care of? What more needs to be done? Are finances holding out or is the financial output greater than expected at this point?

Ongoing monitoring of a plan is especially relevant when working with the elderly chronically ill. Over time, resources are likely to run out, even when the work remains stable, because of the long-term nature of chronic illness and the precarious nature of physical (and sometimes financial) status. Even a bad cold or a case of flu can have a tremendous impact on energy and the ability to carry out daily activities of living. With each major step downward in the illness, new routines and arrangements will have to be worked out in order to accommodate changes in physical and mental abilities.

SUMMARY AND CONCLUSIONS

One of the main problems faced by the elderly chronically ill is how to keep a balance between resource needs and available supply. These resources may be limited due to physical, financial, and social changes that accompany aging and chronic illness. The drastic consequence of an inability to keep a balance between demand and supply is a downward cycle of resource depletion, which in turn has consequences for the well-being and quality of life of the ill elderly. Through careful assessment and planning before clients are discharged from the hospital, or in follow-up home visits, and by means of ongoing monitoring of resources, nurses can assist the elderly to develop strategies that will enable them to use their resources wisely and creatively. The clients so served will have a better chance to secure the time, energy, money, knowledge, and sense of well-being that will allow them to remain actively engaged in life, within the limits imposed by their physical and mental disabilities.

References

Brody, E (1985): Parent care as normative family stress. *Gerontologist*, 25:19–29.

Brody, S, Poulshock, W, & Masciocchi, C (1978): The family caring unit: A major consideration in the long-term system. *Gerontologist, 18*:556–561.

Cluff, L (1981): Chronic disease, function and the quality of care. *J Chron Dis, 34*:299–304.

Corbin, J, & Strauss, A (1985): Managing chronic illness at home: Three lines of work. *Qualit Sociol, 8*:224–247.

Corbin, J, & Strauss, A (1988): *Unending Work and Care.* San Francisco, Jossey-Bass.

Estes, C (1979): *The Aging Enterprise.* San Francisco, Jossey-Bass.

Estes, C, & Lee, P (1986): Health problems and policy issues of old age. *In* Aiken, L, & Mechanic, D (eds): *Applications of Social Science to Clinical Medicine and Health Policy.* New Brunswick, NJ, Rutgers University Press, 335–349.

Estes, C, Newcomer, R, et al. (1983): *Fiscal Austerity and Aging.* Beverly Hills, CA, Sage Publications.

Fengler, A, & Goodrich, N (1979): Wives of elderly disabled men: The hidden patients. *Gerontologist, 19*:175–183.

Gallagher, E (1985): Intervention strategies to assist caregivers of frail elders: Current research status and future directions. *Annu Rev Gerontol Geriatr, 5*:249–282.

Gerson, E (1976): On the quality of life. *Am Sociol Rev, 4*:266–279.

Glaser, B, & Strauss, A (1967): *The Discovery of Grounded Theory: Strategies for Qualitative Research.* Chicago, Aldine.

Goldstein, V, Regnery, G, & Wellin, E (1981): Caretaker role fatigue. *Nurs Outlook, 29*:24–30.

Hooyman, N, Gonyea, J, & Montgomery, R (1985): The impact of in-home services termination on family caregivers. *Gerontologist, 25*:141–145.

Hewner, S (1986): Bringing home the health care. *J Gerontol Nurs, 12*:29–35.

Kart, C, Metress, E, & Metress, J (1978): *Aging and Health: Biological and Social Perspectives.* Menlo Park, CA, Addison-Wesley.

National Center for Health Statistics (1981): Current estimates from the National Health Institute Survey. US 1981 Vital & Health Statistics (Series 10, 141 DHHS No 83–1569). Washington, DC, US Government Printing Office.

Rew, L, Fields, S, LeVee, L, et al. (1987): Affirm: A nursing model to promote role mastery in family caregivers. *Fam Commun Health, 9*:52–64.

Rice, D, & LaPlante, M (1986): The burden of multiple chronic conditions: Past trends and policy implications. Paper presented at the annual meeting of the American Public Health Association, Las Vegas, Nevada.

Shanas, E (1979): The family as a social support system in old age. *Gerontologist, 19*:169–174.

Strauss, A, Corbin, J, Fagerhaugh, S, et al. (1984): *Chronic Illness and the Quality of Life,* 2nd ed. St Louis, CV Mosby.

Strauss, A, & Corbin, J (1988): *Shaping a New Health Care System.* San Francisco, Jossey-Bass.

Vladeck, B, & Firman, J (1983): The aging population and health services. *Ann American Academy of Political and Social Science.* Beverly Hills, CA, Sage Publications, 132–148.

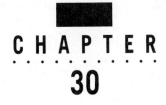

CHAPTER
30

Home Health Care

SATO HASHIZUME, R.N.C., M.S., N.P.

INTRODUCTION

The home, an increasingly significant setting for health care delivery to older people, has been drawing national attention from policy-makers and media sources. The public focus on home health care might suggest that home-delivered services are a recent innovation, but formalized nursing services in the home have been in existence since 1886 (Tinkham, Voorhies, & McCarthy, 1984). Throughout the decades, the home health nurse (variously known as district nurse, public health nurse, visiting nurse, and community health nurse) has been pivotal as the primary care provider. Time has brought new levels of sophistication and technology into the home, but home adaptation of treatment regimens, patient and family instruction, and skillful, caring, creative decision-making have been mainstays of nursing practice.

Contemporary home health nursing service for the elderly homebound patient is discussed in this chapter. As one approach to the comprehensive assessment and provision of quality nursing care to the older patient, a home health nursing systems model is presented. This home health nursing model, based on a synthesis of community health and gerontological nursing practice, is intentionally global to encompass the complex needs of the elderly homebound patient and to emphasize the biopsychosocial parameters that require assessment in the home environment. In the limited space of this chapter it is impossible to sufficiently elaborate on all the essential sections of the framework. Therefore, after presenting the model, this chapter highlights selected components to illustrate those unique challenges and opportunities for nursing assessment and intervention in the setting of the patient's home. For further information on specific content in the model, the reader is referred to other chapters in this textbook and community health nursing references.

The Home Setting

Unlike in any other nursing practice setting, such as the hospital, clinic, or skilled nursing facility, the home health nurse is functioning in the patient's domain. When a home health nurse enters the patient's home, the nurse is in an environment determined by the patient

557

and family. The home reflects the patient's lifestyle, socioeconomic status, and cultural and personal preferences. In health matters, the primary management and control of the patient's care rests not with the nurse but with the patient and family who carry out the prescribed treatment regimen between intermittent home nursing visits. In this transposition, the home health nurse actively collaborates with the patient and family to achieve patient and family care management and independence. Patient and family education and individualized instruction become paramount in the nursing process.

Further, the home setting is unique in offering the home health nurse the opportunity to observe how the elderly patient copes in familiar surroundings with available resources. The home itself, then, is a therapeutic environment inextricably interwoven with the patient's health, and it requires evaluation in tandem with assessment of the patient's needs.

HOME HEALTH NURSING MODEL

Broadly conceived, the home health nursing model encompasses the homebound elderly patient, which is the micro system; the patient's immediate social and environmental supports, constituting the mini system; and the formal community programs and services, which compose the macro system (Fig. 30–1). In this dynamic, multifactorial approach, the individual patient's unique profile of medical problems, functional status, coping strategies, and needs requiring nursing intervention are the initial point of focus. Then, going beyond the individual patient, the ecological framework expands to examine the patient's surroundings for insights into the informal, contextual support structure.

After assessment of the patient's micro and mini system, unmet biopsychosocial needs are identified. If these needs are beyond the scope of nursing practice, the broader community support structure, the macro system, is assessed for available resources and appropriate intervention.

This comprehensive framework extends beyond the current acute-care home health model under the federal program Medicare or through the program for the medically indigent, Medicaid. Many homebound, frail, chronically ill or disabled elderly patients can benefit from home health nursing intervention but do not qualify for limited Medicare and Medicaid benefits. The home health nursing model addresses the needs of homebound elderly patients regardless of funding.

With the focus on the elderly homebound patient's health care problems, this inclusive home health nursing practice model spans the wellness-to-death continuum and has as its goals health promotion, disease prevention, early detection and treatment of illness, rehabilitation, and comfort measures. Along the care continuum from wellness to death, a homebound elderly patient falls into one of three major groups: the acutely ill, the chronically ill, or the terminally ill. This broad care continuum places responsibility on the home health nurse to coordinate the transfer of patients to and from the home with other sites of care (hospital, rehabilitation, or skilled nursing facility), consistent with the acuity and dictates of the patient's medical condition, individual social situation, and preferences.

With the complex, multifocus character of the home health nursing model, the approach should be interdisciplinary, with the home health nurse as the gatekeeper and case coordinator of services. The nurse often enters the home first and therefore must be the first to assess the biopsychosocial environmental needs of the patient. The comprehensive nursing care plan specifies nursing interventions, referrals for other multidisciplinary services, and plans for the coordination of all services provided in the home.

Occasionally, the home health nurse may be the only health care provider with an opportunity to assess and intervene for the patient's benefit. In remote rural areas, limited resources, severe weather conditions, program eligibility, or patient's wishes may dictate and limit the number of visits made to a patient.

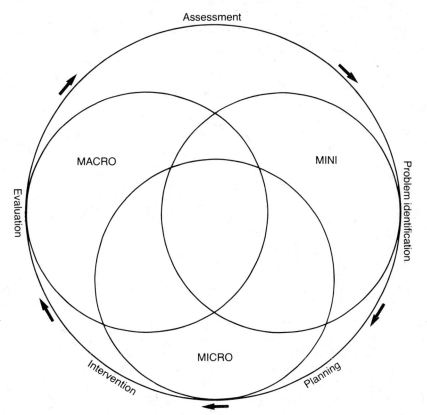

Figure 30–1. Home health nursing systems model.

Miss J, a reclusive 69-year-old single woman, was bedbound, confused, and covered with incontinent excrement when she was admitted to the hospital for severe dehydration, malnutrition, and pneumonia. At the time of her hospital discharge she was rehydrated and continent, and her pneumonia was improved. However, she was very forgetful and weak with an unsteady gait. She insisted on going home alone and very reluctantly agreed to have a home health nurse visit.

After a 20-minute wait, the nurse was allowed into a small cottage where the patient lived with four undisciplined, unhousebroken dogs. The nurse took a nursing history, examined Miss J, obtained her weight, and inspected her medications. A quick glance into the kitchen revealed a table piled high with dirty dishes, open cartons, and cans of spoiled food. The social history revealed that Miss J bred dogs, had no relatives or friends to help her, and had her groceries delivered by a grocer two blocks from her home. She refused homemaker services and insisted she was fine. Of all the problems identified, the nurse decided to emphasize and instruct Miss J on the two major problems that could lead her back to the hospital— poor nutrition and medication noncompliance. Since Miss J wanted to remain in her own home, she seemed receptive. However, as the nurse was leaving, Miss J said she did not need further services from anyone.

At times, the nursing care plan may include consultation with community-based nurse practitioners and clinical nurse specialists. More patients are being discharged from the hospital sooner than in the past with medical conditions and equipment formerly confined to a hospital setting. The patient's care may be highly technical and complex. The home health nurse may work closely with a geriatric or adult nurse practitioner who is skilled in physical assessment and management of chronic illness and special problems of the homebound elderly ill patient. Or the nurse may consult with a community clinical nurse specialist specially trained in respiratory, ostomy, or parenteral therapy management (Meany-Handy, Nowinski & Rickerson, 1985).

Micro System

The nursing assessment of the micro system includes the patient's physical, functional, and mental status and cultural orientation. Although each subsystem of the micro system is presented as an entity, the micro subsystems are dynamically interrelated. This requires the home health nurse to constantly integrate data from each subsystem with the information already gathered, then synthesize the data from the whole micro system to specifically identify problem areas.

Physical Status

The increasing acuity level of the home care patient with earlier discharge from the hospital intensifies the continuing need for the home health nurse to update and expand assessment skills. Physical assessment of the geriatric patient is covered in depth in Unit II and will not be repeated here except to offer a caveat. In general, the patient's eyes, ears, teeth, and feet are neglected in the presence of more pressing problems. Yet, these four vital, functional parts of the body can present disabling conditions that often can be remedied with relatively minor medical, dental, and podiatric interventions. With simple screening tests of

the patient's vision and hearing and inspection of the teeth and feet, along with the patient's history, the home health nurse can find problem areas and refer to the appropriate provider for further evaluation and correction of remedial problems. For instance, an 84-year-old man, profoundly hard of hearing for 2 years, thought his hearing loss was normal for his age. After finding that this patient had not been medically evaluated for hearing loss, the home health nurse referred the patient to a physician who removed deeply impacted plugs of old cotton from both ears, which resulted in restoration of normal hearing.

With this model, other areas of assessment under the physical status are nutrition, medications, sleep, and elimination.

Nutrition. Homebound elderly ill people are likely to be at nutritional risk, with multiple factors interfering with their ability to obtain adequate nutrition. When the home health nurse visits, some elderly patients are in marginal nutritional states that can advance to frank deficiencies with any new physical or emotional stress (Karkeck, 1985). Quality patient care requires assessment of nutritional status, planning of interventions, and monitoring of progress.

The dietary assessment includes a 24-hour dietary recall by the patient or caregiver, measures of height and weight, and an exploration of food practices in relation to the medical, psychological, social, and economic status of the patient (Table 30–1). A visit at mealtime and a tour of food preparation and storage

Table 30–1. DIET HISTORY

Height: _____ Weight: _____

Breakfast: _____ Amts: _____ Lunch: _____ Amts: _____ Dinner: _____ Amts: _____
(or generalized pattern)

Vitamin or dietary supplements: Name: _____ Amt: _____ Frequency: _____
Dietary Preferences:_____
Dietary Restrictions: Prescribed:_____ Self imposed:_____
Medications: Antacids: _____ Laxatives: _____
Dentures: _____ Problems with chewing, swallowing: _____
Food stamps: _____ Meals on Wheels: _____ Other: _____
Meals prepared by: _____

sites furnish objective data, but the patient may view these activities as intrusive. Unless the information is needed on the first visit, it is better to wait until a relationship is established and permission granted.

Most manifestations of nutritional problems are relatively nonspecific. Goode (1984) advises clinicians to develop an "index of suspicion" with respect to nutrition. Generalized malnutrition should be considered if any of the conditions listed in Table 30–2 exists. Mr. B's situation illustrates the multiple interacting medical, psychosocial, and cultural factors contributing to malnutrition.

Mr. B, a 74-year-old married Chinese man, came home from the hospital cachectic, almost nonverbal, and with an open, slow-healing sternal wound requiring dressing changes three times a day. The patient had been in the hospital 3 months following a coronary artery bypass complicated by respiratory arrest with long ventilatory dependency and wound dehiscence. He was recently informed that he had lost his lawsuit for his work-acquired asbestosis and was depressed. He rarely ate solid foods and drank only the Chinese soups his wife prepared.

Major nutritional imbalances that occur in aging persons consist of excessive or insufficient caloric intake relative to activity and excessive intake of fats and sodium. Other common deficiencies include inadequate fiber intake with the attendant problems of constipation and deficient calcium in Caucasian and Oriental women, unless the diet is supplemented with calcium (Goode, 1984). Suboptimal protein consumption is seen in some older people, whereas in others single-nutrient insufficiency is found in response to abstinence from specific categories of food. A patient who avoids fruits and vegetables because of indigestion may have folic acid deficiency. The exclusion of essential nutrients may result from mistaken dietary restrictions or as a side effect of a medically prescribed diet for specific disease conditions.

With dietary assessment information, the home health nurse can evaluate the patient's eating patterns utilizing the widely recognized Dietary Guidelines developed by the Senate Select Committee on Nutrition and Human Needs (1977) (see Table 30–3). These guidelines presume that a sufficiently wide variety of foods is selected within each of the four major food groups.

Federal nutrition programs sponsored by the United States Department of Agriculture

Table 30–2. FACTORS CONTRIBUTING TO MALNUTRITION

Physical	Psychological	Social
Acute or chronic illness	Emotional stress	Inadequate food preparation and storage facilities
Immobility	Loneliness	
Alcohol abuse	Isolation	
Dementia	Depression	Limited finances
Obesity or cachexia	Bereavement	Limited social support
Multiple medications or laxatives		Loss of person who shops and cooks
Edentulous or poorly fitting dentures		

Table 30–3. DIETARY GUIDELINES

Increase carbohydrates to account for 55% to 65% of the caloric intake.

Reduce overall fat intake from 40% to 30% of total energy intake.

Reduce saturated fat intake to 10% of total energy intake; balance with polyunsaturated and monounsaturated fats, which should account for about 10% of energy intake each.

Reduce cholesterol intake to about 300 mg/day.

Reduce sugar intake to account for 15% of total energy intake.

Reduce salt intake to approximately 3 gm/day.

The goals suggest the following changes in food selection and preparation:

Increase intake of fruits, vegetables, and whole grains.

Decrease intake of fatty or processed high-fat meats and increase intake of poultry, fish, and lean cuts of meat.

Decrease intake of foods high in fat and partially substitute polyunsaturated for saturated fat; no fried foods; trim fat and skin from meats.

Substitute low-fat or nonfat milk for whole milk.

Decrease intake of butter fat, eggs, organ meats, and other high-cholesterol sources.

Decrease intake of sugar and foods high in sugar content.

Decrease consumption of salt and foods high in salt content.

Keep alcoholic drinks to 2 per day or less.

(Adapted with permission from Goode, ET (1984): Nutrition. *In* Cassel, CK, & Walsh, JK (eds): *Geriatric Medicine*, vol. 2. New York, Springer-Verlag.)

are available in virtually every United States community for the indigent population, including the elderly homebound. Unfortunately, these programs—the National Food Stamp Program and the Direct Food Distribution Program—pose access problems for persons with reduced ambulatory capacity and limited social supports. A more viable dietary option for many patients at home is Meals on Wheels, a community or privately sponsored nutrition program. For a nominal fee the patient receives a hot noon meal 3 to 5 days a week. Arrangements can be made for additional meals to be delivered at the same time for evening and weekend use. Some Meals on Wheels programs offer special meals for sodium-, fat-, and concentrated carbohydrate–restricted diets. Patients on special diets or those with definite food preferences may not find home-deliverd meals an acceptable alternative. For those patients unable to prepare their own meals and lacking a caregiver, a homemaker service may fill the void. The homemaker, paid either privately or through the local department of social services division for the medically indigent, can shop and prepare the food with the patient's preferences and specific circumstances in mind.

Medications. It has been amply documented that older persons with multiple chronic diseases, high drug exposure, and age-related pharmacokinetic changes are at increased risk for adverse drug reactions and noncompliance to drug regimens (Fedder, 1984; German, Klein, McPhee, et al., 1982.)

The home health nurse is in a strategic position to uncover actual or potential problem areas and to improve medication usage and storage. Nursing assessment of drug use in the patient's home offers the distinct advantage of direct inspection for drug utilization practices, in addition to the patient's or caregiver's report. According to Hammarlund, Ostrom, and Kethley (1985), drug utilization information derived solely from a patient's self-report can be misleading.

Starting with the drug interview, the nurse assesses the patient's or caregiver's knowledge of and compliance with the prescribed drug regimen. The nurse utilizes a 24-hour recall technique to learn which prescribed and over-the-counter medications are ingested or possibly missed. The drug interview covers the following areas (Crichton, Smith, & Demanuele, 1978; Simonson, 1984):

Name of medication
Purpose of medication
Dose of medication
Special times of administration
Method of administration
Duration of therapy
Pertinent side effects
Pertinent adverse effects
Drugs, foods, or activities to avoid
What to do if a dose is missed
Refill information
Storage requirements

After the drug interview, the nurse inspects the medications at their storage site and compares the self-report with the objective data. It is important to see all the medications—current and expired, prescribed and over-the-counter. It is not uncommon for cost-conscious patients to save and store unused drugs in multiple locations. Persistence is required to disclose forgotten, infrequently used, or expired medications. As the nurse inspects the medications, the following potential problem areas should be noted for later discussion with the patient (Simonson, 1984):

Pill count reveals either too many or too few pills left in the bottle in relation to the date of the prescription and the physician's instructions
Label discrepancy—the dose or schedule is changed by the prescriber after the drug was first dispensed, and label has not been updated
Outdated prescriptions dispensed at least 1 year before, or a lapsed expiration date
More than one drug in the container
Duplicate medications—two or more currently used, labeled prescriptions containing the same generic drug
Over-the-counter medications that may interact with the prescribed medication

A couple in their eighties, Mr. and Mrs. Y, was referred to the home health nurse for medication noncompliance. Both were on digoxin but on different dosages. Their digoxin levels were never consistent, and Mr. Y had been hospitalized with altered mental status attributed to digoxin toxicity. With the couple's permission all the current, unused, and expired medications were collected for inspection. A large cache of drugs, some dating back 10 years, was found under the bed, in the kitchen cupboard, bathroom cabinet, bedroom dresser, and in two closets. The couple kept their prescribed and over-the-counter medications together in various shoe boxes and indiscriminately used each other's drugs. Usually, the digoxin was taken when they did not feel well. It was not until the nurse sorted, separated, and placed the prescribed medications in individual prefilled medication compliance aids, wrote out the schedules, and discussed proper utilization that the couple no longer had drug-related problems.

Inappropriate medication use stems from various factors that need to be clearly delineated for effective nursing intervention. Impediments to patient compliance may be related to the patient, to the drug therapy, or to the health professional. Drawn from several sources (Fedder, 1984; Martin & Mead, 1982; Simonson, 1984) and personal experience, selected barriers to compliance and specific nursing interventions are listed in Table 30–4.

The home health nurse's role in fostering appropriate drug utilization through patient education cannot be overemphasized. In order to fulfill his or her role responsibly, the home health nurse must be knowledgeable about the latest drugs on the market. This information can be obtained from a number of references, including the *American Hospital Formulary Service*, the *Physician's Desk Reference* (PDR), *United States Pharmacopeia Dispensing Information* (USPDI), and *Facts and Comparisons*. In addition, the home health nurse will find the family's pharmacist a useful consultant on new or unfamiliar medications, possible drug interactions, and complex medication regimens.

Sleep. Sleep habits vary markedly from one individual to another, but an individual's sleep pattern is generally consistent. Changes occur in sleep patterns of the elderly. The time from the onset of sleep to the first rapid eye movement (REM) activity is decreased, and stage 4,

Table 30–4. BARRIERS TO COMPLIANCE AND INTERVENTIONS TO PREVENT AND TREAT NONCOMPLIANCE

Barrier to Compliance	Nursing Intervention
Patient Related	
Impaired vision	Ask pharmacist to use large type on labels. Affix label on central axis. Use color-coding system.
Impaired hearing	Get patient's attention before speaking. Speak clearly and slowly. Do not shout.
Impaired dexterity	Use nonchildproof medication container.
Memory loss	Write out medication schedule. Use compliance aids (medication boxes, medication calendars). Involve caregiver.
Social isolation	Suggest volunteer home visitor or telephone program.
Drug Therapy Related	
Complex drug regimen	Work with physician and pharmacist to simplify schedule. Use compliance aids.
Cost of drugs	Suggest generic drugs. Discourage use of unnecessary nonprescription drugs. Suggest nondrug alternatives.
Health Professional Related	
Inadequate knowledge about drug use	Provide specific detailed oral and written information about the drug regimen.
Diffidence of patient toward health professionals	Ask about patient's previous experience with health professionals. Allow time for questions and concerns.

the deepest stage of sleep, virtually disappears. As a result of frequent and prolonged waking periods, the total sleeping time is shortened. There may be complaints of difficulty falling asleep, in staying asleep, or of awakening early in the morning.

Sleep disorders may also be present, complicating the normal decrease in sleep time related to the aging process. Sleep research has shown that sleep disorders are due, for the most part, to situational stresses or crises, psychosocial concerns, medical pathophysiology, or drug-related conditions (Malasanos, Barkauskas, Moss, et al., 1986). In assessing the patient at home, a 3- to 5-day time record of sleep/wakefulness and daytime activities will reveal the patient's habits and sleep patterns. A careful history evaluating the factors listed below, along with an observation of the sleeping quarters, will furnish additional data essential for appropriate intervention.

Sleeping environment—bed, bedding, light, noise, ventilation, temperature, privacy
Medical problems—chronic pain, reflux esophagitis, cardiovascular symptoms, respiratory alterations, metabolic disorders, urinary symptoms
Medications taken—sedatives, narcotics, psychotropics, diuretics
Mealtimes—including bedtime snacks, bedtime beverage, alcoholic drinks
Pre-bedtime activities associated with sleep—bath, massage, reading
Daytime activities, exercise, recreation
Mood, mental status
Psychosocial status
Personal beliefs about sleep

In the management of sleep problems, alleviating the offending cause becomes the major concern. For elderly patients complaining of sleep loss without a sleep disorder, an explanation of the normal sleep changes with aging may be all that is necessary. For patients with sleep disorders associated with complicated medical or psychosocial problems, resolution may be more difficult. Possible interventions based on the individualized assessment include (Bender & Howle, 1986; Ebersole & Hess, 1985; Sherman, 1987):

Sleep-conducive physical environment
Regular rising time to promote regular sleep onset time
Discouraging daytime napping
Daily exercise and recreation, avoiding exercise at bedtime
Relaxing bedtime rituals
Positioning, warmth, and alleviation of pain
Attending to psychosocial issues
Consultations regarding medical problems and drug-induced insomnia

Avoiding cigarettes, alcohol, and caffeine prior to sleep
Sparing use of sedatives and hypnotics least disruptive to the sleep cycle

Mr. A complained of "constant turning and tossing in bed, and a crick in the neck." He insisted on stronger pain and sleep medications. His recently evaluated medical problems were stable, he was not depressed, and he was content with his social situation. On inspection of Mr. A's apartment, the home health nurse found that Mr. A slept in an unventilated, dark closet of his studio apartment on a makeshift bed too short for his 6-foot frame. Options such as sleeping on the living room sofa or adding an extension to his bed from the closet into the living room were suggested, and instruction in body mechanics, heat, and range of motion exercises were given. However, the patient, preferring the arrangement of his "bedroom," continued to sleep in his closet and to rely, with only fair results, on various medications for sleep and pain control.

Elimination. Bowel and bladder function of the aged, fraught with social implications, can present problems severe enough to interfere with independence and the ability to remain in one's own home. The sensitive home health nurse can assess and intervene to provide comfort and support, decrease embarrassment of the patient and family, and improve bowel and bladder habits and patterns. (For a detailed discussion on bowel and bladder assessment and intervention, see Chapters 8 to 10.) In this chapter, environmental factors in the home that can affect bowel and bladder function are emphasized. Nursing assessment should include the following:

Patterns of micturition and defecation
Signs and symptoms of urinary tract infection, impaction
High-risk medical problems or conditions—central nervous system lesions, diabetes, immobilization, debilitation
Medications—including laxatives, sedatives, hypnotics, anticholinergics, diuretics
Diet—including amount of fluids, fiber
Mental status, emotional problems
Exercise, recreation
Functional status—timely ambulation to the

bathroom, ability to transfer from a bed to the commode, to handle a bedpan or urinal, to manipulate clothes, to use assistive devices or aid from others

Location of toilet or commode in relation to the patient's activities

Social support system

In the home setting, simple interventions with diet and medications or manipulation of the environment often yield positive results. Interventions based on the assessment of the patient may consist of:

Diet—regular mealtimes, adequate fiber and fluids

Daily exercise

Physical or occupational therapy to improve function

Assistive devices to increase mobility and safety—quad canes, walkers

Bathroom equipment—bars, raised toilet seats, over-the-toilet rails

Clothing—easy to handle and remove, washable

Toilet facilities placed close to patient activities

Consultation on medical problems affecting bowel and bladder function

Appropriate use of medications, laxatives

Mrs. C was an alert, feisty, frail, 99-year-old San Francisco earthquake (1906) survivor who was able to negotiate one flight of stairs to her bedroom and bathroom until she was hospitalized with gastrointestinal bleeding. Mrs. C and her employed 63-year-old daughter thought she had to be placed in a skilled nursing facility because now she required assistance to get out of bed and was incontinent of urine and stool. She wore incontinence pants, which humiliated her and proved difficult for her to manipulate independently. She was willing to try another brand that she could fasten and unfasten herself. Upon digital rectal examination, the nurse found impacted barium, which was removed and solved the problem of incontinent stool. Then a commode was ordered and placed by her bedside with instructions to use it every 2 hours. The patient and her daughter were instructed to encourage the patient to be out of bed as much as possible, drink at least 2 liters of fluid a day, and include fiber-rich foods in her diet. Mrs. C balked at the dietary measures but used the commode and stayed out of

bed for longer periods of time. A physical therapist worked with her to improve her strength and endurance, ambulation, and stair-climbing ability. With renewed confidence and determination, Mrs. C's incontinence improved and she was able to go downstairs again.

Functional Status

Elderly patients living at home are usually more concerned with independent function and how they feel than with the disease they have. To achieve the goal of optimal function and independence, a thorough functional assessment must be performed. In this context, function refers to the performance of daily living tasks or self-care (feeding, dressing, bathing, transferring, and toileting) and the more complex instrumental tasks (shopping, cooking, cleaning house, using the telephone, taking medications, handling money, and transporting self).

In assessing the patient's functional status, the home health nurse makes direct observations of the patient's function in the home environment. Watching patients struggle to answer the door or transfer from the bed to the commode will reveal much more than asking them how well they can transfer and walk. The activities of daily living (ADL) and instrumental activities of daily living (IADL) can be assessed by self-report, but direct observation, although more time-consuming, provides the most accurate information (Harris, 1986).

The functional assessment includes measures of both ADL and IADL. As reviewed by Kane and Kane (1981), several assessment tools are available, but the Katz Index of ADL (1965) and OARS Instrumental ADL (Duke University, 1978), both widely tested and validated, are brief and easy to use in the home. (See Chapter 7 for more details on functional assessment.)

From the assessment of the ADL and IADL, deficits with personal care, cooking, housekeeping, and shopping are defined and the management of these responsibilities is explored. The patient may be independent or may require minimal to maximal assistance with ADL and the more complex IADL. In the home setting, a family member or caregiver may be fulfilling these functions, or assistance may be limited or unavailable. A home health aide or homemaker (depending on specific need, insurance coverage, ability to pay, and length of time required) may supplement the patient's reduced capacities by performing the necessary functions in the home.

Assistive devices, too, may be indicated for patients with diminished function in ADL. A raised toilet seat, grab bar, commode, or walker can mean increased independence for the patient. Since there is a wide variety of devices to suit specific individual requirements, a consultation or referral to a physical or occupational therapist is recommended. Many assistive devices go unused because of inaccurate fit to the individual or lack of training with the device.

Rehabilitation programs in the home are indicated for patients with functional losses following a recent illness. However, before a rehabilitation program can be started, underlying medical problems must be defined and treated. For patients with a history of falls, weakness, and mental status change, a thorough medical evaluation is necessary. Moreover, the functional deficits identified from the ADL and IADL assessment cannot be isolated from the patient's psychosocial status (Fortinsky, Granger, & Seltzer, 1981; Kane & Kane, 1981.) The presence of emotional and social problems closely correlates with decreased functional levels and necessitates assessment and appropriate intervention for optimal rehabilitation.

To establish realistic goals for the rehabilitation candidate, the patient's functional level prior to the most recent episode of illness must be known. Depending on the particular functional deficit, the home health nurse and the physical, occupational, or speech therapist, singly or in a team, assess the functional status of the patient and conduct an individualized rehabilitation program.

Home health nurses have traditionally worked with patients deconditioned by an acute episode of illness to return them to their former activity level. More recently, home health nurses with additional training perform cardiac and respiratory rehabilitation with an emphasis on energy conservation, pacing, and graded activity.

Mr. B, a 72-year-old man with oxygen-dependent, end-stage chronic obstructive pulmonary disease, was extremely anxious after his last exacerbation, which resulted in respiratory arrest and intubation. He had been marginally independent with self-care activities, but now he was bedbound. Even eating caused dyspnea and exhaustion. With consultation and joint home visits with a respiratory clinical specialist, the nurse case manager planned an individualized, incremental, supervised rehabilitation program.

Throughout the nursing treatment period, the nurse closely monitored and educated the patient regarding his cardiopulmonary status (including cough and sputum production), nutrition, and medication compliance. The patient was observed and instructed on the correct use and timing of his bronchodilator inhaler drugs. Then, a step-by-step program of progressive instruction and practice with relaxation exercises, pursed-lip breathing, and coordinated breathing with exercise and ambulation were introduced and reinforced on subsequent visits. To pace the program, the patient's heart and respiration rates were monitored during rest and exercise, and signs and symptoms of oxygen desaturation were observed. Because of early fatigue and poor reserve, progress was slow, but it became measurable in small increments of strength and endurance over a 4-month period of three-times-a-week to biweekly home visits. Mr. B's disease was irreversible, but using the new techniques he could manage his self-care activities, eat a small meal comfortably, and ambulate 30 feet before dyspnea occurred. The rehabilitation strategies allowed Mr. B fuller independence and a sense of control over his breathing and anxiety.

In some home health agencies, physical therapists manage cardiac and respiratory rehabilitation and the nurse monitors medical problems. Physical therapists provide treatment services to improve or maintain range of motion, strength and dexterity of the musculoskeletal system, to teach ambulation and other functional maintenance techniques, and to reduce or relieve pain, swelling, and muscle spasm. The latter treatment modalities are the least familiar to other disciplines.

Mrs. A was a 79-year-old woman with terminal uterine cancer and aggravated cervical osteoarthritis. She developed an immobilizing, extremely painful spasm of her right sternocleidomastoid muscle. Heat and trials of several analgesics proved worthless, and she did not want to be sedated with narcotics. The home health nurse referred the patient to a physical therapist. The physical therapist applied ultrasound for 10 minutes, followed by gentle massage to the affected site. The patient was instructed to alternate 5 minutes of an ice pack with 15 minutes of heat four times a day and as needed to relieve pain. In 5 days the spasm and pain were resolved and the patient was spared a hospitalization.

In contrast to the physical therapist's role, the occupational therapist employs rehabilitation techniques involving the upper extremities, hand function restoration, general coordination, and prosthetic and perceptual training. In addition, functional activities that increase the patient's ability to carry out daily tasks such as toileting, feeding, dressing, grooming, meal preparation, and household chores are an essential part of the occupational therapist's responsibilities. Whenever caregivers are involved with providing personal care, they are trained to assist the patient to resume self-care.

Speech and language pathologists, whose broad range of diagnostic and treatment services is not always appreciated, tend to be underutilized. These specialists provide professional services to stroke, brain-injured, or brain surgery patients to help them relearn speech and language or to improve their swallowing abilities. Patients who have had a laryngectomy are taught an alternative to verbal communication. Parkinson's disease, multiple sclerosis, and amyotrophic lateral sclerosis patients are taught to develop the best of weak and uncoordinated muscles for more intelligible speech or to use an appropriate nonoral communication system.

Mental and Psychological Status

The nurse visiting in the home is in a prime position to identify and assist high-risk patients in obtaining needed care. It has been estimated that 5% of the population over 65 years of age living in the community are either psychotic or have severe mental disturbances; another 15% have mild to moderate degrees of impairment (Lowy, 1980.) Persons over 65 years of age are less likely to seek mental health services than those younger than 65 years, and when they do ask for help it is usually from a general medical provider (Shapiro, 1986). Not infrequently, it is the home health nurse, entering the patient's home for a medical problem, who first observes the patient's emotional upset or altered mental status.

The assessment of the mental and psychological status of the patients begins the moment the nurse steps into the home. Skillful observation of the patient and environment yields pertinent data. It is important to remember that the patient's lifestyle and standards of housekeeping may be quite different from those of the nurse without representing abnormal behavior. (See Chapter 7 for complete details on observations of the patient.)

Appropriate observations of the patient include:

Appearance
Speech—content and rate and flow
Mood
Movement
Affect

Appropriate observations of the environment include:

Physical appearance—neatness, clutter, disrepair, filth
Odors of alcohol, gas leaks, spoiled food, incontinence
Accurate clocks and calendars
Adequate heat (in winter), electricity, water, plumbing
Others in the home—family members, significant others, caregiver
Pets—obvious care or neglect

Along with the observations of the patient and environment, a careful history is taken (either from the patient, if competent, or from a reliable relative or caregiver) to assess when the symptoms began and if and how the symptoms are changing. This helps determine whether the problem is recent or longstanding. Then, a physical examination, including a medication check, is performed to determine if there are signs or symptoms of a medical or medication problem. The interdependence of physical, mental, and social well-being has been amply documented (Habot & Libow, 1980). These observations, integrated with a brief mental status test and findings from the micro and mini systems, provide the home health nurse with data to formulate a plan and intervene appropriately in a timely manner.

Home-delivered services for mental health problems do exist but are fragmented and not universally available (Butler & Lewis, 1982; Lowy, 1980). When a request for mental health services is received, part or all of the evaluation can be done in the home, including an assessment of the person's home situation and living conditions. Some communities have in-home mental health screening and evaluation, 24-hour emergency services, protective services for the functionally limited elderly, and counseling services.

One particularly effective nursing intervention for mental health in the home environment is the life review. Reminiscences, once thought to be a sign of loss of memory and of aging, are considered normal and essential for the older adult confronting the last stage of life and eventual death. The goals of the life review process include a sense of accomplishment, resolution of conflicts, the reconciliation of family members, the transmission of knowledge to the younger generation, and an acceptance of mortal life.

Reminiscence, although usually spontaneous and beneficial, with some patients produces anxiety, guilt, and depression (Butler & Lewis, 1982). For the nurse who is not trained in psychiatry, it is important not to probe or confront the patient with revealed information. If the patient becomes unduly distraught, it is best to seek consultation or suggest that the patient discuss the difficult issues with a specially trained professional.

With these caveats in mind, the home health nurse with ready access to the patient's favorite pictures, scrapbooks, family albums, and mementos can prompt the patient to begin the life narrative. As the patient progresses, the nurse may include the family to help them view and accept the patient's reminiscences as an important, integrative process.

Mrs. M, a 75-year-old Russian immigrant, had been an active woman until she suffered a myocardial infarction. She lived with her daughter, whose home she had maintained until her last hospitalization. Now unable to keep house, she felt worthless and a burden on her daughter. The nurse noticed many unusual Chinese antiques in the home and commented on their beauty. Mrs. M brightened and with animation began to tell of her life in China. The nurse suggested to her that the fascinating stories were an important part of her family history and that they should be saved for the grandchildren who had not heard about her early years. As part of her intervention, the nurse engaged the daughter in a plan to tape-record the anecdotes as Mrs. M related her experiences to her grandchildren. The daughter, who had long before tired of listening to her mother talk about the past, suddenly realized that her mother was a valuable historian for the family. With the daughter's enthusiastic support, the grandchildren became quickly involved. Mrs. M's self-esteem was restored, and the entire family benefited from the patient's life review.

Most homebound patients benefit from reminiscence therapy, but patients who have severe cognitive impairments or who are psychotically depressed, removed from reality, or have never acquired trust are less likely to be influenced by the intervention (Viederman & Perry, 1980).

Cultural Orientation

In the home setting, culturally sensitive nursing becomes imperative when serving elderly patients with diverse cultural values, beliefs, and lifestyles. Culture is an important determinant in health-related decision-making and actions. If the patient's cultural values are different from those of the nurse, the potential for cultural conflict and patient noncompliance with the regimen is high (Leininger, 1984). The goal of cultural assessment is to obtain adequate, appropriate knowledge of the patient's cultural background to help identify cultural divergence that could positively or negatively affect the nursing care plan and assist in devising culturally congruent interventions.

The patient's home is an especially productive setting to learn about the patient's cultural orientation. Significant visual, auditory, and olfactory clues pervade the home atmosphere, offering ideal access to the patient's values and traditions. Moreover, surrounded by familiar possessions, patients are more likely to talk about themselves and their world view.

Used in conjunction with environmental data, a cultural assessment guide provides valuable supplementary information. Tripp-Reimer, Brink, and Saunders (1984) have reviewed a variety of cultural assessment tools. Most of the guides are comprehensive, but in the home setting it may not be desirable or necessary to elicit all the data suggested. Time is limited, and the patient may be too ill, may be in crisis, or may find the questions irrelevant to care. The following data, considered an essential minimum, may suffice:

Ethnic affiliation
Languages spoken and fluency
Religious preferences
Food patterns and preferences
Family patterns and decision-making patterns
Caregiver—languages spoken and fluency
Ethnic health care practices

If adherence to a prescribed treatment is a problem and cultural factors are suspected, further questions may clarify the discrepancies between the patient's and nurse's cultural construction of the causation, effect, and treatment of the illness (Kleinman, Eisenberg, & Good, 1978).

What caused your problem?
Why do you think it started?
What does your sickness do to you?
How severe is your sickness?
What kind of treatment should you receive?
What results do you hope to receive?
What are the problems your illness has caused you?
What do you fear about your illness?

Mrs. C, a 69-year-old southern black woman, had severe peripheral vascular disease with 4-plus pitting edema and slow-healing leg ulcers. Much to the patient's detriment and discomfort, she used kerosene on her ulcers to "draw out the soreness." She had refused elastic stockings, leg elevation, and any type of dressings. The physician had given up. In assessing the patient, the nurse found that the patient was deeply religious and was a respected deaconess in her Southern Baptist church. It was unthinkable not to go to church on Sunday and appear well-dressed. Further, "salves" were an acceptable remedy for "sores." Bandages, too, were fine if the patient did not wear them to church. With this information, the nurse suggested zinc oxide, "a wonderful old remedy for sores." Then, the nurse negotiated the use of Unna boots, which had "wonderful salves right in the dressings." It was agreed that Mrs. C could remove the Unna boots just before going to church on Sunday and would have them replaced by the nurse on Monday. With Mrs. C's compliance with the treatment regimen, the ulcers began to heal for the first time.

An understanding of a patient's behavior may be elusive even with heightened cultural awareness and skillful interviewing. Lipson and Meleis (1985) advise the use of consultants who are bicultural or those who have experience with the culture being considered. These cultural negotiators can interpret differences in language, communication style, value preferences, and lifestyles for both the patient and health professional.

For the non–English-speaking patient in the home environment, it is usually a family member or caregiver who becomes the interpreter. To obtain accurate information, the nurse instructs the interpreter to communicate exactly what the patient and nurse say without adding or subtracting information. Sometimes when the patient and translator carry on a conversation of their own, it is appropriate for the nurse to intervene to check on the content of the discussion. To facilitate a positive relationship with the patient, it is helpful to keep eye contact with the patient, speak directly to the patient, and, if appropriate to the culture, touch or shake hands. Also, a few words in the patient's language can lower barriers.

Mini System

The mini system, composed of proximal social and environmental factors, determines sense of well-being and patients' ability to maintain themselves in their homes. This ecological relationship between a patient and personal social supports becomes particularly vulnerable when an elderly person develops an acute illness with loss of function and independence or a progressive, debilitating chronic illness. An analysis of the patient's mini system yields invaluable data concerning the social support system, housing, finances, and transportation and suggests interventions for identified problems.

Social Support

Recent research validates the premise that adequate social supports do improve the physical and mental health of the elderly person (Antonucci, 1985). In assessing the homebound patient's social support system, the relationship to significant people and relative closeness to the patient are specified. Then, the frequency, quality, and type of social interaction—that is, affective or instrumental support—are noted. The support to the patient may be financial aid or friendship only, temporary respite, or ongoing total physical and emotional support for an elderly, ill, dependent person. This caregiver is generally a family member, but it may be a neighbor, friend, hotel manager, or a paid attendant or homemaker.

Cohen and Rajkowski (1982) caution clinicians not to assume that having family and friends implies intimacy or the ability to provide concrete material assistance and, conversely, that the absence of kin and friends implies such support is lacking.

Mr. M, an 84-year-old single man with congestive heart failure, had lived in the same dingy, cramped single hotel room without bathing or cooking facilities for 18 years. Whenever he became too ill to go to a nearby restaurant for his meals, his hotel manager purchased and brought his meals to his room. The manager also provided and cleaned a pail for Mr. M's toilet needs. Mr. M did not consider the hotel manager his friend. Mr. M always said he had no family or friends.

From the assessment of the social support system, the primary caregiver is identified. The type and degree of caregiver involvement and the willingness and ability to handle the situation currently and in the future require careful evaluation. With the earlier release of hospital patients, caregivers today are doing tasks that were managed before in an acute-care setting. If further instruction in the care of the patient is warranted, the caregiver's motivation and intellectual, psychological, and physical capacity to learn and manage the care should be assessed.

At times, it is the caregiver family member(s) who has the most difficulty coping with the patient's illness. Unless the home health nurse recognizes and addresses the needs and concerns of the family caregiver, optimal care of the patient may not be realized. At worst, the caregiver may abuse the patient or become unable to maintain the patient at home.

For the caregiver who has been carrying a heavy physical and emotional burden in the provision of care, respite becomes a primary consideration. Respite care, medical or social in nature, may be based in the home or in a facility. The services may range from coverage for 2 to 4 hours once a week to 2 or more weeks of continuous 24-hour care (McFarland, Howells, & Dill, 1985). Turning to the formal supports of the macro system, the home health nurse can work with a skilled social worker to find resources, such as a short stay in a skilled nursing facility, a moderately priced homemaker, or an adult day care setting. Unfortunately for the majority of caregivers, adequate financial means for respite are not always available (Archbold, 1983).

When assessing the social support system, the role of pets should not be overlooked. The "significant other" in some older people's life may be a pet. Studies have indicated that pets can be beneficial to the emotional health of the pet's owner. The nonthreatening, unconditional love that a pet provides fulfills the need for giving and receiving affection (Carmack, 1985). Physical health may benefit as well. Walking the dog provides exercise, talking to and stroking a pet promotes relaxation, and feeding an animal may motivate older persons to prepare meals for themselves (Katcher, 1984).

The loss of a beloved pet can result in grief like that for the death of a family member or close friend (Carmack, 1985). Grief reactions, such as anger, despair, helplessness, mental anguish, and deep sorrow, are not uncommon when a close bond exists between the elderly person and a pet. The bereaved patient needs to grieve and be recognized and supported in the loss (Schmall & Pratt, 1986).

Mrs. M, an 85-year-old patient with rheumatoid arthritis, lived alone. The physician requested a skilled nursing visit because the patient was losing weight and "failing to thrive" without apparent medical cause. After the initial history and physical examination, the nurse commented on the handsome, carved soapstone cat on the entry hall table and the large oil painting of a golden Persian cat prominently displayed over the sofa. The patient, bursting into tears, responded that she felt silly crying about the recent death of her 16-year-old cat. The nurse spent most of the visit encouraging the patient to talk about her life with "Ginger." At the end of the visit, the patient stated she felt much better and, for the first time in a month, felt hungry.

Although for many elderly patients owning a pet can be a positive experience, for others the care and maintenance of a pet may be too much for their physical capabilities or too expensive for their limited incomes. For example, Mrs. M felt she could no longer manage a pet, especially a new kitten. The nurse creatively involved one of the neighbors who owned an 8-year-old cat. Much to Mrs. M's delight, the cat visited Mrs. M each morning when the neighbor placed a small plate of cat food on Mrs. M's kitchen floor.

Housing

In evaluating the housing needs of the homebound elderly patient, the physical environment is observed for safety, adequacy of the housing unit, and environmental barriers.

These factors are interrelated, and often an intervention in any area will markedly improve the livability and safety of the home.

In and around the home, there may be high-risk areas—poorly lit stairs, threadbare or loose carpeting, high slippery bathtubs. There may be environmental barriers, such as narrow doorways blocking wheelchair access, several flights of stairs for patients unable to negotiate stairs, and awkwardly placed bathroom fixtures. Some homes may have inadequate heating units, badly leaking roofs, nonfunctional plumbing, or general disrepair. High crime neighborhoods can present risks as well.

The safety of the patient's home can be improved with assistive devices, creative adaptation of the physical space, and home repairs. Some communities have subsidized home repair programs, but these inconsistently funded programs are not widely available (Greenstein, 1985). Physical and occupational therapists are particularly skilled in home safety assessment and environmental modification in the home.

For many frail elderly persons wishing to remain independent in their homes, an inability to contact someone for help when they fall, become ill, or sustain an injury is the greatest dread. The Emergency Response Network (ERN), now found in many cities, allays this fear. The ERN incorporates electronic units connected to home telephones that contact a central response center when given a signal by the patient. The patient wears a small device on a pendant or clip and simply activates the system when there is an emergency (Vanderslice, 1985). A nominal fee, often waived for those who cannot afford to pay, is charged for this service.

Finances

Most elderly persons will disclose the amount of Social Security or pension benefits they receive but have reservations about discussing other income and assets. For the home health nurse's purpose, it is more important to know if the patient feels able to meet basic expenses and is aware of benefits and entitlements.

A major concern for many elderly persons is the high out-of-pocket cost for health care. Surprisingly, there are elders who are unaware of their entitlements or mistakenly believe entitled benefits are automatically received. One 69-year-old man not covered by Medicare said he wrote to Medicare when he turned 65 years old but never heard from the Social Security office so assumed he had coverage. To receive Medicare it is mandatory that the beneficiary apply for the benefit before his 65th birthday. If the initial deadline is missed, application may be made during an open enrollment period held only twice a year. This patient, who lived alone, had a fractured hip and required home physical therapy and a home health aide to advance his therapy and allow him to manage safely at home. The home health nurse referred him to the nearest Social Security office for a mailed Medicare application form. Needed services were provided with the hope of retroactive coverage for the services rendered.

Even with Medicare coverage, beneficiaries find that less than half of their health expenses are covered. Relatively costly supplemental health insurance (Medigap), purchased by three of every four Medicare beneficiaries, covers only 7% of health care expenses (Waldo & Lazenby, 1984). These policies rarely cover hearing aids, eyeglasses, routine foot and dental care, housekeeping, and meal services (McCall, 1985). More recently, long-term care insurance, designed to cover costs associated with catastrophic chronic illness, has been receiving increasing attention (Meiners, 1985). Many elderly patients find these health care coverage issues difficult to understand and turn to the home health nurse for assistance.

Noncovered ongoing home care expenses can drain financial resources. To meet these costs, homeowners who are "house rich and cash poor" have an option wherein they convert part of their home equity into cash without leaving their homes. There are several methods being developed and tested by public, nonprofit, and private sectors. Each has advantages and drawbacks to be weighed

carefully in accordance with the patient's circumstances (Belling, Kenny, & Scholen, 1985). Referral to a program with a reliable financial counselor is essential.

Transportation

The assessment of the homebound patient's support systems includes the patient's transportation requirements. Convenient, affordable, safe transportation may be limited for the homebound elderly patient who is unable to drive. Without adequate transportation, necessary medical appointments may be missed. Already functionally impaired by medical problems, people using public transportation can find it an inappropriate and hazardous albeit affordable mode of transport. Taxicabs, though more convenient, are unrealistic for individuals on a fixed income, and in rural communities neither public transportation nor taxicabs may be available.

In assessing the patient's transportation requirements, safety, accessibility, and affordability are considered in addition to the suitability of transport based on medical acuity and functional status. The following should be considered:

Acuity of medical situation
Functional status—ability to ambulate, to navigate stairs
Use of assistive devices—canes, walkers, wheelchairs
Need for escort
Number of stairs, elevators
Ability to pay, insurance coverage
Destination and distance
Type of transportation required—automobile, taxicab, van with wheelchair access, ambulance with or without emergency equipment

Although unevenly distributed in the United States, there are a number of federal, state and local transportation programs for older people. Funded through the Area Agencies on Aging (AAAs), small buses and vans purchased by service providers provide transportation for the elderly in their communities. The Urban Mass Transit Act provides funding for the purchase of small buses equipped with

Table 30–5. FEDERALLY FUNDED HOME HEALTH SERVICES

Program	Eligibility	Requirements	Coverage
Medicare	Over 65 years Payment into Social Security or Railroad Retirement System	Homebound Needs intermittent skilled care Physician treatment plan	Skilled nursing Physical therapy Speech therapy Occupational therapy Medical social work Home health aide Medical supplies and equipment
Medicaid	Meets income and categorical requirements	Needs intermittent medically necessary care Physician treatment	Nursing care Home health aide Medical supplies and equipment *At state's option:* Physical therapy Speech therapy
Older Americans	Over 60 years Low income		Home delivered meals (indirect) Transportation Home repair Information and referral
Social Services Act	Financial need (varies state to state)		Homemaker/chore services
Veterans Administration	Service-connected disability	Prior hospitalization at VA facility	Same as Medicare

(Adapted from O'Malley, ST: Reimbursement issues. *In* Stuart-Siddall, S (ed): *Home Health Care Nursing: Administrative and Clinical Perspectives*, p. 28. With permission of Aspen Publishers, Inc., © 1986.)

wheelchair lifts for the elderly and the handicapped. Other communities sell low-cost coupons for taxi fares or enlist volunteers to transport the elderly in personal automobiles (Ebersole & Hess, 1985). The home health nurse, independently or with the help of a social worker, can find the available resources and instruct and assist the patient as needed. At times, however, meeting the transportation needs of the homebound patient can be a formidable problem.

Macro System

In the home health nursing model, the macrosystem embodies the formal community supports available to augment a patient's diminished physical and social resources. These reduced capacities may be temporary or permanent, partial or total. The formal supports, then, may be required for a short period during an acute illness or indefinitely for a long-term chronic illness or permanent disability. Single or multiple services may be needed at any time. Many of the available community resources have already been discussed relative to the problems in the micro and mini systems and will not be repeated here.

Within the macro system, the current constraints and benefits of existing programs require review to appropriately select services from a diffuse, fragmented health care delivery system for the elderly. There are four major federal funding sources that provide some form of financing or reimbursement for the delivery of selected components of home health or in-home services: Medicare (Title XVIII); Medicaid (Title XIX); Social Service Amendments (Title XX); and Older Americans Act (Titles III and VII). (See Table 30–5.) Additionally, there are several federal programs that fund, through direct provision, contract purchase, or cash grants, specific limited home-delivered services. In the private sector, voluntary sources, private insurance, and proprietary interests are also involved to varying degrees with a variety of funding arrangements (private purchase, part pay, partial or full insurance reimbursement).

Each community offers services for the older person, but the range, availability, and quality of services differ from community to community (Harrington, Newcomer, & Estes, et al., 1985; Mundinger, 1983; Nassif, 1986; Oktay & Palley, 1981). In rural communities, long travel distances and scarce resources limit health and social services. In urban communities, services abound but are uncoordinated with other senior services and have restricting, often changing admission criteria. Thus, it is essential for home health nurses to become knowledgeable about the specific resources in the particular community where they practice or to have access to social workers and others with whom they can work collaboratively to fill the unmet needs of the patient.

SUMMARY

In this chapter, a dynamic, comprehensive home health nursing systems model was presented. This broad, interactive format allows the home health nurse to assess holistically the elderly homebound patient in the contextual framework of the patient's home and community. In the limited length of this chapter, the focus has been on selected features of the model to illustrate its use in the home setting. It is anticipated that with current trends—the rapid growth of the aging population, shortened hospital stays, emphasis on self-care and independence, improved technology in the home, and patient preference for care in the home (versus in a skilled nursing facility)—the home health nurse will remain a vital catalyst and provider of quality care in the home. This flexible home health nursing model can be adapted to assist the home health nurse in meeting the challenges of the future.

References

Antonucci, TC (1985): Personal characteristics, social support and social behavior. *In* Binstock, R, & Shanas, E (eds): *Handbook of Aging and the Social Sciences* (ed 2). New York, Van Nostrand Reinhold, 94–128.

Archbold, PG (1983): The impact of parent-caring on women. *Family Relations*, 32:39–45.

Archer, SE, & Fleshman, RP (eds) (1985): *Community Health Nursing* (ed 3). Monterey, CA, Wadsworth.

Becker, MH, & Maiman, LA (1980): Strategies for enhancing patient compliance. *J Commun Health*, 6:113–135.

Becker, PM, & Cohen, HJ (1984): The functional approach to the care of the elderly: A conceptual approach. *J Am Geriatr Soc*, 32:923–929.

Belling, B, Kenny, D, & Scholen, K (1985): Home equity conversion: For the 'house rich, cash poor.' *Generations* 9(3):20–21.

Bender, KJ, & Howle, JA (1986): Pharmacotherapy for the disorders of initiating and maintaining sleep. *Resident Staff Phys*, 32(12):33–49.

Brody, EM (1978): The aging of the family. *Ann Am Acad Political Soc Sci*, 438:13–27.

Brody, EM (1985): Parent care as a normative family stress. The Donald P. Kent Memorial Lecture. *Gerontologist*, 25:19–29.

Burke, T, & Faber, S (1982): A man on a complex regimen. *Geriatr Nurs*, 3:41–43.

Butler, R, & Lewis, M (1982): *Aging and Mental Health: Positive Psychosocial Approaches*. St Louis, CV Mosby.

Carmack, BJ (1985): The effects on family members and functioning after the death of a pet. *In* Sussman, MB (ed): *Pets and the Family*. New York, Haworth Press, 149–161.

Caro, FG, & Blank, AE (1984, November): Burden experienced by informal providers of home care for the elderly. Paper presented at the 37th Annual Meeting of the Gerontological Society of America, San Antonio, TX.

Clark, MC, & Gaide, MS (1986): Choosing the right device. *Generations*, 11(1):18–27.

Coe, RM, Wolinsky, FD, Miller, DK, et al. (1984): Complementary and compensatory functions in social network relationships among the elderly. *Gerontologist*, 24:396–400.

Cohen, C, & Rajkowski, H (1982): What's in a friend: Substantive and theoretical issues. *Gerontologist*, 22:261–266.

Crichton, EF, Smith, DL, & Demanuele, F (1978): Patient recall of medication information. *Drug Intell Clin Pharm* 12:591–599.

Duke University Center for the Study of Aging and Human Development (1978): *Multidimensional Functional Assessment: The OARS methodology*. Durham, NC, Duke University.

Ebersole, P, & Hess, P (1985): *Toward Healthy Aging: Human Needs and Nursing Response*. St. Louis, CV Mosby.

Engel, GL (1980): The clinical application of the biopsychosocial model. *Am J Psychiatry*, 137:535–544.

Erickson, R, (1985): Companion animals and the elderly. *Geriatr Nurs* 6:92–96.

Estes, C (1979): *The Aging Enterprise*. San Francisco, Jossey Bass.

Falcone, AR (1983): Comprehensive functional assessment as an administrative tool. *J Am Geriatr Soc*, 31:642–650.

Fedder, DO (1985): Drug use in the elderly: Issues of noncompliance. *Drug Intell Clin Pharm*, 18:158–162.

Fortinsky, RH, Granger, MD, & Seltzer, GB (1981): The use of functional assessment in understanding home care needs. *Med Care*, 19:489–497.

Frownfelter, DL (1978): *Chest Physical Therapy and Pulmonary Rehabilitation: An Interdisciplinary Approach*. Chicago, Year Book.

German, PS, Klein, LE, McPhee, SJ, et al. (1982): Knowledge of and compliance with drug regimens in the elderly. *J Am Geriatr Soc*, 30:568–571.

Goode, ET (1984): Nutrition. *In* Cassel, CK, & Walsh, JK (eds): *Geriatric Medicine: vol. 2*. New York, Springer-Verlag, 156–178.

Greenstein, D (1985): Home repairs programs. *Generations*, 9(3):52–55.

Haber, PAL (1986): Technology in aging. *Gerontologist*, 26:350–357.

Habot, B, & Libow, LS (1980): The interrelationship of mental and physical status and its assessment in the older adult: Mind-body interaction. *In* Birren, JE, & Sloane, RB (eds): *Handbook of Mental Health and Aging*. Englewood Cliffs, NJ, Prentice-Hall, 701–716.

Hammarlund, ER, Ostrom, JR, & Kethley, A (1985): The effects of drug counseling and other educational strategies on drug utilization of the elderly. *Med Care*, 23:165–170.

Harrington, C (1985): Alternatives to nursing home care. *Generations*, 9(4):43–46.

Harrington, C, Newcomer, RJ, Estes, C, et al. (1985): *Long Term Care of the Elderly*. Beverly Hills, Sage Publications.

Harris, BA, Jette, AM, Campion, EW, et al. (1986): Validity of self-report measures of functional disability. *Topics in Geriatric Rehabilitation* 1(1):31–41.

Holt, SW (1986): The role of home care in long term care. *Generations*, 11(2)9–12.

Howell, SA (1985): Home: A source of meaning in elders' lives. *Generations*, 9(3):58–60.

Irwin, S, & Tecklin, JS (eds) (1985): *Cardiopulmonary Physical Therapy, vol I*. St. Louis: CV Mosby.

Jette, A (1986): Functional disability and rehabilitation of the aged. *Top Geriatr Rehabil* 1:1–7.

Kane, RA, & Kane RL (1981): *Assessing the Elderly: A Practical Guide to Measurement*. Lexington, KY, Lexington Books.

Karkeck, JM (1985): *Assessing the Nutritional Status of the Elderly*. Silver Spring, MD, American Society for Parenteral and Enteral Nutrition.

Katcher, AH (1984): Are companion animals good for your health? *Aging*, 346:2–3.

Katz, S (1983): Assessing self-maintenance: Activities of daily living, mobility and instrumental activities of daily living. *J Am Geriatr Soc*, 31:721–727.

Katz, S, Ford, AB, Moskowitz, RW, et al. (1963): Studies of illness in the aged. The index of ADL: A standardized measure of biological and psychosocial function. *JAMA*, 185:914–919.

Kleinman, A, Eisenberg, MD, & Good, B (1978): Culture, illness and care: Clinical lessons from anthropology and cross-cultural research. *Ann Intern Med*, 88:251–258.

Koren, M (1986): Home care—who cares? *N Engl J Med*, 314:917–920.

Leininger, M (1984): Transcultural nursing: An essential knowledge and practice field for today. *Canadian Nurse*, 80(11):41–45.

Lipson, JG, & Meleis, AI (1985): Culturally appropriate care: The case of immigrants. *Top Clin Nurs*, 7(3):48–56.

Lowy, L (1980): Mental health services in the community.

In Birren, JE, & Sloane, RB (eds): *Handbook of Mental Health and Aging*. Englewood Cliffs, NJ, Prentice-Hall, 827–846.

Lundin, DV, Eros, PA, Melloh, J, et al. (1980): Education of independent elderly in the responsible use of prescription medications. *Drug Intell Clin Pharm*, 14:335–342.

Malasanos, L, Barkauskas, V, Moss, M, et al. (1986): *Health Assessment* (ed 3). St. Louis, CV Mosby.

Martin, DC, & Mead, K (1982): Reducing medication errors in a geriatric population. *J Am Geriatr Soc*, 30:258–260.

McCall, N (1985): Health insurance. *Generations*, 9(4):36–39.

McFarland, LG, Howells, D III, & Dill, B (1985): Respite care. *Generations*, 9(3):46–47.

Meany-Handy, J, Nowinski, S, & Rickerson, T (1985): Community health nurses in technologically advanced home care. *In* Archer, SE, & Fleshman, RP: *Community Health Nursing* (ed 3). Monterey, CA, Wadsworth, 452–462.

Meiners, MR (1985): Long term care insurance. *Generations*, 9(4):39–42.

Miller, SJ (1986): Conceptualizing interpersonal relationships. *Generations*, 10(4):6–9.

Mundinger, M (1983): *Home Care Controversy: Too Little, Too Late, Too Costly*. Rockville, MD, Aspen.

Nassif, JZ (1986): There's still no place like home. *Generations*, 11 (2):5–8.

Oktay, J, & Palley, H (1981): Home health and in home service programs for the chronically limited elderly: Some equity and adequacy considerations. *Home Health Care Serv Q*, 2(4):5–28.

O'Malley, ST (1986): Reimbursement issues. *In* Stuart-Siddall, S (ed): *Home Health Care Nursing: Administrative and Clinical Perspectives*. Rockville, MD, Aspen.

Orque, MS, Bloch, B, & Monrroy, LS (1983): *Ethnic Nursing Care: A Multicultural Approach*. St. Louis, CV Mosby.

Ouslander, JG (1981): Urinary incontinence in the elderly. *West J Med*, 135(6):482–491.

Palley, HA, & Oktay, JS (1983): The chronically limited elderly. (Special issue.) *Home Health Care Serv Q*, 4(2):1–142.

Reifler, BV, & Hansen, L (1986): In-home mental health programs. *Generations*, 10(3):52–53.

Rice, DP, & Feldman, JJ (1983): Living longer in the United States: Demographic changes and health care needs of the elderly. *Milbank Memorial Fund Q*, 61(3):362–396.

Roe, DA (1983): *Geriatric Nutrition*. Englewood Cliffs, NJ, Prentice-Hall.

Schmall, VL, & Pratt, C (1986): Special friends: Elders and pets. *Generations*, 10(4):44–45.

Shapiro, S (1986): Are elders underserved? *Generations*, 10(3):14–17.

Sherman, JA (1987): Identifying and treating insomnia in the elderly. *Consult Pharm*, January/February.

Simonson, W (1984): *Medications and the Elderly*. Rockville, MD, Aspen.

Stuart-Sidall, S (ed) (1986): *Home Health Care: Administrative and Clinical Perspectives*. Rockville, MD, Aspen.

Tinkham, CW, Voorhies, EF, & McCarthy, NC (1984): *Community Health Nursing: Evolution and Process* (ed 2). New York, Appleton-Century-Crofts.

Tripp-Reimer, T, Brink, PJ, & Saunders, JM (1984): Cultural assessment: Content and process. *Nurs Outlook,* 32(2):78–82.

Vanderslice, D (1985): Emergency response network. *Generations,* 9(3):55–56.

Viederman, M, & Perry III, S (1980): Use of a psychodynamic life narrative in the treatment of depression in the physically ill. *Gen Hosp Psychiatry,* 3:177–185.

Waldo, D, & Lazenby, H (1984): Demographic characteristics and health care use and expenditures by aged in the United States: 1977–1984. *Health Care Financ Rev,* 6(1):1–29.

Wenger, NK (ed) (1978): *Exercise and the Heart.* Philadelphia, FA Davis.

Williams, TF (1983): Comprehensive functional assessment: An overview. *J Am Geriatr Soc,* 31:637–641.

Zawadski, RT (ed) (1983): Community-based systems of long term care. (Special issue.) *Home Health Care Serv Q,* 4(3/4).

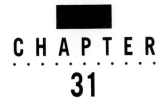

CHAPTER

31

Program Planning and Development

MARILYN D. FRAVEL, R.N., N.H.A.

"Failure of existing rules is the prelude to a
search for new ones."

**Thomas Kuhn, The Structure of Scientific
Revolutions**

HISTORY—LONG-TERM CARE AND GERONTOLOGICAL NURSING

Until as recently as the 1970s long-term care
meant institutional care. Gerontological nurses
worked primarily in institutional settings.
These nurses were faced with a variety of
expectations and limitations related to internal
program management and development from
a number of sources:

1. Those mandated by laws, regulation, and
surveillance
2. Those imposed by reimbursement mechanisms
3. Those defined by administration and
ownership
4. Those required by clients based on their
needs
5. Those imposed by ancillary staff and their
needs
6. Those professional and personal expectations the nurse brought to the career

These factors dictating nursing practice were
often conflicting in their requirements and
heedless of realistic capabilities and priorities.
Institutions sought professional nurses with
a combination of clinical and supervisory skills
who were willing to function at high levels of
responsibility with substantially less remuner-
ation and professional support than their
acute-care counterparts. With few nursing
hour requirements and little budgetary allocation for professional nursing, gerontological
nursing program development was limited to
meeting basic regulatory requirements in institutional settings lacking in resources to provide even quality custodial care. Skilled nursing facilities, as the primary precursors of a

long-term continuum of care, bore nursing's name and presented to the geriatric and general public what has been publicized by the press and designated by a variety of public entities as the "scourge" of geriatric care.

The concept of *long-term care* now includes all levels of medical and social care for elderly and chronically disabled clients and assumes a wide variety of system uses, with constant to intermittent service utilization (Sheldon & Windham, 1984). Gerontological nurses are challenged to participate in the definition of continuums of long-term care. Because of a combined generalist and specialist education and high-profile involvement in care management at most levels of care, the gerontological nurse is well prepared to participate in strategic planning to effect appropriate care.

STRATEGIC MARKET PLANNING

The concept of marketing in a professional health care environment is relatively new. For years, the health care industry was preoccupied with growth and expansion. Health care development was primarily *product-driven* in its orientation—services evolved and were offered by providers based on the products and services available or developing. Program development was geared toward capitalizing on existing, internal skills of the organization. Little emphasis was placed on approaching and consulting potential customers or caregivers. Competition was the prime mover, and "keeping up with the Joneses" the prevailing attitude in health care–dominated planning efforts. Government funding and insurance encouraged and reimbursed this type of program development activity.

In the *sales orientation* to health care planning, emphasis is placed on pushing the product or service. Packaging is important, with less regard for the quality of or need for a product or service. For example, some organizations adopt a sales approach when referrals or admissions decline. Since this approach does not inherently provide for consumer input, it has not affected market planning that assures ongoing utilization of services needed by the community.

The *marketing orientation* to planning places the consumer in the center of the program development process. Emphasis is placed on meeting the needs of the client and client community. Elements of the strategic market planning process include:

1. Market analysis: trend analysis, needs assessment, feasibility study
2. Program planning and implementation: business/resource planning, marketing, management and operation, program evaluation and revision (Commission on Accreditation of Rehabilitation Facilities, 1984)

A marketing orientation to health care planning assumes involvement not only of potential clients but also of their formal and informal caregivers at all intervals of program development (Hillestad & Berkowitz, 1984).

Market Trends and Analysis

Health care providers no longer have the luxury of designing and implementing new programs in self-sufficient isolation. As a society, we are necessarily moving away from a preoccupation with immediate gratification of short-term needs toward long-term planning, with emphasis on deinstitutionalization (including less reliance on government) and self-reliance with a variety of personal options. Health care generalists are more in demand, as strategic planning forces the need for a "common purpose of players and ownership" in program design. Decentralization allows more creative problem-solving on a more personal or local level. The past preference for institutional care is changing to interest in personalized care with decreasing use of professionals. Creation of programs geared toward self-sustenance, self-responsibility, and sharing of oneself as a resource will be required (Naisbitt, 1984).

In 1986, for example, the American Hospital Association published results of its Survey of Hospital Services for the Aging and Chronically Ill. Figure 31–1 illustrates organizational and delivery service changes noted over a 2-year period by responding community-based acute-care hospitals. These changes reflect

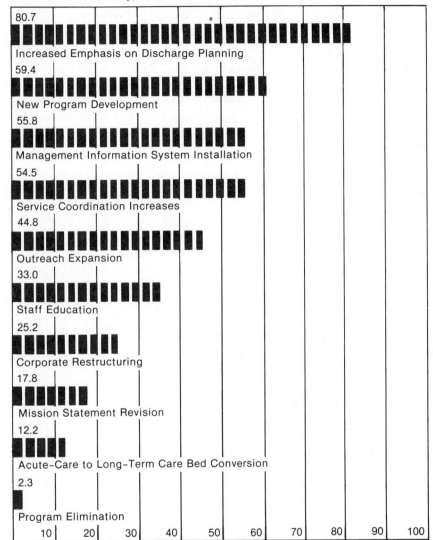

Changes in the Organization and Delivery of
Services to the Elderly, 1983–1985

80.7

Increased Emphasis on Discharge Planning

59.4

New Program Development

55.8

Management Information System Installation

54.5

Service Coordination Increases

44.8

Outreach Expansion

33.0

Staff Education

25.2

Corporate Restructuring

17.8

Mission Statement Revision

12.2

Acute–Care to Long–Term Care Bed Conversion

2.3

Program Elimination

10   20   30   40   50   60   70   80   90   100

%Community Hospitals Reporting   N = 2789

Figure 31–1. Changes in the organization and delivery of services to the elderly, 1983 to 1985. (Redrawn from American Hospital Association, Hospital Research and Educational Trust: *Emerging Trends in Aging and Long-Term Care Services.* Chicago, American Hospital Association, Hospital Research and Educational Trust, 1986, p 10. With permission.)

early institutional response to the need for market-based planning.

Simultaneously, demographic projections of "who's who" in the market of current and potential consumers influence program planning and development efforts:

1. By the year 2020, approximately 31% of the United States population will be at least 55 years old, with the 75-plus age group increasing most dramatically.

2. By the year 2030, 20% of the United States population will be over 65 years of age.

3. Due to advances in medicine and technology, adults with severe injuries and developmental disabilities are living longer.

4. Survival of infants born with multiple disabilities has increased dramatically.

5. An estimated 1 million people in the United States fell below poverty levels in 1986 due to the cost of long-term care services and

the lack of insurance options for the non–Medicaid-reimbursed middle class population.

6. Demands for outpatient long-term care services will start to outweigh inpatient needs. Diminishing government resources and participation by private insurance companies has resulted in requirements for cost efficiency and coordination of services.

7. Restriction of reimbursement for inpatient services will continue and increase.

8. It is estimated that currently 6.6 million people in the United States require long-term care services, with projections of the number rising to 19 million by the year 2040 (American Hospital Association, 1986).

With de-emphasis on unnecessary centralization of services, caregivers will take a more active part in planning and implementing services. As concepts of multidisciplinary care evolve, with objectives specifically tied to client need and expected outcome (Clark & Shyavitz, 1983), the nursing role becomes important in assessment of client needs, program design and care planning on a broader level, and assurance of quality and program evaluation.

Needs Assessment and Feasibility Study

Health as an industry can no longer function in isolation; neither can gerontological nurses. Not only must nurses be concerned with plans of care designed for each client but also with all facets and tenets of the larger client care program (Milch & Martinelli, 1978). Gerontological nurses will be obligated, in addition, to increase professional interactions with non-specialists—non-nursing, nonmedical, and unskilled persons who are all caregivers or participants in planning the continuum of gerontological care. While gerontological nurses frequently assume this responsibility informally, the role will necessarily become formal.

In conducting needs assessment, primary research should also provide for examination of interrelationships between (National Easter Seal Society, 1984):

1. Prevalence of a specific need and problem
2. Geographic area and breakout of "need centers"
3. Program data—other and comparable, competitive, or complementary services provided (internally and externally)
4. Priorities of needs

Methods of primary research for needs assessment should be weighed according to projected efficiency (including cost efficiency and staff time), validity, reliability, and availability for long-term, applicable data (Table 31–1). Needs assessment need not be costly for nurses working in smaller, community-based settings. Inexpensive approaches, such as literature review and minisurveys, can be conducted singly or in combination with other approaches, with moderate accuracy and reliability. Needs assessment will necessarily become an ongoing process (Drachman, 1983). Networking will allow nurses to become more conscious of and educated regarding the whole range of resources available or needed, keeping nursing fingers on the pulse of community health care. Involvement with other nursing and non-nursing organizations maintains a flow of needs assessment data, as do subscriptions to journals and demographic and trend reports. The times are also ripe for more program development partnerships between gerontological nurses who are direct service providers and nursing researchers. Service-providing nurses will take more advantage of research skills and methodologies available through these working relationships. Since nurses are strategically placed throughout the continuum of health services, and with gradually increasing reimbursement for non-institutional nursing services, nurses maintain access to people needing nursing and other services and increasingly will be expected to participate as consultants in planning and educational processes.

As needs assessment data are collected and analyzed and new programs are planned, the feasibility of continuing development of a particular program area is defined. Included in this process are matching a prospective program goal statement with that of the umbrella organization, defining services to be provided, refining admission and evaluative criteria, and

Table 31–1. COMPARISON OF NINE MAJOR TYPES OF PRIMARY RESEARCH

Approach	Cost	Number Staff Needed	Time Needed	Validity (On Average)	Ability to Produce Broad-Ranging Data	Ability to Produce Solid Limited Data	Utility for Regular, Ongoing Assessment
Key informants assessment	Varies by approach	✔	✔	✔	—	+	✔
Service provider assessment	Varies by approach	✔	✔	✔	—	+	✔
Brainstorming ("group think")	+	+	+	—	—	✔	+
Key indicators (analyze and extrapolate available data)	+	✔	+	✔	✔	+	+
Public meetings	✔	✔	+	✔	✔	✔	+
Mini-survey (in comparison to formal survey)	+	+	+	✔	✔	✔	+
Formal survey: • personal interview	—	—	—	✔	—	+	Not practical for regular use
• telephone	—	—	—	+	✔	+	Not practical for regular use
• mail	✔	—	—	+	+	+	Not practical for regular use

+ = strength
✔ = adequate to good
— = poor to adequate
Note: These ratings are rough guides only. Effectiveness depends on numerous variables, from the people involved in "group think" to the number of individuals surveyed in a telephone survey.

(From National Easter Seal Society: *Conducting Needs Assessment: A Program Portfolio Resource Manual.* Chicago, National Easter Seal Society, 1984, p 14. Reprinted with permission.)

allocating financial and human resources, including capital required for start-up and ongoing operations (Clark & Shyavitz, 1983; National Easter Seal Society, 1985).

Business Planning and Marketing

Development of a business plan for the program enables the organization to focus on the new program itself, as well as its relationship to other existing programs. The business plan, as a tool for internal reference, is helpful in defining a needs-oriented marketing plan for expansion of current services to new markets (market development), expanding referrals from current sources (market penetration),

or development of new programs and new service populations (diversification). Four major factors of marketing are considered (National Easter Seal Society, 1984):

1. Product—seeking customer acceptance
2. Price—rate-setting and reimbursement mechanisms
3. Distribution—admission requirements; physical placement of program
4. Communication—methods of promotion of the program to potential clients and to referral and funding sources

The management and operations plan defines the placement of a new program within the existing structure in terms of administration and operations responsibility, staffing, other required resources, program evaluation, and quality assurance (Kotler, 1980).

As shown in Table 31–2, all components of the business plan are translated into the financial plan and summary. Financial goals are summarized with definition of underlying assumptions. Historical financial data for comparison with projections and actual numbers are helpful for ongoing analysis. For new programs or expansion of current programs, the projections may need to be reviewed and revised (based on new assumptions and variable program indicators) as frequently as once a month.

Program Evaluation

A formal system for evaluation of service programs is essential to strategic market planning. Utilization of program data for analysis helps ensure that the organization continues to be market-driven and continually responsive to community needs.

Funding sources of all types, including foundations and third-party payers, are increasingly requiring program evaluation that proves efficiency and effectiveness. With government funding shrinking for all health care programs, programs developed for geriatric clients must be increasingly cost-efficient in response to need (Gaedeke, 1977). A program that is highly *efficient* in operation saves funds and, as a consequence, more resources are available to serve more clients. A program that is *effective* guarantees that measures for quality are in place. Neither efficiency nor effectiveness should be sacrificed in the equation of positive program evaluation (Tucker, 1981).

Table 31–2. SPU FINANCIAL SUMMARY*

Item	Time Periods				
	Historical			Projections	
A. Income					
1. Fee for services					
2. Contributions, subsidy					
3. Other					
4. Total					
B. Expenses					
1. Staff					
2. Fringe benefits					
3. Contracted services					
4. Marketing, promoting					
5. Supplies equipment					
6. Space (rent, utilities, phone)					
7. Other					
8. Administrative overhead					
9. Total					
C. Net gain (loss)					
D. Program utilization (client volume)					

(Modified with permission from National Easter Seal Society: *Developing Program Futures: A Program Portfolio Resource Manual*. Chicago, National Easter Seal Society, 1985, p 55.)

*SPU refers to a unit of organizational structure or analysis for program planning, budgeting, and management.

Program efficiency can be directly related to the productivity of all staff involved in service provision. Standards of productivity are best developed by those who will be required to meet standards or ensure that other staff meet standards. In arriving at definitive productivity standards, a number of factors should be considered:

1. Experience of the organization in providing the service—historical data such as "seasonal" census activity and trends of clients and their compliance with the schedule

2. Standards used by peers in comparable and noncomparable program settings

3. Uncontrollable external variables that alter productivity, such as changes in reimbursement by third-party payers (National Easter Seal Society, 1984).

Productivity standards for analysis of efficiency address expectations regarding time spent on direct client care and documentation of that care, time spent on administrative functions, allocation of subsidized or "free" services—all typically based on labor time available. Frequent, routine review of individual and group productivity promotes timely identification of problems and implementation of resolutions, as well as any need for standards revision.

The operation budget for a program is an essential standard for efficiency and should, in part, be based on staff productivity standards. Review of revenue sources and corresponding expenses pinpoints inefficient operations and areas requiring closer staff analysis and monitoring.

Equally important to include in a program evaluation plan are standards for effectiveness. Standards for effectiveness may be both objective and subjective.

Objective standards are primarily related to continual evaluation of client progress during program participation. The baseline admission clinical profile is measured against the same clinical criteria at intervals during the treatment plan and at client discharge. Although each client is an individual, clients with like diagnoses and admission profiles can be expected, generally, to progress in a broadly similar fashion in terms of functional status. As an example, an initial projected treatment plan can be compared with the actual plan at client discharge to determine the effectiveness of staff planning to determine the relationship of client benefit to duration of treatment.

Subjective evaluation should not be excluded from the program evaluation plan, but should be a formal procedure. Surveys sent to clients after discharge can be designed to determine clients' satisfaction and adherence to their self-care treatment plans. Administrative investigation and tracking of client complaints and positive feedback, based on a well-defined grievance procedure, complements more objective functional status analysis (Kotler, 1979, 1980).

CASES IN NURSING PROGRAM DEVELOPMENT

The following are programs developed by gerontological nurses in two types of long-term care settings. Due to lack of funds specified for development, emphasis was placed on low-cost market/program planning. Whereas professional nurses in management positions assumed administrative responsibility for program design, implementation, and evaluation, other personnel, including ancillary nursing staff, paraprofessionals, rehabilitation professionals, clients, and caregivers, were involved to a high degree in strategic program development.

Client Orientation Program in a Skilled Nursing Facility

An urban, 70-bed, skilled nursing facility had been in operation for nearly 20 years. Historically, the client profile was composed of upper middle class elderly; average length of stay was over 1 year. Many clients had entered the setting requiring custodial, long-term nursing care due to lack of appropriate care alternatives. As alternatives evolved and acute-care hospital stays shortened, strategic planning was required to address operational and client needs for both short- and long-term care and rehabilitation.

Trends

1. Increased admissions
2. Decreased length of stay
3. Change in client profile to one where there was increased rehabilitation potential and residual functional abilities not requiring inpatient long-term care
4. Increased "rapid fire" admissions from acute-care hospitals, with less time for discharge planning
5. Decreased ability by administration in the skilled nursing facility to control and confine "admission hours" to before noon, when the facility staff is best able to process the admission
6. Increased nursing care acuity (sicker patients than was customary) on admission

Trend Analysis

Since client stay had been substantially shortened, evaluation of current admission policies and procedures reflected the need for condensing admission procedures and speeding development of individual plans of care. In the past, longer lengths of stay and lower acuity levels had allowed more time for establishing trust relationships with clients and significant others and allowing clients to adjust to the skilled nursing facility at their own pace. Nursing staff had informally relied on roommates to provide significant (albeit less technical) components of the admission and orientation process (i.e., how to get what you need from individual staff members when you need it). With less time for development of client-to-client relationships, this transition through admission was curtailed.

Needs Assessment

The following needs were identified:
1. Need for revision of admission policies and procedures
2. Need for expansion of staff education and orientation to the admission process (i.e., for those on evening shift and for ancillary nursing staff)
3. Need to shorten the transition and adjustment period from acute-care setting to skilled nursing facility setting
4. Need to address the impact of trends on other clients (roommate turnover and changing roommate roles)
5. Need to address the impact of trends on external participants in planning: family members/caregivers, physicians, acute-care hospital nursing and social service staff

Feasibility

It was clearly feasible not only to revise procedures (formal and informal) to effect a positive client transition, but also to address these needs with groups of clients with like needs, staff and family members, administration in the skilled nursing facility, and external professionals involved in the clients' long-term care planning.

Planning and Management

Nursing administration was assigned the responsibility for addressing policy revision and staff development needs as part of their routine job descriptions. Time was allocated for the professional nursing staff to work on the definition of components of a group-oriented Client Orientation Program. Clients and significant others were encouraged to attend 1-hour sessions two times a week for 3 weeks. Various staff members from all levels of the skilled nursing facility organization were "guest speakers." "Client leaders" who had successfully completed transition training were invited to speak and offered peer support. A professional nursing staff member conducted each session. Program goals emphasized acclimation to the structure, value, and reasons for daily routines; areas of flexibility; "house rules"; problem-solving; and development of trust, channels of communication, and lines of staff authority.

Program costs were minimal. Professional nursing hours increased slightly. Activity room space was used during its normal "down time."

Marketing

Information summarizing the goals, process, and schedule of Client Orientation Sessions was distributed to all referring agencies and care providers along the continuum of care. Comparable information was included in the packet of business papers reviewed with clients and financially responsible parties during the routine administrative portion of the admission process.

Program Evaluation

After a 3-month period, the Client Orientation Program was positively (albeit subjectively) evaluated by participatory clients, caregivers, and staff. Clients who attended sessions were noted to be better prepared to advocate for their own needs and to have more quickly developed relationships with others. They were better able to concentrate on their own physical restoration programs. Also, those "client leaders" and staff members involved became known as expert resources—internal contact persons that new clients used for validation and problem-solving.

As more staff were trained in the technical components of the admission process and psychological components of the transition process, members' need for organizational training during the group sessions lessened, and more time was given to establishing relationships. Also, clients and family members were made increasingly familiar with the program prior to admission and were more aware of and prepared to deal with transition issues on entering the skilled nursing facility.

The nursing management team at this small, free-standing skilled nursing facility effectively defined client needs as a group and effected a program that not only resolved technical, internal operational problems related to admissions, but also promoted a positive transition for elderly clients using this part of the continuum of care. The nurses were able to use their skills of organization, problem-solving, networking, and teaching to address requirements of the strategic planning process and increase quality of service cost-effectively to a defined market of clients.

Comprehensive Outpatient Rehabilitation in a Community Clinic

An urban, nonprofit agency had operated a free-standing outpatient rehabilitation clinic for 15 years. Services included physical therapy, occupational therapy, speech therapy, social services, and disability-specific peer support groups, coordinated by professional staff. The financial status of the agency was poor. The need for an emergent, crisis-oriented, strategic market-based plan was the first priority for the nursing manager, who was also chief executive officer.

Trends

1. Decreased utilization of the clinic over the previous 5 years
2. Increased referrals of chronic-care clients
3. Decreased referrals of clients recovering after orthopedic treatments (a former mainstay of the referral population)
4. Utilization of services primarily by clients residing in the central urban area where the clinic was located
5. Decreased number of clients requiring multiple services
6. Increased average age of clients over the previous 3 years
7. Staff frustration due to lack of strategic planning and staff involvement; preference for caring for the acutely disabled; 70% to 75% professional staff turnover each year; and low salaries and benefits
8. Decreased revenues from fund raising and lack of coordination with client services and programs
9. Lack of reimbursement for occupational therapy and social and nursing services
10. Increased utilization of and reimbursement for home health rehabilitation services
11. Increased competitive specialty physical

therapy clinics (i.e., sports medicine clinics) with high capital expenses

12. Increased need for services for elderly clients

Needs Assessment

Due to time and budgetary constraints, staff relied heavily on their networking capabilities and professional contacts to define community rehabilitation health care needs. A simple survey questionnaire was designed and directed to physicians and other health and social service providers in the larger service area, allowing for specific input regarding the need for clinic services offered and suggestions on other markets needing services or programs.

Seventy percent of respondents were aware of agency services and felt they continued to be needed, although more so by the chronically physically disabled market. Seventy percent of respondents indicated a need for group/day programs tailored to the needs of an elderly population (i.e., social and adult day health care). Ninety percent of respondents emphasized the need for a more comprehensive paratransit system for elderly and physically disabled people, which would, in turn, increase utilization of the clinic. Eighty percent of respondents cited lack of reimbursement for some rehabilitation services as negative factors to be considered in clinic utilization or program design. Interestingly, a number of respondents who had been considered "higher referral potential" resources by the clinic expressed lack of knowledge of clinic services and admission requirements.

Review of the external, competitive environment revealed the presence of three major acute-care hospitals within 2 miles of the clinic, none of which had developed or were in the process of developing structured inpatient rehabilitation units. All three offered outpatient services with minimal staffing and emphasis on orthopedic physical therapy. The clinic was primary provider of inpatient occupational therapy and speech therapy services for one hospital and secondary provider for the other two.

Feasibility

It was determined at the time of the survey that the clinic had lost its two major markets: acute-care, short-term, orthopedically disabled clients; and acute-care, short-term rehabilitation clients who were more easily treated in their own homes due to transportation problems.

While the philosophy and mission statement of the clinic mandated reaching out to serve disabled people regardless of their ability to pay, the clinic's financial status precluded the feasibility of developing all new programs with inherent financial deficits (such as adult day health care). Start-up and operating capital was not readily available. It was also thought that staff burnout and a service hiatus for strategic market planning had negatively affected referrals.

The clinic's board of directors and program administrative staff decided, as a first step, to evaluate the current program in terms of staff appropriateness and productivity, including staffing patterns and program organization and efficiency. It was seen as important to conduct an outreach program to formally disseminate service information to professionals as well as potential client markets. Administration also explored reimbursement mechanisms and, based on an internal comparative projection of data, recommended changing the clinic's status of Medicare certification to that of CORF (Comprehensive Out-Patient Rehabilitation Facility). This certification allowed for Medicare reimbursement of occupational therapy, social services, and nursing services.

Fund-raising and clinical staff worked together to develop specific new program plans for elderly and chronically disabled clients to define start-up and working capital needs. Research regarding foundation and corporate funding sources for new program development was initiated by the nurse executive.

Planning and Management

Staffing problems were addressed immediately and included:

1. Incorporation of all staff in the planning

process, including mission statement revision and changed staff expectations

2. Address of burnout and start of an informal employee motivation program with subsequent personnel changes

3. Redefinition of productivity standards and staffing patterns based on actual clinic utilization

4. Revision and upgrading of salary and benefit schedules

The business/financial plan reflected increased reimbursement projections based on CORF implementation and expected clinic utilization. Professional staff were expected to use most of their time in direct treatment and little in nonprofessional tasks. The boat was rocking—it was sink or swim.

Marketing

The clinic brochure was revised to indicate changes in program emphasis. It was sent to survey respondents, selected physicians, all current referrers (to affect market development and penetration), and to nonhealth agencies serving Medicare beneficiaries (i.e., 20 senior day activity and social centers). A Speakers Bureau was developed; interested staff at all levels were encouraged to be guest lecturers and to include review of clinic services in their presentations. Efforts were initiated to include service information in copy used for the clinic's expansive direct-mail fund-raising campaigns.

Program Evaluation

In less than 1 fiscal year, the following changes in the clinic and organizational status were noted:

1. A 33% increase in overall clinic treatment visits

2. The addition of four full-time clinical staff, based on utilization

3. A 105% increase in Medicare clients served

4. A 205% increase in clients requiring multiple services

5. An 80% decrease in clinical staff turnover

6. A 20% increase in the number of physicians referring directly to the clinic

7. On paper, development of two major and two minor new programs based on community need

Formal post-discharge client surveys showed higher satisfaction with services received at the clinic.

Clinical staff defined specific areas for additional services or adjuncts to the CORF, including:

1. Rehabilitation nursing service and consultation

2. Expanded information and referral services

3. Group treatment methods

4. Caregivers' support group

5. Maintenance exercise program

Clinic staff at all levels participated in the strategic planning process. Needs for new programs and expansion of the CORF program were defined by clients, caregivers, and other service providers and professionals. The combination of a board of directors and staff dedicated to meeting health care needs of the community allowed the planning and transition process to occur rapidly and effectively.

SUMMARY

The changing environment in health care delivery systems and economics challenges policymakers and service providers to become increasingly involved in strategic market planning. Gerontological nurses, by the nature of their generalist specialty, are in an optimal position to assume leadership positions in planning processes. Understanding program development and its close relationship to the nursing process enables gerontological nurses to broaden and better utilize their professional skills.

References

American Hospital Association, Hospital and Research Educational Trust (1986): *Emerging Trends In Aging and Long Term Care Services*. Chicago, American Hospital Association, Hospital and Research Educational Trust.

Clark, RN, & Shyavitz, L (Summer, 1983): Strategies for

a crowded marketplace. *Health Care Manage Rev, 8:*45–51.

Commission on Accreditation of Rehabilitation Facilities (November, 1984): *Market-Based Planning: A Tool for Facilities Serving People with Disabilities.* Tucson, AZ, Commission on Accreditation of Rehabilitation Facilities.

Drachman, DA (Spring, 1983): A community marketing survey of a proposed ambulatory care facility. *J Health Care Marketing, 3:*51–55.

Gaedeke, RM (1977): *Marketing in Private and Public Nonprofit Organizations.* Santa Monica, CA, Goodyear Publishing.

Hillestad, SG, & Berkowitz, EN (1984): *Health Care Marketing Plans: From Strategy to Action.* Homewood, IL, Dow Jones-Irwin.

Kotler, P (January, 1979): Strategies for introducing marketing into non-profit organizations. *J Marketing, 43:*37–44.

Kotler, P (1980): *Marketing Management: Analysis, Planning and Control* (ed 4). Englewood Cliffs, NJ, Prentice-Hall.

Kuhn, T (1970): *The Structure of Scientific Revolutions* (ed 2). Chicago, University of Chicago Press.

Milch, RA, & Martinelli, PA (Fall, 1978): Community health markets: A portfolio perspective. *Health Care Manage Rev, 3:*23–28.

Naisbitt, J (1984): *Megatrends.* New York, Warner Books.

National Easter Seal Society (1984): *Conducting Needs Assessment: A Program Portfolio Resource Manual.* Chicago, National Easter Seal Society.

National Easter Seal Society (1985): *Developing Program Futures: A Program Portfolio Resource Manual.* Chicago, National Easter Seal Society.

Sheldon, A, & Windham, S (1984): *Competitive Strategy for Health Care Organizations.* Homewood, IL, Dow Jones-Irwin.

Tucker, SL (April 1981): Introducing marketing as a planning and management tool. *Hosp Health Serv Admin, 26.*

CHAPTER
32

Nursing Dynamics: Community Care for the Elderly

LINDA CROSSMAN, R.N., M.S.

HISTORY

Nursing Dynamics Corporation (NDC) was established in 1973 in Marin County, California, by a group of community health nurses who sought a vehicle for creating innovative programs and opportunities for independent practice in a variety of settings. Two of its founding members describe the motivating factors in creating the organization.

We were all increasingly impatient with expanding demands to maintain the bureaucracies that kept us from what we considered to be professional nursing. In addition, we shared a number of discontents with a health care delivery system oriented and geared primarily to diagnosis and treatment rather than disease prevention and health promotion. . . . We wanted to be accountable to our clients with a minimum of red tape and bureaucracy. . . . Independent practice was and is the only avenue we could find. . . . (Archer & Fleshman, 1978)

NDC filed its articles of incorporation and was officially incorporated in the state of California on November 15, 1973. In the process of incorporating, one of the first decisions to be made was the type of organization this would be. The options included a nonprofit corporation, a for-profit corporation, a partnership, and sole proprietorship. Consultation with an attorney, which is essential throughout all phases of incorporation, helped the organization's founding members determine that a nonprofit corporation was the most appropriate for its intended purposes for several reasons. Because innovative programs and activities were to be pursued, grants were likely to be an important source of funding. Governmental agencies and private foundations make grants primarily to nonprofit organizations. Also, the types of services planned, such as health counseling, would not receive third-party reimbursement, mak-

589

ing grants and donations necessary for funding these services.

Incorporation and filing for federal and state tax-exempt status are generally straightforward, but they do require the assistance of an attorney, preferably one experienced with nonprofit organizations. Requirements for incorporation may vary between states. NDC's Articles of Incorporation were required to include:

Name of the corporation
Purposes for which the corporation is formed
Location of the principal office
Board of directors composition and means of election
Stipulations of nonprofit status
Process for amending articles

Bylaws also are required, and generally these must cover details concerning:

Membership in the organization
Board of directors and their election and meeting process
Officers
Committees
Records and reports
Amendments

NDC's board of directors was formed during this process. The bylaws specified that all directors must be nurses. This was later to change as the organization evolved, as was the number of board members. The original board members represented a cross-section of nursing practice, with representatives having backgrounds in nursing education, administration, and direct service. All were community health nurses.

One of the first problems encountered by the NDC board was in securing the organization's tax-exempt status under Section 501(c)(3) of the Internal Revenue Service Code (Internal Revenue Service, 1954). This is the classification for most nonprofit service agencies. In order to qualify, the organization must serve the public interest rather than a private interest, such as the organizing individual or shareholders. NDC's experience points out the importance of formulating the organization's statement of purpose in order to meet this requirement. NDC's application was denied based on one of the statements of purpose, which read:

> To act in the capacity of a contracting agent for independent nurses licensed to practice the profession of nursing with foundation groups and organizations, including health maintenance organizations; to provide such nurses with the benefits of group practice while preserving the patient's rights to freedom of choice in the selection of nursing and related health care services.

Although this was considered an important purpose for the organization, the Internal Revenue Service interpreted it to mean that individual nurses, rather than the general public, would derive the benefits of the organization's activities. The board voted to delete this statement. However, the remaining statements clearly indicated NDC's purpose:

> a. The specific and primary activity in which the corporation is engaged is the planning and offering of educational programs with respect to nursing care services in the community and the providing of consultative services to community groups and health organizations with respect to nursing care.
> b. Offer consultative, advisory and administrative services regarding nursing care and nursing care education; to participate with and assist in general community health education.

As a fledgling organization, NDC had minimal assets and, fortunately, was able to find an attorney who believed in the organization's purpose and charged less than his customary fee. However, the cost of these initial organizational tasks is generally in the $3,000 to $7,000 range in California.

The initial programs for the elderly undertaken by NDC were carried out by board members, often assisted by graduate students in community health nursing. They included a hypertension screening and health counseling program offered once a week at the county's major senior center and a series of "remodeling yourself" classes taught in senior centers by community health nurse-dietitian teams. In addition, the local Area Agency on Aging contracted with NDC to conduct a study of ambulatory elderly in a tri-county area, to define health and lifestyle factors affecting their independence. Results, based on the responses of 679 older adults, were used by the Area Agency on Aging, county planning and health departments, and transportation commissions for planning and developing services for older people. Funding for these activities came, as anticipated, from grants and donations, rather than from fee-for-service reimbursement. The board members engaged in providing these services had other sources of income upon which they could rely. And while the services provided did not generate a great deal of income for the organization, they did establish NDC's reputation in the community as an innovator in community health services for the elderly.

Being an innovator often also means risk-taking. NDC demonstrated this in 1976 when the board agreed to serve as the organizational "umbrella" for Marin County's first senior day care program—a service that no other agency in the community was willing to develop. This was, in large part, due to the fact that senior day care was, at that time, a new concept in community care for the elderly, and less than 500 such centers existed in the entire country. However, the need for this service in the community had been well documented by a task force composed of representatives from public and private agencies serving the elderly and concerned older adults. The Area Agency on Aging had also designated grant funds for such a project. Members of NDC's board and the task force collaborated in writing the grant proposal, and the day center was opened in July 1977. From this point on, NDC was to play a significant role in the development of community-based long-term care services for the elderly. This was, and continues to be, an effort guided by nurses with programs for direct client services, education, and research.

DIRECT CLIENT SERVICES

Adult Day Care

Adult day care is a community-based group program designed to meet the needs of func-

tionally impaired adults through an individual plan of care. It is a structured, comprehensive program that provides these adults with a variety of health, social, and related support services in a protective setting during any part of a day, but for fewer than 24-consecutive hours.

Individuals who participate in adult day care attend on a planned basis during specified hours. Adult day care assists its participants to remain in the community, enabling families and other caregivers to continue caring for an impaired member at home (National Institute on Adult Day Care, 1984).

With $21,674 in Title III Older Americans Act funds granted by the local Area Agency on Aging, NDC opened the community's first adult day care center and named it Marin Senior Day Services. Two nurses who had been graduate students of one of NDC's founders served as co-directors. Establishing an adult day care program is a subject worthy of its own text, and there are references available on the subject (National Institute on Adult Day Care, 1984; O'Brien, 1982; Padula, 1983; Weiler & Rathbone-McCuan, 1978). The development of Marin Senior Day Services was typical of how these programs developed throughout the country. Grants covered basic operating expenses, such as salaries, rent, insurance, supplies, and telephone. The program was able to succeed largely because of the support of the community. Volunteers provided much of the staffing support. They were trained by the co-directors to provide "hands-on" care to the frail elderly (e.g., assistance with eating, ambulating, and toileting). The activity program centered around classes provided at no cost through the local community college district and adult education department of the high school district. The noon meal was provided through a federally funded senior nutrition program. Health assessment, counseling, and monitoring were provided by the co-directors. In addition to functioning as nurses, the co-directors served as administrators, supervisors, activity directors, volunteer recruiters, and fundraisers (Carver & Crossman, 1980).

The reputation of NDC's board for innovation was carried on by its first hired staff, the day care co-directors. Soon after the day care center opened, they submitted a proposal for a grant under the federally funded Comprehensive Employment and Training Act (CETA) to train five workers as day care program assistants. The project was funded and provided more stable staffing for the day care program. Curriculum developed by the co-directors, in consultation with other service providers, was a model for training paraprofessionals to work in the newly emerging field of adult day care.

Soon after the day care center opened in 1977, the NDC board, ever on the alert for new funding sources, learned of grants available through the Administration on Aging for model projects. A grant proposal was submitted for developing a continuum of care for the frail elderly in Marin County. Its key components were:

1. A network of adult day care/service centers that would be the focal point for delivering a range of services for the frail elderly

2. A case management model utilizing volunteers to assist the frail elderly and their caregivers in locating appropriate services

3. Education programs and support groups for family members caring for a frail elder

4. Development of in-home services in the community

Although the proposed project was not selected for funding, it did provide the framework for NDC's program development in the ensuing years. Because of funding constraints, NDC had to develop the component of the envisioned model in incremental steps.

In 1979, funding was once again available through the Area Agency on Aging to establish a second senior day care center in Marin County as part of an initiative to develop "focal points" for senior services in specific communities. This provided NDC with the opportunity to implement its decentralized model of adult day care. One of the designated focal points was the northern part of the county. NDC collaborated with two other agencies serving that part of the county, one serving the elderly exclusively and the other a multipurpose social service agency, to develop a coordinated plan for addressing the needs of the elderly in that community. Grant funds were awarded, and NDC opened its second adult day care center in November, 1979.

Nursing Dynamics learned, as do all other nonprofit services agencies, that grants are more readily available for start-up of programs than for ongoing operating support. NDC had to develop other revenue sources to sustain its adult day care centers. The board, staff, and volunteers became much more involved in community fundraising, from running rummage sales and bake sales to soliciting support from service clubs, such as the Rotary and Lions clubs. The importance of such efforts should not be underestimated. Not only do they raise money to support the agency's programs, but they also increase the community's awareness of the needs that exist among the frail elderly, with a possible effect of increasing monetary support. In addition to fundraising, the NDC board began to develop a fee-for-service system. In the early stages, the adult day care program was totally supported by Older Americans Act (Title III), a funding that prohibited fees. However, as the agency began to bring in other revenues, Title III funds were designated to support one component of the program, transportation, and fees were instituted to cover all other services. Instead of a flat fee equivalent to the actual cost of providing the service, $32 per day for social-health maintenance day care and $50 per day for adult day health care, the agency instituted a sliding fee scale, using grants and donations to subsidize the difference between actual cost and a client's ability to pay.

In developing its program, NDC has successfully tapped all available funding resources. The agency took a major step forward in 1980 when a major bequest was made available to the community. NDC had been attuned to the possibility and had prepared a proposal to develop a comprehensive, coordinated, county-wide community-based system of long-term care services. The system included adult day care, home care, and case management. NDC adhered to the principles articulated 3 years earlier in its model project proposal to the Administration on Aging.

However, as often happens with grants, only one component of the proposal was funded— adult day care.

With this grant and continuation grants that were to follow, NDC established a county-wide network of three adult day care centers that serve a total of 115 clients each month and 300 a year. Of an annual operating budget of $780,000, 50% is covered by fees and Medicaid reimbursement. The remaining revenues come from grants and donations.

Home Care

The disabled elderly can certainly benefit from adult day care, and adult day care can be a more cost-effective substitute for home-delivered services when the primary need is for companionship and supervision. However, often the disabled older person needs both services, especially when living alone. Housekeeping, shopping, laundry, and bathing are activities of daily living that adult day care centers cannot do, in most cases. Through the clients served in its adult day care programs, NDC staff were made acutely aware of the problem encountered by the elderly who needed home care but who could not afford prevailing rates charged by for-profit agencies. Instead, NDC found that the frail elderly and their caregivers were seeking independent home care providers in the community who charged lower rates than were customary. NDC became concerned about the lack of quality control measures in this whole process. Elderly individuals and caregivers were not educated as to what to look for in screening providers. There was a particular concern for the elderly living alone who could be subject to abuse and exploitation. NDC's goal was to establish a nonprofit home care agency with services available on a sliding fee scale. However, funding was not available to subsidize the program. With available but limited funds ($26,000), NDC established a home care brokerage service.

Under this program, a registered nurse conducts an individualized assessment of each client who calls requesting a home care provider and then matches him or her with available attendants. All attendants are interviewed and screened by, for example, reference checks by the nurse, who also provides information and referral to other services for clients. Followup and support are provided to both the client and the attendant.

CAREGIVER SUPPORT SERVICES

Support Groups

Agencies committed to serving the frail elderly must consider the family as their clients. Contrary to the myths that families abandon their dependent elders, studies have proved that families continue to be the major providers of care for the disabled elderly (Chappell, 1983; Comptroller General, 1977; Sangel, 1983).

As community health nurses, NDC's board recognized this family resource at the outset. One of the primary purposes of the adult day care program is to provide respite for family caregivers. Soon after the first center opened, a support group was organized for older women caring for disabled spouses. This group constituted the majority of caregivers in the day care population. Their needs were of special concern to the agency because of their age, precarious health status, and level of stress they were experiencing. In establishing this support group, NDC once more demonstrated its innovative approaches to care for the elderly, because such groups were relatively rare in 1977. NDC also was instrumental in starting a national movement that focused attention on the needs of older women caregivers and the universal need for respite care for all caregivers of the frail elderly. The support group's founder and leader was herself an older woman who had cared for her disabled husband for 17 years prior to his death. She was a most effective advocate and organizer, and she gained the interest of the Older Women's League (OWL) in this issue. Ten years later, respite care remains a priority issue for OWL, and a National Caregivers Task Force, involving NDC staff, has been established to promote legislative action. In 1985, a model respite care bill was introduced into the California legislature that would have established demonstration projects for delivering respite care services. A revised version of this bill with a drastically reduced appropriation eventually passed.

As with its adult day care centers, NDC developed a county-wide network of caregiver support groups, expanding from one to three support groups that meet monthly. In addition to the support group for older women, two others meet at the day centers, one during the day and another in the evening to accommodate working caregivers. The groups are facilitated by day center staff, either a nurse or a nurse and social worker team. There is no fee for this service.

The Wives Respite Project

This model project was developed by NDC in response to the concerns repeatedly expressed by members of the wives' support group about the lack of affordable respite care in the community. With a 3-year grant from a local foundation, the project offered low-cost home care and out-of-home respite care for support group members. A major objective of the project was community education, accomplished through production of a videotape and a local conference on the issue of older women as caregivers (Crossman, London, & Barry, 1981). NDC became one of the first organizations in the country to raise the issue of respite care, particularly as it relates to older women caring for spouses. The videotape has been widely disseminated for use at conferences on aging, in university classes, and by agencies interested in developing similar programs. It has been an effective tool for the dissemination of information about this innovative project.

Although the Wives Respite Project ended in 1982, NDC continued to act upon its commitment to continued care for the caregivers. All components of the project were continued with alternative funding sources, with the exception of out-of-home respite care. Day care became increasingly available as a respite service as the agency developed its network of centers, and affordable home care was at least partially addressed through NDC's home care brokerage service. A grant from California's Department of Aging enabled the agency to develop a respite care registry as an adjunct to the home care brokerage service. The legislation that created this demonstration project was directly related to the consciousness-raising among legislators that was accomplished through the respite care bill sponsored by OWL.

The registry provides information on all available resources for respite care in the community, including adult care, home care, and short-term nursing home placement. A major objective of the project is to actively recruit individuals to provide respite care in the home through announcements at colleges, employment offices, and churches.

EDUCATION

Gerontology and geriatrics have not traditionally been a standard part of curricula for health care professionals. Consequently, continuing education for practitioners in this field is important if the elderly are to receive quality care. NDC is certified as a continuing education provider by both the California Board of Registered Nurses and Board of Nursing Home Administrators. NDC offers from one to four courses each year in the community, often co-sponsoring them with other aging service providers. The content for the courses is most often determined by NDC staff who have identified a particular problem among their elderly clients and a need for a better understanding of these problems among those working with the frail elderly. Continuing education programs offered by the agency have included such courses as "Depression and Loss in the Elderly," "Nursing Responses to Common Problems of the Aging," and "Alzheimer's Disease: Where Are We Now? Where Are We Going?"

In addition to its organized training programs, NDC provides fieldwork experience for undergraduate and graduate students in nursing in both direct service and administration. Three of the NDC's program directors did their preceptorships with the agency. NDC's executive director holds an appointment as clinical professor in the School of Nursing at the University of California, San Francisco, and frequently teaches classes on adult day care and long-term care. The expertise of NDC's board and staff also is shared with other health care professionals who invite them for presentations at conferences throughout the country. This serves as a vehicle for encouraging other nurses to build on the agency's experience and advocate for community-based long-term care services.

ADVOCACY

It is evident from NDC's statement of purpose that the agency viewed itself as a change agent. One of the avenues for facilitating or instituting change is advocacy. This has taken several forms for NDC. NDC board and staff members have been active at the local, state, and national level to improve existing services. Locally, board and staff have served on the Mental Health Advisory Board and its advocacy committees. As many as three NDC board members at a given time have served on the county Commission on Aging, advisory body to the Area Agency on Aging, which allocates federal funds to local programs. NDC was instrumental in convening the Marin Section on Aging, a coalition of service providers and interested individuals that meets for information-sharing to improve service coordination. NDC has also played an active role in the formation and work of the local Long Term Care Committee, which has examined alternatives for coordinating and financing long-term care services. At the state and national levels, NDC's executive director has served as president of the California Association of Adult Day Services and chair of the National Institute on Adult Day Care. She also served on the state Long Term Care Review Committee and was elected as a delegate to the 1981 State House Conference on Aging. To support the work of other local organizations providing

services to the elderly, NDC board and staff members have served on advisory committees to the family service agency, a health screening project for seniors, housing projects in the community, and the paratransit coordination council. And finally, NDC has supported cooperative efforts in service provision by its active participation in various community organizations, including the Section on Aging and Long Term Care Committee. One of the best examples of a cooperative effort was NDC's first adult day care center, which coordinated services from the local high school district's adult education department, the Easter Seal Society, the senior nutrition program, county paratransit services, and other community resources to create a low-cost but rich and varied program.

NDC has always maintained a commitment to extending itself beyond the confines of its own programs to promote an improved long-term care delivery system. The involvement of board and staff members in a wide range of advocacy activities has enhanced the visibility of the organization and its credibility while also promoting the ultimate goal of improving services to its client population. These activities have also kept the agency attuned to new developments and trends in the field, which has contributed to more appropriate planning.

ORGANIZATIONAL ISSUES

NDC experienced significant growth as an agency over a 10-year period. Services initially developed were delivered by board members. When the first day center opened in 1977, the agency had two half-time paid staff members and an annual budget of $25,000. In 1987, NDC employed 26 staff members and had an annual budget of $745,000. NDC learned a few valuable lessons during this period. One was that a broad base of community support was essential to the agency. As grants dwindled in size or held constant while the program's operating costs continued to increase, fundraising became a major activity for the board and staff. One of the keys to successful fundraising is a board that consists of individuals who represent a cross-section of the community and who are connected to various sectors, such as local businesses and service organizations. In its early years, NDC's all-nurse board did not have this type of representation. It also lacked board members with areas of expertise needed by a growing nonprofit health and human service organization, for example, legal, banking, and public relations experience. Therefore, in 1986, the organization's bylaws were changed to expand the board from 6 to 15 members and to actively recruit non-nurses. At least 51% of board members now must be recipients of services, relatives of recipients or representatives of community organizations with particular interest in programs for the elderly.

Another lesson learned was the need for board development as an organization expands. NDC originally intended to be an "umbrella agency" for the adult day care program, leaving its operation to staff and an advisory council. However, it soon became apparent that the board, as the legally liable entity for all of its programs, needed to be actively involved in policy- and decision-making. This led to more frequent board meetings (monthly versus quarterly) and the formation of board committees to work with staff on various management issues, such as personnel, budget, fundraising, and planning.

A third significant lesson learned was the importance of long-range planning for an evolving organization. NDC's activities were guided by its mission statement and vision for a coordinated, comprehensive system of long-term care services in the community. However, NDC was only one part of that system, and it was important to define the agency's role within that context. A number of questions arose. Was NDC the appropriate agency to take the lead in developing a comprehensive system? Should NDC focus on the frail elderly or other functionally impaired adults as well? Should NDC develop and administer a county-wide case management system? How would this agency sustain its programs if grant funds were reduced? These were but a few of the issues that had to be addressed.

Long-range planning is not always easy nor often a priority for newly developing nonprofit organizations like NDC, which are intent on identifying and filling unmet needs. The uncertainties of year-to-year funding for an agency highly dependent on grants and fundraising often make it difficult to look ahead. However, a clear definition of the agency's mission and its relationship to other providers in the community is absolutely essential to guide an organization.

SUMMARY

Over a 15-year period, NDC evolved from a small organization primarily involved in education, health promotion programs, and consultation to a major provider of long-term care services in the community. However, the organization has not deviated from the vision of its founders.

The structure of the organization has allowed for a great deal of creativity as well as risk-taking in developing programs directly responsive to the identified needs of the frail elderly. While the agency's clients suffer from chronic diseases and multiple health problems, health promotion and tertiary prevention are still emphasized in care planning and management. Through its direct client services and strong advocacy efforts, NDC successfully created a county-wide network of community-based long-term care services that are directed and managed by nurses. It is just one example of how nurses can take a leadership role in the development and delivery of health care services.

References

Archer, SE, & Fleshman, RP (1978): Doing our own thing: Community health nurses in independent practice. *J Nurs Admin*, 8:44–51.

Carver, C, & Crossman, L (1980): Job-sharing—may be right for you. *Am J Nurs*, 80:676–678.

Chappell, NL (1983): Informal support networks among the elderly. *Res Aging*, 5:77–79.

Comptroller General of the United States (1977): Report to Congress on home health—the need for a national policy to better provide for the elderly. Washington, DC, US General Accounting Office.

Crossman, L, London, C, & Barry, C (1981): Older women caring for disabled spouses: A model for supportive services. *Gerontologist, 21*:464–470.

Internal Revenue Service Code (1954): Section 501(c)(3). Washington, DC, Internal Revenue Service.

National Institute on Adult Day Care (1984): *Adult Day Care Standards*. Washington, DC, National Council on the Aging.

O'Brien, C (1982): *Adult Day Care: A Practical Guide*. Belmont, CA, Wadsworth.

Padula, H (1983): *Developing Adult Day Care: An approach to maintaining independence for impaired older persons*. Washington, DC, National Council on the Aging.

Sangel, J (1983): The family support system of the elderly. *In* Vogel, R, & Palmer, J (eds): *Long-term Care: Perspectives from Research and Demonstrations*. Washington, DC, Health Care Financing Administrations.

Weiler, PG, & Rathbone-McCuan, E (1978): *Adult Day Care: Community Work with the Elderly*. New York, Springer.

CHAPTER
33

Models for Respite Care

LOIS L. MILLER, R.N., M.N.

INTRODUCTION AND DEFINITION

Respite care is temporary care provided to a disabled or frail older person for the purpose of relieving the family member or friend who is the main care provider. Respite care may be informal or formal. This chapter focuses on formal respite care. Formal respite care is pro- vided in the home or in institutions, for a few hours, a full day, several days, or weeks. Care provided to the disabled elderly person ranges from custodial oversight to personal care to complex nursing care.

Nurses encounter many elderly people who are cared for at home by a family member or friend. Caring for a disabled elderly relative can be stressful and can adversely affect the caregiver's physical and emotional health (Cantor, 1983; George & Gwyther, 1986). For- mal support services to families can relieve some of the caregiving burden and allow fam- ilies to continue providing care. Respite care is one of many support services that families may need at various times and to varying degrees. It is important for nurses to be aware of the impact of caregiving on families and the availability, nature, and benefits of respite care and other support services in the community. Nurses can be an information and referral source for families about respite care and fre- quently are active participants in respite care programs. This chapter discusses the devel- opment of respite care in elderly populations, settings for respite care, implementation prob- lems and strategies, response to respite care, the role of nursing in respite care, and social policy issues.

HISTORICAL DEVELOPMENT OF RESPITE CARE

Respite care had its beginning with families of developmentally disabled children (Cohen

& Warren, 1985). Respite care appeared in the mid-1970s in response to a dramatic shift in ways of thinking about and treating the severely disabled. Prior to that time, many developmentally and physically disabled babies were institutionalized, usually for life. Deinstitutionalization of these disabled people began in the late 1960s and meant discharging institution residents and avoiding institutional placement altogether. Families began to assume care responsibilities once provided by institutions. Funding to support families caring for disabled children in the community was slow in coming. Respite care was only one of many necessary supports and the key service identified to prevent caregiver burnout (Sullivan, 1979). The 1970s saw an increase in statewide grass-roots pressure for trial respite projects. By 1980 a definition of respite care was included in the Title XIX Medicaid Home and Community Based Waiver (Cohen & Warren, 1985).

THE NEED FOR RESPITE CARE IN ELDERLY POPULATIONS

The application of the concept of respite care to elderly populations is a development reflective of a growing interest in and understanding of two related factors: (1) the changing demographics of the elderly population and (2) the central role of the family in providing long-term care to the elderly. Increasing numbers of elderly with chronic health problems and functional impairments are living longer, creating an increased need for long-term care. Currently, most of the long-term care for the elderly is provided by family. Family demographics, however, also are changing. Spouse caregivers often experience aging changes and health problems of their own, accompanied by increased dependency and need for care. They may not be able to provide help to the disabled spouse as long as it is needed. In addition, the decline in the size of the family, the entry of more women into the labor market, and the increasingly mobile lifestyle that distributes family members across the country make fewer adult children available to care for their frail elderly parents. Formal support services for families may allow them to continue to provide long-term care and maintain their elderly relatives at home. Respite or periodic relief from caregiving responsibilities is one of many supports that can help families to accomplish these goals.

NURSES AND RESPITE CARE

Nurses working in many settings are confronted by family caregiving situations that could benefit from respite care. Information about and referral to available respite care services can be an important first step in helping families cope with long-term caregiving. Nurses can be instrumental in encouraging families to utilize respite care as a preventive measure rather than waiting until fatigue is too great to continue in the caregiving role.

Nurse clinicians who focus on families can assist them in choosing the most appropriate type of respite care by considering the types of informal and formal respite available, care needs of the elderly care receiver, needs of the caregiver, and financial constraints of the family. Making decisions to use respite care and adjusting to respite care are often difficult processes for families, providing opportunity for nursing intervention. Such interventions may include giving information about effects of long-term caregiving and various respite programs, identifying and discussing feelings associated with respite care use, mediating family conflicts, supporting the decision, seeking alternatives, assisting with negotiation of the systems providing the care, using trial respite care, assisting in planning the respite care, and problem-solving when problems occur. Nurses can also help evaluate both the positive and negative impact of respite care on both the caregiver and care receiver.

Nursing assessment of caregiving families provides the data base necessary for determining respite care needs. It includes assessment of both the primary caregiver and the care receiver. Assessment of the caregiver includes age; health; other responsibilities, including employment and responsibility for other family members; financial resources; length of time in the caregiving role; quality of the relationship with the care receiver; family decision-making; availability of informal respite care from other family members or friends; other formal and informal supports; willingness to use respite care; and evidence of caregiver fatigue. Assessment of the care receiver determines physical and functional abilities; mental status; behavior problems; feelings about using respite care; relationship with the caregiver; adjustment to disability; and living arrangements.

The role of nurses within actual respite care programs is varied and somewhat dependent upon setting. The unique skills of nurses are knowledge of the disease processes afflicting the elderly and resultant care requirements, communication skills, an understanding of social and psychological behavior, and an appreciation of family dynamics. These skills enable nurses to play a pivotal role in planning and coordinating respite programs by matching the respite services of a particular agency or facility with the care needs of elderly. They also enable nurses to be effective problem-solvers and to work with families through all phases of the respite process.

Advanced nursing clinicians, such as clinical nurse specialists and nurse practitioners who have advanced degrees in gerontological nursing, clinical geriatrics, or a related specialty, bring special skills to respite care programs. These clinicians have additional education in selected areas of nursing, expert assessment skills, and usually some research skills. Advanced clinicians can assess the need for and feasibility of a respite care program and plan for the types of clients the program will serve, the types of respite workers needed, and the education of respite workers. They can plan special services for respite clients above minimal care requirements, such as periodic health assessment or monitoring of specific problems. They can provide consultation services in all phases of program planning and implementation, and design educational programs and evaluation measures.

The nurse administrator's role in respite care is determined in part by the setting. Some important considerations for the nurse administrator include planning staff education and training, deciding on the type of respite worker needed, developing policies and procedures, making provision for ongoing conflict resolution, monitoring the cost-effectiveness of the program, and supervising respite care workers. Responsibility for the program should be assigned, whether to the nurse administrator or a respite care coordinator. It is especially important to determine and specify whether there are certain categories of clinical problems the respite care program cannot serve.

SETTINGS FOR RESPITE CARE

Formal respite care may take several different forms. The most basic distinction among these forms is the location of service, which can be either in-home or out-of-home. In-home respite care can include companion-type services or temporary use of combined homemaker and chore service or home health services. Out-of-home respite care includes adult day care and temporary stays in respite group homes, foster homes, nursing homes, rehabilitation centers, hospitals, or other health-related facilities. Other distinctions relate to the content of the service and the type of respite provider. This section describes in-home and out-of-home models, the content of the service, characteristics and needs of the caregiver, types of providers, nurses' role, response to respite care, strengths and limitations, implementation problems and strategies, and examples of representative respite care programs.

Home

Respite care in the home ranges from custodial oversight and general supervision to nursing care, depending on the needs of the older person, the qualifications of the respite care provider, and the length of time the respite care is available. In-home respite care is most often provided for periods up to a few hours during the day, either on a regular or a periodic basis. Less frequently it may be provided during the evening or night hours or for periods of time up to several days or weeks. Caregivers who use in-home respite may be either unable or unwilling to leave their disabled relative unattended and may then depend on brief periods of respite in order to accomplish other activities, such as shopping and appointments. Caregivers may use evening respite to attend meetings, support groups, or diversional activities. Night respite, though not common in the United States, is reported as an option in Sweden. It was designed to help reduce the caregiving burden of attending to idiosyncratic nocturnal patterns, such as sleepwalking and bedwetting. Services include preparing the elderly person for bed, administering medication, turning the person in bed, and incontinence care (Stone, 1985).

Many in-home respite care programs utilize specially trained respite care workers who provide companionship and general supervision. These respite care providers may be either paid or volunteer workers. Lidoff (1983) describes a typical respite companion program in which respite care workers' responsibilities include establishing a relationship with both caregiver and care receiver, clarifying with the caregiver any special needs of the care receiver, socializing, monitoring medications, providing general supervision, and responding to emergencies. Personal care and housekeeping duties are not included. Because of the minimal amount of training these respite care workers receive, they may be inappropriate for clients with complex care needs, except for very brief periods of time.

One role of nurses in in-home respite care is that of respite provider. In-home respite care is provided by nurses when nursing care and professional nursing management are required and minimally trained respite care workers are unable to provide such care. Respite care by nurses may be a secondary benefit to regular home health visits. In other words, caregivers use the time when home health nurses are in the home to shop, run errands,

or just get out of the house. Increased use of nurses as providers of respite care may be required as more people are maintained at home with complex medical technologies such as ventilators, intravenous feedings, and Hickman catheters. Other roles for nurses in in-home respite care include assisting families in making decisions about the use of respite care, evaluating the impact of in-home respite care on both caregiver and care receiver, and assisting with problem-solving in adjustment to respite care workers.

In-home respite care has several advantages. It is more economical than other respite care models, and it does not require the care receiver to adjust to a new environment. Specialized and familiar equipment or supplies are available, and transportation to and from the respite care program need not be arranged. In-home respite care is limited by the generally short time periods it is available. It usually does not help the caregiver who needs several days or weeks of rest. Unless special training has been provided, minimally trained respite care workers are limited to providing care for higher-functioning elderly.

Implementation of in-home respite care generally requires the development of training courses for respite care paraprofessionals. There is, however, no standard system for selection, training, education, or certification. Netting and Kennedy (1985) describe one training program in which criteria for volunteer selection include maturity, honesty, kindness, and a sufficient degree of mental and physical health to assist clients. Initial training sessions include basic information on working with people, improving communication skills, understanding and working with older adults, developing skills in working with ill or disabled people, and basic information on mental health and mental illness.

Ongoing supervision and training of respite care workers help them to do their jobs and contribute to retention (Lidoff, 1983). Regular staff meetings can give them the opportunity to share experiences, discuss problems they face in their work, and learn about topics of concern. If respite clients are severely impaired or have limited ability to communicate, it will be especially important to provide support and motivation to the respite care worker beyond that drawn from the relationship with the client. Training and supervision should emphasize that relieving caregivers is meaningful and worthwhile, even if relating to some clients is not easy or intrinsically satisfying. The peer affirmation derived from group meetings can be a major source of support. While providing needed information and skills, the training sessions also offer an opportunity for ongoing education, which in itself is an attraction to the job.

Many in-home respite care programs use volunteers. Netting and Kennedy (1985) identify several problems when using volunteers. These include maintaining volunteer interest, the need for continual nurturing and recognition of volunteers, recruiting new volunteers, tension between paid staff and volunteers, dealing with caregivers' feelings of guilt at leaving even for brief periods, and dealing with rapid changes in family burden or client functioning. In addition, some elderly require a level of health and personal care that cannot be provided by minimally trained volunteers.

An example of in-home respite care is RESPITE, a nationwide program of the National Council of Catholic Women (NCCW). In this program, Catholic women work through their local churches to offer companionship and care to the elderly in their homes in order to relieve family caregivers (Kane, 1985). The program began in 1983 and has expanded to 4,000 volunteers in 2,200 parishes around the country. Care is provided for up to 4 hours per respite episode and may include assistance with personal care. Volunteers receive 1 day of training. Training topics include distinguishing between normal aging changes and those that can lead to disability and dependence; techniques for assisting with walking, positioning, moving, transferring, feeding, and elimination; learning how to recognize and respond to emergencies; and providing emotional support for the elderly and their families. Outside funding has been obtained for program evaluation. Future plans include the development of training and evaluation manuals.

Nursing Homes

Nursing homes are the most common site of institutional respite care in the United States. Respite care in nursing homes may be an identified program with designated beds and a coordinator, or it may consist merely of an informal practice of admitting a small number of elderly for short periods of time. An elderly care receiver is admitted to a nursing home for several days, weeks, or months, depending on the needs and desires of the individual and his or her family. The individual can expect to receive the same type of care by regular nursing home staff as that for other residents of the nursing home. The nursing home should provide the essentials of care that the elderly individual receives at home. Nursing home respite may be the only option for elderly who have complex care needs requiring professional nursing expertise for 24-hour care. Caregivers may choose nursing home respite in order to stay at home by themselves and rest without the demands of caregiving, to take a trip, or to recuperate from an illness or surgery.

Nurses are the primary providers of respite in this model. The goals of nursing care are to maintain care receivers at their functional level on admission, to provide care consistent with the home routine, and to prevent complications.

The role of nurses in nursing home respite care includes assessment of care receivers and their care needs. Care needs and routines should be discussed with the caregivers and care receivers. Their expectations, as well as the expectations of the nursing home staff, should be clarified and agreement reached about the actual content and process of care that can be realistically delivered. The nurse should assess the relationship between the caregiver and care receiver and determine areas of concern for each about the nursing home admission. On admission the nurse may have to respond to a variety of emotions from both the caregiver and care receiver. Caregivers may feel anxious and guilty and care receivers may feel fearful. Both may need reassurance that the elderly care receiver will be properly taken care of.

Nursing home respite care can be advantageous in several respects. Nursing homes can manage elderly with complex and severe health and personal care problems. Staff who are skilled in this type of care are available. The New York State Foundation for Long Term Care in 1983 reported an unexpectedly helpful role played by nursing home respite care providers as a referral agency, informing and educating families about other support services for home care. In this project, families using home respite care increased from 12% before nursing home respite care to 21% 1 month later.

Nursing home admission also provides the opportunity for health assessment. Care practices and routines of the caregiver can be evaluated and information about new equipment, products, and care techniques shared with the caregiver. Nurick (1983) reports a positive impact of respite care admissions on the nursing home staff because they enjoy dealing with people who will be discharged in short periods of time; they enjoy helping people to go back home.

The major limitation of nursing home respite care is the cost, both to families and to the nursing home. Since Medicare and Medicaid generally do not pay for nursing home respite care, families must assume the total cost. For the nursing home, respite care beds are more expensive because they are often empty due to scheduling problems and because extra staff may be required to manage the additional workload. The use of nursing homes for respite care may be limited by the negative view that many people have about them. The amount of illness and disability seen in nursing homes can be upsetting. Some people may not receive as much attention from nursing home staff as they do at home, and care routines may not be performed in the accustomed manner or time. This can be a source of conflict between the care receiver and the nursing home staff. Additionally, the extra staff time required by some respite care admissions may be resented by the long-term residents.

An implementation problem for nursing home respite care is that it affects many aspects of nursing home routine, staff, other residents, and resources. Ellis and Wilson (1983) found that staff needed to spend more time initially with the respite care client than with other admissions to facilitate the transition. Also, they found that respite care clients were more demanding and required more care than anticipated. Additional staff were provided to the unit with respite care beds. The New York Foundation for Long Term Care (1983) reported an increased cost for respite care beds stemming primarily from income lost by keeping beds vacant for respite care admissions and utilizing extra personnel to accommodate these admissions.

Planning for respite care admissions can be difficult due to the great variety in functional abilities and care needs of elderly clients. Some are relatively independent in activities of daily living (ADL) and merely need supervision, and others have severe ADL deficits accompanied by complex care requirements. Staff must be ready to quickly assess the client and plan the respite care activities shortly after admission. If care requirements are complex, it is useful to have written instructions and care routines from the caregiver. The challenge for nursing homes providing respite care is to carry out care routines as close to those given at home as possible within staffing limitations, and without jeopardizing care to other residents.

Extra staff time may be required for the caregiver, both on admission and discharge and sometimes in between. If a caregiver is ambivalent about the respite care admission, he or she may need reassurance from staff and time to discuss care routines. Some caregivers call frequently, and occasionally a caregiver will visit, sometimes daily, during the respite stay. Although this practice seems to defeat the purpose of respite care, it may be difficult to prevent. Caregivers should be encouraged to use the time off for their own rest and a change in routine.

It is important to consider the timing of the discussion of the nursing home respite care admission with the elderly person. Consideration should be given to the amount of anxiety or concern it is likely to cause and the level of decision-making it requires. Some individuals cope better when they know far in advance and may even benefit from a visit to the nursing home before making a decision. Others manage better if they are not told until a few days before the admission. Families should be advised of potential problems in this area and assisted in determining the best approach.

Despite attempts to make the nursing home respite care admission a positive experience for all concerned, it must be remembered that care routines for the elderly person are interrupted, their expectations may not be met, and adjustment may be a problem even though it is understood that the admission is temporary. There may be resistance and hostility on the part of the care receiver.

Procedures and policies for nursing home respite care vary. Usually, clients cannot have an acute illness when admitted. Additionally, there should be formal plans in case of illness during the stay and plans if the client should require hospitalization. Home visits by nursing home staff or a 1- to 2-day trial admission for the purpose of assessment is used by some programs (Ellis & Wilson, 1983). The New York Foundation for Long Term Care (1983) made the following recommendations for institutional respite care: (1) support at the board and administrative levels is critical; (2) special identity of the program is needed, with one person designated as the director/coordinator for respite care; (3) respite care should be offered to the general population, with flexible admission criteria and aggressive marketing; (4) staff must be oriented to the benefits of respite care and the unique needs of respite care residents; (5) facilities should designate specific beds for respite care and avoid using them for anything else; and (6) single rooms are generally preferred by residents to avoid scheduling problems.

Some Veterans Administration (VA) nursing homes offer respite care, which is free to those veterans who are eligible. The Palo Alto, California, VA established a five-bed respite care unit in 1979, which has since been expanded to ten beds (Delaney & Bleck, 1985; Ellis & Wilson, 1983). The average respite stay is 1 week, and veterans using respite care may participate in all nursing home activities, including physical and occupational therapies. Procedural aspects include a detailed assessment in the home setting, if possible by a nurse or social worker, and an initial 3-day trial visit. Respite care admission is cancelled if the veteran has an acute illness on the day of admission; those with a history of wandering or unprovoked assaultiveness are not eligible.

One Canadian nursing home respite care program is described by MacCourt and Southam (1983). Four beds are available for respite care in the Tache Nursing Center. Any individual who is being managed by the family at home is eligible. The length of stay is flexible and may extend for days or weeks. Frequency of admission may be as often as monthly or as infrequently as yearly. All respite care clients are admitted to the same ward, and all are encouraged to participate in all nursing home activities. The initial interview is conducted by the social worker who, jointly with the family, determines the length of respite stay. A multidisciplinary conference, which includes the caregiver and care receiver, is held on admission to plan the respite stay. Nursing home staff emphasize maintaining the independence of care receivers and discharging them home again. Respite care at Tache is financed by the Manitoba Health Services Commission. Tache is paid a flat per diem rate even when beds are unoccupied and regardless of level of care when occupied.

Hospital

Intermittent hospital admission was the first formal respite care option for the elderly. The practice originated in Great Britain (Delargy, 1957). Review of the literature indicates that hospital respite care is still available in Great Britain (Griffiths & Cosin, 1976; Thorne & Hursey, 1986), but only two examples from the United States have been described (Hasselkus & Brown, 1983; Huey, 1983). Neither of these examples is recent. It seems likely that hospital respite care in the United States is not and will not be an option because the cost is too high, the environment is inappropriate, and most clients do not need the level of care provided by hospitals.

Combination Programs

Combination programs offer a variety of respite care options. They are rarely offered, but they demonstrate the flexibility needed by many families as caregiving situations change. These programs generally combine in-home with out-of-home plans. They also frequently contain a mixture of short-term, several-hour respite care with longer-term respite care of days or weeks. Many of these programs are specially funded and time-limited, so that unless provisions are made for ongoing funding, respite care may be discontinued at the end of the funding period.

Crossman, London, and Barry (1981) describe a combination respite care program that began as a caregiver support group and developed through the caregivers' own advocacy efforts into a funded respite care project. Elements of this project included adult day care, 4 hours of home care by a nurse each week, and 4-day respite weekends that utilized a six-bed adult residential facility. The residential facility was staffed by nurses who were affiliated with the project or day care program.

One British respite care project, developed for elderly with mental illness, combines day care and short-term overnight residential care in a house bought specifically for this purpose (Farries, 1985). This project is staffed by a multidisciplinary group of health care providers. Five elderly people may stay overnight and an additional eight people attend day care.

A number of combination programs were formed as a result of legislation passed by the New York state legislature in 1981, authorizing a large, 3-year demonstration project on respite care (Stone, 1985). Seven individual respite care programs were funded from this legislation, each with different characteristics. One of these projects was operated by the Metropolitan Commission on Aging and Home Aides of Central New York, with head-

quarters in Syracuse. It offered four types of respite care: companion in-home care of 24 hours to a few weeks; homemaker/home health aide in-home care; temporary placement in an adult home; and temporary placement in a nursing home (Cohen & Warren, 1985). Another project funded by this legislation, managed by the Ridgewood-Bushnick Senior Citizen Council in New York City, offered several respite care options and an array of other services. These included information and referral, brief in-home respite care, extended in-home respite care for up to 6 weeks a year, day care, caregiver counseling and training, and support groups (Cohen & Warren, 1985).

Other Settings

Adult day care provides out-of-home respite care for several hours at a time, generally during the day. A number of other strategies to provide respite care are now being reported, but information is sketchy. These strategies include adult foster homes, special respite homes, small facilities developed specifically for respite care, and respite co-ops. Two of these programs will be described here.

Elder Care Share is a project of the Southcentral Michigan Commission on Aging, established to assist families caring for elderly relatives in organizing and operating their own cooperative group in which they provide mutual support and short-term respite care (Stone, 1985). Families train each other to care for their impaired elderly relatives and take turns providing each other with respite. No money is exchanged; care received is "paid for" with care given. The sponsoring agency provides funding and administrative services through its program coordinator. A co-op committee works with the coordinator to establish policies and procedures and to recruit families.

Another example is TempCare, which offers overnight respite care for 1 to 30 days in a converted wing of a parochial school in the Bronx, New York (Stone, 1985). This program features 21 private rooms and a staff of eight but is not licensed as a skilled nursing or health-related facility. Basic services include three meals a day, housekeeping, personal care, and recreational activities. Clients of TempCare may be frail but must be ambulatory and continent. Following initial foundation support, TempCare has operated on a fee-for-service basis, with limited outside funding. For the 1983 to 1984 program year, operating costs were met through a sliding scale system based on $32 per night (Stone, 1985).

Settings for the Cognitively Impaired

Cognitively impaired older adults present special problems in all models of respite care. It is well recognized that cognitively impaired elderly function best in a structured environment with predictable daily routines. The presence of respite care workers in the home, admission to a nursing home, or use of day care changes the daily routine and can cause anxiety reactions or worsening of behavioral problems. For some cognitively impaired elderly, nursing home respite care is not an option because of the extreme anxiety or confusion it can produce. For these people an in-home plan may be best. A home visit or a 24- to 48-hour trial in the nursing home helps nursing home staff assess their ability to manage the person. Nursing homes with identified Alzheimer's disease units and special adult day care for the cognitively impaired are probably more suitable for these elderly. The issue of respite for the cognitively impaired is further complicated in that their caregivers, more often than any others, need respite because of relatively constant demands and frequently interrupted sleep.

RESPONSE TO RESPITE CARE

Unfortunately, at this time the benefits of respite care remain unknown because very little research has been conducted to provide this information. Limited evidence of its benefits exists, primarily as self-reports by family members (Crossman, London, & Barry, 1981; Delargy, 1957; Ellis & Wilson, 1983; Huey, 1983; Packwood, 1980). In an evaluation of an institutional respite care program used by 98 caregivers, Scharlach and Frenzel (1986) reported improved physical and mental health in the caregiver, a better relationship between the caregiver and care receiver, and increased confidence in the caregiver's ability to continue in the caregiving role. The researchers found that involvement in respite was not at the expense of the older client's physical or mental functioning. Montgomery (1986) reports findings of the only study to date that used a controlled experimental design to determine the effects of respite care when compared with several other support services. The objective burden of spouse caregivers who received volunteer respite services was significantly lower than that of spouses who did not receive respite services.

The use of any type of respite care may be a source of conflict between the caregiver and care receiver. The care receiver may resent any attempt by the caregiver to obtain relief. Alzheimer's victims, especially in the early stages, may be very resentful of having someone stay with them while the caregiver goes out. Families may fear the loss of control over their relative's care, that something will go wrong with a substitute caregiver, or that carefully developed, long-standing care routines will not be followed.

There are a number of model-specific responses to respite. Danaher, Dixon-Bemis, and Pederson (1986) reported that in-home respite care was resisted by some families who questioned why somebody would want to come into their home and help. This was especially true when the respite care providers were volunteers. Families expressed a certain amount of embarrassment about exposing their private concerns and problems in dealing with a difficult situation and about letting a stranger see what goes on in their homes. Netting and Kennedy (1985) found that 11 of 40 families turned down in-home respite care because they did not want to leave their relative with a stranger.

As might be expected, nursing home respite

care can be problematic for families for many reasons. Fear of abandonment and rejection by the elderly care receiver and guilt and anxiety on the part of caregivers are not uncommon. Scharlach and Frenzel (1986) reported that 38% of veterans using institutional respite care were resentful of caregivers for leaving. They expressed fears of being abandoned, rejected, or unloved.

There is some early evidence that the use of nursing home respite care may be a major step toward permanent institutionalization. Scharlach and Frenzel (1986) found that 30% of caregivers who used institutional respite reported that they saw placement as more likely as a result of respite care. The New York Foundation for Long Term Care in 1983 reported a surprising 12% of patients institutionalized within 1 month of the use of nursing home respite care. The experience of the break in caregiving may provide caregivers with an opportunity to reevaluate their ability to continue caregiving, with its attendant personal costs. The care receiver may also have an easier than expected adjustment to the institution, thus facilitating the decision for permanent placement.

Expressions of anger by either caregiver or care receiver are responses encountered by respite care workers in some families receiving respite services. This anger may be long-standing, growing out of the caregiving situation, but repressed, with few opportunities for expression. Anger toward respite care staff can occur when care routines are not followed exactly as the caregiver performs them or when unexpected complications occur. Respite care staff can be taught the likely origins of anger and strategies to manage it.

DEMOGRAPHICS

Comprehensive data on the number and scope of respite programs nationwide are not available. However, in one nationwide study, Bursac (1983) reviewed data from 31 states on state-mandated respite programs. Of these states, 33% were engaged in planning activities for respite care, 33% were developing or implementing model demonstration projects, and 33% had included respite care as part of their community-based long-term care programs. The same survey reports that the majority of respite care was provided in the home, whereas institutional settings were the second most frequent providers of respite care. Adult day care and day hospitals were the most frequently cited respite care providers, followed by homemaker/home health aides and home health agencies.

The characteristics of families who use respite services have been documented (Cantor, 1983; Ellis & Wilson, 1983; New York Foundation for Long Term Care, 1983). Montgomery (1986) reports the key characteristics of elderly and caregivers who are likely to use respite services. These characteristics are based on data from 306 families who participated in a study that focused on the impact of a volunteer respite care program on families caring for older members and are similar to those in other studies and program reports.

The average age of care receivers was 81 years. Forty-seven percent were widowed and 46% were married. Forty percent were male, 60% were female. Fifty-seven percent reported their health as fair or not good at all, and 46% were reported to have serious problems with mental impairment.

Most caregivers in this study were female (79%) and were either a child (57%) or spouse (37%) of the disabled person. The median age was 62 years, with adult children averaging 58 years of age and spouses averaging 71 years of age. The majority of caregivers were married and reported their health as good. Thirty-two percent were employed. Approximately 9 hours each week were spent on assisting the elderly relative with body tasks such as bathing and dressing and 17 hours with eating tasks. In addition, 4 hours were spent on financial tasks and 7 hours on movement tasks, such as transportation. Caregivers tended to use few formal supports and frequently were unaware of the availability of respite care.

SOCIAL POLICY AND PLANNING

Policymakers, concerned with the increasing cost of institutional long-term care, are beginning to acknowledge the importance of the family in providing informal long-term care to the elderly. At the same time, many believe that the costs of home care with supportive services are considerably lower than institutional care. The result is an emphasis at federal and state levels on funding services that will make it easier for informal caregivers to care for the elderly in their own homes and delay costly institutionalization. Respite care is one type of service strategy that is being supported by policymakers to achieve this goal. There is, however, little evaluative information about the role of respite care in relieving the stress and burden associated with caregiving or postponing the decision to institutionalize an elderly family member. This lack of data about the effects and role of respite care underscores the need for more research in this area.

Current information on state and federally funded respite care programs is fragmented, reflecting both the emerging nature of respite care as a recognized long-term care service and the lack of clear financing and program development strategies. A number of recent surveys of state respite care policies have provided data on eligibility criteria, legislation, provider eligibility, and financing (Bursac, 1983; Meltzer, 1982; National Council on Aging [NCOA], 1985). Although this information is not comprehensive, it is representative of state-supported respite care in the early 1980s, and is summarized here.

Eligibility for respite care services varies among states. While several states limit eligibility to the mentally retarded/developmentally disabled (MR/DD), others target services only to the frail elderly population. A number of states have developed a generic program that serves a variety of adult disabled groups (i.e., elderly, MR/DD, mentally ill). Other eligibility criteria include those with a high risk of institutionalization, need for supervision, and level of functional limitation. Several programs were developed to meet the particular needs of elderly people with Alzheimer's disease and other dementing illnesses.

The analysis by NCOA (1985) revealed that 15 states had enacted legislation specifically authorizing state support of respite services for families with frail or handicapped elderly members. The content of the legislation ranged from funding for demonstration projects to the inclusion of respite care as an allowable service within a comprehensive community-based care system.

Meltzer (1982) notes that respite care providers are as diverse as the programs themselves. In a survey of 34 states, Bursac (1983) found that although respite care was not licensed by the state, the majority of respite care providers were licensed health care facilities or agencies. Various sources were identified as potential respite providers, including home health agencies, social service agencies, residential health facilities, public agencies, and private not-for-profit corporations.

Although public financing for respite care has until very recently been virtually nonexistent, there are a limited number of federal and state financing sources. Medicaid waivers under Section 2176 of the Omnibus Budget Reconciliation Act of 1981 (PL 97-35) allow states to support the provision of respite care to individuals at risk of institutionalization. The Medicare hospice benefit allows the provision of inpatient respite for periods of no more than 5 days. Other federal sources include Title III of the Older Americans Act and the Social Services Block Grant. A number of states allocate monies, primarily for funding respite demonstration projects.

Emerging Policy Issues

There are several key policy issues surrounding the further development of respite care. One issue is whether to recognize respite care as a formal, distinct service with policies, regulations, and standards. This position is advocated by some to ensure provision of this valuable service. The Older Women's League (OWL) has prepared a model respite bill that establishes an administrative structure for the development and provision of respite care programs at the local level. On the other hand, such structure may dissuade potential respite care providers from participating; these actions may increase administrative costs excessively. In its final report, the New York Foundation for Long Term Care (1983) noted that even though New York is a highly regulated state, it was possible to develop respite care programs with only minor modifications in structure and policy.

Another issue is the gap between the level of care required by an elderly care receiver and the level of respite care provider available. The level of care required by some may be more than trained paraprofessionals can provide (Rabbitt, 1986). A related issue is the length of time per respite episode and the varying time-off needs of caregivers. There is a need for a continuum of respite services, with medical as well as social models.

Perhaps the major issue to be faced by policymakers is how to finance respite care. Presently, financing of respite care is very limited, and most of the cost is borne by the elderly client or caregiver (New York Foundation for Long Term Care, 1983). Some suggested approaches are to expand resources through current programs such as Medicaid or Medicare, to secure coverage by private insurance companies, and to use vouchers to allow the client to choose among a variety of services.

SUMMARY

Respite care is a support service for families caring for chronically ill or disabled elderly members. Although respite care is a recent development, it is becoming increasingly important, since the elderly are living longer with chronic disabilities, requiring long-term management that is usually assumed by the family. Nurses can play a vital role in respite care by referring families for respite services, by assisting families in the process of utilizing respite care, by providing care in a respite care program, and by developing and implementing respite care programs. Respite care is provided in the home of the client, in nursing homes, in adult day care centers, and in other types of facilities. The particular respite care service utilized by the family depends on availability, ability to pay for the service, care needs of the care receiver, the type of respite care provider, and needs of the caregiver. There are strengths and limitations in each setting, and respite care for the cognitively impaired requires special considerations. Although self-reports from families indicate that respite care is beneficial, the decision to use respite care can be a source of family conflict. Many states are in the process of planning and implementing respite care programs. Legislation, eligibility criteria, financing, and provider requirements vary among states. Future directions for respite care will depend on how well respite care is developed and financed.

References

Bursac, K (1983): *An Analysis of a Nationwide Survey of Respite Care Services.* Tucson, Arizona Long Term Care Gerontology Center.

Cantor, MH (1983): Caring for the frail elderly. Paper presented at the 33rd Annual Scientific Meeting of the Gerontological Society of America, San Diego, CA.

Cohen, L, & Warren, RD (1985): *Respite Care: Principles, Programs, and Policies.* Austin, TX, PRO-ED.

Crossman, L, London, C, & Barry, C (1981): Older women caring for disabled spouses: A model for supportive services. *Gerontologist, 21*:464–470.

Danaher, D, Dixon-Bemis, J, & Pederson, SH (1986): Staffing respite programs: The merits of paid and volunteer staff. *In* Montgomery, RJV, & Prothero, J (eds): *Developing Respite Services for the Elderly.* Seattle, Washington University Press, 78–90.

Delaney, N, & Bleck, D (1985): *Inpatient Respite: Nuts and Bolts.* Palo Alto, CA, Veterans Administration Medical Center.

Delargy, J (1957): Six weeks in: Six weeks out. *Lancet,* 1:418–419.

Ellis, V, & Wilson, D (1983): Respite care in the nursing home unit of a veterans hospital. *Am J Nurs, 83*:1433–1434.

Farries, J (1985): Giving carers a much needed break. *Health Soc Serv J, 95*:986–987.

George, LK, & Gwyther, LP (1986): Caregiver well-being: A multidimensional examination of family caregivers of demented adults. *Gerontologist, 26*: 253–259.

Griffiths, RA, & Cosin, LZ (1976): The floating bed. *Lancet,* 1:684–685.

Hasselkus, BR, & Brown, M (1983): Respite care for community elderly. *Am J Occup Ther, 37*:83–89.

Huey, T (1983): Respite care in a state-owned hospital. *Am J Nurs, 83*:1431–1432.

Kane, A (1985): RESPITE's brief history shows nationwide growth. *Health Progress*, July-August:83.

Lidoff, L (1983): *Respite Companion Program Model*. Washington, DC, National Council on Aging.

MacCourt, P, & Southam, M (1983): Respite care provides relief for care-givers. *Dimensions, 60*(12):18–19.

Meltzer, JW (1982): *Respite Care: An Emerging Family Support Service*. Washington, DC, The Center for the Study of Social Policy.

Montgomery, RJV (1986): Researching respite: Beliefs, facts and questions. *In* Montgomery, RJV, & Prothero, J (eds): *Developing Respite Programs for the Elderly*. Seattle, Washington University Press, 18–32.

National Council on Aging (1985): *State Support for Respite Care: Report of an exploratory survey*. Washington, DC, National Council on Aging.

Netting, FE, & Kennedy, LN (1985): Project Renew: Development of a volunteer respite care program. *Gerontologist, 25*:573–576.

New York Foundation for Long Term Care (1983): *Respite Care for the Frail Elderly: A Summary Report on Institutional Respite Research and Operations Manual*. Albany, NY, The Center for the Study of Aging, Inc.

Nurick, L (1983): Respite care services in the nursing home: Findings from a study conducted in New York State. *In Respite Care: New Opportunities*. Conference Proceedings. Tucson, Arizona Long Term Care Gerontology Center.

Packwood, T (1980): Supporting the family: A study of the organization and implications of hospital provision of holiday relief for families caring for dependents at home. *Soc Sci Med 14A*:613–620.

Rabbitt, WJ (1986): The New York respite demonstration program. *In* Montgomery, RJV, & Prothero, J (eds): *Developing Respite Programs for the Elderly*. Seattle, Washington University Press, 33–49.

Scharlach, A, & Frenzel, C (1986): An evaluation of institution-based respite care. *Gerontologist, 26*:77–82.

Stone, R (1985): *Recent Developments in Respite Care Services for Caregivers of the Impaired Elderly*. San Francisco, University of California at San Francisco, Aging Health Policy Center.

Sullivan, RC (1979): The burn-out syndrome. *J Autism Dev Disord, 9*:112–126

Thorne, T, & Hursey, K (1986): Short hospital breaks. *Nurs Times, 82*(21):28–31.

INDEX

Note: Page numbers in *italics* refer to illustrations; page numbers followed by t refer to tables.

SAGINAW COMMUNITY HOSPITAL